T0178367

Statistics for Biology and Health

Series Editors

Mitchell Gail, Division of Cancer Epidemiology and Genetics, National Cancer
Institute, Rockville, MD, USA
Jonathan M. Samet, Department of Epidemiology, School of Public Health, Johns
Hopkins University, Baltimore, MD, USA
B. Singer, Department of Statistics, University of California at Berkeley, Berkeley,
CA, USA

More information about this series at http://www.springer.com/series/2848

Ewout W. Steyerberg

Clinical Prediction Models

A Practical Approach to Development, Validation, and Updating

Second Edition

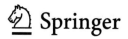 Springer

Ewout W. Steyerberg
Department of Biomedical Data Sciences
Leiden University Medical Center
Leiden, The Netherlands

ISSN 1431-8776   ISSN 2197-5671   (electronic)
Statistics for Biology and Health
ISBN 978-3-030-16401-0   ISBN 978-3-030-16399-0   (eBook)
https://doi.org/10.1007/978-3-030-16399-0

For Aleida, Matthijs, Laurens and Suzanne
For my father Wim

Preface

The first edition of this book was made during the years 2005–2007. Since then quite some new developments have taken place, both in the general scientific direction that prediction research is taking and specific technical innovations. These developments have been addressed as far as possible in the second edition. Many new references have been added. Some detailed material has been moved from print to the web. Many figures have been redrawn in color for better clarity and attractiveness. In all, many changes have been made to nearly every chapter.

Prediction models are important in widely diverse fields, including medicine, physics, engineering, meteorology, and finance. Prediction models are becoming more relevant in the medical field with the increase in biological knowledge on potential predictors of outcome, e.g., from "omics" (including genomics, transcriptomics, proteomics, glycomics, metabolomics). Also, the Big Data era implies we will have increasing access to large volumes of routinely collected data. The number of applications for prediction models will increase, e.g., with targeted early detection of disease, and individualized approaches to diagnostic testing and treatment.

We are moving to an era of personalized evidence-based medicine that asks for an individualized approach to shared medical decision-making. Evidence-based medicine has a central place for meta-analysis to summarize results from randomized controlled trials; prediction models summarize the effects of predictors to provide individualized predictions of the absolute risk of a diagnostic or prognostic outcome. Prediction models and related algorithms will increasingly form the basis for personalized evidence-based medicine and individualized decision-making.

Why Read This Book?

My motivation for working on the first and second editions of this book stems primarily from the fact that the development and applications of prediction models are often suboptimal in medical publications. With this book, I hope to contribute to better understanding of relevant issues and give practical advice on better modeling strategies than are nowadays used.

Issues include the following:

(a) Better predictive modeling is sometimes readily possible, e.g., a large data set with high-quality data is available, but all continuous predictors are dichotomized, which is known to have several disadvantages.

(b) Small samples are used:

- Studies are underpowered, implying unreliable answers to difficult questions such as "Which are the most important predictors in this prediction problem?"
- The problem of small sample size is aggravated by doing a complete case analysis which discards information from nearly complete records. Statistical imputation methods are nowadays available to exploit all available information, especially "multiple imputations."
- Predictors are omitted that should reasonably have been included based on subject matter knowledge. Analysts rely too much on the limited data that they have available in their data set, instead of wisely combining information from several sources, such as medical literature and experts in the field.
- Stepwise selection methods are abundant when researchers apply regression modeling, while these methods are suboptimal, especially in small data sets.
- Modeling approaches are used that require higher numbers. Data-hungry techniques, such as neural network modeling, machine learning or artificial intelligence techniques, should not be used in small data sets.
- No attempts are made towards validation, or validation is done inefficiently. For example, a split-sample approach is followed, leading to a smaller sample for model development and a smaller sample for model validation. Better methods are nowadays available and should be used far more often, specifically bootstrap resampling.

(c) Claims are exaggerated:

- Often, we see statements such as "the independent predictors were identified"; in many instances, such findings are purely exploratory and may not be reproducible; they may largely represent noise.
- Models are not internally valid, with overoptimistic expectations of model performance in new patients.
- One modern machine learning method with a fancy name is claimed as being superior to a more traditional regression approach, while no convincing evidence is presented, and a suboptimal modeling strategy was followed for the regression model. Fair comparisons between well-used statistical methods and machine learning methods are required.
- Researchers are insufficiently aware of overfitting, implying that their apparent findings are merely coincidental.

(d) Poor generalizability:

- If models are not internally valid, we cannot expect them to generalize to new patients.
- Models are developed for each local situation, discarding earlier findings on effects of predictors and earlier models; a framework for continuous improvement and updating of prediction models is required.

In this book, I suggest many small improvements in modeling strategies. Combined, these improvements should lead to better development, validation, and updating of prediction models.

Intended Audience

Readers should have a basic knowledge of biostatistics, especially regression analysis, but no strong background in mathematics is required. The number of formulas is deliberately kept small. The focus is on concepts in prediction research, which are also relevant to computer scientists and data scientists working on prediction in the field of Predictive Analytics.

Usually, a bottom-up approach is followed in teaching regression analysis techniques, starting with the required type of data, model assumptions, estimation methods, and basic interpretation. This book is more top-down: given that we want to predict an outcome, how can we best utilize regression and related techniques?

Three levels of readers are envisioned:

(a) The core intended audience is formed by epidemiologists and applied bio-statisticians who want to develop, validate, or update a prediction model. Both students and professionals should find practical guidance in this book, especially by the proposed seven steps to develop a valid model (Part II).
(b) The second group is formed by clinicians, policy-makers, and healthcare professionals who want to judge a study that presents or validates a prediction model. This book should aid them in a critical appraisal, providing explanations of terms and concepts that are common in publications on prediction models. They should try to read chapters of particular interest, or read the main text of the chapters. They can skip the examples and more technical sections (indicated with*).
(c) The third group includes more theoretical researchers, such as (bio)statisticians and computer scientists, who want to improve the methods that we use in prediction models. They may find inspiration for further theoretical work and simulation studies in this book. Many of the methods in prediction modeling are not fully developed yet, and common sense or intuition underlies some of the proposed approaches in this book. Improvements are welcome!

Other Sources

Many excellent textbooks exist on regression analysis techniques, but these usually do not have a focus on modeling strategies for prediction. The main exception is Frank Harrell's book "Regression Modeling Strategies". He brings advanced biostatistical concepts to practical application, supported by the rms package for R. Harrell's book may, however, be too advanced for clinical and epidemiological researchers. This also holds for the Hastie, Tibshirani, and Friedman quite thorough textbook "The Elements of Statistical Learning". These books are very useful for a more in-depth discussion of statistical techniques and strategies. Harrell's book provided the main inspiration for the presented work here. Another good companion book is the Vittinghoff et al. book on "Regression Methods in Biostatistics".

Various sources at the Internet can be used that explain terms used in this book. Frank Harrell maintains a useful glossary: [http://hbiostat.org/doc/glossary.pdf].

Structure

It has been found that people learn by example, by checklists, and by own discovery. Therefore, many examples are provided throughout the text, including the essential computer code and output. I also suggest a checklist for prediction modeling (Part II). Own discovery is possible with exercises per chapter, with data sets and scripts provided at the book's website: www.clinicalpredictionmodels.org.

Many statistical techniques and approaches are readily possible with any modern software package. Personally, I have worked with SPSS for simple, straightforward analyses. This package is insufficient for more advanced analyses which are essential in prediction modeling. The SAS computer package is more advanced, but may not be so practical for some. A package such as Stata is very suitable. It is similar in capabilities to R software for the key elements of prediction modeling. The R software has several advantages: the software is for free, and innovations in biostatistical methods become readily available. Therefore, R is the natural choice as the software accompanying this book. R software is available at www.cran.r-project.org, with help files and a tutorial.

An important disadvantage of R is a relatively slow learning curve; it takes time and efforts to learn R. Some R commands are provided in this book; full programs can be downloaded from the book's website (www.clinicalpredictionmodels.org). This website also provides a number of data sets that can be downloaded for application of the described techniques. I provide data files in SPSS format that can readily be imported in R and other packages. Many useful R tips and tricks are available on the web.

Leiden, The Netherlands   Ewout W. Steyerberg

Acknowledgements

Many have made small to large contributions to this book and the revision. I'm very grateful to all. Frank Harrell has been a source of inspiration for my research in the area of clinical prediction models, together with Hans van Houwelingen, who has developed many of the theoretical innovations that are presented in this book. I'm grateful to be his successor as a chair of the Department of Biomedical Data Sciences at the Leiden University Medical Center. At the Department of Public Health, Erasmus MC, Rotterdam, Dik Habbema, and René Eijkemans have sharpened my thinking on prediction modeling. Hester Lingsma was very supportive in the last phase of finishing the first edition of this book and has been a wonderful colleague over many years. Lex Burdorf, Daan Nieboer, and Jan Verbeek (Erasmus MC) provided specific comments for the second edition.

My insights in meta-analysis have benefitted from a project with Carl Moons and Thomas Debray (Utrecht). I have enjoyed the vigorous discussions about the evaluation of model performance with Ben van Calster, Michael Pencina, Stuart Baker, and Andrew Vickers, which is reflected in further textual changes in the second edition. Several Ph.D. students, colleagues, and external reviewers provided input and made specific comments on various chapters.

I specifically would like to thank investigators who allowed their data sets to be made available for didactic purposes, including Kerry Lee (Duke University) for the GUSTO-I data, Andrew Maas (Antwerp University) for the IMPACT data, Yolanda van der Graaf (Utrecht University) for the SMART data, and all other investigators and patients who were involved in the studies used in this book. Finally, I thank my family for their love and support over the years, and for allowing me to devote private time to this book.

Leiden, The Netherlands   Ewout W. Steyerberg
February 2019

Contents

About the Author

Ewout W. Steyerberg, Ph.D. worked for 25 years at Erasmus MC, Rotterdam, the Netherlands, before moving to Leiden as Professor of Clinical Biostatistics and Medical Decision Making and Chair at the Department of Biomedical Data Sciences, at Leiden University Medical Center, Leiden, the Netherlands. His research has covered a broad range of methodological and medical topics, which is reflected in hundreds of peer-reviewed methodological and more applied publications. Ewout's methodological expertise is in the design and analysis of randomized controlled trials, cost-effectiveness analysis, and decision analysis. His methodological research focuses on the development, validation, and updating of prediction models, as reflected in this textbook. Medical fields of application include oncology, cardiovascular disease, internal medicine, pediatrics, infectious diseases, neurology, surgery, and traumatic brain injury. His research benefitted from many research grants by various funders, including a fellowship from the Royal Netherlands Academy of Arts and Sciences, and research stays at Duke University (Durham, NC) and Dana-Farber Harvard Cancer Center (Boston, MA).

Chapter 1
Introduction

1.1 Diagnosis, Prognosis, and Therapy Choice in Medicine

Prediction and prognosis are central to many domains of medicine:

- Screening: If we screen for early signs of disease, we may, for example, find cancers early in their course of disease and treat them better than when they were detected later. But whether screening is useful depends on the improvement in prognosis that is achieved compared to a "no screening" strategy. Some cancers may not have caused any impact on life expectancy, while side effects of treatment may be substantial. For example, overdiagnosis is a serious concern in breast cancer screening [90, 365].
- Diagnosis: If we do a diagnostic test, we may detect an underlying disease. But some diseases are not treatable, or the natural course might be very similar to what is achieved with treatment.
- Therapy: New treatments are proposed nearly every day, but their impact on prognosis is often rather limited, despite high hopes at early stages. "Magic bullets" are rare. Treatment effects are often small relative to the effects of determinants of the natural history of a disease, such as the patient's age. The individual benefits need to be considered and exceed any side effects and harms [419].

1.1.1 Predictions for Personalized Evidence-Based Medicine

Physicians and health policy-makers need to make predictions on the likelihood of a diagnosis and the prognosis of a disease in many settings, for example, decision-making on screening for disease, diagnostic workup (e.g., ordering further tests, including possibly risky or expensive tests), and therapy choice (where the benefits of treatment should exceed any burden and risk of harm). Traditionally, the

© Springer Nature Switzerland AG 2019
E. W. Steyerberg, *Clinical Prediction Models*, Statistics for Biology and Health, https://doi.org/10.1007/978-3-030-16399-0_1

probabilities of diagnostic and prognostic outcomes were mostly implicitly assessed for such decision-making. Medicine was much more subjective, relying on expert knowledge. The field of prognosis research has however grown strongly since [238].

How is prognosis research related to recent general scientific developments (Table 1.1)?

- Prediction models are an explicit, empirical approach to estimate probabilities of disease or an outcome of disease. This relates to the "evidence-based medicine" (EBM) movement which aims to use the current best evidence in making decisions about the care of individual patients [413, 481]. Evidence-based medicine applies the scientific method to medical practice [214]. Its laudable intentions are to make clinical practice more scientific and empirically grounded and thereby achieving safer, more consistent, and more cost-effective care [200]. The Cochrane Collaboration has grown internationally and focuses on the synthesis of evidence, mainly using meta-analytic techniques [49].
  Evidence-based medicine has been criticized for a number of reasons, specifically on the issue of being not sufficiently individualized. EBM relies heavily on overall effect estimates from randomized controlled trials (RCTs), as summarized in meta-analyses [270]. There is a natural tension between the average results in clinical studies and individual decisions for real patients, where average results may not apply [200]. This tension is related to the "reference class" problem: to whom do the trial results apply? [300, 468].
- Personalized medicine has been proposed as a new paradigm, with a primary focus on what intervention works for what specific patient [492]. Personalized medicine has been fueled by discoveries in basic science to define variations in human diseases, for example, related to genetic variability in patients' responses to drug treatments [220]. The central goal of personalized medicine is to narrow the reference class to yield more patient-specific effect estimates to support more individualized clinical decision-making [300]. The empirical identification of patient-specific effects is a formidable task, however, with a history of disappointments and failures [240, 284, 658].
- We might hope that the Big Data era opens new avenues. Indeed, the growth in the availability of registries and claims data and the linkages between all these data sources have created a big data platform in health care, vast in both size and scope [504]. The increase in data availability has fueled the development of computer-oriented methods known as "Machine Learning" (ML) [283]. ML claims to make fewer assumptions in prediction modeling than traditional statistical approaches. ML places the data at the forefront, with a more limited role of the data analyst than in traditional statistical analyses. ML encompasses fields such as "data mining," which focuses on exploratory data analysis. It is also connected to artificial intelligence ("AI"), a field where algorithms mimic cognitive functions that humans associate with human minds, such as learning and problem-solving. Machine learning and statistics may both fall in the overall field of "data science," which has seen a spectacular growth in recent years. Predictive analytics may be seen as the subfield of data science where data are used to make predictions, either using more traditional or ML methods [449, 666].

Table 1.1 Concepts and key aspects of recent scientific developments

Concept	Description
Evidence-based medicine (EBM)	An attempt to the conscientious, explicit and judicious use of current best evidence in making decisions about the care of individual patients [413, 481]
Personalized medicine	A form of medicine that seeks to improve stratification and timing of health care by utilizing biological information and biomarkers on the level of molecular disease pathways, genetics, proteomics, and metabolomics [492]. Personalized medicine is related to "stratified medicine" and "precision medicine" [249]
Big Data	Big data in health care implies the availability of registries and claims data and the linkages between all these data sources [504]
Machine Learning (ML)	ML methods claim to make fewer assumptions in data analyses than traditional statistical approaches. ML encompasses fields such as "data mining", which focuses on exploratory data analysis. It is also connected to artificial intelligence ("AI") [283]
Shared Decision-Making (SDM)	In SDM, physicians and patients both actively participate in deciding on choices for diagnostic tests and therapeutic interventions [111]

- A criticism of EBM is that it ignores patients' values and preferences, which are central elements in Shared Decision-Making (SDM) [253]. In SDM, physicians and patients both actively participate in deciding on choices for diagnostic tests and therapeutic interventions [111]. For shared decision-making, adequate communication is required about the patient's options, and their pros and cons, tailored to the specific patient [570].

Clinical prediction models combine a number of characteristics (e.g., related to the patient, the disease, or treatment) to predict a diagnostic or prognostic outcome. Typically, a limited number of predictors are considered (say between 2 and 20) [558]. Clinical prediction models are related to each of the above-described fields. For one, predictions are essential to the individualization of estimates of treatment benefit. By separating those at low versus those at high risk, we can target treatment at the high-risk patients, where the benefits of treatment well exceed any burden of treatment [300]. Prediction models, hence, provide a direct tool for Personalized Medicine [249]. Prediction models will increase in quantity and hopefully also in quality by the increasing access to rich data sets in the Big Data era, using modern techniques where appropriate, for example, for specific tasks such as text recognition and image processing [283]. Predictions from models are also the evidence-based input for shared decision-making, by providing estimates of the individual probabilities of risks and benefits [323].

Scientific publications on modeling for prediction have increased steeply over recent years, to a total of 651,000 over the years 1993–2017. The annual numbers more than doubled per decade: from 7,400 in 1993 to 17,000 in 2003, 39,000 in 2013, and 53,000 in 2017 (Fig. 1.1). These publications especially include fields other than medicine, such as engineering, mathematics, and computer science. Life sciences is only at place 15 of the top research areas (Fig. 1.2).

Fig. 1.1 Annual number of publications with the terms "prediction" and "model" published between 1993 and 2017 as identified at the Web of Science

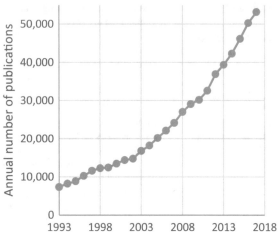

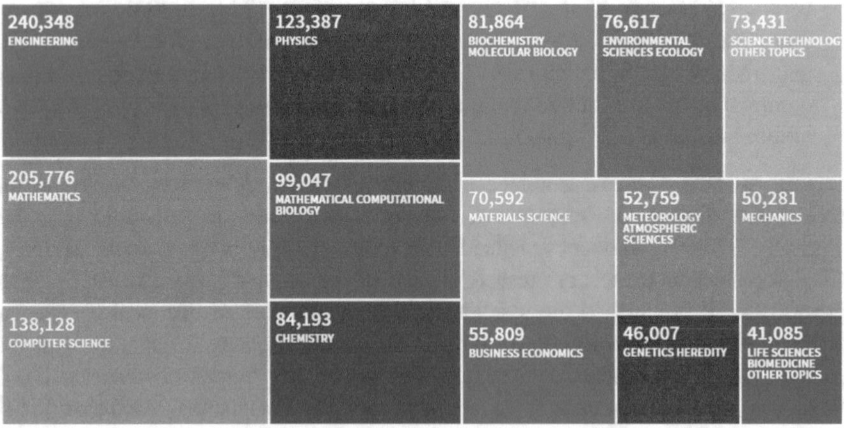

Fig. 1.2 The top 15 scientific fields of publications with the terms "prediction" and "model" published between 1993 and 2017 as identified at the Web of Science

1.2 Statistical Modeling for Prediction

Prediction is primarily an estimation problem. For example,

- What is the likelihood that this patient with hypertension has a renal artery stenosis?
- What is the risk of dying of this patient within 30 days after an acute myocardial information?
- What is the expected 2-year survival rate for this patient with esophageal cancer?

Prediction is also about testing of hypotheses. For example,

- What is the relevance of specific test results in diagnosing renal artery stenosis?
- Is age a predictor of 30-day mortality after an acute myocardial information?
- How important is nutritional status for survival of a patient with esophageal cancer?

Or more general, what are the most important predictors in a certain disease? Are some predictors correlated with each other, such that their apparent predictive effects are explained by other predictor variables? The latter question comes close to etiologic research, where we aim to learn about biology and explain natural phenomena [508].

Statistical models may serve to address both estimation and hypothesis testing questions. In the medical literature, much emphasis has traditionally been given to the identification of predictors. Over 200,000 papers had been published with the terms "predictor" or "prognostic factor" in PubMed by December 2018. The total number of publications with the term "prognostic model" or "prediction model" exceeded 10,000 by that time; so approximately 20 times more prognostic factor studies had been published than prognostic modeling studies [458, 558].

Note that that the prognostic value of a predictor has to be shown in addition to already known, easily measurable predictors [510]. For example, the prognostic value of a new genetic marker would need to be assessed for additional value over classical, well-established predictors [293]. Such evaluations require statistical modeling. Prognostic modeling and prognostic factor studies are, hence, connected [425].

1.2.1 Model Assumptions

Statistical models summarize patterns of the data available for analysis. In doing so, it is inevitable that assumptions have to be made. Some of these assumptions can be tested, for example, whether predictor affects work in an additive way, and whether continuous predictors have reasonably linear effects. Testing of underlying assumptions is especially important if specific claims are made on the effect of a predictor (Chaps. 4, 6, and 12).

Statistical models for prediction have traditionally been discerned in main classes: regression, classification, and neural networks [231]. Machine learning refers to the latter two categories and other methods that claim to make fewer assumptions in the modeling process. The characteristics of alternative modeling approaches are discussed in Chaps. 4 and 6. The main focus of this book is on regression models, which are the most widely used in the medical field [653]. We consider situations where the number of candidate predictor variables is limited, say below 25. This is in contrast to research in areas such as genomics (genetic effects), proteomics (protein effects), or metabolomics (metabolite effects). In these areas, more complex data are generated, with larger numbers of candidate predictors (often >10,000, or even >1 M). Moreover, we assume that subject knowledge is available, from previous empirical studies and from experts on the topic (e.g., medical doctors treating patients with the condition under study).

1.2.2   Reliability of Predictions: Aleatory and Epistemic Uncertainty

Statistical models face various challenges in providing reliable predictions. Reliability means that when a 10% risk is predicted, on average 10% of patients with these characteristics should have the outcome ("calibration", Chaps. 4 and 15) [602]. Such a probabilistic estimate implies that we cannot classify a patient as having a diagnosis or prognosticate an event as unavoidable: we suffer from aleatory uncertainty. Probabilities provide no certainty.

Next to simple, aleatory uncertainty we also suffer from epistemic uncertainty, or systematic uncertainty [527]. For prediction models, the first goal is that predictions need to be reliable for the setting where the data came from internal validity. Here, we suffer from two sources of uncertainty: model uncertainty and estimation uncertainty. Model uncertainty arises from the fact that we usually do not fully prespecify a model before we fit it to a data set [94, 138]. An iterative model building process is often followed. On the other hand, standard statistical methods assume that a model was prespecified. In that utopic case, parameter estimates such as regression coefficients, their corresponding standard errors, 95% confidence intervals, and p-values are largely unbiased. When the structure of a model was at least partly based on findings in the data, severe bias may occur, and underestimation of the uncertainty of conclusions drawn from the model.

Fortunately, some statistical tools have become available which help to study such model uncertainty. Especially, a statistical resampling procedure named "bootstrap resampling" is helpful for many aspects of model development and validation [148]. The bootstrap, hence, is an important tool in prediction research (Chaps. 5 and 17) [673].

Next to internal validity, we may also worry about external validity or generalizability. Epistemic uncertainty includes that the model may not be applicable to a
certain setting: the predictions are systematically incorrect. For example, we may
systematically overestimate risks if we use a model developed in a clinical setting
for a screening setting. The concepts of internal and external validity are central in
this book, with part II focusing on internal validity and part III on external validity.
Intuitive synonyms are reproducibility and transportability, respectively [285].

1.2.3   Sample Size

A sufficient sample size is important to address any scientific question with
empirical data. The first point we have to appreciate is that the effective sample size
may often be much smaller than indicated by the total number of subjects in a study
[225]. For example, when we study complications of a procedure that occur with an
incidence of 0.1%, a study with 10,000 patients will contain only 10 events. The
number 10 determines the effective sample size in such a study. In small samples,
model uncertainty will be large, and we may not be able to derive reliable predictions from a model.

Second, a large sample size facilitates many aspects of prediction research. For
example, large-scale international collaborations are increasingly set up to allow for
the identification of gene–disease associations [269]. Also, more and more observational databases are linked in the current era of Big Data. For multivariable
prognostic modeling, a large sample size allows for selection of predictors with
simple automatic procedures such as stepwise methods with $p < 0.05$ and reliable
testing of model assumptions. An example is the prediction of 30-day mortality
after an acute myocardial infarction, where Lee et al. derived a prediction model
with 40,830 patients of whom 2850 died [329]. This example will be used
throughout this book, with a detailed description in Chap. 22. In practice, we often
have relatively small effective sample sizes. For example, a review of 31 prognostic
models in traumatic brain injury showed that 22 were based on samples with less
than 500 patients [400]. The main challenges are, hence, with the development of a
good prediction model with a relatively small study sample. The definition of
"small" is debatable, while most will agree that challenges arise especially in settings where we have less than 10 events (outcomes per patient) per predictor
variable ("EPV < 10") [422]. On the other hand, having more than 50 events per
variable (EPV > 50) allows for substantial freedom in modeling and will usually
provide for limited model uncertainty [25, 112, 225, 410, 543].

Third, with small sample size we have to be prepared to make stronger modeling
assumptions. For example, Altman illustrated the use of a parametric test (ANOVA)
to compare three groups with eight, nine, and five patients in his seminal text
"Practical statistics for medical research" [8]. With larger samples, we would more
readily switch to a nonparametric test such as a Kruskal–Wallis test. With small
sample size, we may have to assume linearity of a continuous predictor (Chap. 9)

Table 1.2 Stages of development of regression models and implications for modeling approach and required sample size [529]

Predictors known?	Functional form known?	Model parameters known?	Approach	Required sample size
−	−	−	Development from scratch	Very large
+	−	−	Define nonlinearity and interactions	Large
+	+	−	Fit regression coefficients	Moderate
+	+	+	Validation and updating	Moderate

and no interaction between predictors (Chap. 13). We will subsequently have limited power to test deviations from these model assumptions. It, hence, becomes more important what our starting point of the analysis is. From a Bayesian viewpoint, we could say that our prior information becomes more important, since the information contributed by our study is limited.

Finally, we have to match our ambitions in research questions with the effective sample size that is available [226, 227, 529]. When the sample size is very small, we should only ask relatively simple questions, while more complex questions can be addressed with larger sample sizes. A question such as "What are the most important predictors in this prediction problem" is more complex than a question such as "What are the predictions of the outcome given this set of predictors" (Chap. 11). Table 1.2 lists questions on predictors (known or determined from the data?), functional form (nonlinearity and interactions known or determined from the data?), and regression coefficients (known or determined from the data?) and the consequence for the required sample size in a study. A validation study asks least from the data, since the prediction model is fully specified (predictors, functional form, and model parameters), although sample size needs again to be adequate to draw reliable conclusions [643] (Table 1.2).

1.3   Structure of the Book

This book consists of four parts. Part I provides background on developing and applying prediction models in medicine. Part II is central for the development of internally valid prediction models, while part III focuses on applicability in external settings and advanced issues related to model modification and model extension ("updating"). Part IV is practical in nature with a detailed description of prediction modeling in two case studies, some lessons learned for model development, and a description of medical problems with publicly available data sets.

1.3.1   Part I: Prediction Models in Medicine

This book starts with an overview of various applications of prediction models in clinical practice and in medical research (Chap. 2). Next, we note that the quality of a statistical model depends to a large extent on the study design and quality of the data used in the analysis. A sophisticated analysis cannot salvage a poorly designed study or poor data collection procedures. Data quality is key to a good model. Several considerations are presented around the design of cohort studies for prognostic models, and cross-sectional studies for diagnostic models (Chap. 3). Various statistical techniques can be considered for a prediction model, which each have their strengths and limitations. An overview of more and less flexible models for different types of outcomes is presented in Chap. 4. Unfortunately, prediction models commonly suffer from a methodological problem, which is known as "overfitting". This means that idiosyncrasies in the data are fitted rather than generalizable patterns [225]. A model may, hence, not be applicable to new patients, even when the setting of application is very similar to the development setting. Statistical optimism is discussed with some potential solutions in Chap. 5. Chapter 6 discusses considerations in choosing between alternative models. It also presents some empirical comparisons on the quality of predictions derived with alternative modeling techniques.

1.3.2   Part II: Developing Internally Valid Prediction Models

The core of this book is a proposal for seven steps to consider in developing internally valid prediction models with regression analysis. We present a checklist for model development, which is intended to give a structure to model building and validation.

In Chaps. 7–18, we discuss seven modeling steps.

(1) A preliminary step is to carefully consider the prediction problem: what are the research questions, what is already known about predictors? Next, we consider the data under study: how are the predictors defined, what is the outcome of interest? An important issue is that missing values will occur in at least some of the predictors under study. We discuss and propose approaches to deal with missing values in Chaps. 7 and 8.

(2) When we start on building a prediction model, the first issue is the coding of predictors for a model; several choices need to be considered on categorical variables and continuous variables (Chaps. 9 and 10).

(3) We then move to the most thorny issue in prediction modeling: how to specify a model (Chaps. 11 and 12). What predictors should we include, what are the

pros and cons of stepwise selection methods, and how should we deal with assumptions in models such as additivity and linearity?

(4) Once a model is specified, we need to estimate model parameters. For regression models, we estimate coefficients for each predictor or combination of predictors in the model. We consider classical and more modern estimation methods for regression models (Chaps. 13 and 14). Several techniques are discussed which aim to limit overfitting of a model to the available data.

(5) For a specified and estimated model, we need to determine the quality. Several statistical performance measures are commonly used, as discussed in Chap. 15. Most relevant to clinical practice is whether the model is useful; this can be quantified with some more novel performance measures, firmly based on decision theory (Chap. 16).

(6) Since overfitting is a central problem in prediction modeling, we need to consider the validity of our model for new patients. It is easier to perform retrodiction than prediction of the future. In Chap. 17, we concentrate on statistical techniques to evaluate the internal validity of a model, i.e., for the underlying population that the sample originated from. Internal validation addresses statistical problems in the specification and estimation of a model ("reproducibility") [285], with a focus on how well we can separate low from high-risk patients.

(7) A final step to consider is the presentation of a prediction model. Regression formulas can be used, but many alternatives are possible for easier applicability of a model (Chap. 18).

1.3.3   Part III: Generalizability of Prediction Models

Generalizability (or external validity) of a model relates to the applicability of a model to a plausibly related setting [285]. External validity of a model cannot be expected if there is no internal validity. Steps 1–7 in Part II support the development of internally valid prediction models. Second, the performance may be lower when a model is applied in a new setting because of genuine differences between the new setting and the development setting. Examples of a different setting include a hospital different from the development hospital, in a more recent time period, and in a different selection of patients. Generalizability can be assessed in various ways, with different study designs. We systematically consider patterns of invalidity that may arise when externally validating a model (Chap. 19).

To improve predictions for a new setting, we need to consider whether we can make modifications and extension to the model. Various parsimonious modeling techniques are available to achieve such updating (Chap. 20). When several settings are considered, we may use more advanced updating methods, including random effect models and Empirical Bayes methods. Moreover, we may specifically be interested in ranking of providers of care (Chap. 21).

1.3.4   Part IV: Applications

A central case study in this book is provided by the GUSTO-I trial. Patients enrolled in this trial suffered from an acute myocardial infarction. A prediction model was developed for 30-day mortality in relation to various predictors [329]. Overfitting is not a concern in the full data set (n = 40,830 patients, 2850 died within 30 days). Modeling is more challenging in small parts of this data set, where some are made publicly available for applying the concepts and techniques presented in this book. We discuss the logistic regression model developed from the GUSTO-I patients in Chap. 22.

A further case study concerns a survival problem. We aim to predict the occurrence of secondary cardiovascular events among a hospital-based cohort. The seven steps to develop a prediction model are systematically considered (Chap. 23).

Finally, we give some practical advice on the main issues in prediction modeling and describe the medical problems used throughout the text and available data sets (Chap. 24).

Each chapter ends with a few questions to test insight in the material presented. Furthermore, practical exercises are available from the book's website (www.clinicalpredictionmodels.org), involving work with data sets in R software (www.cran.r-project.org).

Part I
Prediction Models in Medicine

Chapter 2
Applications of Prediction Models

Background In this chapter, we consider several areas of application of prediction models in public health, clinical practice, and medical research. We use several small case studies for illustration.

2.1 Applications: Medical Practice and Research

Broadly speaking, prediction models are valuable both for medical practice and for research purposes (Table 2.1). In public health, prediction models may help to target preventive interventions to subjects at relatively high risk of having or developing a disease. In clinical practice, prediction models may inform patients and their treating physicians on the probability of a diagnosis or a prognostic outcome. Prognostic estimates may, for example, be useful for planning of an individual's remaining lifetime in terminal disease, or give hope for recovery if a good prognosis is expected after an acute event such as a stroke. Classification of a patient according to his/her risk may also be useful for communication among physicians.

In the diagnostic workup, predictions can be useful to estimate the probability that a disease is present. When the probability is relatively high, treatment is indicated; if the probability is low, no treatment is indicated and further diagnostic testing may be considered necessary. In therapeutic decision-making, treatment should only be given to those who benefit from the treatment. The patients with highest benefit may usually be those at highest risk [298]. In any case, those at low risk have little to gain from any treatment. Any harm, such as the burden of treatment, or the risk of a side effect, may then readily outweigh any benefits. The claim of prediction models is that better decisions can be made with a model than without one.

In research, prediction models may assist in the design of intervention studies, for example, to select high-risk patients and, in the analysis of randomized trials, to

E. W. Steyerberg, *Clinical Prediction Models*, Statistics for Biology and Health, https://doi.org/10.1007/978-3-030-16399-0_2

Table 2.1 Some areas of application of clinical prediction models

Application area	Example in this chapter
Public health	
Targeting of preventive interventions	
Incidence of disease	Models for (hereditary) breast cancer
Clinical practice	
Diagnostic workup	
Test ordering	Probability of renal artery stenosis
Starting treatment	Probability of deep venous thrombosis
Therapeutic decision-making	
Surgical decision-making	Replacement of risky heart valves
Intensity of treatment	More intensive chemotherapy in cancer patients
Delaying treatment	Spontaneous pregnancy chances
Research	
Inclusion in a RCT	Traumatic brain injury
Covariate adjustment in an RCT	Primary analysis of GUSTO-III
Confounder adjustment with a propensity score	Statin effects on mortality
Case-mix adjustment	Provider profiling

adjust for baseline risk. Prediction models are also useful to control for confounding variables in observational research, either in traditional regression analysis or with approaches such as "propensity scores" [466, 479]. Several areas of application are discussed in the next sections.

2.2   Prediction Models for Public Health

2.2.1   *Targeting of Preventive Interventions*

Various models have been developed to predict the future occurrence of disease in asymptomatic subjects in the population. Well-known examples include the Framingham risk functions for cardiovascular disease [674]. The Framingham risk functions underpin several current policies for preventive interventions. For example, statin therapy is only considered for those with relatively high risk of cardiovascular disease. Similarly, prediction models have been developed for breast cancer, where more intensive screening or chemoprophylaxis can be considered for those at elevated risk [171, 173].

2.2.2   *Example: Prediction for Breast Cancer*

In 1989, Gail et al. presented a by-now famous risk prediction model for developing breast cancer [171]. The model was based on case–control data from the Breast Cancer Detection Demonstration Project (BCDDP). The BCDDP recruited 280,000 women from 1973 to 1980 who were monitored for 5 years. From this cohort, 2,852 white women developed breast cancer and 3,146 controls were selected, all with complete risk factor information. The Gail model risk projections are hence applicable to women who are examined about once a year. The model includes age at menarche, age at first live birth, number of previous biopsies, and number of first-degree relatives with breast cancer. Individualized breast cancer probabilities were calculated from information on relative risks and the baseline hazard rate in the general population. The calculations accounted for competing risks (the risk of dying from other causes).

The predictions were validated later on other data sets from various populations, with generally favorable conclusions [415]. Practical application of the original model involved cumbersome calculations and interpolations. Hence, more easily applicable graphs were created to estimate the absolute risk of breast cancer for individual patients for intervals of 10, 20, and 30 years. The absolute risk estimates have been used to design intervention studies, to counsel patients regarding their risks of disease, and to inform clinical decisions, such as whether or not to take tamoxifen to prevent breast cancer [172].

Other models for breast cancer risk include the Claus model, which is useful to assess risk for familial breast cancer [101]. This is breast cancer that runs in families but is not associated with a known hereditary breast cancer susceptibility gene. Unlike the Gail model, the Claus model requires the exact ages at breast cancer diagnosis of first- or second-degree relatives as an input.

Some breast cancers are caused by a mutation in a breast cancer susceptibility gene (BRCA), referred to as the hereditary breast cancer. A suspicious family history for hereditary breast cancer includes many cases of breast and ovarian cancers, or family members with breast cancers under age 50. Simple tables have been published to determine the risk of a BRCA mutation based on specific features of personal and family history [168]. Another model considers the family history in more detail (BRCAPRO [418]). It explicitly uses the genetic relationship in families and is therefore labeled as a Mendelian model. Calculations are based on Bayes' theorem.

Risk models may have two main roles in breast cancer: prediction of breast cancer in asymptomatic women and prediction of the presence of a mutation in a BRCA gene. These models not only have some commonalities in terms of predictors but also some differences (Table 2.2) [98, 169]. Various measures are possible to reduce breast cancer risk, including behavior (e.g., exercise, weight control, and alcohol intake), prophylactic surgery, and medical interventions (e.g., tamoxifen use).

Table 2.2 Risk factors in four prediction models for breast cancer: two for breast cancer incidence, two for the presence of mutation in BRCA1 or BRCA2 genes [169]

Risk factor	Gail model [171]	Claus model [101]	Myriad tables [168]	BRCAPRO model [418]
Woman's personal information				
Age	+	+	+	+
Race/ethnicity	+			
Ashkenazi Jewish			+	+
Breast biopsy	+			
Atypical hyperplasia	+			
Hormonal factors				
Age at menarche	+			
Age at first live birth	+			
Age at menopause	+			
Family history				
First-degree relatives with breast cancer	+	+	Age <50/ $\geq$ 50	Age for all affected
Second-degree relatives with breast cancer		+	Age <50/ $\geq$ 50	Age for all affected
First or Second degree with ovarian cancer			+	Age for all affected
Bilateral breast cancer				+
Male breast cancer				+
Outcome predicted	Incident breast cancer		BRCA1/2 mutation	

2.3   Prediction Models for Clinical Practice

2.3.1   Decision Support on Test Ordering

Prediction models may be useful to estimate the probability of an underlying disease, such that we can decide on further testing. When a diagnosis is very unlikely, no further testing is indicated, while more tests may be indicated when the diagnosis is not yet sufficiently certain for decision-making on therapy [263]. Further testing usually involves one or more imperfect tests (sensitivity below 100%, specificity below 100%). Ideally, a gold standard test is available (sensitivity = 100%, specificity = 100%). In practice, many reference tests are not truly "gold", while they are used as definitive in determining whether a subject has the disease. The reference test may not be suitable to apply in all subjects suspected of the disease because it is burdensome (e.g., invasive) or costly.

2.3.2   *Example: Predicting Renal Artery Stenosis*

Renal artery stenosis is a rare cause of hypertension. The reference standard for diagnosing renal artery stenosis, renal angiography, is invasive and costly. We aimed to develop a prediction rule for renal artery stenosis from clinical characteristics. The rule might be used to select patients for renal angiography [314]. Logistic regression analysis was performed with data from 477 hypertensive patients who underwent renal angiography. A simplified prediction rule was derived from the regression model for use in clinical practice. Age, sex, atherosclerotic vascular disease, recent onset of hypertension, smoking history, body mass index, presence of an abdominal bruit, serum creatinine concentration, and serum cholesterol level were selected as predictors. The diagnostic accuracy of the regression model was similar to that of renal scintigraphy, which had a sensitivity of 72% and a specificity of 90%. The conclusion was that this clinical prediction model can help to select patients for renal angiography in an efficient manner by reducing the number of angiographic procedures without the risk of missing many renal artery stenoses. The modeling steps summarized here will be described in more detail in Part II.

An interactive Excel program is available to calculate diagnostic predictions for individual patients. Figure 2.1 shows the example of a 45-year-old male with recent onset of hypertension. He smokes, has no signs of atherosclerotic vascular disease, has a BMI <25, no abdominal bruit is heard, serum creatinine is 112 μmol/L, and serum cholesterol is not elevated. According to a score chart (See Chap. 18), the sum score was 11, corresponding to a probability of stenosis of 25%. According to exact logistic regression calculations, the probability was 28% [95% confidence interval 17–43%].

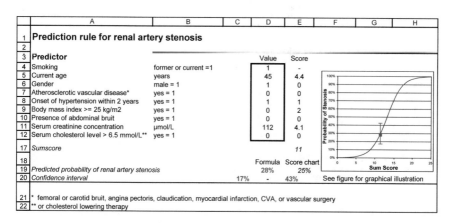

Fig. 2.1 Prediction rule for renal artery stenosis as implemented in an Excel spreadsheet [314]

2.3.3   Starting Treatment: The Treatment Threshold

Decision analysis is a method to formally weigh pros and cons of decisions [263]. For starting treatment after diagnostic workup, a key concept is the treatment threshold. This threshold is defined as the probability where the expected benefit of treatment is equal to the expected benefit of avoiding treatment. If the probability of the diagnosis is lower than the threshold, no treatment is the preferred decision, and if the probability of the diagnosis is above the threshold, treatment is the preferred decision [420]. The threshold is determined by the relative weight of false-negative versus false-positive decisions. If a false-positive decision is much less important than a false-negative decision, the threshold is low. For example, a risk of 0.1% for overtreatment versus a benefit of 10% for correct treatment implies a close to 1% threshold (odds 1:100, threshold probability 0.99%) [263]. On the other hand, if false-positive decisions confer serious risks, the threshold should be higher. For example, a 1% harm associated with overtreatment implies a threshold of 9.1% (odds 1:10, Fig. 2.2). Further details on the threshold concept are discussed with the assessment of performance of prediction models with decision curves [648] (Chap. 16).

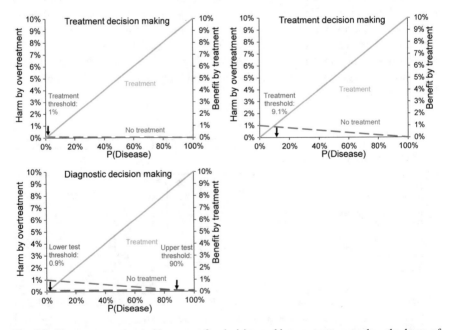

Fig. 2.2 The treatment threshold concept for decision-making on treatment when the harm of overtreatment is 0.1% (upper left panel) or 1% (upper right panel). If a reference test with perfect sensitivity and specificity is available with a constant 0.1% risk of harm, this test would be indicated between 0.9 and 90% probability of disease (lower left panel). The probability of disease may be estimated by a clinical prediction model

Note that a single treatment threshold applies only when all diagnostic workup is completed, including all available tests for the disease. If more tests can still be done, a more complex decision analysis needs to be performed to determine the optimal choices on tests and treatments. We then have two thresholds: a low threshold to identify those receiving no treatment and no further testing; and a higher threshold to identify those who would be treated without further testing (Fig. 2.2). In between are those who would benefit from further testing [263]. This approach is used for decision-making in the diagnosis of Deep Venous Thrombosis (DVT) using ultrasound and D-dimer testing [488].

2.3.4 *Example: Probability of Deep Venous Thrombosis

The Wells clinical prediction rule combines nine signs, symptoms, and risk factors to categorize patients as having low, moderate, or high probability of DVT [664]. This rule stratifies a patient's probability of DVT much better than individual findings [665]. Patients with a low pretest probability (for example, "score ≤ 1") can have DVT safely excluded, either by a single negative ultrasound result, or a negative plasma D-dimer test. Patients who are at increased pretest probability ("score > 1") require both a negative ultrasound result and a negative D-dimer test to exclude DVT [663]. A possible diagnostic algorithm is shown in Fig. 2.3 [488].

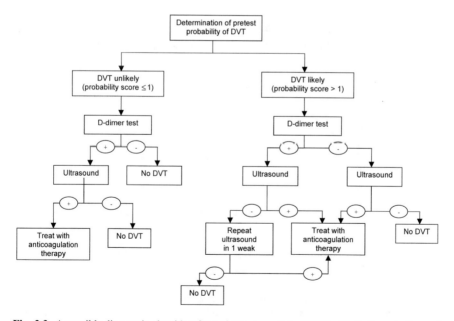

Fig. 2.3 A possible diagnostic algorithm for patients suspected of DVT with D-dimer testing and ultrasound imaging [488]. The pretest probability comes from a clinical prediction model, such as developed by Wells [663], or another predictive algorithm [665]

2.3.5   Intensity of Treatment

Prognostic estimates are also important to guide decision-making once a diagnosis is made. Decisions include, for example, more or less intensive treatment approaches. The framework for decision-making based on prognosis is very similar to that for based on diagnostic probabilities as discussed before.

A treatment should only be given to a patient if a substantial gain is expected, which exceeds any risks and side effects (Fig. 2.4). A classical case study considers anticoagulants and risk of atrial fibrillation [184]. Anticoagulants are very effective in reducing the risk of stroke in patients with non-rheumatic atrial fibrillation. However, using these drugs increases the risk of serious bleedings. Hence, the risk of stroke has to outweigh the bleeding risk before treatment is considered. Both risks may depend on predictors. Similar analyses have been described for the indication for thrombolytics in acute MI [60, 86].

We illustrate this approach to decision-making in a case study of testicular cancer patients: which patients are at sufficiently high risk to need more intensive chemotherapy, which may be more effective, but is also more toxic? [615].

2.3.6   *Example: Defining a Poor Prognosis Subgroup
in Cancer

As an example, we consider high-dose chemotherapy (HD-CT) as first-line treatment to improve survival of patients with non-seminomatous testicular cancer

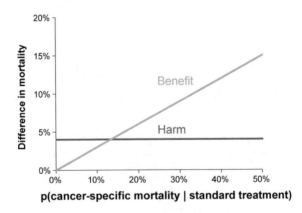

Fig. 2.4 Graphical illustration of weighing benefit and harm of treatment. *Benefit* of treatment (reduction in absolute risk) increases with cancer-specific mortality (relative risk set to 0.7). *Harm* of treatment (excess absolute risk, e.g., due to toxicity of treatment) is assumed to be constant at 4%. Net benefit occurs only when the cancer-specific mortality given standard treatment is above the threshold of 11% [615]

[615]. Several non-randomized trials reported a higher survival for patients treated with HD-CT as first-line treatment (including etoposide, ifosfamide, and cisplatin) with autologous stem cell support, compared to standard-dose (SD) chemotherapy (including bleomycin, etoposide, and cisplatin). However, HD-CT is related to a higher toxicity, during treatment (e.g., granulocytopenia, anemia, nausea/vomiting, and diarrhea), shortly after treatment (e.g., pulmonary toxicity), and long after treatment (e.g., leukemia and cardiovascular disease). HD-CT should therefore only be given to patients with a relatively poor prognosis.

We can specify the threshold for such a poor prognosis group by weighing expected benefit against harms. Benefit of HD-CT treatment is the reduction in absolute risk of cancer mortality. Benefit increases linearly with risk of cancer mortality if we assume that patients with the highest risk have most to gain. Harm is increase in absolute risk of treatment mortality (e.g., related to toxicity) due to treatment. The level of harm is the same for all patients, assuming that the toxicity of treatment is independent of prognosis. Patients are candidates for more aggressive treatment when their risk of cancer mortality is above the threshold, i.e., when the benefit is higher than harm (Fig. 2.4).

2.3.7 Cost-Effectiveness of Treatment

Cost-effectiveness of treatment directly depends on prognosis. Treatments may not be cost-effective if the gain is small (for patients at low risk) and the costs high (e.g., for all patients the same drug costs are made). For example, statin therapy should only be given to those at increased cardiovascular risk [160]. And more aggressive thrombolysis should only be used in those patients with an acute myocardial infarction who are at increased risk of 30-day mortality [86]. Many other examples can be found, where the relative benefit of treatment is assumed to be constant across various risk groups, and the absolute benefit hence increases with higher risk [630].

In Fig. 2.4, we assume a constant harm and a risk-dependent benefit. The latter relies on a valid prognostic model in combination with a single relative effect of treatment. Extensions of this approach can be considered, with more reliability if larger data sets are modeled [298, 300, 630]. Specifically, we search for differential treatment effects among subgroups of patients. The assumption of a fixed relative benefit is then relaxed: some patients may respond relatively well to a certain treatment and others do not. Patient characteristics such as age, or the specific type of disease, may interact with treatment response. Effects of drugs are affected may be the drug metabolism, which is, e.g., mediated by cytochrome P450 enzymes and drug transporters [141]. Researchers in the field of pharmacogenomics aim to further understand the relation between an individual patient's genetic makeup (genotype) and the response to drug treatment, such that response can better be predicted. Cost-effectiveness will vary depending on the likelihood of response to treatment.

Note that in the absence of a biological rationale, subgroup effects may be largely spurious [300, 658]. And even if a biological rationale is present, huge sample sizes are needed for sufficient statistical power of subgroup analyses. These far exceed the sample sizes required for the detection of a main effect of a treatment. In the optimal case, the sample size needs to be four times as large to detect an interaction of the same size as the main effect [81]. If we assume that the interaction is half the size of the main effect, a 16 times larger sample size is needed [175]. See also http://www.clinicalpredictionmodels.org/doku.php?id=additional:chapter02.

2.3.8   Delaying Treatment

In medical practice, prediction models may provide information to patients and their relatives, such that they have realistic expectations of the course of disease. A conservative approach can sometimes be taken, which means that the natural history of the disease is followed. For example, many men may opt for a watchful waiting strategy if a probably unimportant ("indolent") prostate cancer is detected [295, 349]. Or women may be reassured on their pregnancy chances if they have relatively favorable characteristics.

2.3.9   *Example: Spontaneous Pregnancy Chances

Several models have been published for the prediction of spontaneous pregnancy among subfertile couples. A "synthesis model" was developed for predicting spontaneous conception leading to live birth within 1 year after the start of follow-up based on data from three previous studies [261]. This synthesis models hence had a broader empirical basis than the original models. It has later been revised [47]. The predictors included readily available characteristics such as the duration of subfertility, women's age, primary or secondary infertility, percentage of motile sperm, and whether the couple was referred by a general practitioner or by a gynecologist (referral status). The chance of spontaneous pregnancy within 1 year can easily be calculated. First, a prognostic index score is calculated. The score corresponds to a probability, which can be read from a graph (Fig. 2.5).

For example, a couple with a 35-year-old woman (7 points), 2 years of infertility (3 points), but with one child already (secondary infertility, 0 points), normal sperm motility (0 points), and directly coming to the gynecologist (secondary care couple, 0 points), has a total score of 10 points (*circled scores* in Fig. 2.5). This corresponds to a chance of becoming pregnant resulting in live birth of around 42%.

Most couples who have tried for more than 1 year to become pregnant demand immediate treatment [261]. Most couples overestimate the success of assisted reproduction, such as in vitro fertilization, and underestimate the related risks. The estimated spontaneous pregnancy chance leading to live birth can be a tool in advising such couples. If the chances are low, e.g., below 20%, there is no point in

							Subfertility Score
Woman's age (years)	21-25	26-31	32-35	36-37	38-39	40-41	
Score	0	3	(7)	10	13	15	....
Duration of subfertility (years)	1	2	3-4	5-6	7-8		
Score	0	(3)	7	12	18		....
Type of subfertility	Secondary		Primary				
Score	(0)		8				....
Motility (%)	≥ 60	40-59	20-39	0-19			
Score	(0)	2	4	6			....
Referral status	Secondary-care		Tertiary-care				
Score	(0)		4				....
			Prognostic Score (Sum)				....

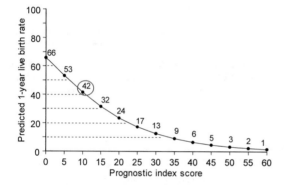

Fig. 2.5 Score chart to estimate the chance of spontaneous pregnancy within 1 year after intake resulting in live birth. Upper part: calculating the score; lower part: predicting 1-year pregnancy rate [261]. The subfertility scores for the example couple are circled, which implies a prognostic score of 10 points, corresponding to a 42% chance of spontaneous pregnancy within 1 year resulting in live birth

further waiting, and advising the couple to quickly undergo treatment is realistic. In contrast, if the chances are favorable, e.g., above 40%, the couple should be encouraged to wait for another year because there is a substantial chance of success.

2.3.10 Surgical Decision-Making

In surgery, it is typical that short-term risks are taken to reduce long-term risks. Short-term risks include both morbidity and mortality. The surgery aims to reduce long-term risks that would occur in the natural history. Acute situations include surgery for trauma and conditions such as a ruptured aneurysm (a widened artery). Elective surgery is done for many conditions, and even for such planned and well-prepared surgery, the short-term risk and burden are never null. In oncology,

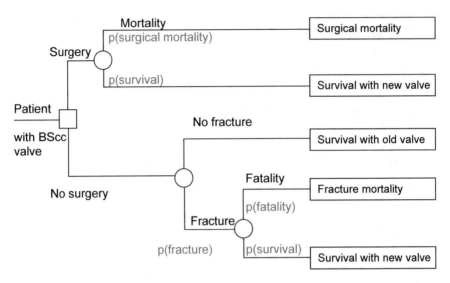

Fig. 2.6 Schematic representation of surgical decision-making on short-term versus long-term risk in replacement of a risky heart valve ("BScc"). Square indicates a decision, circle a chance node. Predictions ("*p*") are needed for four probabilities: surgical mortality, long-term survival, fracture, and fatality of fracture

increased surgical risks typically lead to the choice for less risky treatments, e.g., chemotherapy or radiation, or palliative treatments. For example, in many cancers, older patients and those with comorbidity do undergo surgery less often [277].

Many prognostic models have been developed to estimate short-term risks of surgery, e.g., 30-day mortality. These models vary in complexity and accuracy. Also, long-term risks have been modeled explicitly for various diseases, although it is often hard to find a suitable group of patients for the natural course of a disease without surgical intervention. As an example, we consider a surgical decision problem on replacement of risky heart valves (Fig. 2.6). Prognostic models were used to estimate surgical mortality, individualized risk of the specific valve, and individual survival [549, 611].

2.3.11   *Example: Replacement of Risky Heart Valves*

Björk–Shiley convexo-concave (BScc) mechanical heart valves were withdrawn from the market in 1986 after reports of mechanical failure (outlet strut fracture). Worldwide, approximately 86,000 BScc valves had been implanted by then. Fracture of the outlet strut occurs suddenly and is often lethal [610]. Therefore, prophylactic replacement by another, safer valve, may be considered to avert the risk of fracture. Decision analysis is a useful technique to weigh the long-term loss of life expectancy due to fracture against the short-term surgical mortality risk

(Fig. 2.6). The long-term loss of life expectancy due to fracture risk depends on three aspects:

(1) the annual risk of fracture, given that a patient is alive;
(2) the fatality of a fracture;
(3) the annual risk of death (survival).

This long-term loss of life expectancy has to be weighed against the risk of surgical mortality. If the patient survives surgery, the fracture risk is assumed to be reduced to zero. Predictive regression models were developed for each aspect, based on the follow-up experience from 2,263 patients with BScc valves implanted between 1979 and 1985 in The Netherlands [549]. We considered 50 fractures that had occurred during follow-up and 883 patients who died (excluding fractures).

The risk of fracture is the key consideration in this decision problem. The low number of fractures makes predictive modeling challenging, and various variants of models have been proposed. A relatively detailed model included four traditional predictors (age, position (aortic/mitral), type (70° opening angle valves had higher risks than 60° valves), and size (larger valves had higher risks)), and two production characteristics [549]. The fatality of a fracture depended on the age of the patient and the position (higher fatality in aortic position). Survival was related to age, gender, position of the valve, and time since implantation. Surgical risk was modeled in relation to age and the position of the valve. This was a relatively rough approach, since many more predictors are relevant, and a later prediction model was much more detailed [619].

The results of this decision analysis depended strongly on age: replacement was only indicated for younger patients, who have lower surgical risks, and a higher long-term impact of fracture because of longer survival (Table 2.3). Also, the position of the valve affects all four aspects (surgical risk, survival, fracture, and fatality). Before, results were presented as age thresholds for eight subgroups of valves: by position (aortic/mitral), by type (70°/60°), and by size (large/small) [611]. The more recent analysis was so detailed that individualized calculations were necessary, which were performed for all patients who were alive in the Netherlands in 1998. The recommendations from this decision analysis were rather well followed in clinical practice [620].

2.4 Prediction Models for Medical Research

In medical research, prediction models may serve several purposes. In experimental studies, such as randomized controlled trials, prognostic baseline characteristics may assist in the inclusion and stratification of patients and improve the statistical analysis. In observational studies, adequate controlling for confounding factors is essential.

Table 2.3 Patient characteristics used in the decision analysis of replacement of risky heart valves [549]

Characteristic	Surgical risk	Survival	Fracture	Fatality| fracture
Patient related				
Age (years)	+	+	+	+
Sex (male/female)		+		
Time since implantation (years)		+		
Valve related				
Position (aortic/mitral)	+	+	+	+
Opening angle (60°/70°),			+	
Size (<29 mm or >=29 mm)			+	
Production characteristics			+	
Type of prediction model	Logistic regression	Poisson regression	Poisson regression	Logistic regression

2.4.1   Inclusion and Stratification in a RCT

In randomized clinical trials (RCTs), prognostic estimates may be used for the selection of subjects for the study. Traditionally, a set of inclusion and exclusion criteria are applied to define the subjects for the RCT. Some criteria aim to create a more homogeneous group according to expected outcome. All inclusion criteria have to be fulfilled, and none of the exclusion criteria. Alternatively, some prognostic criteria can be combined in a prediction model, with selection based on individualized predictions. This leads to a more refined selection.

Stratification is often advised in RCTs for the main prognostic factors [18, 687]. In this way, balance is obtained between the arms of a trial with respect to baseline prognosis. This may facilitate simple, direct comparisons of treatment results, especially for smaller RCTs, where some imbalance may readily occur. Prediction models may refine such stratification of patients, especially when many prognostic factors are known. We illustrate prognostic selection with a simple example of two predictors in traumatic brain injury.

2.4.2   *Example: Selection for TBI Trials

As an example, we consider the selection of patients for RCTs in Traumatic Brain Injury (TBI). Patients above 65 years of age and those with nonreacting pupils are often excluded because of a high likelihood of a poor outcome. Indeed, we find a higher than 50% mortality at 6-month follow-up in patients fulfilling either criterion (Table 2.4). Hence, we can simply select only those less than 65 years with at least one reacting pupil (Table 2.5, part A). We can also use a prognostic model for more efficient selection that inclusion based on separate criteria. A simple logistic

Table 2.4 Analysis of outcome in 7143 patients with severe or moderate traumatic brain injury according to reactive pupils and age dichotomized at age 65 years [364]

	>=1 reactive pupil		Nonreactive pupils	
	<65	>=65 years	<65	>=65 years
6-month mortality	926/5101 (18%)	159/284 (56%)	849/1644 (52%)	97/114 (85%)

Table 2.5 Selection of patients with 2 criteria (age and reactive pupils) in a traditional way (A) and according to a prognostic model (probability of 6-month mortality < 50%, B)

		A: Traditional selection		B: Prognostic selection		
		<65	>=65 years	<30	30–75	>=76 years
Pupillary reactivity	No reactivity	Exclude	Exclude	Include	Exclude	Exclude
	>=1 pupil	Include	Exclude	Include	Include	Exclude

regression model with "age" and "pupils" can be used to calculate the probability of mortality in a more detailed way. If we aim to exclude those with a predicted risk over 50%, this leads to an age limit of 30 years for those without any pupil reaction, and an age limit of 76 years for those with any pupil reaction (Table 2.5, part B). So, patients under 30 years of age can always be included, and patients between 65 and 75 years can be included if they have at least one reacting pupil, if we want to include only those with <50% mortality risks (Table 2.5).

2.4.3   Covariate Adjustment in a RCT

Even more important is the role of prognostic baseline characteristics in the analysis of a RCT. The strength of randomization is that comparability is created between treated groups both with respect to observed *and unobserved* baseline characteristics (Fig. 2.7). No systematic confounding can hence occur in RCTs. But some observed baseline characteristics may be strongly related to the outcome. Adjustment for such covariates has several advantages [174, 233, 241, 243, 441, 463]:

(1) to reduce any distortion in the estimate of treatment effect occurred by random imbalance between groups
(2) to increase the statistical power for detection of a treatment effect.

Remarkably, covariate adjustment works differently for linear regression models and generalized linear models (e.g., logistic, Cox regression, Table 2.6).

(1) For randomized clinical trials, the randomization guarantees that the bias in the estimated treatment effect is zero a priori, without distortion by observed or unobserved baseline characteristics. However, random imbalances may occur,

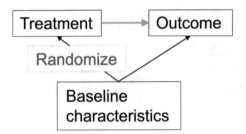

Fig. 2.7 Schematic representation of the role of baseline characteristics in a RCT. By randomization, there is no systematic link between baseline characteristics, observed or unobserved, and treatment. Baseline characteristics are still important, since they are commonly prognostic for the outcome

Table 2.6 Comparison of adjustment for predictors in linear and generalized linear models (e.g., logistic regression) in estimation and testing of treatment effects, when predictors are completely balanced

Method	Effect estimate	Standard error	Power
Linear model	*Identical*	*Decreases*	*Increases*
Generalized linear model	*Further from zero*	*Increases*	*Increases*

generating questions such as: What would have been the treatment effect had the two groups been perfectly balanced? We may think of this distortion as a bias a posteriori since it affects interpretation similarly as in observational epidemiological studies.

Regression analysis is an obvious technique to correct for such random imbalances. When no imbalances have occurred for predictors considered in a regression model, the adjusted and unadjusted estimates of the treatment effect would be expected to be the same. This is indeed the case in linear regression analysis. Remarkably, in generalized linear models such as logistic regression, the adjusted and unadjusted estimates of a treatment effect are not the same, even when predictors are completely balanced [174] (see Questions 2.3 and 22.2). Adjusted effects are expected to be further from zero (neutral value, odds ratio further from 1). This phenomenon has been referred to as the "non-collapsibility" of effect estimates [210], or a "stratification effect". It does not occur with linear regression [537].

(2) With linear regression, adjustment for important predictors leads to an improvement in precision of the estimated treatment effect since part of the variance in the outcome is explained by the predictors. Contrarily, in generalized linear models such as logistic regression, the standard error of the treatment effect always increases with adjustment [463]. In linear regression, adjusted analyses provide more power to the analysis of treatment effect since the standard error of the treatment effect is smaller. For a generalized linear model such as logistic regression, the effect of adjustment on power is not so

straightforward. It has however been proven that the expected value of the treatment effect estimate increases more than the standard error. Hence, the power for detection of a treatment effect is larger in an adjusted logistic regression analysis compared to an unadjusted analysis, similar to linear regression models [463].

2.4.4 Gain in Power by Covariate Adjustment

The gain in power by covariate adjustment depends on the correlation between the baseline covariates (predictors) and the outcome. For continuous outcomes, this correlation can be indicated by Pearson's correlation coefficient (r). The sample size can be reduced with $1 - r^2$ to achieve the same statistical power with a covariate adjusted analysis as an unadjusted analysis [441]. A very strong predictor may have $r = 0.7$ (r^2 50%), e.g., a baseline covariate of a repeated measure such as blood pressure, or a questionnaire score. The required number of patients is then roughly halved. The saving is less than 10% for $r = 0.3$ (r^2 9%) [441].

Similar results have been obtained in empirical evaluations with dichotomous outcomes, where Nagelkerke's R^2 [403] was used to express the correlation between predictor and outcome [241, 243, 537]. The reduction in sample size was slightly less than $1 - R^2$ in simulations for mortality among acute MI patients [537] and among TBI patients (Table 2.7) [242,589].

2.4.5 *Example: Analysis of the GUSTO-III Trial

The GUSTO-III trial considered patients with an acute myocardial infarction [3]. The primary outcome was 30-day mortality. The protocol prespecified a prognostic

Table 2.7 Illustration of reduction in sample size with adjustment for baseline covariates with dichotomous outcomes

Application area	Correlation baseline—outcome	Reduction in sample size
Acute MI: 30-day mortality [537]		
Age adjustment	R^2 13%	12%
17 predictor adjustment	R^2 25%	19%
Traumatic brain injury: 6 month mortality [242]		
3 predictor model	R^2 30%	25%
7 predictor model	R^2 40%	30%

model for the primary analysis of the treatment effect. This model combined age, systolic blood pressure, Killip class, heart rate, infarct location, and age-by-Killip-class interaction. These predictors were previously found to comprise 90% of the prognostic information of a more complex model for 30-day mortality in the GUSTO-I trial [329]. As discussed above, there are quite some strong arguments for wider use of such covariate adjustment [286].

2.4.6   Prediction Models and Observational Studies

Confounding is the major concern in epidemiological analyses of observational studies, where we aim to estimate causal effects. When treatments are compared, groups are often quite different because of a lack of randomization. Subjects with specific characteristics are more likely to have received a certain treatment than other subjects ("confounding by indication") [63]. If these characteristics also affect the outcome, a direct comparison of treatments is biased and may merely reflect the lack of initial comparability ("confounding"). In addition to treatment, other factors can also be investigated for their etiologic effects. Often, randomization is not possible, and observational studies are the only possible design. Dealing with confounding is an essential step in such analyses.

Regression analysis is a commonly used method to control the imbalances between treatment groups, e.g., with logistic or Cox regression [63]. Many baseline characteristics can be simultaneously adjusted for (Fig. 2.8). In contrast to RCTs, we can only balance baseline characteristics that are observed, ideally without measurement error. We should especially be worried about any unknown covariates that may nevertheless act as confounders by their association with both treatment choice and outcome.

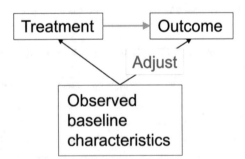

Fig. 2.8 Schematic representation of adjustment for baseline characteristics in an observational study. By adjustment, we aim to correct for the systematic link between observed baseline characteristics and outcome, hence answering the question: what is the treatment effect if observed baseline characteristics were similar between treatment groups?

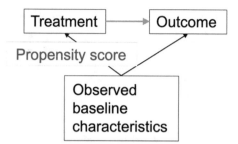

Fig. 2.9 Schematic representation of propensity score adjustment for baseline characteristics in an observational study. The propensity score estimates the probability of receiving treatment. By subsequent adjustment for the propensity score, we mimic an RCT, since we removed the systematic link between baseline characteristics and treatment. We can however only include observed baseline characteristics. We have no control over unobserved characteristics

2.4.7   Propensity Scores

Adjustment with regression analysis is problematic when the outcome is relatively rare. This may lead to biased and inefficient estimates of the difference between groups in the adjusted analysis [91]. An alternative is to use a propensity score, which is especially attractive in the setting of rare outcomes [72]. The propensity score defines the probability that a subject receives a particular treatment ("Tx") given a set of confounders: p(Tx | confounders). For calculation of the propensity score, the confounders are usually used in a logistic regression model to predict the treatment, without including the outcome [82,479]. The propensity score is subsequently used in a second stage as a summary confounder (Fig. 2.9). Common approaches in this second stage are matching on propensity score, stratification of propensity score (usually by quantile), and inclusion of the propensity score with treatment in a regression model for the outcome [117].

Empirical comparisons provided no indication of superiority of propensity score methods over conventional regression analysis for confounder adjustment [503,574]. In contrast, simulation studies suggest a benefit of propensity scores in the situation of few outcomes relatively to the number of confounding variables [91].

2.4.8   *Example: Statin Treatment Effects

Statins have been studied in RCTs and observational studies for their effect on the occurrence of acute myocardial infarction (AMI). A propensity score analysis was performed for members of a Community Health Plan with a recorded LDL >130 mg/dl at any time between 1994 and 1998 [499]. Members who initiated therapy with a statin were matched using propensity scores to members who did not initiate statin therapy. The propensity score predicted the probability of statin initiation. Scores

Table 2.8 The effect of statins on the occurrence of acute myocardial infarction [499]

	Confounders	N with AMI	HR [95% CI]
Unadjusted	–	325 versus 124	2.1 [1.5–3.0]
Propensity score adjusted	52 main effects, 6 quadratic terms	77 versus 114	0.69 [0.52–0.93]

were estimated using a logistic regression model that included 52 variables and 6 quadratic terms (Table 2.8). Statin initiators were matched to non-initiators with a similar propensity to receive treatment (within a 0.01 caliper of propensity). Initiators for whom no suitable non-initiator could be found were excluded, leaving 2901 matched initiators out of 4144 initiators (70%). The 4144 statin initiators had a higher prevalence of established coronary heart disease risk factors than unmatched non-initiators. The follow-up of these unmatched cohorts identified 325 AMIs in the statin initiator group and 124 in the non-initiator group (hazard ratio 2.1, Table 2.8). The propensity score-matched cohorts ($2 \times n = 2901$) were found to be very similar with respect to 51 of the 52 matched baseline characteristics. There were 77 cases of AMI in statin initiators compared with 114 in matched non-initiators (hazard ratio 0.69). The authors conclude that statin use in the members of this Community Health Plan was beneficial on the occurrence of AMI, but rightly warn that predictors that are not part of the model may remain unbalanced between propensity score-matched cohorts, leading to residual confounding.

2.4.9   Provider Comparisons

Another area of application of prediction models is in the comparison of outcomes from different hospitals (or other providers of care) [62]. The quality of healthcare providers is being compared by their outcomes, which are considered as performance indicators. Simple comparisons between providers may obviously be biased by differences in case-mix, for example, academic centers may see more severe patients, which accounts for poorer outcome on average. Prediction models are needed for case-mix adjustment in such comparisons. Another problem arises from the fact that providers may be relatively small and that multiple comparisons are made (see Chaps. 4 and 21).

2.4.10   *Example: Ranking Cardiac Outcome

New York State was among the first to publicly release rankings of outcome of coronary artery bypass surgery by surgeon and hospital. Such cardiac surgery report cards have been criticized because of their methodology [183]. Adequate risk adjustment is nowadays better possible with sophisticated prediction models. An example is a prediction model for 30-day mortality rates among patients with an acute myocardial infarction [317]. The model used information from administrative claims but was aimed to support profiling of hospital performance. They analyzed 140,120 cases discharged from 4664 hospitals in 1998. They compared the model from claims data with a model using medical record data and found high agreement. They also found adequate stability over time (data from years 1995 to 2001). The final model included 27 variables and had an area under the receiver operating characteristic curve of 0.71. The authors conclude that this administrative claims-based model is as adequate for profiling hospitals as a medical record model.

Rather than focusing on individual hospitals, we may also evaluate more general trends in quality of care. For example, we may evaluate the decrease in 30-day mortality rates among patients with an acute myocardial infarction from 1995 to 2006 [316]. The 30-day mortality decreased from 19% in 1995 to 16% in 2006, while the prognostic profile worsened somewhat, with a mean age increase from 77 in 1995 to 79 years in 2006, and higher prevalence of coexisting illnesses such as hypertension, diabetes, renal disease, and chronic obstructive pulmonary disease. The risk-standardized mortality rate decreased from 18.8% in 1995 to 15.8% in 2006 (odds ratio, 0.76), with less variation between hospital outcomes in 2006 [316]. Chapter 21 provides a more in-depth discussion of this research area.

2.5   Concluding Remarks

Many more areas of potential application of prediction models may exist than discussed here, including public health (targeting of preventive interventions), clinical practice (diagnostic workup, therapeutic decision-making, shared decision-making), and research (design and analysis of RCTs, confounder adjustment in observational studies). Obtaining predictions from a model has to be separated from obtaining insights into the disease mechanisms and pathophysiological processes [508]. Often, prediction models serve the latter purpose too, but the primary aim considered in this book is reliable outcome prediction.

Questions

2.1. Examples of applications of prediction models

   (a) What is a recent application of a prediction model that you encountered? Search PubMed [http://www.ncbi.nlm.nih.gov/sites/entrez] if nothing comes to mind.
   (b) How could you use a prediction model in your own research or in your own clinical practice?

2.2. Cost-effectiveness
   How could prediction models contribute to targeting of treatment and increasing cost-effectiveness of medical care?

2.3. Covariate adjustment in a RCT
   What are the purposes of covariate adjustment in a RCT? Explain and distinguish between logistic and linear regression.

2.4. Propensity score

   (a) What is the definition of a propensity score?
   (b) Explain the difference between adjustment for confounders through regression analysis and through a propensity score.
   (c) When is a propensity score specifically appropriate? See papers by Braitman and by Cepeda et al. [72, 91].

Chapter 3
Study Design for Prediction Modeling

Background In this chapter, we consider several issues in the design of studies for prediction research. These include the selection of subjects or patients for a cohort study, strengths, and limitations of case series from a single center, from registries, or randomized controlled trials. We further discuss issues in choosing predictors and outcome variables for prediction models. An important question is often how large a study needs to be for sufficient statistical power. Power considerations are given for studying effects of specific predictors and for developing a prediction model that can provide reliable predictions and validation of prediction model performance. We refer to several case studies for illustration.

3.1 Studies for Prognosis

Prognostic studies are inherently longitudinal in nature, most often performed in cohorts of patients, who are followed over time for an outcome (or "event" or "end point") to occur [238]. The cohort is defined by the presence of one or more particular characteristics, e.g., having a certain disease, living in a certain place, having a certain age, or simply being born alive.

Several types of cohort studies can be used for prognostic modeling. The most common type may be a single-center retrospective cohort study (Table 3.1). For example, patients are identified from hospital records between certain dates. These patients were followed over time for the outcome, but the investigator looks back in time (hence, we may use the label "retrospective study" [638]).

© Springer Nature Switzerland AG 2019
E. W. Steyerberg, *Clinical Prediction Models*, Statistics for Biology and Health, https://doi.org/10.1007/978-3-030-16399-0_3

Table 3.1 Study designs for prognostic studies

Design	Characteristics	Strengths	Limitations
Retrospective	Often single-center studies	Simple, low costs	Selection of patients Definitions and completeness of predictors Outcome assessment not by protocol
Prospective, RCT/trial	Often multicenter	Well-defined selection of patients Prospective recording of predictors Prospective assessment of outcome according to protocol	Poor generalizability because of stringent in- and exclusion criteria
Registry	Complete coverage of an area/participants, e.g. covered by insurance	Simple, low costs Prospective recording of predictors	Outcome assessment not by protocol
Case–control	Efficient when the outcome is relatively rare	Simple, low costs	Selection of controls critical Definitions and completeness of predictors Outcome assessment not by protocol

3.1.1   Retrospective Designs

Strengths of a retrospective study design include its simplicity and feasibility. It is a design with relatively low costs, since patient records in a single center can often easily be searched, especially with modern hospital information systems or electronic patient records. A limitation is the correct identification of patients, which has to be done in retrospect. If some information is missing, or was incorrectly recorded, this may lead to a selection bias. Similarly, the recording of predictors has to have been reliable to be useful for prediction modeling. Finally, the outcome assessment has to be reliable. This may be relatively straightforward for hard end points such as survival, where some deaths will be known from hospital records. But additional confirmation of vital status may often be required from nationwide statistical bureaus for a complete assessment of survival status. Other outcomes, e.g., related to functional status, may not be available at the time points that we wish to analyze. Finally, single-center studies may be limited by their sample size, which is a key problem in prediction research.

3.1.2 *Example: Predicting Early Mortality in Esophageal Cancer

As an example, we consider outcome prediction in esophageal cancer. A retrospective chart review was performed of 120 patients treated in a single institution between January 1, 1997, and December 31, 2003 [326]. The patients had palliative treatment, which means therapy that relieves symptoms, but does not alter the course of the disease. A stent was placed in the esophagus because of malignancy-related dysphagia (difficulty in swallowing). The authors studied 30-day mortality, which occurred in an unspecified number of patients (probably around 10%, $n = 12$). Predictors were nutritional status (low serum albumin levels, low BMI) and performance status (WHO class, which ranges from normal activity to 100% bedridden) [326].

3.1.3 Prospective Designs

In a prospective study, we can better check specific inclusion and exclusion criteria. The investigators age with the study population (hence, the label "prospective study"). We can use clear and consistent definitions of predictors and assess patient outcomes at predefined time points. Prospective cohort studies are therefore preferable to retrospective series.

Prospective cohort studies solely for prediction modeling are rare. A more common design is that prediction research is done in data from randomized clinical trials (RCTs), or from prospective before–after trials. The strengths are in the well-defined selection of patients, the prospective recording of predictors, usually with quality checks, and the prospective assessment of outcome. Sample size is usually reasonably large. A limitation of data from (randomized) trials may be in the selection of patients. Often stringent inclusion and exclusion criteria are used, which may limit the generalizability of a model developed on such data. On the other hand, RCTs are often performed in multiple centers, sometimes from multiple countries or continents. Benefits of the multicenter design include that consensus has to be reached on definition issues for predictors and outcome, and that generalizability of findings will be increased. This is in contrast to single-center studies, which only reflect associations from one specific setting.

A topic of debate is whether we should only use patients from an RCT who are randomized to a conventional treatment or placebo (the "control group"). If we combine randomized groups, we assume that no specific subgroup effects are relevant to the prognostic model. This may generally be reasonable. The prognostic effect of a treatment is usually small compared to prognostic effects of other predictors (see GUSTO-I example in Chap. 22). If the prediction model is intended to support decision-making on treatment, the easiest and quite reasonable solution is to include treatment as a main effect [299, 300].

3.1.4   *Example: Predicting Long-term Mortality in Esophageal Cancer

In another study of outcome in esophageal cancer, data from an RCT ("SIREC", $n = 209$ [255]) were combined with other prospectively collected data ($n = 396$) [548]. Long-term mortality was studied after palliative treatment with a stent or radiation ("brachytherapy"). A simple prognostic score was proposed that combined age, gender, tumor length, presence of metastases, and WHO performance score.

3.1.5   Registry Data

Prognostic studies are often performed with registry data, for example, cancer registries, or insurance databases. Data collection is prospective but not primarily for prediction research. The level of detail may be a limitation for prognostic analyses. For example, the well-known US-based cancer registry (Surveillance, Epidemiology and End Results, SEER) contains information on cancer incidence, mortality, and patient demographics and tumor stage. It has been linked to the Medicare database for information on comorbidity [305] and treatment (surgery [108], chemotherapy [661], radiotherapy [652]). Socioeconomic status is usually based on median income as available at an aggregated level [35]. SEER-Medicare does not contain detailed information on performance status, which is an important factor for medical decision-making and for survival. Also, staging may have some measurement bias [156].

Another problem may occur when reimbursement depends on the severity that is scored for a patient. This may pose an upward bias on the recording of comorbidities in claims databases.

The outcomes for prognostic analyses in registry data may suffer from the same limitations as retrospective studies, since usually no predefined assessments are made. Outcomes are therefore often limited to survival, although other adverse events can sometimes also be derived [143, 523]. Strengths of prognostic studies with registry data include large sample sizes and representativeness of patients (especially with population-based cancer registries). Available large databases may especially be useful for studying prognostic relations of a limited number of predictors with survival.

3.1.6   *Example: Surgical Mortality in Esophageal Cancer

The SEER-Medicare database was used to analyze 30-day mortality in 1327 patients undergoing surgery for esophageal cancer. Predictive patient characteristics included age, comorbidity (cardiac, pulmonary, renal, hepatic, and diabetes), pre-operative radiotherapy or combined chemoradiotherapy, and a relatively low hospital volume, which were combined in a simple prognostic score. Validation was done in another registry and in a hospital series [560].

3.1.7 Nested Case–Control Studies

A prospectively designed, nested case–control study is sometimes an efficient option for prediction research. A case–control design is especially attractive when the outcome is relatively rare, such as incident of breast cancer [171]. For example, if 30-day mortality is 1%, it is efficient to determine predictors in all patients who died, but, for example, 4% of the controls (1:4 case–control ratio). A random sample of controls is used as comparison for the cases. Assessment of predictors is in retrospect, which is a limitation. If a prediction model is developed, the average outcome incidence has to be adjusted for final calculation of probabilities, while the regression coefficients might be based on the case–control study [171].

3.1.8 *Example: Perioperative Mortality in Major Vascular Surgery

An interesting example is the analysis of perioperative mortality in patients undergoing major vascular surgery [442]. Predictors were determined in retrospect from a detailed chart review in all cases (patients who died) and in selected controls (patients who did survive surgery). Controls had surgery just before and just after the case. Hence, a 1:2 ratio was achieved for cases against controls.

3.2 Studies for Diagnosis

Diagnostic studies are most often designed as a cross-sectional study, where predictive patient characteristics are related to an underlying diagnosis. The study group is defined by the presence of a particular symptom or sign that makes the subject suspected of having a particular (target) disease. Typically, the subjects undergo the index test and subsequently a reference test to establish the "true" presence or absence of the target disease, over a short time span.

3.2.1 Cross-sectional Study Design and Multivariable Modeling

Ideally, a diagnostic study considers a well-defined cohort of patients suspected of a certain diagnosis, e.g., an acute myocardial infarction [308]. Such a diagnostic study then resembles a prognostic cohort study. The cohort is here defined by the *suspicion* of having (rather than *actually* having) a disease. The outcome is the underlying diagnosis. The study may therefore be labeled cross-sectional, since the predictor–outcome relations are studied at a single point in time. Several characteristics may be predictive of the underlying diagnosis. For a model, we should start with considering simple characteristics such as demographics, and symptoms and signs obtained from patient history. Next, we may consider simple diagnostic tests, and finally invasive and/or costly tests [386]. The diagnosis (presence or absence of the target disease) should be established by a reference test. The result of the reference test is preferably interpreted without knowledge of the predictor and diagnostic test values. Such blinding prevents information or incorporation bias [387].

A common problem in diagnostic evaluations includes incomplete registration of all predictive characteristics. Moreover, not all patients may have undergone the entire diagnostic workup, especially if they are considered as at low risk of the target disease. Also, outcome assessment may be incomplete, if a test is used as a gold standard which is selectively performed [450]. These problems are especially prominent in diagnostic analyses on data from routine practice [411]. Prospective studies are, hence, preferable, since these may use a prespecified protocol for systematic diagnostic workup and reference standard testing.

3.2.2 *Example: Diagnosing Renal Artery Stenosis*

A cardiology database was retrospectively reviewed for patients who underwent coincident screening abdominal aorta angiography to detect occult renal artery stenosis. In a development set, stenosis was observed in 128 of 635 patients. This 20% prevalence may be an overestimate if patients underwent angiography because of suspicion of stenosis [456].

3.2.3 *Case–Control Studies*

Diagnostic studies sometimes select patients on the presence or absence of the target disease as determined by the reference test as executed conform routine care. Hence, patients without a reference standard are not selected. In fact, a case–control study is performed, where cases are those with the target disease, and controls those without. This design has a number of limitations, especially related to the representativeness of the selected patients for all patients who are suspected of the diagnosis of interest. This is different from a nested case–control study. Selection bias is another important limitation. Indeed, empirical evidence is now available on the biases that may arise in diagnostic studies, especially by including nonconsecutive patients in a case–control design, nonrepresentative patients (severe cases compared to healthy controls), and when data are collected retrospectively [337, 480, 670].

3.2.4 *Example: Diagnosing Acute Appendicitis*

C-reactive protein (CRP) has been used for the diagnosis of acute appendicitis. Surgery and pathology results constituted the reference test for patients with a high CRP. Patients with a low CRP were not operated on and clinical follow-up determined whether they were classified as having acute appendicitis. As low-grade infections with low CRPs can resolve spontaneously, this verification strategy fails to identify all false-negative test results. Hence, the diagnostic performance of CRP may be overestimated [337].

3.3 Predictors and Outcome

3.3.1 Strength of Predictors

For a well-performing prediction model, strong predictors have to be present. Strength is a function of the association of the predictor with the outcome ("effect size"), and the distribution of the predictor. For example, a dichotomous predictor with an odds ratio of 2.0 is more relevant for a prediction model than a dichotomous predictor with an odds ratio of 2.5, when the first predictor is distributed in a 50:50 ratio (50% prevalence of the predictor), and the second 1:99 (1% prevalence of the predictor). Similarly, continuous predictors have to cover a wide range to make them relevant for prediction.

When some characteristics are considered as key predictors, these have to be registered carefully, with clear definitions and preferably no missing values. This is usually best possible in a prospective study, with a protocol and prespecified data collection form.

3.3.2 Categories of Predictors

Several categories of predictors have been suggested for prediction models [225]. These include

- demographics (e.g., age, sex, race, education, socioeconomic status),
- type and severity of disease (e.g., principal diagnosis, presenting characteristics),
- history characteristics (e.g., previous disease episodes, risk factors),
- comorbidity (concomitant diseases),
- physical functional status (e.g., Karnofsky score, WHO performance score), and
- subjective health status and quality of life (psychological, cognitive, psychosocial functioning).

The relevance of these categories will depend on the specifics of the application. Investigators tend to group predictors under general headings, see, for example, the predictors in the GUSTO-I model (Chapt. 22) [329]. Of note, definitions of predictors may vary from study to study [681]. For example, socioeconomic status (SES) can be defined in many ways, considering a patient's working status, income, and/or education. Also, SES indicators are sometimes not determined at the individual level, but, for example, at census tract level ("ecological SES", e.g., in analyses of SEER-Medicare data [35, 538]). Race/ethnicity can be defined in various ways, and sometimes be self-reported rather than determined by certain predefined rules. Comorbidity definitions and scoring systems are still under development. Variations in definitions are serious threats to generalizability of prediction models [16, 355]. Initiatives have been taken to define "Common Data Elements", which should improve the comparability of predictors across studies [686].

Another differentiation is to separate the patient's condition from his/her constitution. Condition may be reflected in type and severity of disease, history characteristics, comorbidity, physical, and subjective health status. Constitution may especially be related to demographics such as age and gender. For example, the same type of trauma (reflected in patient condition) affects patients of different ages differently (constitution) [260, 343].

In the future, genetic characteristics will be used more widely in a prediction context. Inborn variants of the human genome, such as polymorphisms and mutations, may be considered as indicators of the patient's constitution. Other genetic characteristics, for example, the genomic profile of a malignant tumor, may better be thought of as indicators of subtypes of tumors, reflecting condition.

3.3.3 Costs of Predictors

Predictors may require different costs, in monetary terms, but also in burden for a patient. In a prediction context, it is evident that information that is easy to obtain should be considered before information that is more difficult to obtain. Hence, we should first consider characteristics such as demographics and patient history, followed by simple diagnostic tests, and finally invasive and/or costly tests. Expensive genetic tests should, hence, be considered for their incremental value over classical predictors rather than alone [293]. Such an incremental evaluation is well possible with predictive regression models, where a model is first considered without the test, and subsequently a model with the test added [531].

3.3.4 Determinants of Prognosis

Prognosis can also be viewed in a triangle of interacting causes (Fig. 3.1). Predictors may be separated as related to environment (e.g., socioeconomic

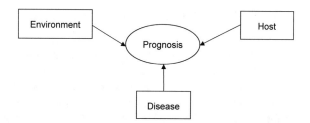

Fig. 3.1 Prognosis may be thought of as determined by predictors related to environment, host, and disease [237]

conditions, health care access and quality, climate), the host (e.g., demographic, behavioral, psychosocial, premorbid biologic factors), and disease (e.g., imaging, pathophysiologic, genomic, proteomic, metabolomic factors) [237].

3.3.5 Prognosis in Oncology

For prognosis in oncology, it has been proposed to separate factors related to the patient, the tumor and to treatment (Fig. 3.2) [239]. Examples of patients characteristics include demographics (age, sex, race/ethnicity, SES), comorbidity, and functional status. Tumor characteristics include the extent of disease (e.g., reflected in TNM stage), pathology, and sometimes values of tumor markers. Treatment may commonly include (combinations of) surgery, chemotherapy, and radiotherapy.

3.4 Reliability of Predictors

3.4.1 Observer Variability

We generally prefer predictors that are well-defined and reliably measured by any observer [73, 355]. In practice, observer variability is a problem for many measurements [73]. Disciplines include, for example, pathologists, who may unreliably score tissue specimens for histology, cell counts, coloring of cells, and radiologists, who, for example, score X-rays, CT scans, MRI scans, and ultrasound measurements. This variability is typically quantified with kappa statistics [321]. The interobserver and intraobserver variability can be substantial, which will be reflected in low kappa values. Such measurement error poses challenges to the generalizability of a prediction model.

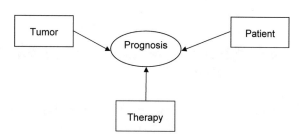

Fig. 3.2 Prognosis of a patient with cancer may be thought of as determined by predictors related to the tumor, the patients, and therapy [239]

3.4.2 *Example: Histology in Barrett's Esophagus

Barrett's esophagus is a premalignant condition. Surgery is sometimes performed in high-grade dysplasia, whereas other physicians defer radical treatment until adeno-carcinoma is diagnosed. The agreement between readings of histology in Barrett's esophagus for high-grade dysplasia or adenocarcinoma was only fair, with kappa values of around 0.4 [412]. The agreement between no dysplasia and low-grade dysplasia had been reported as even lower [516]. Because of observer variability, sometimes a central review process is organized, where 1 expert reviews all readings. This should be done independently and blinded for previous scores. Subsequently, a rule has to be determined for the final score, for example, that only the expert score is used, or that an additional reader is required in case of disagreement. Also, consensus procedures can be set up with experts only, for example, with scoring by two experts, and involvement of the third if these disagree [301]. Some use the unreliability of classical pathology as an argument for using modern biomarkers [319].

3.4.3 Biological Variability

Apart from observer variability, some measurements are prone to biological vari-ability. A well-known example is blood pressure, where a single measurement is quite unreliable. Usually, at least two measurements are made, and preferably more, with some spread in time. Again, definitions have to be clear (e.g., position of patient at the measurement, time of day).

3.4.4 Regression Dilution Bias

The effect of unreliable scoring by observers, or biological variability, generally is a dilution of associations of predictors with the outcome. This has been labeled "regression dilution bias," and methods have been proposed to correct for this bias [334]. A solution is to repeat unreliable measurements, either by the same observer (e.g., use the mean of 3 blood pressure measurements) or different observers (e.g., double reading of mammograms by radiologists). Practical constraints may limit such procedures.

3.4.5 *Example: Simulation Study on Reliability of a Binary Predictor

Suppose we have a binary predictor which has value 0 or 1 in truth, but that we measure the predictor with noise. Suppose two observers make independent

Table 3.2 Sensitivity and specificity for observers in determining the true predictor status (sensitivity = specificity = 80%)

		True predictor status	
		0	1
		N (col%)	N (col%)
Observer	0	750 (80%)	187 (20%)
	1	187 (20%)	750 (80%)

Table 3.3 Agreement between observer 1 and observer 2 (kappa = 0.36)

		Observer 2	
		0	1
Observer 1	0	637	300
	1	300	637

Table 3.4 Association with outcome for the true predictor status and observed predictor status (by observer 1 or 2, Table 3.3)

		Outcome		Odds Ratio	c statistic
		0	1		
		N (row%)	N (row%)		
True predictor status	0	625 (67%)	312 (33%)	4.0	0.67
	1	312 (33%)	625 (67%)		
Observer	0	562 (60%)	375 (40%)	2.25	0.60
	1	375 (40%)	562 (60%)		

judgments of the predictor. Their judgments agree with the true predictor status with sensitivity of 80% (observer scores 1 if true = 1) and specificity of 80% (observer scores 0 if true = 0, Table 3.2). If both observers score the predictor independently and without correlation, the observers agree with each other with a kappa of only 0.36 (Table 3.3).

The true predictor status predicts outcome well, with an odds ratio of 4. The observed predictor status has a diluted predictive effect, with odds ratio of 2.25. Similarly, the discriminative ability is diluted (c statistic decreases from 0.67 to 0.60, Table 3.4, see later chapters for definition of c).

3.4.6 Choice of Predictors

In etiologic research, we may often aim for the best assessment of a predictor. We will be concerned about various information biases that may occur. In the context of a prediction model, we can be more pragmatic [390]. If we aim to develop a model that is applicable in daily practice, we should use definitions and scorings that are in line with daily practice. For example, if medical decisions on surgery are made considering local pathology reports, without expert review, the local pathology report should be considered for a prediction model applicable to the local setting. As illustrated, such less reliable assessments will affect the performance of a prediction model, since prognostic relations are disturbed. If misclassification is at random, a dilution of the relation occurs (Table 3.4). In practice, prediction models tend to include predictors that are quite readily available, not too costly to obtain, and can be measured with reasonable precision. Caution is needed if a prediction model is applied in a context with different precisions in measurement, since such a difference will impact on a model's generalizability [355].

3.5 Outcome

3.5.1 Types of Outcome

The outcome of a prediction model should be relevant, either from an applied medical perspective or from a research perspective. From a medical perspective, "hard" end points are generally preferred. Especially mortality is often used as an end point in prognostic research. Mortality risks are relevant for many acute and chronic conditions, and for many treatments. In other diseases, nonfatal events may be more relevant, including patient-centered outcomes such as scores on quality of life questionnaires, or wider indicators of burden of disease (e.g., absence from work) (Table 3.5) [237].

Table 3.5 Examples of prognostic outcomes [237]

Prognostic outcome	Example	Characteristics
Fatal events	All-cause, or cause-specific	Hard end point, relevant in many diseases, but sometimes too infrequent for reliable statistical modeling
Nonfatal events	Recurrence of tumor, cardiovascular events (e.g., myocardial infarction, revascularization)	Somewhat softer end point, reflecting decision-making by physicians, increases sample size for analysis
Patient-centered	Symptoms, functional status, health-related quality of life, utilities	Subjective end point, focused on the patients themselves; often used as secondary end point
Wider burden	Absence from work because of sickness	Especially of interest from an economical point of view

3.5.2   Survival End Points

Survival end points are often considered in prediction models, either with a relatively short follow-up (e.g., 30-day mortality) or with longer follow-up (where some patients will have censored observations) [100]. When cause-specific mortality is considered, a reliable assessment of the cause of death is required. If cause of death is not known, relative survival can be calculated [219]. This is especially popular in cancer research. Mortality in the patients with a certain cancer is compared with the background mortality from the general population. The difference can be thought of as mortality due to the cancer.

The pros and cons of relative survival estimates are open to debate. Some have proposed to also study conditional survival for patients already surviving for some years after diagnosis, or relative survival for other time periods. These measures may sometimes be more meaningful for clinical management and prognosis than 5-year relative survival from time of diagnosis [185, 276]. Others have proposed that median survival times are better indicators of survival than 5-year relative survival rates, especially when survival times are short [417], with differences in survival time as the effect measure rather than a measure of relative risk such as the hazard ratio [474, 593].

3.5.3   *Examples: 5-Year Relative Survival in Cancer Registries

Five-year relative survival was studied for patients enrolled in the SEER registry in the period 1990–1999 [185]. The 5-year relative survival rate for persons diagnosed with cancer was 63%, with substantial variation by cancer site and stage at diagnosis. Five-year relative survival increased with time since diagnosis. For example, for patients diagnosed with cancers of the prostate, female breast, corpus uteri, and urinary bladder, the relative survival rate at 8 years after diagnosis was over 75%.

Similar analyses were performed with registry data from the Eindhoven region, where it was found that patients with colorectal, melanoma skin, or stage I breast cancer could be considered cured after 5–15 years. For other tumors, survival remained poorer than the general population [276].

3.5.4   Composite End Points

Sometimes, composite end points are defined, which combine mortality with nonfatal events. Composite end points are especially popular in cardiovascular research (see also Chap. 23). For example, the Framingham models have been used to predict incident cardiovascular disease in the general population. A popular

Framingham model (the Wilson model) defines cardiovascular events as fatal or nonfatal myocardial infarction, sudden death, or angina pectoris (stable or unstable) [674]. Composite end points have the advantage of increasing the effective sample size, and hence the power for statistical analyses, at the price of having to assume similar prognostic associations for each of the end point components.

3.5.5 *Example: Composite End Points in Cardiology

A prediction model was developed in 949 patients with decompensated heart failure. The outcomes were 60-day mortality and the composite end point of death or rehospitalization at 60 days. The discriminatory power of the model was substantial for the mortality model (c statistic 0.77) but less for the composite end point (c statistic 0.69) [159]. These findings are in line with prediction of acute coronary syndromes, where predictive performance was better for mortality than for a composite end point of mortality or myocardial (re)infarction [59]. The case study in Chap. 23 also considers a composite end point.

3.5.6 Choice of Prognostic Outcome

The choice of a prognostic outcome should be guided by the context, but the outcome should be measured as reliably as possible. Prediction models may be developed with pragmatic definitions of predictors, since this may resemble the future use of a model. But the outcome should be determined with similar rigor as in an etiologic study or randomized clinical trial. In the future, decisions are to be based on the predictions from the model. Predictions, hence, need to be based on robust statistical associations with an accurately determined outcome.

   If there is a choice between binary and continuous outcomes, the latter are preferred from a statistical perspective, since they provide more power in the statistical analysis. Also, ordered outcomes have more power than binary outcomes. In practice, binary outcomes are however very popular, making logistic regression and Cox regression the most common prediction models in medicine [653].

3.5.7 Diagnostic End Points

The outcome in diagnostic research naturally is the underlying disease, which needs to be defined according to a reference standard [64, 65, 308, 387]. The reference standard can sometimes be anatomical, e.g., findings at surgery. Other definitions of a reference standard may include blood or spinal fluid cultures (e.g., in infectious diseases), results of high-quality diagnostic tests such as angiography (e.g., in coronary diseases), or histological findings (e.g., in oncology). Methods are still under development on how to deal with the absence of an acceptable reference standard. In such situations, the results of the diagnostic test can, for example, be related to relevant other clinical characteristics and future clinical events in latent class analyses [636].

The relevance of the underlying diagnosis may be high when treatment and prognosis depend directly on the diagnosis. Often a diagnosis covers a spectrum of more and less severe disease, and longer term outcome assessment would be desirable. This is especially relevant in the evaluation of newer imaging technology, which may detect disease that remained previously unnoticed [350].

3.5.8 *Example: PET Scans in Esophageal Cancer

In esophageal cancer, positron emission tomography (PET) scans provide additional information on extent of disease compared to CT scanning alone. However, the clinical relevance of the additionally detected metastases can only be determined in a comparative study, preferably a randomized controlled trial. Diagnosing more metastases is not sufficient to make PET/CT clinically useful [637].

3.6 Phases of Biomarker Development

Pepe has proposed a phased approach to developing predictive biomarkers, in particular, for early detection of cancer (Table 3.6) [431]. These phases are also relevant to the development and improvement of prediction models, which may add novel biomarkers to traditional clinical characteristics. The development process begins with small studies focused on classification performance and ends with large studies of impact on populations. The aim is to select promising markers early while recognizing that small early studies do not answer the ultimate questions that need to be addressed (Table 3.6).

As an example, Pepe considers the development of a biomarker for cancer screening. Phase 1 is exploratory and may consider gene expression arrays or protein mass spectrometry that yields high-dimensional data for biomarker discovery. Reproducibility between laboratories is an aspect to consider before moving on to phase 2, where a promising biomarker is compared between population-based cases with cancer and population-based controls without cancer. Phase 3 is a more thorough evaluation in a case–control study to determine if the marker can detect subclinical disease. In phase 4, the marker may be applied prospectively as a screening test in a population. Finally, the overall impact of screening is addressed in phase 5 by measuring effects on clinically relevant outcomes such as mortality and healthcare costs.

Table 3.6 Phases of development of a biomarker for cancer screening [431].

Phase	Objective	Study design
1 Preclinical exploratory	Promising directions identified	Case–control (convenient samples)
2 Clinical assay and validation	Determine if a clinical assay detects established disease	Case–control (population-based)
3 Retrospective longitudinal	Determine if the biomarker detects disease before it becomes clinical. Define a "screen positive" rule	Nested case–control in a population cohort
4 Prospective screening	Extent and characteristics of disease detected by the test; false referral rate	Cross-sectional population cohort
5 Cancer control	Impact of screening on reducing the burden of disease on the population	Randomized trial

The study design implications are shown in Table 3.6; in the exploratory Phase 1, it may be acceptable to use "convenient samples", which will likely lead to spectrum bias in the assessment of the biomarker. In phase 2, population-based samples are desired for a simple case–control design. In phase 3, we require samples taken from cancer patients before their disease became clinically apparent. A nested case–control study design can be efficient for data from a cohort study. For phase 4, a prospective cohort study is required to determine the characteristics and treatability of early detected disease. Finally, an RCT is desired for unbiased assessment of the impact of screening.

3.7   Statistical Power and Reliable Estimation

An important issue is how large a study needs to be for sufficient statistical power to address the primary research question, and reliable estimation of parameters for a prediction modeling. Note that sample size in a binary prediction context depends on the combination of the number of events and the distributions of predictors; we should be especially worried about "sparse data" [209]. Power considerations are discussed below for studying effects of a specific predictor, and for developing a prediction model that can provide reliable predictions.

3.7.1   Sample Size to Identify Predictor Effects

We may primarily be interested in the effect of a specific predictor on a diagnostic or prognostic outcome. We may then aim to test the effect of this predictor for statistical significance. This leads to similar sample size considerations as for testing of treatment effects, e.g., in the context of an RCT. Sample size calculations are

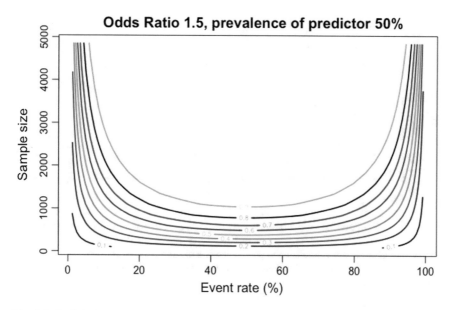

Fig. 3.3 Statistical power corresponding to sample sizes for event rate (incidence of the outcome) ranging from 0 to 100%. A binary predictor was considered with 50% prevalence and odds ratio 1.5

straightforward for such univariate testing. The required sample size is determined by choices for the acceptable Type I and Type II error. The Type I error is usually set at 5% for statistical significance. The Type II error determines the power. It may, e.g., be set at 20% for 80% power. Other considerations include the variability of the effect estimate. For binary predictors of a binary outcome, the prevalence of the predictor and the incidence of the outcome ("event rate") are important. Finally, the magnitude of the effect determines the required sample size, with larger sample size required to detect smaller effects.

For illustration, we consider the statistical power for a binary predictor of a binary outcome (Fig. 3.3). We find that the required sample size increases steeply with a very low or very high event rate, while the sample size is reasonably constant for event rates between 20 and 80%. With an odds ratio of 1.5, 80% power requires approximately 2000 subjects at a 10% incidence of the outcome (200 events), 1000 subjects at 20% incidence (200 events), and 800 subjects at 50% incidence (400 events). So, with low event rates, the number of events is the dominant factor.

Next, we illustrate that statistical power is also directly related to the prevalence of a binary predictor (Fig. 3.4). We consider odds ratios from 1 to 3, as may often be encountered in medical prediction research. In a sample size of 500 subjects, 250 with and 250 without the outcome, 80% power is reached with prevalences of 16% and 5.5% for odds ratios of 2 and 3, respectively. Odds ratios of 1.2 and 1.5 require larger sample sizes than $n = 500$: 3800 and 800 at 50% prevalence, respectively. With a 10% event rate, the power is substantially lower (Fig. 3.4, right panel). An

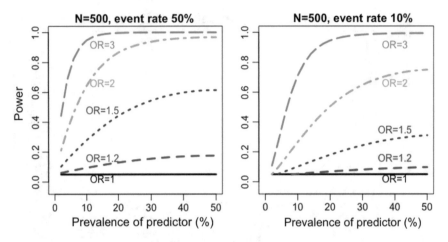

Fig. 3.4 Statistical power in relation to prevalence of a binary predictor, for odds ratios from 1 to 3 in samples with 500 subjects. Incidences of the outcome were 50% (left panel) and 10% (right panel)

odds ratio of 3 then requires 18% instead of 5.5% prevalence of the predictor for 80% power. Without an effect (OR = 1), statistical significance is by definition expected in 5%.

3.7.2   Sample Size for Reliable Modeling

Instead of focusing on predictors, we can focus on the reliability of predictions that are provided by a prediction model. Sample size requirements for prediction models have often been formulated as "at least 10 events per variable" (EPV). Technically, we should consider the degrees of freedom (*df*) of candidate predictors for the model. The EPV concept assumes each variable has 1 *df*. Note that data-driven selection of predictors from a set of candidate predictors does not improve the EPV value. Moreover, we need to consider the total sample size, or the ratio between events and nonevents [634]. If the event rate is 50%, the statistical power for a given number of events is less than for a low event rate such as 10%. With 100 events, the total sample sizes would be 200 and 1000, respectively. In the design of case–control studies, a rule of thumb is that the statistical power does not increase much if the number of controls in increased above 4:1; so, below a 20% event rate (event: nonevent ratio 1:4), the number of events would be the dominant factor. This pattern was confirmed by Fig. 3.3. So, for probability estimates between 20 and 80%, a higher EPV would apply than for more extreme event rates.

Relatively low EPV values may apply for regression analyses where we want to adjust for confounding. The idea is that it is better to include some potential confounders, even if the EPV values drop to lower values, than to risk bias in the predictor of interest [206]. Regression analysis can technically well be performed with lower EVP values, although some type of shrinkage might be considered, e.g., using Firth regression (see Chap. 13) [634]. Adjusted analyses with correction for confounding may, hence, be performed with EPV less than 10 [654].

For prediction, many suggested a minimum of 10 to 20 EPV for obtaining any reasonably reliable predictions [226, 421, 422, 543]. Medical prediction models that are constructed with EVP less than 10 are commonly overfitted and may perform poorer than a simpler model which considers fewer candidate predictors. Limiting the number of candidate predictors may increase the EVP to at least 10 (see further illustration in Chap. 24). For prespecified models, statistical shrinkage may not be required with EPV of at least 20 (Chap. 13) [543]. EPV values for data-driven selection of predictors from a larger set of candidate predictors may be as large as 50 (events per candidate predictor, see Chap. 11). Even higher EPV values, exceeding 200, may be required for stable model estimation with some flexible machine learning algorithms, such as random forests and neural networks [612].

The EPV rules may be criticized for several reasons, including the following:

- in addition to number of events, the number of nonevents is also relevant, specifically for event rates between 20 and 80% [635];
- the distribution and magnitude of predictor effects (see 3.8.1), and the number of events for each category of categorical predictors are also relevant aspects [460, 635].

Riley et al. proposed three criteria for sample size calculations in planning prognostic analyses with binary or time-to-event outcomes [460]:

(1) Small optimism in predictor effect estimates; defined by a shrinkage factor of ≥ 0.9 (see Chap. 13);
(2) Small difference in the apparent and adjusted Nagelkerke R^2; defined as 0.05 (see Chap. 4);
(3) Precise estimation of the mean predicted outcome value (model intercept), e.g., defined with a margin of error of ± 0.1 (see 3.8.2).

These criteria can be used for a specific context, with a number of candidate predictors and a model's anticipated R^2. We might then propose the samples size that meets all criteria. As with any sample size calculation, we need to make estimates for each of these parameters, e.g., informed by previous studies. Some boundaries are rather arbitrary, e.g., a shrinkage factor of 0.8 rather than 0.9 might be acceptable to many, and would lead to a lower sample size requirement for this criterion.

The idea of limiting the expected shrinkage was already put forward by Harrell et al., i.e., fit a full prediction model including all candidate predictors, examine the strength of the model fit (model χ^2), and then consider how many degrees of freedom might be spent in the modeling process [227]. Harrell also proposed earlier that we may want to estimate at least the average risk with reasonable precision. The lower limit might be 96 events, for a margin of error of ± 0.1 in estimating risk in the range of 20–80% event rate. To achieve a margin of error of ± 0.05 around $p = 0.5$ one needs $n = 384$ (192 events) [229]. Again, such limits (± 0.1, or ± 0.05) are rather arbitrary.

Table 3.7 Sample size considerations for development and validation of prediction models

Study aim	Sample size considerations
Predictor effects	Perform sample size calculation with anticipated effect size, prevalence of predictor, and event rate (*see 3.7.1*)
Model development	At least 100 events; consider the number of candidate variables to increase the sample size according to the EPV >10 rule if the event rate is <20%; or perform specific calculations [460]
Model validation	Single setting: At least 100 events Multiple settings: Aim for >50 groups

Overall, tentative advice might be as follows (Table 3.7):

- Aim for at least 100 events as a minimum for reliable estimation of the average risk;
- Aim for at least 10 EPV, and preferably 20, for reliable prediction modeling if the event rate is <20% and higher EPV values if the event rate is between 20 and 80%;
- Allow specific circumstances to increase the required sample size, such as the modeling of predictors with low prevalence, using proposed formulas [154, 460].

Note that once the data are available, we should adapt our modeling strategy to maximize chances for a reliable prediction model that is at least internally valid (read part II of this book). Sparse data may occur even with relatively favorable EPV [209]. In current practice, many prediction models are developed with fewer than 100 events, and with EPV values below 10 [666]. This may contribute to waste in prediction research [271].

3.7.3   Sample Size for Reliable Validation

Similar to model development studies, external validation studies also require substantial sample sizes. One perspective is to test claims of similar performance: what is the statistical power to detect a clinically relevant deterioration in model performance? Simulations suggested that validation studies should include at least 100 events, and preferably more (details in Chap. 19) [533, 643]. This number was confirmed in other studies [423], and also when the perspective was taken that we want a reliable estimate of performance [104]. As with model development, model validation practice is currently not adhering to this minimum number of events guidance, contributing to research waste in prediction research [103, 533].

As an extension of a single validation, it is highly relevant to examine the external validity of a prediction model across a range of settings [30, 31, 451]. Multilevel (or *random effect*) models may then be used (see Chap. 21). Accurate estimation of model parameters and variance components of multilevel logistic regression models may require at least 50 groups with 50 subjects [381]. For validation, our aim is also to obtain a reliable estimate of the between-setting heterogeneity [31, 539]. Such a heterogeneity estimate is more dependent on the number of settings ("groups") than the number of individuals per group [522]. Technically, a minimum of five groups may be required for modeling, while some suggest a minimum of 10 [522], and simulation studies support a minimum of 50 groups for low bias in estimation of the heterogeneity [360].

In sum, single external validation study needs at least 100 events to be meaningful. Assessment of between-setting heterogeneity in validity requires a large number of settings, preferably 50 or more (Table 3.7).

3.8 Concluding Remarks

Prognostic studies are ideally designed as prospective cohort studies, where the selection of patients and definition of predictors is prespecified. Data from randomized clinical trials may often be useful, although representativeness of the included patients for the target population should be considered as a limitation. Data may also be used from retrospective designs, registries, and case–control studies, each with their strengths and limitations. Diagnostic studies are usually cross-sectional in design and should prospectively select all patients who are suspected of a disease of interest. In practice, designs are still frequent where patients are selected based on a reference test which is not performed in all patients.

Predictors may be defined pragmatically and cover the relevant areas in a disease. The outcome of a prediction model should be measured with high accuracy. Hard end points such as mortality are often preferred.

With any study design, we should aim for large sample size for reliable testing and estimation of predictor effects, reliable model building, and reliable assessment of model performance. At least 100 events may be required for any model development or validation, and more for detailed modeling and addressing more refined research questions. A development sample with 100 events corresponds to EPV=10 with 10 candidate predictors. More than 100 events are needed if more than 10 candidate predictors are considered. Higher sample sizes are desired for multi-setting validation, with data from many different settings if claims about generalizability are made.

Questions

3.1 Cohort studies
One could argue that both diagnostic and prognostic studies are examples of cohort studies.

(a) What is the difference between diagnostic and prognostic outcomes in such cohorts?
(b) What is the implication for the statistical analysis?

3.2 Prospective vs. retrospective designs (Sect. 3.2).
Prospective study designs are generally seen as preferable to retrospective designs. What are the pros and cons of prospective versus retrospective designs?

3.3 Accuracy of predictors and outcome (Sects. 3.5 and 3.6)

(a) Why do we need to be more careful with reliable assessment of outcome than assessment of predictors?
(b) What is the effect of imprecise measurement of a predictor? See recent work by Luijken et al. [355]

3.4 Composite end points (Sect. 3.5.4)
Composite end points are often motivated by the wish to increase statistical power for analysis. What is the price that we pay for this increase in terms of assumptions on predictive relations? See a JCE paper for a detailed discussion [186].

3.5 Statistical power (Figs. 3.3 and 3.4)

(a) What is the required total sample size for 50% power at 10%, 30% or 50% incidence of the outcome in Fig. 3.3?
(b) What is the similarity between Figs. 3.3 and 3.4 with respect to the ranges of the event rate and prevalence, and the associated statistical power?

3.6 Study design: epidemiologic and statistical aspects
Suppose we can do a single-center study with 2000 patients, where 400 (20%) will have the event of interest. Alternatively, we can do a multicenter study with three centers, each contributing 500 patients. Among the 1500, we expect 300 events (20% average event rate).

(a) Which design would you prefer? Explain why weighing epidemiological considerations (such as generalizability) and statistical considerations (such as standard error).
(b) What if the alternative to 2000 with 400 events would be 10 centers with 30 events each (300 events in total)?

Chapter 4
Statistical Models for Prediction

Background In this chapter, we consider statistical models for different types of outcomes: binary, unordered categorical, ordered categorical, continuous, and survival data. We discuss common statistical models in medical research such as the linear, logistic, and Cox regression model. We consider simpler approaches and more flexible extensions, including regression trees and neural networks. We also discuss competing risks and the concept of dynamic prediction modeling. We focus on the most relevant aspects of these models in a prediction context. All models are illustrated with case studies. In Chap. 6, we will discuss aspects of choosing between alternative statistical models for the same type of outcome.

4.1 Continuous Outcomes

Continuous outcomes have traditionally received most attention in texts on regression modeling, with the ordinary least square model ("linear regression") as the reference statistical model [653]. Continuous outcomes may be common in many scientific fields, such as engineering, psychology, and economy, but are not so often considered for prediction models in the medical field.

The linear regression model can be written as

$$y = \alpha + \beta_i * x_i + \text{error},$$

where α is the model intercept, and β_i refers to the set of regression coefficients that relate one or more predictors x_i to the outcome y. The error is calculated as observed y—predicted y (or $y - \hat{y}$). This difference is also known as the *residual* for the prediction of y. We estimate the regression coefficients a for the intercept α and b_i for the regression coefficients β_i.

© Springer Nature Switzerland AG 2019
E. W. Steyerberg, *Clinical Prediction Models*, Statistics for Biology and Health, https://doi.org/10.1007/978-3-030-16399-0_4

The outcome y is, hence, related to a linear combination of the x_i variables with the estimated regression coefficients b_i. This use of a simple sum, or linear combination, is an important property, which is also seen in *generalized* linear models, such as the logistic regression model.

4.1.1 *Examples of Linear Regression

An example of a medical outcome is blood pressure. We may want to predict the blood pressure after treatment with an anti-hypertensive or other intervention [312, 628]. Also, quality of life scales may be relevant to evaluate [313]. Such scales are strictly speaking only ordinal, but can for practical purposes often be treated as continuous outcomes. A specific issue is that quality of life scores have ceiling effects, because minimum and maximum scores apply.

4.1.2 Economic Outcomes

Health economics is an important field where continuous outcomes are considered, such as length of stay in hospital, or length of stay at a specific ward (e.g., the intensive care unit), or total costs for patients [378]. Cost data are usually not normally distributed. Such economic data have special characteristics, such as patients without any costs (zero), and a long tail because some patients having considerable costs. We might consider the median as a good descriptor of the typical outcome. We are, however, mostly interested in the mean costs, since the expectation is what matters most from an economical perspective.

4.1.3 *Example: Prediction of Costs

Many children in moderate climates suffer from an infection by the respiratory syncytial virus (RSV). Some children, especially premature children, are at risk of a severe infection, leading to hospitalization. In a Dutch study, the mean RSV hospitalization costs were 3,110 Euros in a cohort of 3,458 infants and young children hospitalized for severe RSV disease during the RSV seasons 1996–1997 to 1999–2000 in the Southwest of The Netherlands [454]. RSV hospitalization costs were higher for some patient categories, e.g., those with lower gestational age or lower birth weight, and younger age. The linear regression model had an adjusted R^2 of 8%. This indicates a low explanatory ability for predicting hospitalization costs of individual children. However, the model could estimate the anticipated mean hospitalization costs of groups of children with the same characteristics. These predicted costs were used in decision analyses of preventive strategies for severe RSV disease [61].

4.1.4 Transforming the Outcome

An important issue in linear regression is whether we should transform the outcome variable. The residuals $(y - \hat{y})$ from a linear regression should have a normal distribution with a constant spread ("homoscedasticity"). This can sometimes be achieved by a log transformation for cost data, but other transformations are also possible. As Harrell points out, transformations of the outcome may reduce the need to include transformations of predictor variables [225]. Care should be taken in backtransforming predicted mean outcomes to the original scale. Predicted medians and other quantiles are not affected by a monotone transformation, but the mean is. The lognormal distribution can be used for the mean on the original scale after a log transformation, but a more general, nonparametric, approach is to use "smearing" estimators [443].

4.1.5 Performance: Explained Variation

In linear regression analysis, the total variance in y is labeled the total sum of squares ("TSS"). TSS is the sum of variability explained by one or more predictors ("model sum of squares," MSS) and the error ("residual sum of squares," RSS):

$$TSS = MSS + RSS = var(\text{regression on } x_i) + var(\text{error})$$
$$= \Sigma(\hat{y} - \text{mean}(y))^2 + \Sigma(y - \hat{y})^2$$

The estimates of the variance follow from the statistical fit of the model to the data, which is based on the analytical solution of the least squares formula. This fit minimizes the error term in the model and maximizes the variance explained by x_i. Better prediction models explain more of the variance in y. R^2 is defined as MSS/TSS [653].

To appreciate values of R^2, we consider six hypothetical situations where we predict a continuous outcome y, which has a standard normal distribution (N(0, 1), i.e., mean 0 and standard deviation (SD) 1) with one predictor x (N(0, 1)). The regression coefficients for x are varied in simulations, such that R^2 is 95, 50, 20, 10, 5, and 0% (Fig. 4.1). We note that an R^2 of 95% implies that observed outcomes are always very close to the predicted values, while gradually relatively more error occurs with lower R^2 values. When R^2 is 0%, no association is present.

To appreciate R^2 further, we plot the distributions of predicted values ($\hat{y}$). The distribution of $\hat{y}$ is wide when R^2 is 95%, and very small when R^2 is 5%, and a single line when R^2 is 0% (Fig. 4.2). The distribution of y is always normal with mean 0 and standard deviation 1.

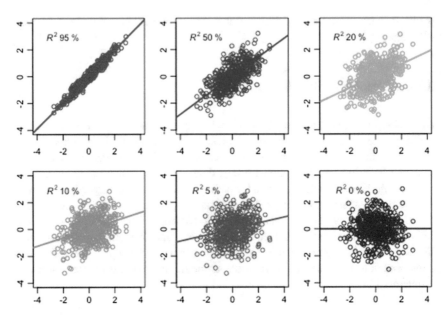

Fig. 4.1 Linear regression analysis with regression models with $y = \beta * x + \text{error}$, where SD $(y) = \text{SD}(x) = 1$. The outcome y is shown on the y-axis, x on the x-axis

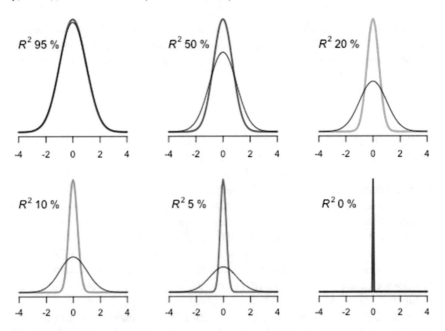

Fig. 4.2 Probability density functions for observed and predicted values ("fitted values", $\hat{y}$), corresponding to Fig. 4.1. For the first graph ($R^2 = 95\%$), the distribution of predicted values (thick red line) is close to the distribution of observed y values (thin line), while for the last graph all predictions are the average ($\hat{y} = 0$)

4.1.6 More Flexible Approaches

The generalized additive model (GAM) is a more flexible variant of the linear regression model [231, 653]. A GAM allows especially for more flexibility in continuous predictors. It replaces the usual linear combination of continuous predictors with a sum of smooth functions to discover potential nonlinear effects:

$$y = \alpha + f_i(x_i) + \text{error},$$

where f_i refers to functions for each predictor, e.g., loess (or "lowess") smoothers.

Loess smoothers are based on locally weighted polynomial regression [102]. At each point in the data set, a low-degree polynomial is fit to a subset of the data, with data values near the point where the outcome y is considered. A polynomial is fitted using weighted least squares, giving more weight to nearby points and less weight to points further away. The degree of the polynomial model and the weights can be chosen by the analyst.

The estimation of a GAM is more computationally demanding than for simple linear models, but this is no limitation anymore with modern computer power and software. A GAM assumes that the outcome is already appropriately transformed, and then automatically estimates the transformation of continuous predictors to optimize relations with the outcome.

An even more flexible approach is to transform y and X simultaneously to maximize the correlation between the transformed y and the transformed X [225, 231]:

$$g(y) = \alpha + f_i(x_i) + \text{error},$$

where g refers to a transformation of the outcome y, and f_i refers to functions for each predictor. For cost data, several other specific approaches have been proposed [378].

4.2 Binary Outcomes

Binary outcomes are most common for diagnostic (presence of disease) or prognostic research questions (e.g., mortality, morbidity, complications, see Chap. 2). The logistic regression model is the most widely used statistical technique for such binary outcomes. The model is flexible in that it can incorporate binary, categorical and continuous predictors, nonlinear transformations, and interaction terms. Many of the principles of linear regression also apply for logistic regression, which is an example of a *generalized* linear model. As in linear regression, the binary outcome y is linked to a linear combination of a set of predictors and regression coefficients β_i. We use the logistic link function to restrict predictions to the interval <0, 1>. The model is stated in terms of the probability that $y = 1$ ("$p(y = 1)$"), rather than the outcome y directly.

Specifically, we write the model as a linear function in the logistic transformation (logit), where $\text{logit}(p(y = 1)) = \log(\text{odds}(p(y = 1)))$, or $\log(p(y = 1)/(p(y = 1) + 1))$:

$$\text{logit}(p(y = 1)) = a + b_i * x_i = lp,$$

where logit indicates the logistic transformation, a is an estimate for the intercept α, b_i are the estimated regression coefficients for β_i, x_i are the predictors, and lp is the linear predictor.

The coefficients b_i are usually estimated by standard maximum likelihood in a logistic regression approach, but this is not necessarily the case. For example, we will discuss penalized maximum likelihood methods to shrink the b_i for predictive purposes (Chap. 13). Many variants of shrinkage and penalization have been proposed over recent years, including the LASSO and elastic net [581, 689].

The interpretation of the coefficients b_i is as for any regression model: the coefficient relates to 1 unit difference in x_i, while the other predictors in the model are constant. We should be careful in not interpreting a regression coefficient as *causing* a difference in outcome; we only estimate association. When we consider a single predictor in a logistic model, b_i is an unadjusted, or univariate association; with multiple predictors, it is an "adjusted" association. The exponent of the regression coefficient (e^b) indicates the odds ratio, so the ratio of the odds of the binary outcome y.

Predicted probabilities can be calculated by backtransforming:

$$p(y = 1) = e^{lp}/\left(1 + e^{lp}\right) = 1/\left(1 + e^{-lp}\right).$$

The quantity $\exp(lp)$, or e^{lp}, is the odds of the outcome. The logistic function has a characteristic sigmoid shape, and is bounded between 0 and 1 (Fig. 4.3). We note that a lp value of 0 corresponds to a probability of 50%. Low lp values correspond to low probabilities (e.g., $lp = -4$, $p = 2\%$), and high lp values correspond to high probabilities (e.g., $lp = +4$, $p = 98\%$).

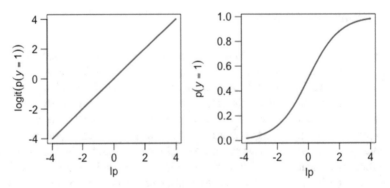

Fig. 4.3 Illustration of the logistic function. The linear predictor lp is related to the predicted probability $p(y = 1)$ as $\text{logit}(p(y = 1)) = lp$, and $p(y = 1) = 1/(1 + \exp(-lp))$

Fig. 4.4 Predicted probabilities of a 0/1 outcome by six logistic models according to a normally distributed x variable. The predictive strength varied, with Nagelkerke's R^2 decreasing from 87% to 0%

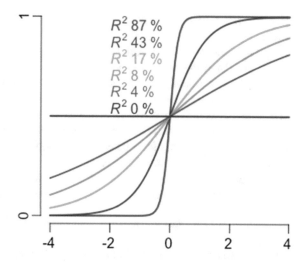

R^2 87 %
R^2 43 %
R^2 17 %
R^2 8 %
R^2 4 %
R^2 0 %

4.2.1 R^2 in Logistic Regression Analysis

The linear regression examples showed how R^2 is related to the relative spread in predictions. When predictions cover a wider range, the regression model better predicts the outcome. This concept also applies to dichotomous outcomes, e.g., analyzed with a logistic regression model. Better prediction models for dichotomous outcomes have a wider spread in predictions, i.e., predictions close to 0% and close to 100%.

To illustrate this concept, we use the same simulated data as for the examples of linear regression models, but we now dichotomize the outcome y (if y < 0, yd = 0, else yd = 1). The relation between a standard normal variable X and six hypothetical dichotomized outcomes *yd* is shown in Fig. 4.4.

4.2.2 Calculation of R^2 on the Log-Likelihood Scale

Where the linear model is optimized with least squares estimation, the logistic model is usually optimized by maximum likelihood. The likelihood refers to the probability of the data given the model and enables estimation of parameters in various nonlinear models. The logarithm of the likelihood (log-likelihood, LL) is usually used for convenience in numerical estimation. The LL is calculated as the sum over all subjects of the distance between the natural log of the predicted probability p for the binary outcome to the actually observed outcome y:

$$LL = \Sigma y * \log(p) + (1 - y) * \log(1 - p),$$

where y refers to the binary outcome and p the predicted probability for each subject.

If $y = 1$, the probability should be high (ideally 100%), such that $\log(p)$ gets close to 0. Then the term $(1 - y)$ drops out. If $y = 0$, the term $(1 - y) = 1$, and p should be low (ideally 0%), such that $\log(1 - p)$ gets close to zero. A perfectly fitting model would have a LL of zero; hence, we aim to maximize the LL. Another term is deviance, defined as -2LL, which we try to minimize, similar to minimizing the residual sum of squares (RSS) for linear regression. Note that perfect predictions cannot be made, unless a fully deterministic model is identified. The LL is, hence, usually negative for a fitted logistic regression model and the deviance positive. A better model will have an LL or deviance closer to zero.

As reference we may consider the LL of a model with average predictions:

$$LL_0 = \Sigma y * \log(\text{mean}(y)) + (1 - y) * \log(1 - \text{mean}(y)),$$

where LL_0 refers to the log-likelihood of the null model, and mean(y) is the average probability of the binary outcome y. The LL_0 is negative, unless mean(y) is 0 or 1.

We can quantify the performance of a prognostic model by comparison with the null model. We multiply by -2, since the difference on the -2 LL (or deviance) scale is a likelihood ratio statistic (LR), which follows a χ^2 distribution:

$$LR = -2(LL_0 - LL_1),$$

where LL_1 refers to the model with predictors, and LL_0 to the null model, and LR is the likelihood ratio. The LR statistic can be used for univariate analysis, and also for testing the joint importance of a larger set of predictors in the model ("global LR statistic") [225]. We can also easily make comparisons between nested submodels, which contain a subset of the predictors in the full model. For example, we can compare models with and without age as a predictor to determine the LR for age, or compare models with and without a block of predictors, e.g., with and without a set of patient history characteristics. Statistical testing is straightforward between such nested models, since the LR statistic follows a χ^2 distribution.

We may use LR to estimate the explained variability by a model (R^2). R^2 values would ideally enable a direct comparison across predictors, irrespective whether the predictor was categorical or continuous and independent of the sample size. The absolute value of the LR depends on n, the number of patients, similar to the sum of squares in linear regression analysis. Moreover, we need to define an R^2 measure relative to a null model without predictors, with -2 LL_0, as the reference value. Nagelkerke proposed to define R^2 as follows:

$$R^2 = \left(1 - e^{(-(LR))}\right) / \left(1 - e^{(-2 * LL0)}\right).$$

This definition scales R^2 between 0 and 100% [403]. For a perfect model, $LR = +2LL_0$, and $R^2 = 100\%$. The relation between the LR statistic and

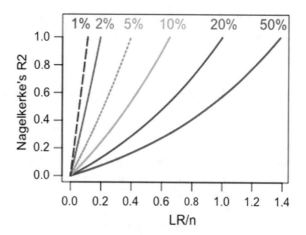

Fig. 4.5 Relation between Nagelkerke's R^2 and the likelihood ratio (*LR*) statistic (divided by sample size, *n*) for event rates of 1–50%. We note a reasonably linear relation. Largest LR values are possible with an event rate of 50%

Nagelkerke's R^2 is more or less linear; absolute values of the LR statistic depend on the event rate, in addition to the sample size *n* (Fig. 4.5).

We will use the Nagelkerke definition of R^2 throughout this book, although quite some alternative R^2 definitions are possible [7]. The scaling between 0 and 100% makes it a natural measure to indicate how close we are with our predictions to the observed 0 and 1 outcomes (Fig. 4.6). The calculation is based on the LL scale, which is the scale used in the fitting process to optimize the model. The calculation

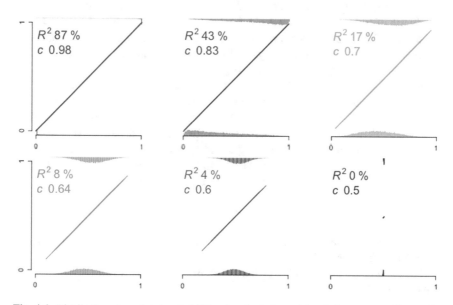

Fig. 4.6 Distribution of predicted probabilities from logistic models relating *y* to a predictor *x* for observed outcomes 0 or 1. The *y* variable was created from the linear regression example in Fig. 4.1 by dichotomization, and the average event rate was 50%. Discrimination is indicated by the *c* statistic (equivalent to the area under the receiver operating characteristic curve, see Chap. 15)

includes the LR, which is the theoretically preferred quantity for testing of significance in logistic models [225].

4.2.3   Models Related to Logistic Regression

Logistic regression can be viewed as an improvement over linear discriminant analysis, which is an older technique [221]. Discriminant analysis usually makes more assumptions on the underlying data, for example, multivariate normality, which is not the case in logistic regression. For logistic regression, the outcome y needs to follow a binomial distribution. This assumption is violated when correlations between outcomes exist, for example, because of grouping of patients within hospitals, or multiple events within the same subject. Generalized estimation equations (GEE) are an extension of logistic regression for correlated data [653]. Multilevel, or random effect, models have become more and more common in recent analyses of correlated binary outcome data (see Chap. 21).

4.2.4   Bayes Rule

Bayes rule has often been used in a diagnostic context for the prediction of the likelihood of an underlying disease [263, 430]. A prior probability of disease $(p(D))$ is considered before information becomes available (e.g., from history taking, or from a diagnostic test, denoted as predictor x). The information is used to calculate a posterior probability of disease $(p(D|x))$.

This approach has been followed with some success in the 1970s by De Dombal in deriving diagnostic estimates for patients with abdominal pain [121]. Probabilities were estimated with a Bayesian approach, where the prior probability of a diagnosis was updated with information from a large database. This database contained data on the prevalence of signs and symptoms according to the outcome diagnosis. This information can be summarized with diagnostic likelihood ratios (LR). The diagnostic LR for a specific sign or symptom x is

$$LR(x) = p(x|D)/p(x|!D)$$

where D indicates the presence of disease (determined by a reference standard), and !D indicates no disease.

The combination of a prior probability of disease and LR is straightforward with Bayes' formula:

Odds$(D|x)$ = Odds(D) * LR(x), where
Odds(D) is the prior odds of disease, calculated as $p(D)/(1 - p(D))$.

In logit form the formula reads as:

$$\text{logit}(D|x) = \text{logit}(D) + \log(LR(x))$$

This looks very similar to the univariate logistic model shown before. The intercept α is replaced by logit(D), the prior probability of disease, and $\beta_1 * x_1$ is replaced by $\log(LR(x))$. The term "$\log(LR(x))$" has been referred to as "weight of evidence," since it indicates how much the prior probability changes by evidence from a test [528].

For a test with a positive or negative result, there is a simple relation between LR and OR:

$$OR = LR(+)/LR(-), \text{ and}$$

$$\log(OR) = \text{coefficient} = \log(LR(+)/LR(-)) = \log(LR(+)) - \log(LR(-)),$$

where LR(+) and LR(−) are the LRs for positive and negative test results, respectively.

In a logistic model with one predictor representing the test (+ or − result), the intercept α reflects the logit(y | test −). When the test is positive, the change in log odds is given by the coefficient, and the logit(y) = intercept + coefficient.

4.2.5 Prediction with Naïve Bayes

Bayes rule is a general scientific approach to handle conditional probabilities, e.g., to obtain p(D|x) from p(x|D). The quantity p(x|D) can sometimes easier be estimated than p(D|x). For example, sensitivity and specificity of a dichotomous test are estimated conditional on disease status. For prediction, we are, however, interested in p(D|x).

We can use a simple method to estimate posterior probabilities for combinations of signs and symptoms [121]: the posterior probability after considering $x1$ is used as the prior when considering $x2$; the posterior probability after considering $x2$ is used as the prior when considering $x3$; etc. This approach is valid if $x1$, $x2$, etc. are conditionally independent. Usually, positive correlations are present which makes that the effect of $x2$ is smaller once $x1$ has already been considered, compared to considering $x2$ unconditionally: $LR_{x2|x1} < LR_{x2}$ [279].

The sequential application of Bayes' rule is equivalent to using the univariate logistic regression coefficients in a linear predictor. Because of its simplicity and mathematical incorrectness, Naïve Bayes is sometimes referred to as "Idiot's Bayes".

The linear predictor reads like

$$lp_k = \beta_{1,u} * x_1 + \beta_{2,u} * x_2 + \cdots + \beta_{p,u} * x_p,$$

where the subscript u indicates univariate estimates for the regression coefficients.

Such a naïve Bayes approach may have remarkably good discriminative ability.[525] Also, the method has been applied in modeling the effects of genetic markers, where robustness in modeling is required at the expense of accepting some bias in coefficients [511].

4.2.6   Calibration and Naïve Bayes

The main problem with Naïve Bayes estimation is that correlations between the predictors are ignored. In the case of positive correlations, the effects of predictors are overestimated and predictions will be too extreme. Both too low and too high predictions arise. This is reflected in a regression coefficient for the linear predictor ("calibration slope", β_{cal}) below 1 in the model: $y \sim lp_u$, where lp_u is the linear predictor based on univariate coefficients.

A simple approach is to correct this calibration problem with a single coefficient for lp_u: $\text{logit}(y) = \alpha + \beta_{cal} * lp_u$.

In terms of multivariable OR (OR_m) or multivariable LR (LR_m), the exponent can be used for ease of notation: $OR_m = OR_u{}^{\beta_{cal}}$ or $LR_m = LR_u{}^{\beta_{cal}}$. The idea of calibration of the linear predictor comes back in Chaps. 15 and 20.

4.2.7   *Logistic Regression and Bayes

The diagnostic likelihood ratio (LR) can be used mathematically correct in a multivariable context. The key trick is to rescale test results. Instead of a 1 for positive and a 0 for negative, the univariate log(LR) values can be filled in for the test results [525]. In a multivariable model, the joint effects for the test results are subsequently estimated. Coefficients for the rescaled test results reflect the degree of correlation between test results from different tests. If there were no correlations, the coefficients of each test would be close to 1.

Multivariable diagnostic LRs can also be calculated by comparing models with and without the test of interest. The model without the test is the prior, and the model with the test included provides the posterior probabilities [279]. Subtracting these two equations provides the LRs.

4.2.8   Machine Learning: More Flexible Approaches

Naïve Bayes estimation is an example of a simpler method than logistic regression. A more flexible alternative model is a generalized additive model (*GAM*), as was already discussed for linear regression models [231, 653].

Another class of alternative approaches is nowadays known as Machine Learning techniques. These typically require less involvement from the analyst to develop a prediction model and aim to learn more directly from the data, without assuming some type of underlying statistical model [80]. A typical example is to consider generalized *non*linear models. Here, the outcome is no longer related to a mathematically simple, linear combination of estimated regression coefficients and predictor values (the linear predictor, *lp*). Instead, nonlinear combinations of

Fig. 4.7 A simple neural network with four input variables (predictors $x1 - x4$), one hidden layer with three nodes, and one output layer (outcome y)

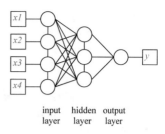

input   hidden   output
layer   layer   layer

predictors are possible. Generalized nonlinear models are commonly implemented as neural networks. Neural networks are often presented as fancy tools, "that represent the way our brain works," but it may be more useful to consider them as nonlinear extensions of linear logistic models [587, 588].

The most common neural network model is the multilayer perceptron (Fig. 4.7). In such a network, the neurons are arranged in a layered configuration containing an input layer, usually one "hidden" layer, and an output layer. The values of input variables (patient characteristics) are imported into the network via the input layer and multiplied with the weights of the connections. These multiplied values constitute the input of the next (hidden) layer, from where the process is continued to produce the output variables (e.g., risk of mortality) in the output layer.

A neural network does not use any preliminary information about the links between the input and output variables; the relations between input and output variables are determined by the data. It is, hence, not easily possible to explicitly force external knowledge into a model, e.g., that an age effect should be monotonically increasing. Neural networks learn iteratively from examples; the errors from the initial prediction for the patients are fed back into the network and the weights are adjusted to minimize the error for the second time predictions are made and compared to the actual outcome. The process from input to output layer is repeated many times. However, to prevent "overtraining", the repetitions are usually stopped before the network is fully trained to the data [543, 587]. This concept relates to shrinkage and penalization for regression models (Chap. 13).

The hidden layer makes the network more flexible to recognize patterns in the data compared to a standard logistic regression model. The number of hidden layers and number of nodes are chosen by the analyst. A neural network without a hidden layer is equivalent to a logistic regression model [587, 588].

4.2.9 Classification and Regression Trees

Recursive partitioning, or Classification And Regression Tree ("CART"), methods have been promoted as strong tools for prediction modeling and may be considered as key machine learning methods. Recursive partitioning is a statistical method to construct binary trees [76]. The method is based on statistically optimal splitting ("partitioning") of the patients into pairs of smaller subgroups. Splits are based on cut-off levels of the predictors, which produce maximum separation among two subgroups and a minimum variability with these subgroups with respect to the outcome. The predictor causing the largest separation is situated at the top of the tree, followed by the predictor causing the next largest separation, and so on. Splitting continues until the subgroups reach a minimum size or until no improvement can be obtained [76].

Many variants of tree-based method exist. The algorithms to construct single trees vary. Moreover, multiple trees may be constructed from a data set with permutations or resampling approaches, known as "random forests". Random forests generate predictions by running a subject through multiple trees, with averaging of the result [79].

*4.2.10   *Example: Mortality in Acute MI Patients*

We fit a tree in patients with an acute myocardial infarction (MI). We again use a sample which contains 785 patients, of whom 52 died by 30 days (Chap. 22). We consider the predictors age (continuous) and Killip (4 categories, Fig. 4.8).

4.2.11   Advantages and Disadvantages of Tree Models

An advantage of a tree is its simple presentation. Some claim that a tree represents how physicians think: starting with the most important characteristic, followed by another characteristic depending on the answer on the first, etc. Indeed, humans are remarkably quick in pattern recognition based on a few clues. However, humans

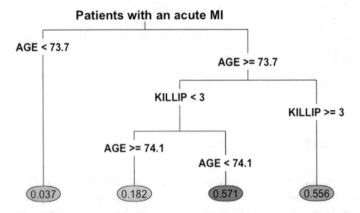

Fig. 4.8 Tree fitted in a subsample of GUSTO-I ("sample4") with age and Killip class as predictors. The terminal nodes are labeled with 30-day mortality as a fraction, e.g., 0.037 indicates 3.7% mortality among those younger than 74 years

have typically been outperformed by systematic prediction methods in experiments where a balanced, quantitative judgment was required, such as estimation of a probability based on a set of characteristics [354]. So, the fact that a tree may represent human thinking for classification does not argue in favor of the method for prediction. A true advantage may be that interaction effects are naturally incorporated in a tree, while a standard logistic regression model usually starts with main effects. So, when multiple, high-order interactions are expected in a huge data set, and only categorical predictors are considered, a tree might theoretically be a good choice. Such situations may be rare in medical data, but may possibly be encountered in other areas of research.

Disadvantages of trees can be noted by considering a tree as a special case of linear logistic regression. First, all continuous variables have to be categorized, which implies a loss of information. As illustrated in Fig. 4.8, age is considered with rather strange splits at different places in the tree, while the age effect could well be approximated with a single, simple, linear term in a logistic model (see Chap. 6). Moreover, these cut-points are determined from a search over all possible cut-points, which is well known to lead to overfitting in a prediction context [12].

Further, the tree assumes interactions between all predictors. After the first split, this interaction is of the first order, i.e., $x1 * x2$. At the second level, second-order interactions are assumed ($x1 * x2 * x3$). In regression analysis, it is common practice to include main effects of predictors when interactions are considered; this principle is not followed in tree modeling. A higher order interaction term is included to model the effect of a predictor in a specific branch, and simply omitted from the other branches. A predictor is typically selected in one branch of the tree and not in another. This poses a clear risk of testimation bias (Chap. 5): predictors are selectively considered when their effects are relatively large, and not if their effects are small [267].

4.2.12 Trees Versus Logistic Regression Modeling

Trees have three distinctive characteristics compared to a logistic regression model when we consider a set of potential predictors.

(1) In a logistic model, a default strategy is to include all predictors as main effects. This model can be extended with interaction terms if the statistical power to examine these is sufficient. It is rare to study interaction terms that are more complex than considering three variables (second-order). In contrast, trees by default assume that higher order interactions are present and cannot model the main effects.

(2) Continuous variables should not be categorized in regression models [472]. Trees do so by necessity, which causes a loss of information.

(3) We should be very cautious in using stepwise selection methods in a logistic model [563]. Small data sets lack sufficient power to select relevant predictors

(Chap. 11) [225]. A tree, however, always needs to be selective in the inclusion of predictors and quickly runs out of cases within branches. Limited power is a major problem in the development of trees: trees are data-hungry [612].

As an example, we can write the tree in Fig. 4.8 as

$$lp = \beta_1 * age < 73.7 + \beta_2 * Killip < = 2 * age > = 74.1 +$$
$$\beta_3 * Killip > = 3 * age = [73.7, 74.1] + \beta_4 * Killip > = 3 * age > 73.7$$

We estimate four parameters which identify the four terminal nodes.

In a logistic regression model, we could combine Killip class 3 and 4 (representing "shock"), and omit the interaction of Killip with age:

$$lp = \alpha + \beta_1 * age + \beta_2 * Killip = 1 + \beta_3 * Killip = 2 + \beta_4 * Killip > 2.$$

Even simpler, we could include Killip as a linear rather than as a categorized predictor:

$$lp = \alpha + \beta_1 * age + \beta_2 * Killip.$$

We could extend this model to allow for age * Killip interaction:

$$lp = \alpha + \beta_1 * age + \beta_2 * Killip + \beta_3 * age * Killip.$$

When we fit these models in small parts of GUSTO-I and validate the performance in the full data set, we note substantially better performance for the simple logistic regression models, in line with a large comparative study [153]. Other empirical comparisons also show poor performance of tree models for prediction in a number of medical prediction problems [20, 23, 29, 612, 613].

4.2.13 *Other Methods for Binary Outcomes

Various other methods are available or under development. Such methods include multivariate additive regression splines ("MARS") models. These form a kind of hybrid between generalized additive models and classification trees [170]. MARS models aim to find low-order additive structure as well as interactions between risk factors.

A support vector machine (SVM) constructs hyperplanes in a multidimensional space that separates cases of different class labels. An SVM supports both regression and classification tasks and can handle multiple continuous and categorical variables [639]. Specialized texts are available that discuss these and other statistical models for binary data [231].

Table 4.1 Characteristics of some statistical models for binary outcomes

Categories	Interactions	Linearity	Selection	Estimation
Linear logistic regression	Possible	Flexible	Flexible	Standard ML or penalization
Naïve Bayes	No	Often categories for diagnostic tests	Flexible	Univariate effects (+ calibration slope)
GAM	Possible	Highly flexible	Flexible	Nonparametric, close to penalized ML
GLNM, neural net	Assumed	Highly flexible	Flexible	Backpropagation, early stopping to prevent overfitting
Trees	Assumed	Categorization	Assumed	Various splitting methods, cross-validation

4.2.14   Summary of Binary Outcomes

In sum, logistic regression provides a quite flexible model to derive predictions for binary data. Interactions and nonlinearity can be incorporated. Some other methods, such as GAM, neural nets (GNLM), MARS, can be seen as extensions, with the default linear logistic model as a special case. Naïve Bayes is a simplified version of logistic regression, ignoring correlations between predictors. Trees can be seen as special cases of logistic regression, requiring categorizations of continuous variables and assuming higher order interactions (Table 4.1).

4.3   Categorical Outcomes

Categorical outcomes without a clear ordering are common in diagnostic medical problems. The diagnostic process starts with considering presenting signs and symptoms of a patient. This leads the physician toward a set of differential diagnoses. Each diagnosis has a probability given the patient's clinical and nonclinical profile. Usually, one of these differential diagnoses is defined as the working diagnosis or target disease, to which the diagnostic workup is primarily directed. Consequently, diagnostic studies commonly focus on the ability of tests to include or exclude the presence of this target disease. The alternative diagnoses (which may direct different treatment decisions) are thus included in the outcome category "target disease absent." After dichotomization of the diagnostic outcome, we may develop diagnostic prediction rules with logistic regression analysis. This focus on the target disease is a simplification of clinical practice.

4.3.1 Polytomous Logistic Regression

Several studies discussed the use of polytomous (or *multinomial*) logistic regression to accommodate simultaneous prediction of three or more unordered outcome categories [44, 605, 671]. The model for j outcome categories can be written as

$$\text{Logodds}(y = j \text{ versus } y = reference) = \alpha_j + \beta_{i,j} * x_i = lp_j$$

where $j - 1$ models are fitted each with separate sets of intercept α and regression coefficients β_i. We illustrate the polytomous model for prediction of three diagnostic outcome categories in a detailed case study.

4.3.2 Example: Histology of Residual Masses

After chemotherapy, patients with nonseminomatous testicular germ cell tumor may have residual masses of metastases [566]. These residual masses may contain benign tissue, mature teratoma, or cancer cells. Surgery is not necessary for benign tissue. Mature teratoma can grow and, hence, cause problems during follow-up. The most serious diagnosis is residual cancer, where a direct benefit from surgery is plausible.

We consider three outcome categories with varying therapeutic benefit: no benefit for benign tissue, some for teratoma, and most benefit for surgical removal of residual cancer [50]. We have previously proposed to weigh the benefit as 1:3:8 based on expert estimates of the prognosis of unresected versus resected masses [557]. This ordering in severity of the outcome was not used in the modeling, since biological knowledge was available that implied that prognostic relations would be very different for each histology. For example, some histologies are known to produce certain tumor markers while others do not. Masses with teratoma masses are not expected to decrease substantially in size by chemotherapy, while cancer is usually responsive. Hence, a substantial decrease would make residual cancer unlikely.

Polytomous logistic regression analysis requires that one of the outcome categories is chosen as the reference category. For the other outcome categories, the polytomous logistic regression analysis fits submodels that compare the outcome categories with the chosen reference. Thus, for each outcome category, different regression coefficients are estimated for each predictor. These submodels together comprise the polytomous model and can be used to estimate the probability of the presence of each diagnostic outcome. In our example study, the reference diagnosis was viable cancer. Hence, we fitted a polytomous regression model, consisting of two submodels, one for benign tissue compared to viable cancer and one for mature teratoma compared to viable cancer. These models take a similar form as the binary logistic model:

$$\text{Logit(benign vs. cancer)} = \alpha_b + \beta_{1,b}x_1 + \beta_{2,b}x_2 + \cdots + \beta_{p,b}x_p = \beta_{i,b}X = lp_b;$$
$$\text{Logit(teratoma vs. cancer)} = \alpha_t + \beta_{1,t}x_1 + \beta_{2,t}x_2 + \cdots + \beta_{p,t}x_p = \beta_{i,t}X = lp_t.$$

The subscript b indicates that we predict the odds of benign tissue, and subscript t for teratoma with p predictors.

The interpretation of the regression coefficients is similar as for dichotomous logistic regression, i.e., the log odds of the outcome (benign tissue or mature teratoma) relative to cancer per unit change in the predictor values. The probabilities of benign and teratoma tissue can be calculated by

$$P(\text{benign tissue}) = \exp(lp_b)/[1 + \exp(lp_b) + \exp(lp_t)]$$
$$P(\text{mature teratoma}) = \exp(lp_t)/[1 + \exp(lp_b) + \exp(lp_t)]$$

As probabilities need to sum to 1, the probability of cancer can then be calculated by

$$P(\text{cancer}) = 1 - P(\text{benign tissue}) - P(\text{mature teratoma})$$

We fitted a multivariable polytomous logistic regression model with six predictors to enable estimation of the probabilities of benign tissue, mature teratoma, and viable cancer. Variable selection was not applied; we simply included all six predictors.

4.3.3   *Alternative Models

For comparison reasons, we may fit consecutive multivariable dichotomous logistic models. In our example, we make one model to predict benign tissue (vs. mature teratoma or viable cancer). The second, consecutive, model aimed to predict the odds of mature teratoma versus viable cancer in patients who did not have benign tissue.

$$\text{Logit(benign vs. teratoma/cancer)} = \alpha_b + \beta_1 x_1 + \beta_2 x_2 + \cdots + \beta_p x_p = \beta_i X = lp;$$
$$\text{Logit(teratoma vs. cancer)} = \alpha_t + \beta_{1,t}x_1 + \beta_{2,t}x_2 + \cdots + \beta_{p,t}x_p = \beta_{i,t}X = lp_t.$$

The latter formula is identical to a previous formula for the polytomous model, but the coefficients are estimated differently. In the polytomous model, all coefficients are estimated jointly. In the consecutive logistic model, a selection of patients is made to estimate the second set of coefficients.

With these two binary logistic models, the diagnostic probabilities are calculated by

$$P(\text{benign tissue}) = \exp(lp)/(1 + \exp(lp))$$
$$P(\text{mature teratoma}) = (1 - P(\text{benign tissue})) * \exp(lp_t)/[1 + \exp(lp_t)]$$
$$P(\text{cancer}) = 1 - P(\text{benign tissue}) - P(\text{mature teratoma})$$

In our example, we use the same six predictors, but in principle we could select different predictors for lp and lp_t. Also, we could have considered different transformations of the continuous predictors LDH, mass size, and reduction in size.

In both approaches, 14 parameters were estimated: two intercepts (α) and two sets of six regression coefficients ($\beta_{1:6}$). The performance of the two approaches was very similar according to discrimination (area under ROC curve) and R^2 measures [50]. Further discussion of approaches to unordered outcomes is provided elsewhere [469, 566, 604].

4.3.4   *Comparison of Modeling Approaches

We illustrate the alternative modeling approaches with data from 1094 men with testicular cancer, of whom 425 (39%) had benign tissue, 535 (49%) mature teratoma, and 134 (12%) viable cancer at postchemotherapy surgery [645]. Table 4.2 shows the distributions of the six predictors across the three diagnostic outcome categories and in the total study population.

Table 4.2 Distribution of predictors across outcome categories in the study sample (n = 1094) [645].

	Benign	Mature teratoma	Viable cancer	Total
	N (%)	N (%)	N (%)	N (%)
Predictors				
No teratoma in primary tumor	279 (55)	170 (34)	54 (11)	503 (46)
Normal AFP level	200 (59)	112 (33)	27 (8)	339 (31)
Normal HCG level	184 (49)	154 (41)	40 (10)	378 (35)
Standardized value of LDH[a]	1.5 (0.39–70)	1.2 (0.12–21)	1.8 (0.34–64)	1.4 (0.12–70)
Postchemotherapy size (mm)[a]	18 (2–300)	30 (2–300)	40 (2–300)	28 (2–300)
Reduction in size (%)[a]	60 (−150 to 100)	20 (−150 to 100)	43 (−250 to 100)	43 (−250 to 100)
Outcome				
Histology at resection	425 (39)	535 (49)	134 (12)	1094 (100)

[a]Median (range)

AFP: alpha-fetoprotein; HCG: human chorionic gonadotropin; LDH: lactate dehydrogenase

Table 4.3 Results of the multivariable polytomous and consecutive dichotomous logistic regression analysis [50]. Values represent odds ratios with 95% confidence intervals

Predictor	Polytomous regression		Consecutive dichotomous regression	
	Benign versus cancer	Teratoma versus cancer	Benign versus other	Teratoma versus cancer
No teratoma in primary tumor	2.2 (1.4–3.3)	0.66 (0.44–0.99)	3.0 (2.2–4.0)	0.61 (0.40–0.92)
Normal AFP serum level	2.8 (1.7–4.6)	0.94 (0.57–1.5)	2.9 (2.1–4.0)	0.90 (0.54–1.5)
Normal HCG serum level	1.4 (0.9–2.3)	0.72 (0.46–1.1)	1.9 (1.3–2.6)	0.70 (0.44–1.1)
Standardized LDH (log)	1.2 (0.8–1.6)	0.58 (0.42–0.78)	1.7 (1.4–2.2)	0.60 (0.44–0.81)
Postchemotherapy mass size (sqrt)	0.79 (0.71–0.88)	0.91 (0.84–0.99)	0.85 (0.77–0.92)	0.89 (0.82–0.98)
Reduction in mass size (per 10%)	1.14 (1.06–1.22)	0.97 (0.92–1.02)	1.18 (1.12–1.24)	0.96 (0.92–1.0)

The odds ratios for the predictors are shown in Table 4.3, considering a polytomous regression model, and a consecutive logistic model. We note that the odds ratios for teratoma versus cancer differ slightly between these modeling approaches. The odds ratios for necrosis versus cancer are larger for most predictors than for necrosis versus other histology.

4.4 Ordinal Outcomes

Ordinal outcomes are quite common in medical and epidemiological studies. Often, such scales are either simplified to binary outcomes or treated as continuous outcomes. As an example, we consider the Glasgow Outcome Scale (GOS) [577]. This scale has five levels (Table 4.4).

Table 4.4 Definition of the Glasgow outcome scale

Category	Label	Definition
1	Dead	Dead
2	Vegetative	Unable to interact with environment; unresponsive
3	Severe disability	Conscious but dependent
4	Moderate disability	Independent, but disabled
5	Good recovery	Return to normal occupational and social activities; may have minor residual deficits

This scale has often been dichotomized as mortality versus survival, or an unfavorable (GOS 1, 2, or 3) versus favorable (GOS 4 or 5) outcome. However, we can also explore the use of full GOS. A practical consideration is that the GOS 2 category is very small and that some may debate whether vegetative state is better than death. Therefore, we combine the adjacent GOS categories 1 and 2, such that an outcome with four ordered levels is formed.

4.4.1   Proportional Odds Logistic Regression

A standard logistic regression model can be used for each of the three possible dichotomous categorizations of the GOS: 12 (dead/vegetative) versus 345, 123 versus 45 (favorable), and 1234 versus 5 (good recovery). A straightforward extension of the logistic model is the proportional odds logistic model [371]. Here, a common set of regression coefficients is assumed across all levels of the outcome, and intercepts are estimated for each level. So, in our example, we have three intercepts α, but only one set of β coefficients, instead of three sets of β coefficients when fitting a polytomous logistic model. The common set of β coefficients can be thought of as a pooled estimate over the three separate sets of β coefficients estimated at each possible dichotomization. As an example, we consider a simple model with age (linear), motor score, and pupillary reactivity (categorical) in a model to predict 6-month outcome in data from two RTCs in traumatic brain injury [259].

An advantage of the proportional odds model is its parsimony in dealing with an ordered outcome. The price we pay is the assumption of proportionality of the odds. This assumption is equivalent to saying that any cut-point on the outcome scale would lead to the same logistic regression coefficient. The model further has very similar assumptions as of the usual logistic model. We can graphically check the proportionality assumption in univariate analyses for each predictor (Fig. 4.9). Distances between points should be identical on the logit scale for each category of a predictor. The assumption of proportional odds can formally be assessed with a score test. We can also develop binary logistic models by each categorization, and check for systematic trends in the estimated odds ratios (Fig. 4.10). There is con-siderable overlap in patients between such evaluations, but clear deviations from proportional odds should become visible. In our example, the ORs per catego-rization are reasonably constant, and the proportional odds ratio provides an attractive summary measure over the three potential categorizations.

4.4.2   *Relevance of the Proportional Odds Assumption in RCTs

We might wonder how crucial the proportional odds (PO) assumption is to the interpretation of the PO odds ratio as a summary of a treatment effect. Recent

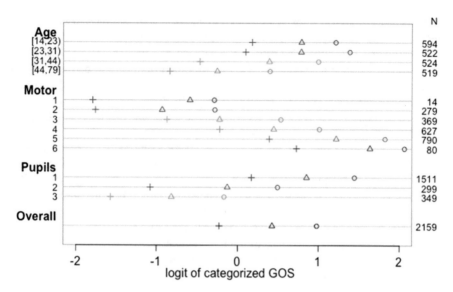

Fig. 4.9 Assessment of the proportional odds assumption for each of three predictors (univariate analysis) to predict for GOS at 6 months after traumatic brain injury. Data from the Tirilazad trials (n = 2159). The circle, triangle, and plus sign correspond to the GOS categorizations 12 versus 345, 123 versus 45, and 1234 versus 5. For example, the overall logit of the last categorization is −1, or a probability of 27% (589/2159 patients). The proportional odds assumption is well satisfied, since the horizontal distance between the points is constant within each category

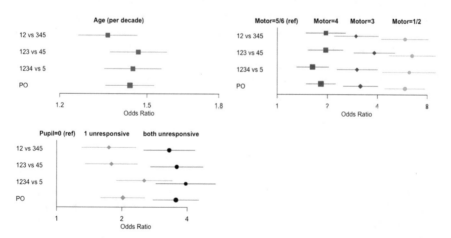

Fig. 4.10 Assessment of the proportional odds assumption for each of three predictors (multivariable analysis) to predict for GOS at 6 months after traumatic brain injury. GOS categorizations were 12 versus 345, 123 versus 45, and 1234 versus 5. The proportional odds (PO) assumption is well satisfied, since the odds ratios are similar for each categorization of the outcome, with the PO estimate as a summary with slightly lower variability (smallest confidence intervals)

randomized controlled trials (RCTs) in top medical journals have used the PO model for their primary analysis, but have varied in their emphasis on testing of the PO assumption [48, 264]. One such trial evaluated decompressive craniectomy for traumatic intracranial hypertension, and did not report the PO ratio because the PO assumption was violated; surgery strongly reduced mortality at the cost of more vegetative state and severe disability [264]. Instead, the authors reported a descriptive analysis, ignoring the ordering in the outcome. The overall trial result was difficult to interpret.

One might argue that the crucial point is the ordering of the outcomes dead, vegetative state, and severe disability. If there is agreement that these adjacent scores represent increasingly favorable outcomes, statistical testing of the PO assumption may be considered largely redundant [502]. For transparency, the binary odds ratios for each cut-off of the ordinal outcome should be presented, as in Fig. 4.10. If there is consensus on the ordering, the PO ratio can be presented and interpreted as a summary estimate of the treatment effect, regardless of violation of the PO assumption. The exception might be when odds ratios are qualitatively different for some cut-offs.

4.5 Survival Outcomes

Survival, or time-to-event, analysis is appropriate for outcomes that occur during follow-up. The most straightforward outcome is to consider death from any cause. A key characteristic of such survival data is that the follow-up of patients is typically incomplete. For example, some patients may have been followed for 1 year, others for 3 years, etc., while we may be interested in estimates of 5-year survival. Patients with such incomplete data are called censored observations. Because of censoring, logistic regression for the outcome (as a binary variable) is inappropriate. One could think of linear regression on the survival time (a continuous outcome), but again censoring makes such an analysis usually inappropriate.

4.5.1 Cox Proportional Hazards Regression

In medical and epidemiological studies, the Cox proportional hazard model is most often used for survival outcomes [113]. It is the natural extension of the logistic model to the survival setting. Indeed, the Cox model is equivalent to conditional logistic regression, with conditioning at times where events occur [325]. In the logistic model, we use an intercept in the linear predictor, while in the Cox model a baseline hazard function is used. So, baseline risk in the logistic model is given by an intercept, and in the Cox model by the baseline hazard function, which can be seen as a time-dependent intercept. The hazard function indicates the risk of the event of interest during follow-up. It is nonparametric in the Cox model. As for the logistic model, simpler and more extensive methods exist, which can be seen as special cases or extensions of the Cox model [579].

The Cox regression model is often stated as a function of the hazard function [653]:

$$\lambda(t|X) = \lambda(t)e^{\beta X},$$

where $\lambda(t)$ is the hazard at time t, and βX is the linear predictor, $\beta_1 x_1 + \beta_2 x_2 + \cdots + \beta_p x_p$.

The linear predictor is usually centered at the mean values of the predictors, and $e^{\beta X}$ then indicates the hazard ratio compared to the average risk profile. Note that the linear predictor relates to the log of the hazard:

$$\log(\lambda(t|X)) = \log(\lambda(t)) + \beta_1 x_1 + \beta_2 x_2 + \cdots + \beta_p x_p$$

The Cox regression model is semi-parametric. It makes a parametric assumption on the effect of predictors, i.e., proportionality of effect during follow-up. The hazard function $\lambda(t)$ is nonparametric. This is commonly considered an advantage of the model when we focus on the effect of predictors. Regression coefficients β_i can readily be estimated by the partial likelihood, and shrinkage or penalization can be done (Chap. 13). The quantity e^{β} is the hazard ratio, similar to how we calculate the odds ratio from a logistic regression coefficient.

4.5.2 Prediction with Cox Models

When we want to make predictions, we need to consider the risk over time, for example, using the cumulative hazard, or survival function. The standard formulation of the predicted survival at time t, given a set of predictors X, is as

$$S(t|X) = S(t)^{e(\beta X)},$$

where $S(t|X)$ denotes the predicted survival at time t, given a set of predictors X; $S(t)$ is the baseline survival, usually estimated at the mean values of the predictors; and βX is the linear predictor.

The baseline survival is estimated from the nonparametric hazard function as

$$S(t) = e^{-\Lambda(t)},$$

where $\Lambda(t)$ is the cumulative hazard at time t.

Note that $\log(\Lambda(t))$ can range between [−inf and +inf]; $\Lambda(t)$ [0, inf]; $S(t)$ [1, 0]. This is very similar to the behavior of quantities in logistic regression: logit, odds, and probability. The baseline survival in the development data determines the precise time points where we can make predictions for. This is not very natural for application of the model in new subjects.

4.5.3 Proportionality Assumption

The effect of predictors is assumed to be constant in time on a relative scale, or more precisely stated: the hazards are assumed to be proportional. The proportionality assumption can be assessed in a number of ways, including graphical and analytical methods. A general approach is to calculate interval-specific hazard ratios. With proportional hazards, the hazard ratio should be similar across any interval considered. Follow-up time can also be considered as a continuous variable, where assessing interaction with log(time) may be useful [225]. Specific tests for nonproportionality can also be used [495].

If we find that the effect of a predictor is (strongly) nonproportional, we can modify the survival model. We might stratify for categorical variables in the baseline hazards. For example, we could estimate baseline hazards for males and females separately if sex has a nonproportional effect on survival, or stratify by cohort in a meta-analysis context. For continuous predictors, e.g., age, we could specify interactions with log(time). Nonproportionality can also be visualized with a fully nonparametric approach, i.e., with Kaplan–Meier curves.

4.5.4 Kaplan–Meier Analysis

Kaplan–Meier analysis is a nonparametric approach to survival outcomes [288]. It adequately deals with censored data and provides attractive graphs on the relation between predictor values and the outcome over time. The method can be seen as the extension of a cross-table to survival data. More technically, it can be interpreted as a Cox model with stratification of the baseline hazard to all predictor levels. For example, we could make a Cox model with sex as a stratification variable for the baseline hazard, without any other variables, which is equivalent to a Kaplan–Meier analysis with sex as a predictor. Also, testing in a Kaplan–Meier analysis is usually done with a log-rank test, which is equivalent to the score test in the Cox model.

Kaplan–Meier analysis often has a role in prognostic modeling as an initial step in the analysis, i.e., to show univariate relations graphically or to compute survival fractions at a certain time of follow-up. Also at the end of a modeling process, Kaplan–Meier curves are often used to present the predictions from the model (Fig. 4.11). It is then necessary to group patients by their predictions, since Kaplan–Meier analysis cannot handle continuous predictors. Kaplan–Meier curves are for survival analysis what cross-tables are for binary or categorical outcomes.

Fig. 4.11 Cumulative incidence of neurofunctional impairment among three risk groups based on the Cox proportional hazards model in Table 4.6 [115]

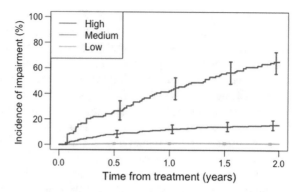

Table 4.5 Multivariable hazard ratios from Cox proportional hazard analysis [115]. Three risk groups could be formed based on the presence of no, one, or two unfavorable predictive characteristics, since the hazard ratios were very similar

Predictor	Hazard Ratio [95% CI]
Leprosy group (MB vs. PB)	7.5 (5.3–11)
Nerve-function loss at registration	8.1 (5.7–12)

4.5.5   *Example: Impairment After Treatment of Leprosy

Nerve-function impairment (NFI) commonly occurs during or after chemotherapy in leprosy. It is the key pathological process leading to disability and handicap. A simple clinical prediction rule was developed with 2510 patients who were followed up for 2 years in Bangladesh [115]. In total, 166 patients developed NFI (Kaplan–Meier 2-year estimate: 7.0% [95%CI 6.0–8.0%]. A Cox regression model was proposed with two strong predictors (Table 4.5). Patients with no, one, or two unfavorable predictive characteristics had 1.3% (95% CI 0.8–1.8%), 16% (12–20%), and 65% (56–73%) risks of developing NFI within 2 years of registration, respectively, according to Kaplan–Meier curves (Fig. 4.11). This example illustrates the combination of Cox regression for modeling and inversed Kaplan–Meier curves for model presentation in a survival context.

4.5.6   Parametric Survival

Whereas Kaplan–Meier analysis represents a more nonparametric approach, parametric survival models are less flexible than Cox regression in their dealing with the baseline hazard function. Parametric models typically assume proportionality of the predictor effects, but a more smoothed baseline hazard over time. Examples of parametric models include the exponential model (or Poisson model, using a constant hazard), and the Weibull model (two parameters to let the hazard increase or decrease monotonically over time). The exponential and Weibull model can also be seen as examples of accelerated failure time (AFT) models. Here, the effects of predictors are not viewed as multiplicative on the hazards scale, but as multiplicative on the time axis (or additive at the log-time axis). Other examples of AFT models are the lognormal and log-logistic model [225, 653].

Regression coefficients in exponential or Weibull models are hazard ratios after exponentiating. In AFT models, they represent a change in the log-time. The advantage of parametric survival models is their concise, parsimonious formulation, and smoothing of the underlying hazard. This makes these models especially attractive for prediction purposes. Extrapolation is readily possible with parametric models, but not with Cox or Kaplan–Meier analysis because of their nonparametric nature. Predictions at the end of the follow-up are unstable with Cox or Kaplan–Meier analysis, and more robust with parametric methods; at the price of making the assumption that the baseline hazard is modeled well. For estimation of the effect of predictors, the Cox model may often be more suitable, since this model is less restrictive than an exponential or Weibull model. Other variants include the log-logistic model, which may be useful in situations where predictors work especially during an early, acute phase of the hazard, which would show as non-proportional hazards in a Cox model [225]. Finally, some of the more flexible methods for binary data have also been extended to survival models, but are not commonly used yet (e.g., neural networks) [231].

4.5.7   *Example: Replacement of Risky Heart Valves

In Chap. 2, we presented an overview of the decision dilemma on Björk–Shiley convexo-concave (BScc) mechanical heart valves [610]. Poisson regression model was constructed to estimate survival and the risk of strut fracture [549]. Poisson regression was especially useful to disentangle the effects of increasing age of the patient during follow-up from the increasing time since implantation of the valve during follow-up. The follow-up time was divided into yearly intervals, each with an age and time since implantation. Time since implantation started at zero and increased in steps of 1 year during follow-up. Age started at the age at implantation and also increased in steps of 1 year during follow-up. The Poisson model could easily estimate the effects of both predictors, which would have been more complicated in a traditional Cox regression analysis. Moreover, extrapolation to longer time since implantation was readily possible with the Poisson model.

4.5.8   Summary of Survival Outcomes

In sum, the Cox regression model provides a default framework for prediction of long-term prognostic outcomes (Table 4.6). Kaplan–Meier analysis provides a

Table 4.6 Common statistical models for survival outcomes

Categories	Proportionality	Baseline hazard
Cox proportional hazards regression	Assumed	Nonparametric
Kaplan–Meier	No	Nonparametric
Exponential and Weibull	Assumed	Parametric
Lognormal, log-logistic	No, multiplicative in time	Parametric

nonparametric method but requires categorization of all predictors. It is the equivalent of cross-tables for binary or categorical outcomes in a survival context. Parametric survival models may be useful for predictive purposes because of their parsimony and robustness, for example, at the end of follow-up, or even beyond the observed follow-up. In survival analysis, repeated events may occur, that are correlated because of underlying frailty in individual patients. This asks for extensions of the Cox model when modeling repeated events within the same patients [517, 579].

4.6   Competing Risks

Prediction of outcomes other than overall mortality is often of interest and may be more complex than a standard survival analysis situation. For example, when we predict impairment after treatment of leprosy (Sect. 4.5.5), some patients might die before the impairment is noted. Death precludes the observation of the event of interest; it is a competing risk to the event of interest (impairment). Similarly, we may be interested in various different events after replacement of heart valves, such as mechanical fracture (Sect. 4.5.7), but also infection (endocarditis) and thrombotic events; if these lead to explantation of the valve, these events are competing with each other, similar to the risk of death of other causes [446].

4.6.1   Actuarial and Actual Risks

We may focus on the event of interest in a "cause-specific analysis." The effect of a predictor is then analyzed with traditional Kaplan–Meier analysis or Cox regression analysis while simply censoring all other events. This has been labeled an "actuarial risk" analysis [212, 213]. It assumes a world where the competing risks are absent. This perspective may be of interest when we aim for a causal interpretation of the effect of predictors on the event of interest [309]. For example, when we aim to reduce a specific event by a specific treatment, the relative effect may well be estimated by a traditional actuarial analysis.

For prediction of absolute risks, especially long-term risks, or risks in the elderly, it is not appropriate to ignore the competing risks [309]. Definitions of "actual risk" acknowledge that competing risks may preclude the observation of the event of interest. Actual risk can be described by the cumulative incidence function (CIF), which can be estimated in different ways [445].

4.6.2   Absolute Risk and the Fine & Gray Model

In many clinical studies, competing risks have been ignored, i.e., patients experiencing competing events were censored at the time of these events, and standard Cox regression was applied both for estimation of effects of predictors and making risk predictions. For prediction of absolute risk, the approach is only adequate when competing risks are rare. Many papers included traditional Kaplan–Meier curves in presenting absolute risk estimates in the presence of competing risks. This is inappropriate [445].

A technically correct approach is to combine the cause-specific hazards model for the event of interest with a model for the competing event to estimate the absolute risk. The formula for this combination is complicated. It is, hence, not possible to present this combination of cause-specific hazards models in an easy format to clinicians for estimation of absolute risk. The currently most common regression model in a competing risk setting is an extension of the Cox model, as proposed by Fine & Gray [163].

Here, a subdistribution hazard is defined for the event of interest that incorporates the disturbing influence of the competing events. Patients who experience a competing event, such as death, are not censored but remain in the risk set. This is equivalent to defining an infinite censoring time for competing events, or a censoring time beyond the last observed failure time. By having more subjects at risk, the actual risk estimate is lower than the actuarial risk. The difference will be substantial if many competing events occur before the event of interest, so relatively early during follow-up.

Predictors are modeled for the subdistribution hazard, assuming proportional effects at that scale. The regression coefficients reflect the impact of the predictor on the cumulative incidence. If the regression coefficient for a predictor is positive (i.e., a subdistribution hazard ratio greater than 1.0), higher values of a covariate imply a higher predicted cumulative incidence at every time point. The coefficients for the subdistribution hazard may be quite different from the cause-specific coefficients (estimated with censoring for the competing event), as illustrated below. Technically, the coefficients are not compatible, since the cause-specific and subdistribution hazard models each assume proportionality of effects, which cannot simultaneously be true. The Fine & Gray model provides a straightforward formula to calculate predicted absolute risks at a specific time point based on the cumulative subdistribution baseline hazard and the estimates of the regression coefficients [22].

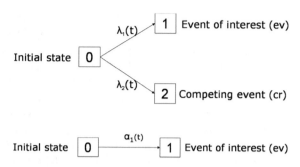

Fig. 4.12 Competing risks as multistate model with cause-specific hazards $\lambda_1(t)$ and $\lambda_2(t)$ and as a Fine & Gray competing risks model with the subdistribution hazards approach $\alpha_1(t)$. For example, the event of interest ("ev") may be the incidence of coronary heart disease, and the competing event ("cr") mortality from other causes

4.6.3   Example: Prediction of Coronary Heart Disease Incidence

As an example, we consider the incidence of coronary heart disease (CHD) prediction in women without CHD (initial state, Fig. 4.12). We analyze 4144 women, aged 55–90 years as enrolled in the Rotterdam study [676]. We define CHD occurrence as the event of interest, with death from other causes as the competing event (Fig. 4.12). The median follow-up was 12 years, during which 465 CHD events occurred and 1263 women died of other causes.

We compare cause-specific models for CHD and other mortality, with the Fine & Gray model for the subdistribution hazard of CHD (Table 4.7). Cause-specific

Table 4.7 Cause-specific models for CHD (event of interest) and other mortality (competing risk), and Fine & Gray model for the subdistribution hazard of CHD (Event of interest) [676].

Predictor	cHR for CHD	HR for non-CHD death	sHR for CHD
Age (per decade)	2.2 [2.0–2.5]	3.6 [3.4–3.9]	1.6 [1.5–1.8]
Blood pressure medication (at 120 mmHg)	1.7 [1.3–2.3]	1.2 [1.0–1.4]	1.7 [1.3–2.2]
Systolic blood pressure (per 10 mmHg, no medication)	1.1 [1.1–1.2]	1.0 [1.0–1.1]	1.1 [1.1–1.2]
Systolic blood pressure (per 10 mmHg, medication)	1.1 [1.0–1.1]	1.0 [1.0–1.1]	1.1 [1.0–1.1]
Diabetes	1.5 [1.2–1.9]	1.3 [1.1–1.5]	1.4 [1.1–1.8]
Total cholesterol/HDL (log)	2.5 [1.9–3.4]	0.6 [0.5–0.8]	2.7 [2.0–3.7]
Current smoker	2.0 [1.6–2.5]	1.9 [1.7–2.2]	1.7 [1.4–2.2]

cHR: cause-specific hazard ratio (censoring lost to follow-up and non-CHD death); HR: hazard ratio (censoring lost to follow-up and CHD); sHR subdistribution hazard ratio (censoring lost to follow-up; keeping non-CHD death in the risk set). Note that a statistical interaction term was included for medication*systolic blood pressure

hazard ratios (cHRs) for the event of interest (CHD) were very similar to the subdistribution HRs (sHRs) from the Fine & Gray model for predictors that did not clearly affect non-CHD death, i.e., predictors related to blood pressure, or the presence of diabetes. In contrast, age and smoking status were also strong predictors for non-CHD death. Hence, cHRs for CHD were larger than the sHRs.

Of specific interest is the effect of age. In a cause-specific analysis, the cHR was 2.2 per decade older, while the HR for non-CHD death was larger (HR = 3.6). Hence, age was stronger associated with the competing event than the event of interest. So, the impact of age on the cumulative incidence of CHD was rather moderate (sHR = 1.6). This example illustrates that the sHRs can be interpreted directly in terms of the cumulative incidence function, and that they depend on both the hazards for CHD and other mortality.

Absolute risk predictions differed substantially between actuarial (censoring competing events) and actual estimates (combining cause-specific models, or Fine & Gray model). Actuarial risks classified 761 (18%) of the women as high risk (>20% 10-year risk) compared with only 342 (8%) according to the Fine & Gray model. This illustrates the substantial overestimation of absolute risk that can occur if actuarial approaches (censoring of competing risks in Kaplan–Meier or Cox models) are interpreted as providing actual risk estimates. The discriminative ability of the different models was similar, with a c index for actual risk prediction of 0.70 [0.68–0.73] [675] (See Chap. 15 for more discussion on performance measures).

4.6.4   Multistate Modeling

Rather than using cause-specific Cox regression models or a Fine & Gray model, we may also consider the use of a simple multistate model to estimate predictor effects and make absolute risk predictions (Table 4.8) [445]. Multistate models are considered useful when several events are of interest. Transition probabilities are specified between states, e.g., from healthy to CHD, from healthy to death, and from CHD to death, with model estimation methods common to survival modeling, such as cause-specific Cox models [126]. Multistate models are very flexible and can also be used to make dynamic predictions.

Table 4.8 Characteristics of models for competing risk modeling

Categories	Hazard ratio interpretation	Prediction
Cause-specific hazard models	Effect on event of interest, ignoring competing risks	Need to combine multiple models
Fine & Gray subdistribution hazard	Impact on cumulative incidence of event of interest	Directly possible
Multistate model	Effect on event of interest	Multiple (intermediate) events, dynamic in time

4.7 Dynamic Predictions

The focus in this book is on making predictions from a defined start point where baseline predictors are measured. Dynamic predictions may, however, also be of interest. For example in survival after a cancer diagnosis, patients may be interested in their prognosis given that they survived for some time without recurrence of disease. Their survival estimate will then be higher than at the time of diagnosis. This pattern can well be illustrated with relative survival curves [276]. Similarly, a bone marrow transplant recipient may not have had graft versus host disease for some time. He/she will have a better prognosis than at the time of receiving the transplant. A simple method to analyze the impact of such an intermediate event is to use a time-dependent variable in a Cox regression model. More elegant models are available that are better suited for dynamic prediction [622].

4.7.1 Multistate Models and Landmarking

A multistate model is very useful if we aim to predict the flow of subsequent events, including intermediate states. It can also be used to estimate the cumulative probability for a final state, incorporating time-dependent information, such as not being in an intermediate state for some time. Several examples are provided in a tutorial and recent textbooks [180, 445, 622].

For prediction, an interesting approach is to use the concept of "landmarking". Landmarks are fixed points in time during follow-up. We consider patients at risk at the landmark time (removing those with earlier events or censoring before the landmark) and update the predictor information, including intermediate events that may have occurred. Prediction models can be fitted at each landmark, but stacking of landmark data sets allows for more flexibility in modeling [625]. Fewer parameters may be needed for a landmark model than for a multistate model, and predictions are more easily obtained [445].

4.7.2 Joint Models

Another situation is that continuous measurements of disease activity are available during follow-up. An example is the prediction of mortality in human immunodeficiency virus (HIV)-infected patients based on their longitudinal CD4 cell count measurements [461]. Another example is monitoring of diabetes patients by their blood sugar levels (Hb1Ac measurements). We may be interested in predicting complications of diabetes, such a diabetic foot, based on the dynamic HbA1c pattern [369].

The predictive role of a continuous, dynamic marker can well be modeled with a joint model, which combines a model for longitudinal data (for a repeatedly measured predictor) with time-to-event data (for prediction of the event of interest). Dynamic survival probabilities can be estimated for future subjects based on their available longitudinal measurements and a fitted joint model [462].

Technically, we need to define an appropriate model to describe the evolution of the marker in time for each patient. This is typically done using a mixed model, which at least allows for subject-specific baseline levels of the marker. Next, the estimated evolutions of the marker are used in a Cox regression model to predict the event of interest. The marker level is not assumed constant in time but follows a dynamic pattern. The hazard for the event of interest can be related to the current marker value but also the change in time (slope of the trajectory) or the area under the curve [369].

Joint models are of interest for personalized predictions since they utilize random effects and therefore have an inherent subject-specific nature. This may allow to better tailor decisions to individual patients, i.e., personalize screening, rather than using the same screening rule for all [462, 585].

4.8   Concluding Remarks

Regression models are available for several types of outcome that we may want to predict from a start point ("$t = 0$"), such as continuous outcomes, binary, unordered categorical, ordered categorical, survival, and competing outcomes. The corresponding default regression models are the linear, logistic, polytomous, proportional odds, Cox, and Fine & Gray regression models, respectively. Both more and less flexible methods are available. Flexible methods may fit particular patterns in the data better but may on the other hand lead to overfitting (Chap. 5). It is therefore not immediately clear whether a more flexible model is to be preferred in a specific prediction problem (Chap. 6).

Special types of data can be encountered that require specific types of analyses. Correlated outcome data may occur by the design of a study, for example, by clustering within patients, or per hospital. Dynamic predictions pose more complex challenges, where multistate, landmarking, and joint models may be useful. Both the specification of such models and the evaluation of performance are more complex than considering prediction from a baseline start point $t = 0$.

Questions

4.1. Explained variation

   (a) What is the difference between explained variation in linear and logistic regression models?

   (b) Is the choice of scale for explained variation more natural in linear or logistic regression models?

4.2. Categorical and ordinal outcomes

   (a) What is the proportionality assumption in the proportional odds model?

   (b) Mention at least one way how the proportionality assumption can be checked?

   (c) Would the proportionality assumption hold in the testicular cancer case study (Table 4.3)?

   (d) We could also make two logistic regression models for the testicular cancer case study, with one model for benign versus other and another model for cancer versus other. What would be the problem with predictions from these models?

4.3. Parametric survival models

   (a) Why may we label the Cox regression model "semi-parametric"?

   (b) Do you agree that Kaplan–Meier analysis is a fully nonparametric model?

   (c) Why is the Weibull model attractive for making long-term predictions? At what price?

4.4. Competing risks

   (a) Why are actuarial risks higher than actual risks?

   (b) The effect of high cholesterol is strong for coronary heart disease (cHR = 2.5, Table 4.7), but seems slightly protective for other mortality (HR = 0.6). Explain why the impact on the cumulative incidence is very large then (sHR = 2.7)?

Chapter 5
Overfitting and Optimism in Prediction Models

Background If we develop a statistical model with the main aim of outcome prediction, we are primarily interested in the validity of the predictions for new subjects, outside the sample under study. A key threat to validity is overfitting: the data under study are well described, but predictions are not valid for new subjects. Overfitting causes optimism about a model's performance in new subjects. After introducing overfitting and optimism, we illustrate overfitting with a simple example of comparisons of mortality figures by hospital. After appreciating the natural variability of outcomes within a single center, we turn to comparisons across centers. We find that we would exaggerate any true patterns of differences between centers, if we would use the observed average outcomes per center as predictions of mortality.

A solution is presented which is generally named "shrinkage". Estimates per center are drawn towards the average to improve the quality of predictions. We then turn to overfitting in regression models and discuss the concepts of selection and estimation bias. Again, shrinkage is a solution, which now draws predictions towards the average by reducing the estimated regression coefficients to less extreme values. Bootstrap resampling is presented as a central technique to correct overfitting and quantify optimism in model performance.

5.1 Overfitting and Optimism

To derive a prediction model, we use empirical data from a sample of subjects, drawn from a population (Fig. 5.1). The sample is considered to be drawn at random. The data from the sample are only of interest in that they represent an underlying population [13]. We use the empirical data to learn about patterns in the population, and to derive a model that can provide predictions for new subjects from this population. In learning from our data, an important threat is that the data under study are well described, but that the predictions do not generalize to new

© Springer Nature Switzerland AG 2019
E. W. Steyerberg, *Clinical Prediction Models*, Statistics for Biology and Health, https://doi.org/10.1007/978-3-030-16399-0_5

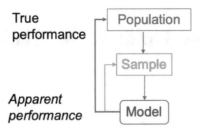

Fig. 5.1 Graphical illustration of optimism, which is defined as the difference between true performance and apparent performance. The apparent performance is determined on the sample where the model was derived from; true performance refers to the performance in the underlying population. The difference between apparent and true performance is defined as the optimism of a prediction model

subjects outside the sample. We may capitalize on specifics and idiosyncrasies of the sample. This is referred to as "overfitting". In statistics, overfitting is sometimes defined as fitting a model that has too many parameters, or as the "curse of dimensionality" [231]. For prediction models, we may define overfitting more precisely as fitting a statistical model with too many effective degrees of freedom in the modeling process. The analyst usually takes substantial freedom in the modeling process, which implies that the effective degrees of freedom are larger than the degrees of freedom of the finally developed model [34]. Effective degrees of freedom are used by estimation of the coefficients in a regression model, but also by searching for the optimal model structure [685]. The latter may include procedures to search for important predictors from a larger set of candidate predictors, optimal coding of predictors, and consideration of potential nonlinear transformations.

Overfitting leads to a too optimistic impression of model performance that may be achieved in new subjects from the underlying population. Optimism is defined as true performance minus apparent performance, where true performance refers to the underlying population, and apparent performance refers to the estimated performance in the sample (Fig. 5.1). Put simply, optimism means that "what you see may not be what you get" [34].

5.1.1   Example: Surgical Mortality in Esophagectomy

Surgical resection of the esophagus (esophagectomy) may be performed for subjects with esophageal cancer. It is among the surgical procedures that carry a substantial risk of 30-day mortality (see also Fig. 6.2) [164, 274]. Underlying differences in quality between hospitals may affect the 30-day mortality. Key questions are whether we can identify the better hospitals, and whether we can predict the mortality for a typical subject in a hospital (Chap. 21) [338].

5.1.2 Variability Within One Center

We first illustrate the variability of mortality estimates within a single center, according to different sample sizes. For esophagectomy, we assume 10% as the average mortality, based on analyses of the SEER-Medicare registry data, where mortality exceeded 10%: 221 of 2031 elderly patients had died within 30 days after surgery, or 10.9% [95% CI 9.6%–12.3%] [560].

For illustration, we assume that case-mix is irrelevant, i.e., that all patients have the same true mortality risks. The observed mortality rate in a center may then be assumed to follow a binomial distribution (Fig. 5.2). When the true mortality is 10% in samples of $n = 20$ patients, around 30% of these samples will contain two deaths (observed mortality 10%). With larger sample sizes, observed mortalities are more likely close to 10%; e.g., when $n = 200$, mortality is estimated as between 8 and 12% in 71% of the samples.

5.1.3 Variability Between Centers: Noise Versus True Heterogeneity

We need to appreciate this variability when we want to make predictions of mortality by center. For example, consider that 50 centers each reported mortality in 20 subjects, while the true mortality risk was 10% for every patient in each center. The distribution of the observed mortality is as in Fig. 5.2: 12% of the centers will have 0% mortality, and 13% will report a 20% or higher mortality. An actual realization is shown in Fig. 5.3. A statistical test for differences between centers should be nonsignificant for most of such comparisons (for 95% of the cases when $p < 0.05$ is used as criterion for statistical significance, given that there are no true differences).

Of more interest is the situation that the true mortality varies by center. This can be simulated with a heterogeneity parameter, often referred to as τ (tau). If we simply assume a normal distribution for the differences across centers, we write true mortality $\sim N(10\%, \mathrm{sd} = \tau)$. With $\tau = 1\%$, 95% of the centers have a mortality

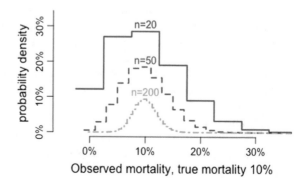

Fig. 5.2 Observed mortality in relation to sample size. When the true mortality is 10% in samples of $n = 20$ patients, around 30% of these samples will contain two deaths (mortality 10%). With larger sample sizes, observed mortalities are more likely to be close to 10%

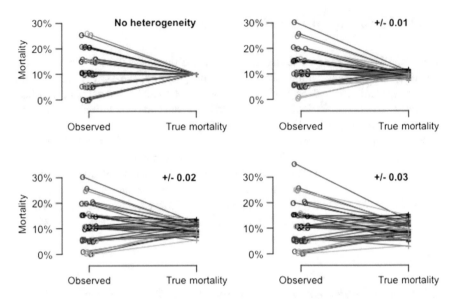

Fig. 5.3 Estimated and true mortality for 50 centers which analyzed 20 subjects each, while the average mortality was 10% for all (upper left panel), 10% ± 1% (upper right panel), 10% ± 2% (lower left panel), 10% ± 3% (lower right panel)

between 8 and 12%, while setting τ to 2% implies that 95% of the centers have a mortality between 6 and 14%. This underlying heterogeneity causes the mortality to have more variability than expected from the binomial distribution with a single true mortality of 10%. This is recognized in the distributions of Fig. 5.3. Differences between centers can be tested and will be identified as significant depending on the magnitude of the heterogeneity (τ) and the sample size (number of centers, sample size per center, see also Chap. 21).

5.1.4 Predicting Mortality by Center: Shrinkage

We recognize that the estimated mortalities are too extreme as predictions compared to the distribution of the true mortalities (Fig. 5.3). Predictions other than 10% are by definition too extreme when there is no heterogeneity. Too extreme predictions also occur when there is underlying variability across centers (e.g., true mortality between 5 and 15%). Per center, the estimated mortality is an unbiased estimator of the true mortality in each center. But the overall distribution of estimated mortality suffers from the low numbers per center, which makes that chance severely affects our predictions.

The phenomenon in Fig. 5.3 is an example of regression to the mean [394]. It is a motivation for shrinkage of predictions to the average, a principle which is also important in more complex regression models [109, 627]. We should shrink the

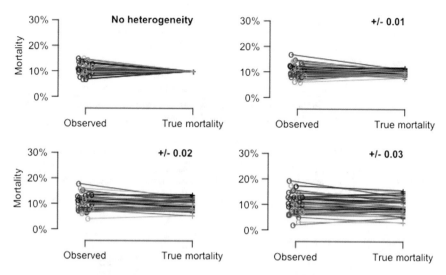

Fig. 5.4 Estimated and true mortality for 50 centers which had 200 subjects each, while the average mortality was 10% for all (upper left panel), 10% ± 1% (upper right panel), 10% ± 2% (lower left panel), 10% ± 3% (lower right panel)

individual center's estimates towards the overall mean to make better predictions overall.

We can also say that predictions tend to be overfitted: they point at very low and very high-risk hospitals, while the truth will be more in the middle. The identification of extreme hospitals will be unreliable with small sample size. With larger sample size, e.g., 200 subjects per center, the overfitting problem is much less (Fig. 5.4). Empirical Bayes and random effects methods have been proposed to make better predictions for such situations (see Chap. 21) [33, 626].

5.2 Overfitting in Regression Models

5.2.1 Model Uncertainty and Testimation Bias

Overfitting is a major problem in regression modeling. It arises from two main issues: model uncertainty and parameter uncertainty (Table 5.1). Model uncertainty is caused by specification of the structure of our model, such as which characteristics are included as predictors, driven by information of the data set under study. The model structure is therefore uncertain. This model uncertainty is usually ignored in the statistical analysis, which falsely assumes that the model was pre-specified [94, 138, 252].

The result of model uncertainty is selection bias [41, 110, 267, 484, 541]. Note that selection bias here refers to the bias caused by selection of predictors from a

Table 5.1 Causes and consequences of overfitting in prediction models

Issue	Characteristic
Causes of overfitting	
Model uncertainty	The structure of a model is not predefined, but determined by the data under study. Model uncertainty is an important cause of overfitting
Parameter uncertainty	The predictions from a model are too extreme because of uncertainty in the effects of each predictor (model parameters)
Consequences of overfitting	
Testimation bias	Overestimation of effects of predictors because of selection of effects that withstood a statistical test
Optimism	Decrease in model performance in new subjects compared to performance in the sample under study

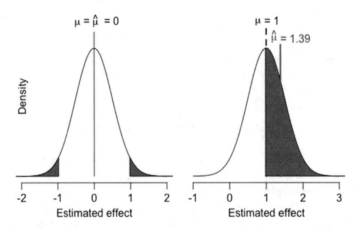

Fig. 5.5 Illustration of testimation bias. In case of a noise variable, the average of estimated regression coefficients is zero, and 2.5% of the coefficients is below −0.98 (1.96*SE of 0.5), and 2.5% of the coefficients is larger than +0.98 (1.96*SE of 0.5). In case of a true coefficient of 1, the estimated coefficients are statistically significant in 52%. For these cases, the average of estimated coefficients is 1.39 instead of 1 (39% testimation bias)

larger set of predictors, in contrast to the selection of subjects from an underlying population in standard epidemiological texts. Suppose that we investigate 20 potential predictors for inclusion in a prognostic model. If these are all noise variables, the true regression coefficients are zero ($\mu = 0$). On average, one variable will be statistically significant at the $p < 0.05$ level. The estimated effect will be relatively extreme, since otherwise the effect would not have been statistically significant. If this one variable is included in the model, it will have a quite small or quite large effect (Fig. 5.5, left panel). On average, the estimated effect ($\hat{\mu}$) of such a noise variable is still zero.

If some of the 20 variables are true predictors, they will sometimes have a relatively small and sometimes a relatively large effect. If we only include a predictor when it has a relatively large effect in our model, we are overestimating the effect of such a predictor. This phenomenon is referred to as *testimation bias*: because we test first, the effect estimate is biased [41, 94]. Testimation bias is related to phenomena such as "Winner's curse" [267] and regression to the mean [94].

In the example of a predictor with true regression coefficient 1 and SE 0.5, the effect will be statistically significant if estimated as lower than $-1.96*SE = -0.98$ (virtually no estimated coefficients), or exceeding $+1.96*SE = +0.98$ (52% of the estimated coefficients, Fig. 5.5, right panel). The average of the estimated coefficients in these 52% cases is 1.39 rather than 1. Hence, a bias of 39% occurs. In formal terms, we can state if b significant, then $b = b$, else $b = 0$. Instead of considering the whole distribution of predictor effects, we only consider a selected part.

Testimation bias is a pervasive problem in medical statistics and predictive modeling [225]. The bias is large for relatively weak effects, as in common in medical research [541]. Selection bias is not relevant if we have a huge sample size, or consider predictors with large effects, since these predictors will anyway be selected for a prediction model. Neither does selection bias occur if we prespecify the prediction model ("full model") [225].

5.2.2   Other Modeling Biases

A well-known problem in prediction research is bias by selection of an "optimal" cut-point for a continuous predictor [12, 155, 472]. The optimal point may be poorly reproducible, and the effect of the predictor is exaggerated.

A similar problem occurs if we examine different transformations for predictor variables as a check for linearity. For example, we may add a square term to a linear term for a continuous predictor variable and omit the square term if not statistically significant. Even if the square term was omitted, the fascinating finding was that we should use two degrees of freedom for this predictor rather than one [197].

More subtle biases creep in when we less formally assess alternative model specifications. For example, we may consider different transformations of the outcome variable in a linear model and visually judge the best transformation for use in further modeling. Or we examine different coding variants of a categorical predictor, with merging of groups with what we consider to have "similar outcomes." These issues are discussed in more detail in Chaps. 9 and 10 on coding of predictors, and Chaps. 11 and 12 on selection of predictors.

5.2.3   Overfitting by Parameter Uncertainty

It appears that even when the structure of our model is fully prespecified, predictions are too extreme when multiple predictors are considered. This is because parameters, such as regression coefficients, are estimated in the model with uncertainty. This surprising finding has been the topic of much theoretical research [109, 627]. An intuitive explanation is related to how we create a linear predictor in regression models. Hereto, the regression coefficients of multiple predictors are multiplied with the predictor values. With default estimation methods (i.e., least squares for linear regression, and maximum likelihood for logistic or Cox regression), each of the coefficients is estimated in a (nearly) unbiased way. But each coefficient is associated with uncertainty, as reflected in the estimated standard error and 95% confidence interval. This uncertainty makes that we tend to overestimate predictions at the extremes of a linear predictor, i.e., low predictions will on average be too low, and high predictions will on average be too large. This is again an example of regression to the mean. We can shrink coefficients towards zero to prevent this overfitting problem [109, 225, 627].

This overfitting problem is related to "Stein's paradox": biased estimates rather than unbiased estimates are preferable in multivariable situations to make better predictions [147, 530]. Shrinkage introduces bias in the multivariable regression coefficients, but if we shrink properly the gain in precision of our predictions more than offsets the bias. The issue of bias–variance trade-off is central in prediction modeling [231], and will be referred to throughout this book. Estimation with shrinkage methods is discussed in more detail in Chap. 13, including modern variants such as LASSO and elastic net [581, 689].

5.2.4   Optimism in Model Performance

Overfitting can visually be appreciated from the distributions of estimated mortality as in Figs. 5.3 and 5.4, but also from model performance measures. For example, we may calculate Nagelkerke's R^2 for a logistic model that includes 20 centers (coded as a factor variable, with 19 dummy variables indicating the effect of 19 centers against a reference hospital). If the true mortality in all hospitals was 10%, the estimated R^2 was 9.4% when each hospital contained 20 subjects (Table 5.2). In fact, R^2 was 0%, since no true differences between centers were present. The estimated 9.4% is based on pure noise. We refer to the difference between 9.4 and 0% as the optimism in the apparent performance (Fig. 5.1). With larger sample sizes, the optimism decreases, e.g., to 0.1% for 20 centers with 2000 subjects each (total 40,000 subjects, 4,000 deaths). Statistical testing of the between center differences was by definition not significant in 95% of the simulations. We might require statistical significance of this overall test before trying to interpret between center differences (Chap. 21).

When true differences between centers were present (e.g., a range of 6–14% mortality, $\tau = 2\%$), the true R^2 was close to 1% ($n = 2000$). With small sizes per center, the estimated R^2 was 10.1%, which is again severely optimistic (Table 5.2).

A well-known presentation of optimism is to visualize the trade-off between model complexity and model performance [231]. We illustrate this trade-off in Fig. 5.6, where we considered a simple linear regression model with 1–10

Table 5.2 R^2 for a logistic model predicting mortality in 20 centers. True mortality was 10% in the first series of simulations, and R² reflects pure noise. True mortality varied between 6 and 14% (τ = 2%) in the second series of simulations

True mortality (%)	Sample size	$R^2_{apparent}$ (%)	R^2_{adj} (%)	$R^2_{bootstrap}$ (%)
10	20 * n = 20	9.4	−0.1	NA
	20 * n = 200	1.0	0	−0.5
	20 * n = 2000	0.1	0	0
10 ± 2	20 * n = 20	10.1	0.3	NA
	20 * n = 200	1.9	0.9	0.3
	20 * n = 2000	1.0	0.9	0.8

*Nagelkerke's R^2 calculated in logistic regression models [403], averaged over 500 repetitions. $R^2_{apparent}, R^2_{adj}, R^2_{bootstrap}$ refer to the apparent, adjusted, and bootstrap-corrected estimates of R^2, respectively. The R^2_{adj} included "LR−df" instead of "LR" in the formula. Note that not all coefficients could directly be estimated, since some hospitals had 0% estimated mortality with n = 20; for these we used 1% as the estimated mortality (adding 1 subject as dead, with a weight of 1% * 20 = 0.2). Bootstrapping with these weighted samples was not readily possible

predictors, with strong to weak effects. The model performance is evaluated by the mean squared error (mean$(y − \hat{y})^2$) for the underlying population (internal validation), and for a population where the true regression coefficients were slightly different (external validation). The true model had coefficients of 1; at external validation the true coefficients were 1.5 for 5, and 0.5 for 5 predictors. With 50 subjects per sample for estimation of the model (1000 simulations), we note that the apparent performance improves with more predictors considered, even if the predictors are pure noise (Fig. 5.6, left panel). With 10 true predictors, the internal and

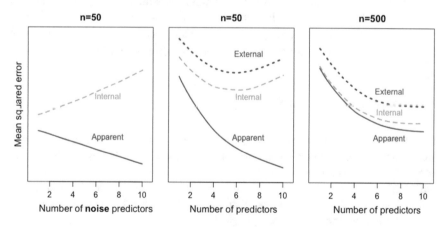

Fig. 5.6 Mean squared error of predictions from three linear regression models with increasing complexity (means of 1000 simulations). Left: 10 noise predictors, n = 50: Apparent performance improves with more predictors, but internal performance increasingly deteriorates. Middle: 10 true predictors with decreasing strength: Internal performance worsens as with noise predictors, with an optimum at six predictors. External performance follows the same pattern as internal performance, for a true model with slightly different effects of the 10 predictors. Right: with n = 500, the statistical optimism in performance (Internal−Apparent) is 1/10 of that with n = 50

external performance does not improve after six predictors are included. Overfitting appears less of a problem for 10 times larger sample sizes ($n = 500$).

5.2.5   Optimism-Corrected Performance

In linear regression analysis, an adjusted version of R^2 is available, which compensates for the degrees of freedom used in estimation of a model. Such an adjusted version can also be considered for Nagelkerke's R^2, which we consider, e.g., for logistic and Cox models. We could subtract the degrees of freedom used to estimate the LR of the model in the calculation:

$$R^2_{adjusted} = \left(1 - e^{(-(LR-df)/n)}\right) / \left(1 - e^{(-2LL0/n)}\right),$$

where LR refers to the difference in log-likelihood (LL) of the model with and without the predictor, df are the degrees of freedom of the predictors in the model, n is the sample size, and LL0 is the log-likelihood of the null model (without predictors).

This adjusted version is not standard in most current software, however. When we apply this formula for the simulated center outcome as shown in Figs. 5.3 and 5.4, the average $R^2_{adjusted}$ for noise differences is 0, with approximately half of the adjusted R^2 values being negative (Table 5.2). The adjustment made the R^2 estimates a bit conservative for small samples. For example, when true differences existed, the adjusted R^2 was 0.3% rather than 0.9% (Table 5.2).

A more general optimism correction is possible with bootstrapping, which is explained in the next section. In Table 5.2, bootstrap-corrected performance was more conservative than the $R^2_{adjusted}$ formula, which may be caused by the fact that the optimism in R^2 does not follow a fully normal distribution [535].

5.3   Bootstrap Resampling

Bootstrapping may allude to a German legend about Baron Münchhausen, who was able to lift himself out of a swamp by pulling himself up by his own hair. In later versions of the legend, he was using his own bootstraps to pull himself out of the sea which gave rise to the term "bootstrapping". In statistics, bootstrapping is a method for estimating the sampling distribution of an estimator by resampling with replacement from the original sample [673].

Bootstrapping mimics the process of sampling from the underlying population [148]. Since we only have a sample from the population, this sampling is not truly possible, similar to the legend about Baron Münchhausen. Bootstrap samples are drawn with replacement from the original sample to introduce a random element. The bootstrap samples are of the same size as the original sample, which is important for the precision of estimates obtained in each bootstrap sample.

Table 5.3 Illustration of five bootstrap samples drawn with replacement from the ages of five subjects. For easier interpretation, age values were sorted per sample

Original sample ages (years)	Bootstrap samples ages (years)
20, 25, 30, 32, 35	20, 20, 30, 32, 35
	20, 25, 25, 30, 35
	20, 25, 30, 30, 32
	25, 32, 35, 35, 35
	30, 30, 32, 35, 35
	…

For illustration, we consider the simple case of the age of five subjects who are 20, 25, 30, 32, and 35 years old. Some subjects may not be included in a specific bootstrap sample, others once, others twice, etc. Bootstrap samples might look like Table 5.3.

5.3.1   Applications of the Bootstrap

Bootstrapping is a widely applicable, nonparametric method. It can provide valuable insight into the distribution of a summary measure from a sample. Bootstrap samples are repeatedly drawn from the data set under study, and each analyzed as if they were an original sample [148].

For some measures, such as the mean of population, we can use a statistical formula for the standard deviation $\left(SD = \sqrt{var} = \sqrt{\left[(x_i - mean(x))^2 / (n-1) \right]} \right)$. We can use the SD to calculate 95% confidence intervals (95% CI) as $+/-1.96 * SE = +/-1.96 * SD/\sqrt{(n)}$. The bootstrap can be used to calculate SD for any measure. For the mean, the bootstrap will usually result in similar SE and 95% CI estimates as obtained from the standard formula. For other quantities, such as the median, no SE or 95% CI can be calculated with standard formulas, but the bootstrap can. See elsewhere for extensive illustrations [225].

5.3.2   Bootstrapping for Regression Coefficients

The bootstrap can assist in estimating distributions of regression coefficients, such as standard errors and confidence intervals. The bootstrap can be useful in estimating distributions of correlated measures such as the difference between an adjusted and an unadjusted regression coefficient [653]. In the latter case, two regression coefficients are estimated in each bootstrap sample. The difference is calculated in each sample, and the distribution over bootstrap samples can be interpreted as the sampling distribution. Confidence intervals can subsequently be calculated with three methods:

1. Normal approximation: the mean and SE are estimated from the distribution (note: the SD over bootstraps is the SE of the mean).
2. Percentile method: quantiles are simply read from the empirical distribution. For example, 95% confidence intervals are based on the 2.5% and 97.5% percentile, e.g., the 50th and 1950th bootstrap estimate out of 1999 replications.
3. Bias-corrected percentile method: Bias in estimation of the distribution is accounted for, based on the difference between median of the bootstrap estimates and the sample estimate ("BCa") [148].

For reliable estimation of distributions, large numbers of replications are advisable, e.g., at least 1999 for method 2 and 3. Empirical p-values can similarly be based on bootstrap distributions, e.g., by counting the number of estimates smaller than zero for a sample estimate larger than zero (giving a one-sided empirical p-value) [148].

5.3.3   Bootstrapping for Prediction: Optimism Correction

A very important application of bootstrapping is in quantifying the optimism of a prediction model [94, 148, 225, 627]. With a simple bootstrap variant, one repeatedly fits a model in bootstrap samples and evaluates the performance in the original sample (Fig. 5.7).

The average performance of the bootstrap models in the original sample can be used as the estimate of future performance in new subjects. A more accurate estimate is, however, obtained in a slightly more complicated way [148]. The bootstrap is used to estimate the optimism: the decrease in performance between performance in the bootstrap sample (Sample*, Fig. 5.7) and performance in the original sample. This optimism is subsequently subtracted from the original estimate to obtain an "optimism-corrected" performance estimate [225].

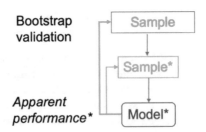

Fig. 5.7 Schematic representation of bootstrap validation for optimism correction of a prediction model. Sample* refers to the bootstrap sample which is drawn with replacement from the sample (the original sample from an underlying population). Model* refers to the model constructed in Sample*

5.3.4 Calculation of Optimism-Corrected Performance

Optimism-corrected performance is calculated as

Optimism-corrected performance = Apparent performance in original sample − Optimism,

where

Optimism = Bootstrap performance − Test performance.

The exact steps are as follows:

1. Construct a model in the original sample; determine the apparent performance on the data from the sample used to construct the model;
2. Draw a bootstrap sample (Sample*) with replacement from the original sample (Sample, Fig. 5.7);
3. Construct a model (Model*) in Sample*, replaying every step that was done in the original sample, especially model specification steps such as selection of predictors. Determine the bootstrap performance as the apparent performance of Model* in Sample*;
4. Apply Model* to the original sample without any modification to determine the test performance;
5. Calculate the optimism as the difference between bootstrap performance and test performance;
6. Repeat steps 1–4 many times, at least 200, to obtain a stable mean estimate of the optimism;
7. Subtract the mean optimism estimate (step 6) from the apparent performance (step 1) to obtain the optimism-corrected performance estimate.

Note that the original sample is used for testing of the model (Model*), while it contains largely the same subjects as the bootstrap sample (Sample*). Although this may seem invalid, both theoretical and empirical research support this process. Alternative bootstrap validation procedures have been proposed. Specifically, we could limit the assessment of performance of the models from the bootstrap sample to subjects from the original sample who were not included in the bootstrap sample. On average, 63.2% of the subjects are selected in a bootstrap sample, leaving on average 36.8% of the subjects for testing of a model from the bootstrap sample. The simplest variant is the out-of-sample bootstrap, where we take the mean of the performance in the unselected subjects. Other variants are the 0.632 and 0.632 + methods, where a weighted mean performance is estimated based on apparent performance and out-of-sample performance [149]. These bootstrap variants may have only limited advantages over the optimism correction procedure described above in specific settings [547, 576, 662]. The bootstrap has several advantages over simplistic approaches such as split-sample validation, or "single-repetition holdout" [576], which should be avoided (Chap. 17) [533].

We can apply the bootstrap approach to any performance measure, including the R^2, c-statistic, and calibration measures such as calibration slope (Chap. 15). A strong aspect of the bootstrap is that we can incorporate various complex steps from a modeling strategy. This is important if exact distributional results are virtually impossible to obtain, such as for common selection algorithms [438]. The bootstrap can, hence, give insight into the relevance of both model uncertainty, including both testimation bias and parameter uncertainty. In practice, it may be hard to fully validate a prediction model, including all steps made in the development of the model. For example, automated stepwise selection methods can be replayed in every bootstrap sample, leading to reasonably correct optimism-corrected performance estimates [535]. But more subtle modeling steps usually cannot fully be incorporated, such as choices on coding and categorization of predictors. The optimism-corrected estimate may then be an upper bound of what performance can be expected in future subjects. Only a fully specified modeling strategy can be replayed in every bootstrap sample.

It is often useful to calculate the optimism of a "full model", i.e., a prediction model including all predictors without any fine-tuning such as deleting less important predictors. The optimism estimate of such a full model may be a guide for further modeling decisions [225]. If the optimism is substantial, it is a warning that we should not base our model only on the data set at hand. Incorporating more external information may improve the future performance of the prediction model in such a case [218].

5.3.5   *Example: Stepwise Selection in 429 Patients

As an example, we consider a sample of 429 patients from the GUSTO-I study, which studied 30-day mortality in patients with acute myocardial infarction (details in Chap. 24). We first fitted a model with eight predictors, as specified in the TIMI-II study ("full model") [395]. This model had a Nagelkerke R^2 of 23% as apparent performance estimate. In 200 bootstrap samples, the mean apparent performance was 25% (Table 5.4). When the models from each bootstrap sample were tested in

Table 5.4 Example of bootstrap validation of model performance, as indicated by Nagelkerke's R^2 in a subsample of the GUSTO-I database (Sample5, $n = 429$)

Method	Apparent (%)	Bootstrap (%)	Test (%)	Optimism (%)	Optimism-corrected (%)
Full eight-predictor model	22.7	24.7	17.2	7.6	15.1
Stepwise, three predictors $p < 0.05$	17.6	18.7	12.7	5.9	11.7
Stepwise model falsely assumed to be prespecified	17.6	18.2	15.4	2.9	14.7

the original sample, the R^2 decreased substantially (to 17%). The optimism, hence, was 25%−17% = 8%, and the optimism-corrected R^2 23%−8% = 15%.

We can follow a backward stepwise selection procedure with $p < 0.05$ for factors remaining in the model (Chap. 11). This leads to inclusion of only three predictors (age, hypotension, and shock). The apparent performance drops from 23 to 15% by excluding five of the eight predictors. The stepwise selection was repeated in every bootstrap sample, leading to an average apparent performance of $R^2 = 18\%$. R^2 dropped to 12% when models were tested in the original sample (optimism 6%, optimism-corrected R^2 9%). When we falsely assume that the three-predictor model was prespecified, we would estimate the optimism as 3% rather than 6%. This discrepancy illustrates that optimism by selection bias may be as important as the optimism due to parameter uncertainty if a model is selected based on the same data.

We note that the apparent performance in the bootstrap samples was higher than the apparent performance in the original sample (Table 5.4). This pattern is often noted in bootstrap model validation. It may be explained by the fact that some patients appear multiple times in the bootstrap sample. Hence, it is easier to predict the outcome, reflected in higher apparent performance. Further, we note that the optimism is smaller after model specification by stepwise selection (6% instead of 8%). The optimism-corrected performance of the stepwise model is clearly lower than the performance of the full eight-predictor model. This pattern is often noted. A full model will especially perform better than a stepwise model when the stepwise selection eliminates several variables that are close to statistically significant while they have some true predictive value. When a small set of dominant predictors is present, including only these would logically be sufficient; a procedure such as LASSO might work well [581]. The bootstrap would show that the key predictors are nearly always selected and that other variables are most often excluded; the optimism would be relatively small and optimism-corrected performance similar to that of a full model. The leprosy case study is such an example (see Chap. 2). In the case that many noise variables are present in the full model, a selected submodel performs better than a full model. Careful preselection of candidate predictors is, hence, advisable, based on subject knowledge (literature, expert opinion), to prevent that pure noise variables are considered in the modeling process.

5.4 Cost of Data Analysis

The development of a prediction model for outcome prediction is a constant struggle in weighing better fit to the data against generalizability outside the sample. This has aptly been labeled the "cost of data analysis" [157]. The more we incorporate from a specific data set in a model, the less the model may generalize [138]. On the other hand, we do not want to miss important patterns in the data, such as a clearly nonlinear relation of a predictor to the outcome. A prediction model where underlying model assumptions are fulfilled will provide better predictions than a model where assumptions are violated. It is therefore considered natural to assess such assumptions as linearity of continuous predictor effects and additivity of effects (Chap. 12). However, if we test all assumptions of a model and iteratively adapt the model to capture even small violations, the model will be very specific for the data analyzed [94, 157].

5.4.1 *Degrees of Freedom of a Model

If we fit a statistical model to empirical data, it is common to consider the degrees of freedom (df) as a measure of model complexity, and the capacity for overfitting. The degrees of freedom reflect the number of dimensions in which a random vector may vary. For example, a 2×2 cross-table has 1 df, since we can vary only one number once the marginals of the table are fixed. Modeling strategies typically cost more degrees of freedom than reflected in the final fit of a selected model. Various authors have proposed more general definitions for the *effective* degrees of freedom of a method [146]. Generalized degrees of freedom (GDF) of a model selection and estimation procedure indicate the risks of overfitting that is associated with a modeling strategy. For example, Ye showed that a stepwise selection strategy that selected a model with five predictors (apparent $df = 5$), had GDF 14.1 [685]. A regression tree with 19 nodes (apparent $df = 19$), had GDF of 76.

An essential part of Ye's approach is to determine the apparent performance of a model when developed with pure noise. In Table 5.2 and Fig. 5.6, we note that the optimism in performance in the pure noise simulations was indeed very similar to the optimism when some true effects were present.

5.4.2 Practical Implications

In the development of prediction models, we have to be aware of the cost of all data analysis steps. We need to balance what we take from external information versus what we aim to learn from the data. The appropriateness of a modeling strategy is indicated by the generalizability of results to outcome prediction for new patients. Some practical issues are relevant in this respect.

- Sample size: with a small sample size, we have to be prepared to make more assumptions; the power to detect deviations from modeling assumptions will anyway be small. If deviations from assumptions are detected, and the model is adapted, testimation will occur and the validity of predictions for new patients may not necessarily be improved (Chap. 13).

- Robust strategies: some modeling strategies are more "data hungry" than other strategies [612]. For example, fitting a prespecified logistic regression model with age and sex uses only 2 *df*. If we test for linearity of the age effect, and interactions between age and sex, we spend more effective *df*. If we use a method such as regression tree analysis, we search for cut-points of age, and model interactions by default, making the method more data hungry than logistic regression (Chap. 4). Similarly, stepwise selection asks more of the data than fitting a prespecified model. Not only do we want to obtain estimates of coefficients, but we also want to determine which variables to include as predictors (Chap. 11).
- Bootstrap validation: Some suggest that the bootstrap can assist in determining an appropriate level of fine-tuning of a model to the data under study [487]. However, when many alternative modeling strategies are considered, the bootstrap results may become less reliable in determining the optimal strategy, since the optimum may again be very specific for the data under study. The bootstrap works best to determine optimism for a single, predefined strategy [225].

5.5   Concluding Remarks

In science, and in prediction modeling research specifically, we need to seek a balance between curiosity and skepticism. On the one hand, we want to make discoveries and advance our knowledge, but on the other hand, we must subject any suggested discovery to stringent tests, such as validation, to make sure that chance has not fooled us. It has been demonstrated that our scientific "discoveries" are often false, especially if we search hard and explore a priori unlikely hypotheses [266]. Overfitting and the resulting optimism in performance assessments are important concerns in prediction models.

Questions

5.1   Overfitting and optimism

    (a)   What is overfitting and why is it a problem?

    (b)   What are the two main causes of overfitting? What is the difference and can you give some examples?

5.2   Shrinkage for prediction (Figs. 5.3 and 5.4)
    A solution against the consequence of overfitting is shrinkage. For example, estimates per center can be drawn towards the average to improve the quality of predictions in Fig. 5.3 and 5.4.

    (a)   Is the required shrinkage more, or less, in Fig. 5.4 compared to Fig. 5.3?

    (b)   Is the underlying true heterogeneity more, or less, in Fig. 5.4 compared to Fig. 5.3?

5.3   Optimism in performance (Fig. 5.6)

    (a)   Verify that the optimism in apparent performance in the linear regression model is 2.8 with six noise predictors, $n = 50$; 2.8 with six true predictors, $n = 50$; 0.3 with six true predictors, $n = 500$.

    (b)   Explain why $n = 500$ leads to 1/10 of the optimism noted with $n = 50$.

5.4   Bootstrapping (Sect. 5.3)

    (a)   How can a bootstrap sample be created? How is this done with the sample command in R?

    (b)   How can the test sample for the 0.632 bootstrap variant by selected in R?

    (c)   How can bootstrapping be used to derive optimism-corrected estimates of model performance, addressing the two main causes of overfitting.

Chapter 6
Choosing Between Alternative Models

Background Any scientific model will have to make simplifying assumptions about reality. Nevertheless, statistical models are important tools to learn from patterns in underlying data. A good model can be used to make accurate predictions for future subjects. We discuss some general issues in choosing a type of model in a prediction context, with illustration in a case study on modeling age–outcome relations in medicine. We also summarize results from some empirical comparisons of alternative models, including classical regression and modern methods related to machine learning approaches.

6.1 Prediction with Statistical Models

In a pure prediction context, statistical models are merely seen as practical tools than as theories about how the world works. As long as the model predicts well, we are satisfied. This relates to the famous quote "All models are wrong, but some are useful" [68]. Although regression models are formulated as models of cause and effect ("y depends on x"), there need not be any causal relation at all, for example, because some intermediate causal factor was not recorded. We, hence, simply use the terms "predictor" and "outcome".

On the other hand, a statistical model may generalize better to new settings if causal effects are modeled, or at least relations that reflect biology, rather than mere associations. Careful modeling can provide important insights into how a combination of predictors is related to an outcome. For inference and hypothesis testing, fulfillment of assumptions becomes more important than for prediction. Prediction is primarily an estimation problem, while insight in effects of predictors is related to hypothesis testing (Chap. 1) [508].

With a good model, we can make predictions for future subjects, test hypotheses, and estimate the magnitude of effects of predictors. It is a philosophical question whether a true, underlying model exists. Many have argued that the notion of a "true model" is false [94]. Indeed, would it be imaginable that natural processes can fully be captured in a model containing relatively few variables, which are related in a mathematically simple way? Many subtle nonlinear and interactive effects probably play a role. Predictors may be unobservable or not yet discovered, or predictive effects may be too small to detect empirically. Therefore, a statistical model can only be an approximation to underlying patterns, based on the limited number of predictors that is known to us. Recent attempts to define biomarkers, and assessment of various "omics" measurements (genomics, proteomics, metabolomics, glycomics, etc.) will not change this limitation of any prediction model.

6.1.1 Testing of Model Assumptions and Prediction

If our primary aim is to make good predictions, we should not place too much emphasis on unobservable, underlying assumptions. It is a standard procedure nowadays to test model assumptions such as nonlinearity and additivity, or proportionality of hazards (see Chaps. 4 and 13). Such testing may be valuable but only to the extent that adaptations to the model lead to better predictions. When assumptions are met, the model will provide a better approximation to reality and hence predict better [225, 227]. Statistically significant violations of underlying assumptions do not mean that a prognostic model predicts poorly [80, 222, 508].

In a prediction context, we are lucky that we can directly measure the observed outcomes and compare these to what is predicted. This allows for direct statistical assessment of model quality with performance measures such as calibration and discrimination. Whether the underlying assumptions of the prediction model are true can never be known, since regression coefficients are unobservable; they can only be estimated.

6.1.2 Choosing a Type of Model

Some general suggestions have been made on the type of model to be used in prognostic research, with a focus on regression analysis [225].

- The mathematical form should be reasonable for the underlying data. For example, models should not give predictions that are below 0% or above 100% for binary outcomes or survival probabilities.
- The model should use the data efficiently. Regression models need to make assumptions, but they pick up general patterns in the data better than a simple cross-tabulation approach. Cross-tables quickly run out of numbers, and hence would provide unstable predictions. Similarly, survival outcomes should be analyzed with methods that use all available information.
- Robustness is preferred over flexibility in capturing idiosyncrasies. For prediction, we aim to model patterns that generalize to future subjects. Very flexible approaches will require large data sets, while medical prediction problems are often addressed with relatively small data sets.

- The results of the model should be transparent and presentable to the intended audience. In some fields, fully computerized models may be acceptable (e.g., neural networks), but in other fields insight in the underlying model is an advantage (e.g., effects of predictors in regression models).

In the current Big Data era, these requirements may be relaxed at some points, for example, with respect to efficient use of data, and allowing for more flexibility in modeling. Also, computerized presentation may nowadays be acceptable to some, although others may still object to black-box algorithms [181]. Also, practical issues play a role, such as familiarity of analysts and their readers with a method. A major requirement of any model is of course that it adequately answers the research question, since we know that all models will miss some aspects of the underlying natural process by their relative simplicity and the relative sparseness of data.

We will first look at some empirical support for relatively simple regression models as tools to capture the prognostic effect of age. This is followed by a brief discussion of some head-to-head comparisons between modeling techniques, including machine learning techniques.

6.2 Modeling Age–Outcome Relations

The effect of age on outcome is important in many medical prediction problems. Together with gender, age is an obvious demographic characteristic to consider in the prediction of an outcome. On the one hand, age represents the biological phenomenon of aging, with a decrease in the performance of biological systems. Observed age effects do, however, not necessarily represent pure biological relations, since many comorbid conditions may be present [440]. Moreover, selection may have occurred, e.g., making that very old patients only undergo surgery when in relatively good condition. Nevertheless, it is of interest to study how increasing age is related to outcome. Specifically, we consider the modeling of age-related mortality with logistic regression.

6.2.1 *Age and Mortality After Acute MI

Within the GUSTO-I data set (details in Chap. 24), Lee et al. found that the relation between age and 30-day mortality after an acute myocardial infarction (MI) was reasonably linear [329]. We can examine the relation between age and outcome in more detail by adding age^2, and a restricted cubic spline with five knots (4 *df*, including the linear term, see Chap. 9). We find that there is relatively limited gain by adding nonlinear transformations (Table 6.1). Graphical inspection (Fig. 6.1) suggests that the differences between the transformations are at the lower ages (below age 50), where limited data are available. It may be that the age–mortality relation is somewhat stronger above age 50 than below age 50 years; a linear spline

Table 6.1 Transformations of age as a predictor of 30-day mortality in the GUSTO-I dataset

Transformation of age	df	LR statistic	Nagelkerke R^2 (%)
Linear	1	2099	12.6
Add age^2	2	2112	12.7
rcs, 5 knots	4	2122	12.7
Linear spline with change point at age 50 years	2	2119	12.7
Dichotomize at age 65 years	1	1463	8.9

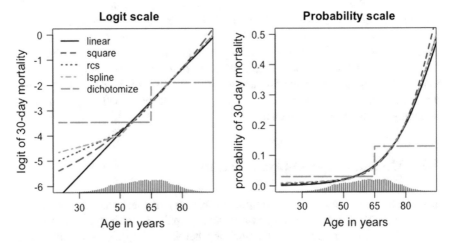

Fig. 6.1 The relation between age and 30-day mortality among 40,830 patients with acute myocardial infarction in the GUSTO-I data set. The distribution of the ages of the patients is shown at the bottom of the graph. Note the enormous range in mortality with age, since a logit of -6 means a probability of 0.2% and a logit of 0 means 50%

with a change point at age 50 captures this pattern. We hereto model a linear spline with two linear pieces connected at age 50 years. A really bad idea would be to dichotomize age at 65 years [472]. Such dichotomization would lose 30% of the prognostic information compared to the linear model (LR statistic 1463/ 2099 = 70%, Table 6.1). At the probability scale, differences between the continuous transformations were all minor, with the main difference with a dichotomized version of age (Fig. 6.1). Overall, assuming a linear effect was quite reasonable for modeling the effect of age for mortality after acute MI in this large data set.

6.2.2   *Age and Operative Mortality

Another example considers modeling of operative mortality in relation to age for 1.2 million elderly patients in the Medicare system [164]. Patients were between 65 and 99 years old, and who were hospitalized between 1994 and 1999 for major elective

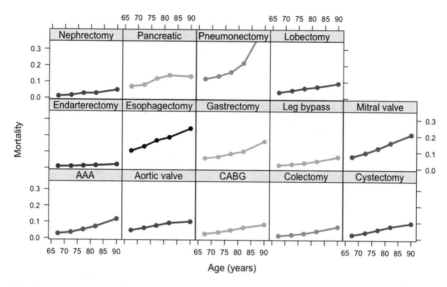

Fig. 6.2 Operative mortality by surgical procedure according to age in 1.2 million elderly patients in the Medicare system [164]

surgery (six cardiovascular procedures and eight major cancer resections, 14 types of procedures in total). Operative mortality was defined as death within 30 days of the operation or death before discharge and occurred in over 38,000 patients.

The mortality risk in this huge, nationwide, representative series varied widely between procedures. Not surprisingly, it was higher than that reported in many published series from specialized centers. Operative mortality clearly increased with age. Operative mortality for patients 80 years of age and older was more than twice that for patients 65–69 years of age (Fig. 6.2).

These data can be used to illustrate the fit of alternative logistic regression models for the relation between age and mortality. Since the data were reported in 5-year categories, we assign an average age per age category to study age as a continuous variable. We assume age to be at midpoints for the first two categories (67.5 and 72.5 years) and at 77.2, 82.0, and 90.0 years for the other three categories.

The simplest logistic regression model assumes a single age effect across categories: mortality ~ procedure + age 10, where mort indicates operative mortality (0/1), procedure is a categorical variable for the 14 levels of procedures, and age10 is age coded per 10 years.

We can test whether the age effect differs by procedure by adding the interaction term "procedure * age10":

$$\text{mortality} \sim \text{procedure} + \text{age}10 + \text{procedure} * \text{age}10$$

The smallest age effect was found for Endarterectomy (OR 1.4 per decade, Fig. 6.3), followed by Gastrectomy (OR 1.5 per decade). The strongest age effects were found for Nephrectomy and Cystectomy (OR 2.1 and 2.2 per decade, Fig. 6.3).

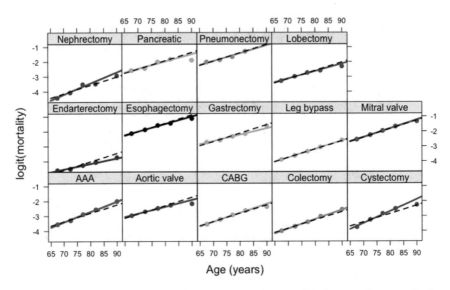

Fig. 6.3 Logit scale presentation of two logistic regression models for operative mortality by surgical procedure according to age, based on analysis of 1.2 million elderly patients in the Medicare system [164]. Dots are the observed mortality rates by type of surgery and age category. Solid lines indicate a model with procedure * age interaction. Dotted lines indicate a common effect for age across surgeries ("mortality ~ procedure + age10")

Table 6.2 Age and operative mortality in 1.2 million elderly patients in the Medicare system [164]

Model	Age 10	LR statistic	Nagelkerke R^2 (%)
procedure + age10	1.75	16,841	5.62
... + procedure * age10	1.44–2.23	16,936	5.66
... + age10^2	1.74	16,843	5.62

The improvement in model fit obtained by this model extension was relatively small (Table 6.2). The likelihood ratio improved by 95, which was only 0.6% of the total model chi-square including this interaction. The explained variation (Nagelkerke R^2) increased by 0.04%.

We can also assess nonlinearity in the age effect by adding a square term $(age10^2)$ to the simplest model:

$$\text{mortality} \sim \text{procedure} + \text{age10} + \text{age10}^2$$

Remarkably, adding such a square term made virtually no contribution to the model fit (χ^2 increased by 2). All code for this analysis is at www.clinicalpredictionmodels.org.

In conclusion, the age—outcome relations were reasonably linear for these surgical procedures. Moreover, we may assume that the effect is in the order of an odds ratio of 1.75 per decade, or a doubling in odds per 12.5 years (dotted lines in Fig. 6.3). Both results may be useful as prior knowledge when we model the effect of age, especially when we are dealing with a relatively small data set. As a starting point we may assume linearity on the logistic scale, and an age effect between 1.5 and 2.2 per decade, the latter depending on the surgical procedure.

6.2.3 *Age–Outcome Relations in Other Diseases

Many studies described the relation between age and outcome in other diseases. We performed a meta-analysis in traumatic brain injury, where again a linear transformation was adequate, although adding the square term of age provided a somewhat better fit [260]. Remarkably, many studies had dichotomized age after searching for an optimal cut-off, which is nonsensical from a biological perspective.

Among seriously ill-hospitalized adults, age had a linear effect that differed slightly by diagnosis, similar to the evaluation of operative procedures described above [307]. Other studies also support a more or less linear association between age and outcome.

Remarkably, for some studies, especially smaller ones, the authors concluded from a statistically nonsignificant age effect that age was not related to outcome. This is a clear illustration of interpreting the absence of evidence as evidence of absence [11].

6.3 Head-to-Head Comparisons

Several studies have described head-to-head comparisons of alternative methods. Especially, attention has been given to alternative methods to predict binary outcomes. Main classes of statistical methods include regression modeling, trees, and neural networks [231]. Machine learning may include the latter techniques (trees, neural networks), deep learning techniques, support vector machines (SVMs), and some techniques that are extensions of traditional statistical methods, such as the LASSO and elastic net. Some published comparisons on medical prediction problems were in favor of regression-based techniques, and some in favor of more modern approaches such as neural networks.

A problem in many comparisons is that one of the comparators is not developed with state-of-the-art methods, while the other is. For example, computer scientists often have been working on variants of neural networks, which were shown to do better than logistic models if the latter were derived with simplistic, suboptimal techniques [497]. Methodological problems were especially severe for comparisons of methods to predict survival outcomes [496]. Kaplan–Meier and Cox regression can deal adequately with survival data, but ad hoc approaches have usually been followed for other techniques.

Moreover, any comparison should include a fair validation procedure. Studies comparing a suggested new method to existing methods are often biased in favor of the new method. A positive development is the competition between modelers on the same data set. A fascinating example on the influence of the analyst is a study where one data set was analyzed by 29 teams regarding the question whether soccer referees are more likely to give red cards to dark-skin players than to light-skin players. The teams came up with odds ratios from 0.9 to 2.9 [509]. Such neutral comparison studies are needed, which are dedicated to the comparison itself: they do not aim to demonstrate the superiority of a particular method and thus are not designed in a way that may increase the probability to observe incorrectly this superiority [66].

The quality of predictions obtained with a model may depend on various factors [377]. There may be intrinsic properties of the prediction problem that make a method more or less suited. For example, the strategy to fit a full model, i.e., without data-driven selection of predictors, may especially work well if a limited number of well-known predictors is available [225]. This is very different from prediction with "omics", where thousands of characteristics with small effects may be present. Also, the actual implementation of the method as a computer program may vary in combination with the skills of the user.

6.3.1 StatLog Results

An important historical example of a systematic comparison of statistical modeling approaches is the StatLog project [377]. Different approaches to classification were studied. Table 6.3 summarizes some results for data sets with a binary outcome, both from medical and nonmedical applications. It appears that logistic regression performs quite well across all examples. More flexible techniques such as trees and neural networks only had advantages in larger data sets. In the medical context, data sets are often relatively small, especially with respect to number of events, and the predictive information is relatively limited, leading to an unfavorable signal-to-noise ratio [222, 231].

Table 6.3 Error rates for problems with binary outcomes in the StatLog project [377]

Data set	N dev	Predictors	Logistic	Naïve Bayes	Tree (CART)	Neural network
Nonmedical						
Credit management	15,000	7	0.030	0.043	NA	0.023
Australian credit	690	14	0.141	0.151	0.145	0.154
German credit	1000	24	0.538	0.703	0.613	0.772
Cut (letters in text)	11,220	20	0.046	0.077	NA	0.043
	11,220	50	0.037	0.112	NA	0.041
Belgian Power	1250	28	0.007	0.062	0.034	0.017
Instability	2000	57	0.028	0.089	0.022	0.022
Medical						
Heart disease	270	13	0.396	0.374	0.452	0.574
Diabetes	768	8	0.223	0.262	0.255	0.248
Tsetse	3500	14	0.117	0.120	0.041	0.065

NA: Not available

6.3.2 *Cardiovascular Disease Prediction Comparisons

Several simulation studies have been performed with the GUSTO-I database. A variety of modern learning methods has been compared, including logistic regression, Tree, GAM, and MARS methods [153]. Logistic regression can be considered as a classic prediction method. The other methods have more flexibility in capturing interaction terms or nonlinear terms and may be referred to as adaptive nonlinear methods. These methods require data sets of substantial size, which is the case in GUSTO-I. Because of the huge size, a large independent test set ($n = 13,610$) could be kept separate from the development set.

- Four different logistic regression models were considered [153], containing

(1) age and Killip class;
(2) age, Killip class, and interactions between age and Killip classes;
(3) 17 covariates as included in an earlier model [329], but no interactions and no nonlinear (spline) terms;
(4) 17 covariates, some of the interactions and nonlinear (spline) terms [329].

- A classification tree, constructed using 17 predictors.
- A generalized additive logistic regression model ("GAM"). The model contained smoothing splines with 4 degrees of freedom for the variables age, height, weight, pulse rate, systolic blood pressure, and time to treatment. No interaction terms were included.
- Multivariate additive regression splines (MARS) is a kind of hybrid between generalized additive models and classification tree [170]. MARS models of degree 1 (additive) and 17 (all interactions allowed) were considered.

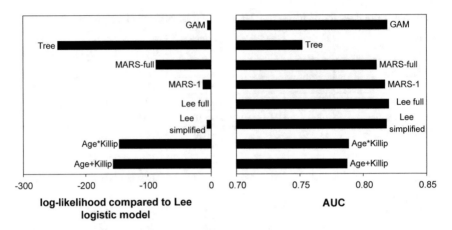

Fig. 6.4 Performance of alternative prediction models in a test part of the GUSTO-I data set (*n* = 13,610 patients with acute MI) [153]. Results are shown for four logistic regression models, two variants of MARS models, a classification tree, and a GAM. In the left panel, the log-likelihood is compared to the Lee full model; in the right panel, the area under the ROC curve (or *c*-statistic) is shown. Age + Killip: main effects; Age * Killip: main and interaction effects; Lee simplified: a simplified version of Lee model; Lee full: Lee et al. model [329]. We note that the Lee full model performed best according to both performance criteria

The performance in the test set of 13,610 patients was remarkable (Fig. 6.4). The most basic logistic model had a *c*-statistic of 0.787, which improved substantially when more predictors were considered (Lee et al. logistic model variant 3 and 4, *c* around 0.82). The performance of Lee et al. traditional logistic model [329] could not be improved by any other method. A similar performance was found for the GAM and additive MARS model. The more flexible variant of the MARS model (with all interactions allowed) had a *c*-statistic of 0.81 (0.01 lower). The tree performed worst, with a *c*-statistic of 0.75. Results were similar when the log-likelihood was used as a measure for predictive performance (Fig. 6.4).

The authors also examined various variants of multilayer neural networks using advanced backpropagation algorithms and various approaches to prevent overfitting (weight decay, early stopping, bagging) [153]. None of these methods led to a better predictive performance than the traditional logistic regression model. The authors suggest that adaptive nonlinear methods may be most useful in problems with higher signal-to-noise ratio, which may occur in the engineering and physical sciences. Adaptive nonlinear algorithms might have limited applicability in clinical settings.

Similar conclusions were reached by Austin et al., who studied large data sets of patients with either congestive heart failure (*n* = 15,848) or acute myocardial infarction (*n* = 16,230). Specifically, traditional and modern tree-based methods did not offer improvements over logistic regression [23, 29].

6.3.3 *Traumatic Brain Injury Modeling Results*

The performance of various modeling strategies was studied in predicting outcome in traumatic brain injury patients [612, 613]. We analyzed individual patient data

Table 6.4 Median apparent and cross-validated c-statistics (or AUC, Chap. 15) over analyses in 15 cohorts containing 11,026 TBI patients [613]

Validation	LR	CART	RF	SVM	NN
Apparent	0.812	0.744	0.750	0.833	0.878
Cross-validated	0.757	0.666	0.735	0.732	0.674
Optimism	0.055	0.078	0.015	0.101	0.204

from 15 cohorts including 11,026 patients that were brought together in the context of the IMPACT project (http://www.tbi-impact.org/). We predicted 6-month mortality, which occurred on average in 25% of the patients. We used default settings with five statistical modeling techniques: logistic regression (LR), classification and regression trees, random forests (RFs), support vector machines (SVM), and neural nets. These techniques, hence, cover classical statistical methods and machine learning type of approaches (RF, SVM).

For external validation, a model developed on one of the 15 data sets was applied to each of the 14 remaining sets. This process was repeated 15 times for a total of 630 validations. The c-statistic was used to assess the discriminative ability of the models. For a model with 10 predictors, 14 df, the LR models performed best (median validated c, 0.76), followed by RF and SVM models (median validated AUC value, 0.74 and 0.73, respectively, Table 6.4). The single tree models showed poor performance (median validated AUC value, <0.7). The SVM and NN approaches had large optimism (Table 6.4). Further analyses also showed that very large sample sizes were needed for RF and SVM to reach stable results, in contrast to logistic regression [612]. Overall, this study confirms the pattern described for cardiovascular disease modeling (Sect. 6.3.2), i.e., that nonlinear and nonadditive relations may not be pronounced enough in medical prediction problems to make modern prediction methods beneficial (Table 6.4).

6.4 Concluding Remarks

We should recognize that true models do not exist, and that any model only approximates relations between predictors and outcome. A model will only reflect underlying patterns, and hence should not be confused with reality. This is also shown in René Margritte's famous painting "La trahison des images" (The Treachery of Images, http://en.wikipedia.org/wiki/The_Treachery_of_Images). This painting shows a pipe, with the words "Ceci n'est pas une pipe" (This is not a pipe) painted below the pipe. Indeed, the painting is not a pipe; it is only an image of a pipe.

Nevertheless, statistical models that better approximate reality closer are better for predictive purposes, as well as for inference on effects of predictors. If we derive models from empirical data, the sample size needs to be sufficient for the complexity of the model that is fitted. For flexible models, empirical results illustrate that nonlinear effects and interactions may need to be quite strong before an advantage is obtained over relatively simple regression models. In medical prediction problems, the signal-to-noise ratio may be relatively low. This makes regression analysis an appropriate default approach in many clinical prediction models.

Questions

6.1 Reasonable modeling approaches
    In traumatic brain injury, the Glasgow Outcome Scale is a 5 point, ordered
    scale. It is common to determine the GOS at 6-month post-injury. A researcher
    proposes to use linear regression analysis to analyze relations for predictors
    with this scale. What are pros and cons of this approach for estimation of
    predictive effects, and for making predictions?

6.2 Predictions from cross-tabulations (Fig. 6.2)
    A researcher might argue that the observed mortality as shown in Fig. 6.2 can
    directly be used for predictive purposes, similar to the cross-tabulation pro-
    vided in an analysis of genetic mutation risks among 10,000 women [168].
    What are pros and cons of this approach?

6.3 GUSTO-I results (Sect. 6.3)
    More flexible methods performed worse than a logistic regression model in the
    GUSTO-I case study. What results would you expect for the comparison in
    Fig. 6.4 with

    (a) Smaller sample sizes for model development (e.g., 1,000 rather than
        23,000 patients)?
    (b) Larger sample sizes for model development (e.g., 10,000,000 rather than
        23,000 patients).

Part II
Developing Valid Prediction Models

In Part I, we presented a number of issues that are relevant to the context of prediction model development and application. We summarize these issues as preliminaries for model development in the checklist below. In Part II, we focus on the development of prediction models that are valid for the population from which the sample originates. Generalizability to other, plausibly related, populations is discussed in Part III. We will discuss seven steps of model development in the following chapters (7–18).

Checklist for developing valid prediction models

Step	Specific issues	Chapter
General considerations		
Research question	Aim: predictors / prediction?	1
Intended application?	Clinical practice / research?	2
Outcome	Clinically relevant?	3
Predictors	Reliable measurement? Comprehensiveness	3
Study design	Retrospective/prospective? Cohort; case-control	3
Statistical model	Appropriate for research question and type of outcome?	4 and 6
Sample size	Sufficient for aim?	2 to 6
7 modeling steps		
1. Preliminary	Missing values	7 and 8
2. Coding of predictors	Continuous predictors Combining categorical predictors Restrictions on candidate predictors	9 and 10
3. Model specification	Appropriate selection of main effects? Assessment of assumptions (distributional, linearity and additivity)?	11 and 12
4. Model estimation	Shrinkage included? External information used?	13 and 14
5. Model performance	Appropriate statistical measures used? Clinical usefulness considered?	15 16
6. Model validation	Internal validation including model specification and estimation? External validation?	17
7. Model presentation	Format appropriate for audience	18
Validity		
Internal: overfitting	Sufficient attempts to limit and correct for overfitting?	4 to 18
External: generalizability	Predictions valid for plausibly related populations?	19 to 21

Chapter 7
Missing Values

Background Missing data are a common problem in medical research. We may encounter missing values of predictor values (X) and for the outcome (y) that we want to predict. Traditional complete case analysis suffers from inefficiency, selection bias of subjects, and other limitations when developing a prediction model. We briefly review the theoretical background on mechanisms of missingness of predictor values and how these may affect prediction models. We further concentrate on imputation methods as a solution, where a completed data set is created by filling in missing values for the statistical analysis. Special attention is given to the specification of an imputation model, which is the essential step in imputation. Multiple imputation is a method is to generate completed data sets multiple times, while single imputation is more straightforward and may be sufficient for some prognostic research questions. Several examples are provided. Chapter 8 presents a case study of dealing with missing values in a meta-analysis of individual patient data on prognosis in traumatic brain injury. Tentative guidelines are provided on how to deal with missing data in relation to the research question.

7.1 Missing Values and Prediction Research

Missing data are a common and increasingly recognized problem in medical scientific research. In this chapter, we focus on missing values of predictors X, assuming that true predictor values are hidden by the missing values [347]. We also consider missingness of the outcome y. Standard statistical software for regression analysis deletes subjects with any missing value from the analysis. With such a complete case analysis, all subjects with a missing value for any potential predictor or the outcome are excluded [207, 347]. An "available case analysis" will consider subjects with complete data for a specific predictor, but who may have missing values for other covariates that are not considered in the specific model. With such

© Springer Nature Switzerland AG 2019
E. W. Steyerberg, *Clinical Prediction Models*, Statistics for Biology and Health, https://doi.org/10.1007/978-3-030-16399-0_7

an analysis, numbers may, therefore, vary per analysis. Both complete case and available case analysis discard information from subjects who have information on some (but not all) predictors. They are hence statistically inefficient, as further illustrated below. For simplicity, we use the term complete case (CC) analysis further onwards.

7.1.1 Inefficiency of Complete Case Analysis

As an example, we consider a data set with 500 subjects. Among these, 100 events occur. We aim to estimate regression coefficients for a prediction model consisting of 5 predictors $x1 - x5$. In the case of complete data, we have 20 events per variable. Such a situation is commonly thought to be sufficient for reliable estimation of the regression coefficients in a model. Suppose, however, that each predictor has 10% missing data and that each patient has at most 1 missing value. Hence, each patient has at least 4 values of the predictors recorded (Table 7.1). A CC analysis will ignore 5 * 10% = 50% of the subjects and will leave only 250 subjects for estimation of the regression model. The number of events per variable drops to 10:1, which is commonly thought of as a lower limit for reliable modeling.

Table 7.1 Hypothetical missing data pattern: 250 subjects have partially complete data (missing data indicated with NA), and 250 have fully complete data (indicated with +). Among the X variables, only 250/2500 = 10% of the information is missing, while a complete case analysis would drop to 50%

ID	$x1$	$x2$	$x3$	$x4$	$x5$	y
1	NA	+	+	+	+	+
...	NA	+	+	+	+	+
50	NA	+	+	+	+	+
51	+	NA	+	+	+	+
...	+	NA	+	+	+	+
100	+	NA	+	+	+	+
101	+	+	NA	+	+	+
...	+	+	NA	+	+	+
150	+	+	NA	+	+	+
151	+	+	+	NA	+	+
...	+	+	+	NA	+	+
200	+	+	+	NA	+	+
201	+	+	+	+	NA	+
...	+	+	+	+	NA	+
250	+	+	+	+	NA	+
251	+	+	+	+	+	+
...	+	+	+	+	+	+
...	+	+	+	+	+	+
500	+	+	+	+	+	+
Total	450	450	450	450	450	500

The information available is 250 complete cases (250 * 5 = 1250 predictor values) + 250 incomplete cases (250 * 4 = 1000 predictor values). Of the required 500 * 5 = 2500 predictor values, 2250 or 90% are available. The approach of using only 50% of the information instead of 90% is quite inefficient: 10% of the required values are missing, but 50% of the subjects are discarded. Admittedly, the inefficiency is less if multiple missing values occur within the same patient, which is a more realistic situation. The general message is that CC analysis discards valuable information from incomplete records.

7.1.2 Interpretation of CC Analyses

In addition to inefficiency, there are further concerns with complete case ("CC") analyses in the presence of missing data. When different models are compared, it is impossible to interpret results when the numbers of subjects vary across the analyses. For example, when a univariate odds ratio is based on 450 subjects for each X variable in Table 7.1, we cannot interpret the change in the odds ratio of an adjusted analysis performed on 250 subjects, due to missing values for 200 of the 450 subjects. Differences between univariate and adjusted analysis may arise because of the correlation between the predictors or because of a selection of subjects due to missing values. This problem would not occur if we would analyze the same 250 patients in both univariate and adjusted analysis. Other problems include a cumbersome comparison of p-values between analyses. Neither can the performance of different models be compared when they are based on different numbers of subjects.

Another concern is that bias may arise due to systematic differences between subjects with complete and subjects with missing data. It appears that bias will especially occur in the estimated regression coefficient for a predictor when missingness in X is associated with the outcome y [594]. This issue will be discussed in Sect. 7.2.

7.1.3 Missing Data Mechanisms

Different mechanisms may lead to missing data (Table 7.2) [347, 478, 600]. It is important to consider these, since approaches to handle missing data in the statistical analysis rely on assumptions on the mechanism.

Missing values can occur completely at random (MCAR). Examples of MCAR mechanisms include administrative errors that occur at random, such as accidents in laboratories (e.g., spilling of material, handling errors, breakdown of equipment), or postal mail that is lost. MCAR is a strict assumption and can be tested. With a MCAR mechanism, the incomplete population is a random sample from the complete population; hence subjects with missings are fully representative of the population with complete data.

Table 7.2 Three types of missing data mechanisms for predictors

Label	Missing mechanism	Description
MCAR	Missing completely at random	Administrative errors, accidents
MAR	Missing at random	Missingness related to known patient characteristics, time or place ("MAR on x"), or to the outcome ("MAR on y")
MNAR	Missing not at random	Missingness related to the value of the predictor, or to variables not available in the analysis

In medical data, missing values often occur specifically in certain types of subjects. If we can fully observe the variables that are associated with missingness, we have a Missing At Random situation (MAR). This means that the probability of a missing value on a predictor ("missingness") is independent of the values of the predictor itself, but depends on the observed values of other variables. The MAR assumption is fulfilled if missingness is only related to measured values in the data set and not to unmeasured variables. MAR examples include more missing values in older subjects, subjects from a certain region, or from an earlier calendar time. Also, the design of a study may intentionally leave values missing for some type of subjects, which is by definition a MAR mechanism. For example, we may choose not to measure a lab value in younger subjects.

With a MAR mechanism, the subjects with complete predictor and outcome values are not representative anymore for the population where we want to generalize to. We will illustrate how a CC analysis affects estimates of the regression coefficients and the estimated performance (see Sect. 7.2).

A problematic situation arises when data are Missing Not At Random (MNAR). A MNAR mechanism implies that the missingness depends on the true values of the variable, or on other variables that are not observed. Examples include selective nonresponse on certain questions (e.g., sexual orientation, income), or clinical condition (e.g., missing if a severe condition is present, which is not measured accurately).

7.1.4 Missing Outcome Data

In diagnostic research, partial verification may often occur, i.e., that a subset of patients is not verified by the reference ("gold") standard and is excluded from the analysis. If predictors of verification are known, we may consider this a MAR situation for the outcome (Table 7.3) [123].

In prognostic research, we may be interested in a single outcome at a specific point in time. This outcome may be missing in some subjects, e.g., 6-month functional status after suffering from traumatic brain injury. Missingness makes that

Table 7.3 Examples for three types of missing data mechanisms for outcomes

Label	Example
MCAR	Administrative censoring because of the end of follow-up
MAR	Drop out of follow-up, related to observed patient characteristics
	Partial verification by a reference standard in diagnostic research
MNAR	Missingness related to the outcome status, or to variables not available in the analysis

we cannot analyze the relation between predictors and this outcome, while this relation is of primary interest. If we know a patient's functional status at 3 or 12 months, we might think about procedures to include patients with such information in the analysis.

In survival analysis, the outcome for a patient can be missing in several situations. Follow-up time is nearly always insufficient to observe the outcome for all subjects. Survival analysis techniques deal with this situation by considering these incomplete observations as "censored". Censoring is a valid approach if censoring is non-informative. If all subjects were followed until the date of closure of a study this assumption may be fully reasonable ("administrative censoring", a MCAR situation). If subjects drop out before the end of the study, we may assume non-informative censoring, conditional on the predictors in the analysis model [273]. This is a variant of the MAR assumption. The assumption is that any mechanisms giving rise to censoring of individual subjects are observed in the data. For example, in clinical studies, the continuation of follow-up should not depend on a participant's medical condition beyond what is captured by predictors. We have a MNAR situation if follow-up outcomes are selectively missing while the reasons for missingness cannot be captured fully by variables in the data. For example, in a study of contralateral breast cancer incidence, we may be able to identify women with an event since they return to the hospital, while it is unclear how many women are still at risk for the event. A specific situation is that competing risks preclude the observation of the outcome of interest, e.g., patients die before contralateral breast cancer is diagnosed (Chap. 4).

7.1.5 Summary Points

Missing data mechanisms can be described as MCAR, MAR and MNAR (Tables 7.2 and 7.3). Missing data may arise in predictors X and the outcome y. Missing data lead to

- inefficient and potentially biased analyses of prediction research questions,
- difficulties in interpretation when analyses differ in numbers of subjects.

7.2 Prediction Under MCAR, MAR and MNAR Mechanisms

For illustration, we consider a simple linear regression model where a continuous outcome y depends on two predictors ($x1$ and $x2$):

$y = \beta_1 x1 + \beta_2 x2 + \text{error}$, with

$x1$ and $x2$ independent standard normal variables (distributed $N(0, 1)$); regression coefficients β_1 and β_2 both 1, and the error distributed as $N(0, 1)$.

We perform a set of simulations for this simple model to illustrate the impact of missing value patterns in a complete case (CC) analysis, followed by imputation. We created missing values for 50% of the $x1$ values in four scenarios, followed by three scenarios with 50% missings in the y variable. A simple linear regression analysis is performed to estimate coefficients b1 and b2, and the explained variance by the model (R^2). The R code is available at http://www.clinicalpredictionmodels. org/.

7.2.1 Missingness Patterns

We created four missing data patterns for the $x1$ variable.

1. We first created 50% missing values in $x1$ fully at random to simulate an MCAR situation. The correlation between $x2$ and $x1$ was zero in the original data and in the random sample (Fig. 7.1). The distributions of $x1$ and $x2$ remained identical to the complete data (mean 0, SD 1, Table 7.4).
2. Of more interest is the situation of "MAR on x". We consider the situation that missingness of $x1$ depends on $x2$, with $x1$ only known for higher values of $x2$ (Fig. 7.1). On average, the $x2$ values were +0.623 higher among those with complete $x1$ values compared to the original data (Table 7.4). This is equivalent to $R^2 = 39\%$ (0.623^2).
3. Next, missingness of $x1$ was made dependent on y ("MAR on y"), with $x1$ only known with lower values of y. This selection created some minor correlation between $x1$ and $x2$ ($R^2 = 2\%$), while the variables were independent from each other in the original data. The mean values of $x1$ and $x2$ were -0.36 each, while they were 0 in the original data. The standard deviation (SD) was smaller (0.93 rather than 1, Fig. 7.1 and Table 7.4).
4. Finally, we consider a MNAR situation, where missingness of $x1$ depends on the values of $x1$. We simulate that $x1$ is only known with higher values of $x1$ (mean +0.62, SD 0.78, Table 7.4). The mean and standard deviation of $x2$ were unaffected by this missingness pattern.

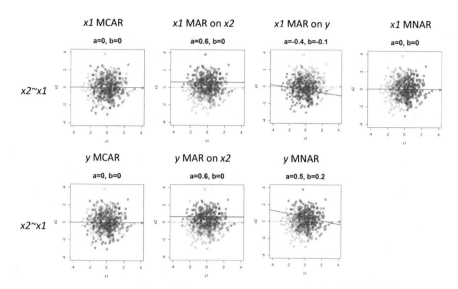

Fig. 7.1 Illustration of patterns of missingness for two continuous predictors $x1$ and $x2$. Original data are marked with a green X. Complete data under MCAR, MAR and MNAR are red circles. Plots show results for $n = 500$

Table 7.4 Descriptives of $x1$ and $x2$ under seven mechanisms for missing values

Missing mechanism	Mean(x1)	SD(x1)	Mean(x2)	SD(x2)
Missing x1				
x1 MCAR	0	1.00	0	1.00
x1 MAR x2	0	1.00	0.62	0.78
x1 MAR y	−0.36	0.93	−0.36	0.93
x1 MNAR	0.62	0.78	0	1.00
Missing y				
y MCAR	0	1.00	0	1.00
y MAR x2	0	1.00	0.62	0.78
y MNAR	0.42	0.91	0.42	0.91

In addition, three more missing data patterns we created for the y variable.

5. We first created missing values in y fully at random to simulate an MCAR situation. The correlation between $x2$ and $x1$ was zero in the original data and in the random sample (Fig. 7.1).
6. A "MAR on x" situation was created in an identical way as for the $x1$ variable, with identical impact on the $x2$ values: these were +0.62 higher among those with complete y values compared to the original data, with less variability in $x2$ (Table 7.4).

7. Finally, in a MNAR situation, missingness of y depended on the values of y. We simulated that y is only known with higher values of y (mean y +1.25; mean $x1$ +0.42; mean $x2$ +0.42; less variability in $x1$ and $x2$, Fig. 7.1 and Table 7.4).

7.2.2 Missingness and Estimated Regression Coefficients

We consider two univariate, or marginal, models $y \sim x1$ and $y \sim x2$, and the full model $y \sim x1 + x2$. In the original data, the estimated regression coefficients b1 and b2 are on average 1 in each of these models, since $x1$ and $x2$ were generated as independent $N(0, 1)$ variables. We consider the seven missing data patterns as described above (Sect. 7.2.1). We fit models in the complete cases: a CC analysis.

Missings in $x1$:

1. MCAR: Obviously, the estimated regression coefficients b1 and b2 are on average 1 in the subjects with complete data (Fig. 7.2).
2. MAR on x: the estimated coefficient b1 remains unaffected in the model $y \sim x1$ in the subjects with complete data (Fig. 7.1). Remarkably, the intercept is +0.6 higher than 0. This +0.6 higher intercept reflects that we estimated this model in data with relatively high $x2$ values (+0.62, Fig. 7.1, Table 7.5). Indeed, the values of $x2$ were +0.6 higher than in the complete data (Table 7.4), and the regression coefficient β_2 was 1, exactly explaining the +0.6 higher intercept.

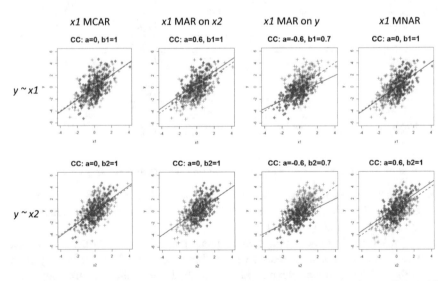

Fig. 7.2 Impact of patterns of missingness in $x1$ on estimated univariate regression coefficients b1 and b2 in the models $y \sim x1$ and $y \sim x2$. Original data are marked with +. Complete data under MCAR, MAR and MNAR are red circles. Plots show results for $n = 500$

Table 7.5 Regression coefficients under various missing value mechanisms, corresponding to Fig. 7.2. The marginal models are: $y \sim x1$, and $y \sim x2$. We note biased estimates (in **bold**) in analyses of complete cases (CC) and analyses of completed cases (with imputation, Sect. 7.3). Results are based on simulations with 500,000 records

Missing mechanisms	Complete cases (CC)				Completed cases (imputation)			
	a	b1	a	b2	a	b1	a	b2
Missing x1								
x1 MCAR	0.00	1.00	0.00	1.00	0.00	1.00	0.00	1.00
x1 MAR on x2	**0.62**	1.00	0.00	1.00	0.00	1.00	0.00	1.00
x1 MAR on y	**−0.83**	**0.70**	**−0.83**	**0.70**	0.00	1.00	0.00	1.00
x1 MNAR	0.00	1.00	**0.62**	1.00	**−0.45**	**1.13**	0.00	1.00
Missing y								
y MCAR	0.00	1.00	0.00	1.00	0.00	1.00	0.00	1.00
y MAR on x2	**0.62**	1.00	0.00	1.00	0.00	1.00	0.00	1.00
y MNAR	**1.01**	**0.58**	**1.00**	**0.58**	**0.74**	**0.63**	**0.74**	**0.63**

The estimated intercept and coefficient b2 remained unaffected in the model $y \sim x2$ for those with $x1$ available. In the full model $y \sim x1 + x2$, no bias arises, since we appropriately condition on $x2$ when estimating the coefficient b1 for $x1$ (Table 7.5).

3. MAR on y: Bias arises if missingness of $x1$ depends on y, with $x1$ only known with lower values of y. Remarkably, the bias is exactly the same for b1 and b2, with intercept −0.6 and coefficient 0.7 (Fig. 7.2). In the full model, the intercept was −0.48, b1 and b2 both 0.83 (Table 7.6). So, missingness of $x1$ in relation to y, independent of $x2$, caused bias in both b1 and b2.

A correlation between missingness of a predictor and the outcome, hence, poses a serious problem in prediction modeling. Note, however, that if we measure all predictors prospectively, before the outcome is known, such a dependency cannot occur in a direct way. We register the predictors before the outcome [594]. This holds both for diagnostic and prognostic problems. If an association between missingness of predictors X and outcome y is noted in a prospective study, the explanation must be through other predictors, including predictors that are further down the causal pathway. If these predictors are not measured, we have an MNAR rather than a MAR situation.

4. MNAR: if missingness of $x1$ depended on the values of $x1$, no bias arose in the models $y \sim x1$ or $y \sim x1 + x2$. These findings may be surprising to some, but are in line with the principle of conditioning in regression modeling: estimates of b1 and b2 are conditional on $x1$, and hence selection on $x1$ does not affect these regression coefficients. In the model $y \sim x2$, the regression coefficient was estimated correctly as 1.0, while the intercept (+0.6) reflected that the subjects with complete data had higher $x1$ values (Tables 7.4 and 7.5).

In sum, regression coefficients b1 and b2 in this simple example remained unbiased under various missing data generating mechanisms for $x1$. Bias in the CC analysis arose in the situation of "MAR on y", for example, that $x1$ was only known for lower values of y.

Missings in y:

5. As expected, under MCAR, the estimated regression coefficients b1 and b2 are on average 1 for the subjects with complete data (Tables 7.5 and 7.6).
6. With y MAR on $x2$, results are identical to $x1$ MAR on $x2$, with an intercept of +0.62 in the model $y \sim x2$, because of high $x2$ values (Fig. 7.1, Table 7.5). In the full model, no bias arises, since we appropriately condition on $x2$ when estimating the coefficient b1 (Table 7.6).
7. Under MNAR, missingness of y depended on the values of y. Severe bias arose in the models $y \sim x1$, $y \sim x1$, and $y \sim x1 + x2$. These findings are in contrast to the findings for MNAR of the $x1$ variable.

In sum, missing values in y have a similar impact on regression coefficients of predictors as missing X variables under a MAR mechanism. MNAR in y causes severe bias though. As we will see below, imputation of missing values does not work well under MNAR. Hence, MNAR in y is to be avoided at all costs, i.e., selective missingness of outcome, not related to predictors or other observed variables that can be modeled in an imputation model.

Table 7.6 Regression coefficients and model performance under various missing value mechanisms. The full model is considered: $y \sim x1 + x2$. We note biases (in **bold**) in regression coefficients of complete cases (CC) and analyses of completed cases (with imputation, Sect. 7.3), under different missing value mechanisms. CC leads to the underestimation of model performance under all missing mechanisms

Missing mechanisms	Complete cases (CC)				Completed cases (imputation)			
	a	b1	b2	R^2 (%)	a	b1	b2	R^2 (%)
Missing $x1$								
$x1$ MCAR	0.00	1.00	1.00	67	0.00	1.00	1.00	66
$x1$ MAR on $x2$	0.00	1.00	1.00	**62**	0.00	1.00	1.00	66
$x1$ MAR on y	**−0.48**	**0.83**	**0.83**	55	0.00	1.00	1.00	66
$x1$ MNAR	0.00	1.00	1.00	62	**−0.45**	**1.15**	1.00	**61**
Missing y								
y MCAR	0.00	1.00	1.00	67	0.00	1.00	1.00	66
y MAR on $x2$	0.00	1.00	1.00	**62**	0.00	1.00	1.00	66
y MNAR	**0.64**	**0.73**	**0.73**	49	**0.74**	**0.63**	**0.63**	54

7.2.3 Missingness and Estimated Performance

As noted above, patterns of missingness impact on estimates of the model intercept and the regression coefficients. Missingness also impacts on the estimated model performance. For the simple linear model $y \sim x1 + x2$ we consider the R^2 values to indicate explained variability by the model (Table 7.6). As expected, MCAR has no impact on the estimated R^2 value ($R^2 = 67\%$). MAR on $x2$ (either for $x1$ or for y) leads to the estimation of performance with a narrower distribution of $x2$ values, and hence lower explained variability ($R^2 = 62\%$). Similarly, MNAR for $x1$ leads to the estimation of performance with a narrower distribution of $x1$ values ($R^2 = 62\%$).

Biased regression coefficients were found in the CC analysis if $x1$ was MAR on y, with lower R^2 ($R^2 = 55\%$). This lower performance is attributed to a narrower distribution of $x1$ and $x2$ values (Table 7.4) and smaller regression coefficients b1 and b2 (Table 7.6). Even lower performance was found if the outcome y was selective missing (MNAR for y, $R^2 = 49\%$).

7.3 Dealing with Missing Values in Regression Analysis

Multiple imputation (MI) has become the dominant approach in medical research to deal with missing values (Fig. 7.3). MI is a specific imputation method, where missing values are filled in ("imputed") multiple times. MI methods make efficient use of all available data, i.e., they do consider the information from incomplete cases. Obviously, they cannot know the values of the missing data. Making educated guesses makes sense though. An alternative is to consider maximum

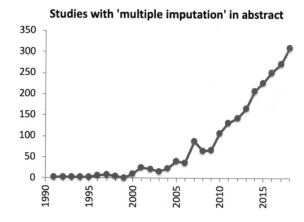

Fig. 7.3 Studies in PubMed with the term "multiple imputation", published between 1990 and 2018. We note a remarkable increase since 1990, with for example 41 publications in 2005, and 226 in 2015. Earlier publications on multiple imputation can be found in the methodological literature

Studies with 'multiple imputation' in abstract

likelihood (ML) approaches, which also exploit all available information in the data, accounting for the missingness of some information for some subjects. Both MI and likelihood methods are generally preferred over a CC analysis. Both methods have theoretical and empirical support [347, 478, 489, 600]. Further focus here is on imputation methods as a practical approach to missing values in prediction research [532, 600].

7.3.1 Imputation Principle

Imputation methods substitute the missing values with plausible values so that the completed data can then be analyzed with standard statistical techniques. In some data sets, we may find a characteristic or combination of characteristics that closely defines the predictor with missing values, for example, when variables are strongly related to the same underlying phenomenon. For example hematocrit ("ht") and hemoglobin ("Hb") are both red blood cell indices. If we aim to include Hb in a prognostic model, it is easy to estimate Hb from ht for patients that have both measurements (Fig. 7.4). The predicted Hb can subsequently be filled in for those patients with ht available but Hb missing. This is an example of a regression imputation approach (Table 7.7). In this example, it appears that the correlation between Hb and ht is very strong.

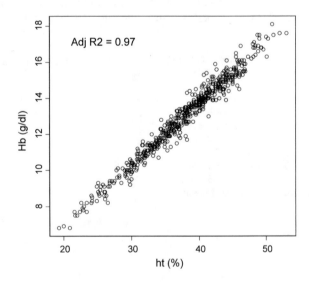

Fig. 7.4 Correlation between hematocrit (ht) and hemoglobin (Hb) in 566 patients with traumatic brain injury. The final imputation model included ht (t statistic 123, $p < 0.001$) and gender (t statistic 2.6, $p = 0.01$), which had a similar adjusted R^2 statistic as the model with ht alone (0.97)

Table 7.7 Approaches to dealing with missing values, including imputation methods

Label	X/Y used?	Approach
CC	–	Complete case analysis; subjects with missing values are excluded from the analysis
CM	X	Single imputation with the conditional mean. The conditional mean can e.g. be estimated with a regression model
SI	X + Y	Single imputation with a random draw from the predictive distribution from an imputation model ("stochastic regression imputation")
MI	X + Y	Multiple imputation with a random draw from the predictive distribution from an imputation model, repeated e.g. 20 times

7.3.2 Simple and More Advanced Single Imputation Methods

Simple imputation methods include the substitution of a missing value of a continuous predictor with the mean, or the most frequent category for a categorical predictor. Such simple methods ignore potential correlation of the values of predictors among each other and are hence suboptimal. Further, they lead to an underestimation of variability in the predictor values among subjects.

Regression imputation [152], or "conditional mean imputation" [347], does consider the correlation among predictors. An imputation model is made to predict the missing values (see, for example, Fig. 7.4). Expected values can then be imputed reflecting the correlations in the data. An alternative is to take a random draw from the distribution of predicted values ("stochastic regression imputation" [152]). The random element reflects that the imputed values are not certain, which is especially important in the case of relatively uncertain predicted values.

Simple, conditional mean, and stochastic regression imputation methods are examples of *single* imputation methods. In contrast, Rubin proposed a *multiple* imputation method for handling missing data [478].

7.3.3 Multiple Imputation

With multiple imputation, m completed data sets are created instead of a single completed data set. Missing values are imputed m times using m independent draws from an imputation model. As with (stochastic) regression imputation, the imputation model aims to reasonably approximate the true distributional relation between the missing data and the available information. This means that for each variable with missing data, a conditional distribution for the missing data can be specified given other data [136].

A challenge with imputation models is that we may want to predict missing values for one predictor, using other predictors which also have missing values.

This may well be solved with data augmentation methods, which follow an iterative process of an imputation step, which imputes values for the missing data, and a posterior step, which draws new estimates for the model parameters based on the previously imputed values [489]. This process continues until convergence. The final imputed values are used as the first imputed dataset. The whole process is repeated with different starting values to obtain m imputed datasets. The variation among m imputations reflects the uncertainty with which the missing values can be predicted from the observed data [489, 600].

After creating m completed data sets, m analyses are performed by treating each completed data set as a real complete data set. Standard procedures and software can be used, as we would for a data set without any missing values.

Finally, the results from the m complete-data analyses are combined, for example, to obtain the estimates of regression coefficients and performance esti-mates, while properly taking into account the uncertainty in the imputed values. Point estimates of regression coefficients and other normally distributed quantities are simply the average over the m imputed data sets. These estimates could in principle also have been obtained in a large stacked data set instead of m separate data sets. The variance of the estimates (e.g., regression coefficients, performance measures) is the average of the variance as estimated within the m imputed data sets plus the variance between these m data sets. The latter element is an essential difference between single (conditional mean or stochastic) regression imputation, or analysing a stacked data set, and multiple imputation. MI takes the uncertainty into account that is caused by having to estimate an imputation model. The formula for MI results is relatively straightforward. For an estimated regression coefficient b, the variance over M imputed datasets is

$$\mathrm{Var(b)} = \ \mathrm{var(b)\ within}\ m + \ (1+1/M)\ \mathrm{var(b)\ between}\ m$$
$$= \ \mathrm{mean(var(b_m))} \ + \ (1+1/M)(1/(M-1)) \ \Sigma \ (b_m - \mathrm{mean(b)})^2,$$

where $m = 1 \ldots M$ imputed data sets.

This formula (or closely related variants) is implemented in many software packages that can perform MI. The number M for the imputed data sets is usually set to 5 or 10, although $M = 20$ may be a better default. If $M = 10$, the mean–variance estimates within the m imputed data sets are the dominant factor in the formula, since the term $(1 + 1/M)$ becomes 1.1 and the "between imputation" variance is usually much smaller than the "within imputation" variance. Some suggest that M should be as large as the average percentage missing values; so for 20%, $M = 20$ [600]. Setting $M = 1$ makes MI a single stochastic regression imputation procedure (SI). In small data sets, M may need to be set to higher values than in larger data sets, e.g. 50, since the differences between analyses in different imputed data sets will be larger [600].

The most important step in any imputation procedure is the definition of the imputation model to make the MAR assumption reasonable. We discuss this step in more detail, largely following others [600, 601, 669].

7.4 Defining the Imputation Model

The imputation model aims to approximate the true distributional relation between the unobserved data and the available information. The imputation model is an explicit attempt to model the MAR process. Imputation models can be specified for each potential predictor with missing data, irrespective of the quantity of missing data. Two modeling choices usually have to be made: the form of the model (e.g., linear, logistic, polytomous, Chap. 4), and the set of variables that enter the model, including potential transformations.

For binary predictor variables (e.g., the presence or absence of a patient characteristic) it is convenient to use a logistic regression model, for categorical variables with three or more ordered levels a polytomous logistic model and for continuous variables a linear regression model. A problem may arise when imputations are outside the observed range of values. In such cases, it may be reasonable to truncate imputed values, so that they remain within plausible ranges; or use a predicted mean matching approach, which prevents such imputations [600].

7.4.1 Types of Variables in the Imputation Model

The variables in the imputation model can be differentiated into various categories. All predictors that appear in the prediction model ($y \sim X$) should be included in the imputation model. Failure to do so may bias the analysis. This is known as the principle of congeniality, i.e., that the imputation model is at least as rich as the prediction model.

Next, some variables that do not appear in the prediction model may serve as auxiliary variables. For example, calendar time or geographic site may be associated with missingness and should be considered for the imputation model. Finally, we need to include the outcome. This may appear a bit circular, since the aim of a prediction model is to predict the outcome. However, not including the outcome in the imputation model may cause substantial bias in the MI analysis of prognostic effects, even in the MCAR situation [385]. Severe dilution of the predictive effects may occur if the outcome is not included in the MI procedure. For example, if 50% of the data is MCAR, omitting the outcome in the imputation model for that predictor approximately halves the estimated regression coefficient.

Imputation of the outcome remains controversial, although some examples have been given where efficiency gains may be obtained. As always with imputation, these gains come at the price of assuming that the imputation model is reasonable. An interesting proposal is to perform multiple imputation for the outcome, followed by deletion of the imputed outcome (MID) [656]. When there is something wrong with the imputed y values, MID protects the regression estimates from these problematic imputations, while estimation of the X imputations has benefited from the full data structure. MID may offer somewhat more efficient estimates than an MI strategy that deletes records with missing y from the start of the modeling process.

It has been observed that including many variables in the imputation model tends to make the MAR assumptions more plausible. Putting in noise variables does not harm the imputation process [106], unless computational problems arise because of multicollinearity and inclusion of many predictors with missing data [99]. It is, therefore, generally convenient to include all predictors, some auxiliary variables, and the outcome in the imputation model for an MI procedure.

7.4.2 *Transformations of Variables

A difficult topic is how transformations among X variables and between X and y should be handled. Current software for MI deals with this issue in different ways. The `mice` function assumes linearity of associations among X variables and between X and y in the default setting. Specific forms of imputation models can be specified by the user, using, for example, $x + x^2$ for some X variables. In contrast, the `aregImpute` function searches for spline transformations among variables such that the correlations are maximized. If nonlinear associations are present, this may be of advantage. However, it is inefficient in the case of truly linear associations. The default settings can be changed such that aregImpute resembles mice. Indeed, very similar results in simulations between mice and aregImpute have been found when linearity was enforced (using the identity function ("I") in `aregImpute`).

Note that the principle of congeniality should be respected; if a nonlinear analysis of a specific x variable is planned, the imputation model should be flexible for this predictor. Similarly, if interactions are considered in the regression model, the imputation model also needs to include these. A straightforward approach is to transform, then impute—i.e., calculate the interactions or squares in the incomplete data and then impute these transformations like any other variable [657]. This "transform-then-impute" method yields good regression estimates, even though the imputed values may be inconsistent with one another. We should not aim to correct inconsistent imputations of x and x^2 [657].

7.4.3 Imputation Models for SI and MI: X and y

For single imputation with the conditional mean (e.g., from a regression model), only the predictor variables should be used in the imputation model [594]. If the outcome y is also used in the imputation model, we exaggerate the strength of relations between predictors and outcome in the prediction model. In contrast, stochastic regression imputation should be performed with the outcome y. This is because a random element is added to the predicted values from the imputation model, similarly to an MI procedure (see Table 7.7).

7.4.4 Summary Points

Imputation models for a multiple imputation (MI) procedure need to include

- all predictors and the outcome considered in the prediction model;
- auxiliary variables, related to the predictors, but not included in the prediction model;
- outcomes related to the outcome considered in the prediction model.

7.5 Success of Imputation Under MCAR, MAR and MNAR

7.5.1 Imputation in a Simple Model

Multiple imputation was applied in the simple regression model $y \sim x1 + x2$, where seven types of missing data were generated (four for $x1$, three for y, Sect. 7.2). We consider estimates of regression coefficients (bias) and estimates of predictive performance (R^2).

Overall, MI gave good results in this simple simulation study: regression coefficients were at least as well estimated as a CC analysis (Tables 7.5 and 7.6), and performance was estimated as $R^2 = 66\%$ rather than $R^2 = 67\%$ (Table 7.6). Under MNAR for $x1$, CC analysis was unbiased for the regression coefficients, but underestimated predictive performance for the original, complete data. With imputation, regression coefficients were quite biased. So, this simulation confirms that MNAR is a situation that MI cannot handle well.

7.5.2 Other Simulation Results

White and Carlin evaluated various models of the form $y \sim x1 + x2$, similar to the model described above [667]. They confirmed the results with respect to bias for linear models, and also considered logistic regression models. Overall, they found MI superior to CC across a wide range of settings.

Under MCAR, MI was more efficient than CC for linear but not logistic regression. For other missing data mechanisms, bias might arise in one or both methods, but bias tended to be smaller for MI than for CC. Data analysts should aim to understand the nature of their missing data as much as possible; and perform both CC and MI. If it seems plausible that both CC and MI may be valid, MI results should be preferred because of the greater efficiency.

7.5.3 *Multiple Predictors

In prediction models, we usually study more than 2 predictors. We reconsider the situation of Table 7.1, where 250 subjects have 1 missing value, and 250 have fully complete data for 5 predictors. Regression coefficients were set to 1 for all 5 predictors.

A CC analysis uses only 250 subjects. Regression coefficients are unbiased, but have considerably more variability than the estimates from an MI procedure (Table 7.8). The conditional mean (CM) and stochastic SI procedures perform quite similar to MI. All approaches correctly estimate the predictive performance as an adjusted R^2 around 35%.

Table 7.8 Regression under different missing value mechanisms, and the effect of single and multiple imputation procedures. Results are means over 1000 repetitions of samples with 500 subjects. The square root of the mean squared error was highlighted in bold for the strategy with the best result in dealing with missing values

	Table 7.1 b ± SE; sqrt(MSE)	Adj R^2	Mix of mechanisms b ± SE; sqrt(MSE)	Adj R^2
X correlated	10% missing (total 50%)		20% missing (total 75%)	
Original data, no missings ($n = 500$)		35%		35%
b1	1.00 ± 0.18; 0.18		1.00 ± 0.18; 0.18	
b2	1.01 ± 0.19; 0.19		1.00 ± 0.19; 0.19	
b3	1.00 ± 0.19; 0.20		1.00 ± 0.19; 0.19	
b4	0.99 ± 0.19; 0.20		1.00 ± 0.19; 0.20	
b5	1.00 ± 0.20; 0.20		1.00 ± 0.20; 0.20	
Complete case analysis ($n = 250$)		35%		19%
b1	1.00 ± 0.26; 0.26		0.66 ± 0.36; 0.49	
b2	1.03 ± 0.27; 0.27		0.66 ± 0.38; 0.51	
b3	0.98 ± 0.27; 0.27		0.69 ± 0.33; 0.45	
b4	1.00 ± 0.28; 0.28		0.68 ± 0.33; 0.47	
b5	1.00 ± 0.28; 0.28		0.67 ± 0.39; 0.52	
Conditional mean with X ($n = 500$)		33%		27%
b1	0.99 ± 0.19; **0.19**		1.08 ± 0.21; 0.23	
b2	1.01 ± 0.20; **0.21**		0.75 ± 0.23; 0.32	
b3	0.99 ± 0.21; **0.21**		1.05 ± 0.23; 0.24	
b4	0.98 ± 0.21; **0.21**		1.07 ± 0.24; 0.25	
b5	0.99 ± 0.21; **0.22**		1.03 ± 0.28; 0.29	
SI with $X + y$ ($n = 500$)		36%		35%
b1	1.00 ± 0.18; 0.22		1.03 ± 0.18; 0.25	
b2	1.01 ± 0.19; **0.21**		1.02 ± 0.19; 0.30	
b3	1.00 ± 0.19; 0.23		1.03 ± 0.19; 0.27	
b4	1.01 ± 0.19; 0.22		1.03 ± 0.20; 0.27	
b5	1.00 ± 0.20; 0.23		1.02 ± 0.23; 0.34	

(continued)

Table 7.8 (continued)

	Table 7.1 b ± SE; sqrt(MSE)	Adj R^2	Mix of mechanisms b ± SE; sqrt(MSE)	Adj R^2
MI with $X + y$ ($n = 500$)		35%		35%
b1	1.00 ± 0.19; **0.19**		1.03 ± 0.22; **0.22**	
b2	1.02 ± 0.20; **0.21**		1.02 ± 0.26; **0.26**	
b3	1.00 ± 0.21; **0.21**		1.02 ± 0.23; **0.24**	
b4	0.99 ± 0.21; **0.21**		1.03 ± 0.23; **0.24**	
b5	0.99 ± 0.21; **0.22**		1.02 ± 0.28; **0.29**	

SI: Single imputation, i.e., the first set of imputations from a multiple imputation (MI) procedure
The true model was: $y = x1 + x2 + x3 + x4 + x5$ + error
For the 10% missing example, all X variables were independent standard normal, and error $N(0, 4)$.
10% MCAR per variable were created as in Table 7.1
For the 20% missing example, X variables were correlated
$x1 \sim N(0, 1)$; $x2 \sim 0.2 * X1 + N(0, 0.98)$; $x3 \sim 0.2 * X1 + 0.16 * x2 + N(0, 0.97)$
$x4 \sim 0.2 * x1 + 0.16 * x2 + 0.14 * x3 + N(0, 0.96)$
$x5 \sim 0.2 * x1 + 0.16 * x2 + 0.14 * x3 + 0.12 * x4 + N(0, 0.95)$; error $\sim N(0, 4)$. For each
X variable, 20% missings were created, with MCAR for $x1$; MAR on y for $x2$; MAR on $x1$ for $x3$;
MAR on $x2$ for $x4$; and MNAR for $x5$. Covariances of missingness were set at 50%

A more complex situation was also simulated. More missing values were created (20% versus 10%), with more complex missing value mechanisms for correlated $x1$ – $x5$ (covariance 0.2 for all). MCAR was used for $x1$; MAR on y for $x2$; MAR on $x1$ for $x3$; MAR on $x2$ for $x4$; and MNAR for $x5$. A CC analysis led to biased estimates for all regression coefficients, which can be attributed to the MAR on y mechanism for $x2$. Hence, MAR on y for only one of the five predictors was sufficient to bias all coefficients. Also, the variability was considerable, since only 25% of the subjects were included in the CC analysis. MI did quite well overall. SI was a next best, with a slightly poorer estimation of the regression coefficients. In the conditional mean (CM) analysis, the regression coefficient b2 for $x2$ was underestimated, but less so than with a CC analysis. Coefficients b3–b5 were well estimated. Both the CC and CM analyses underestimated the predictive performance (adjusted R^2 19% and 27% instead of $R^2 = 35\%$).

7.6 Guidance to Dealing with Missing Values in Prediction Research

We provide some guidance for dealing with missing values and imputation in prediction research, based on previous research, findings in simulations, and practical considerations.

7.6.1   *Patterns of Missingness*

As a preliminary step, it is recommended to investigate the missing data patterns.

1. We need to examine how many missing values occur for each potential predictor; this examination is part of the basic approach to any data analysis. Missing values are easily noted when examining frequency distributions of the predictors.
2. We want to know whether predictor values are correlated with missingness of other predictors; this determines how well we may be able to impute a missing value, and how useful the remaining information on subjects without missing values is. We may also study associations with auxiliary variables, such as calendar time and geographic site.
3. Regression trees and logistic regression analysis can be used to assess associations between predictor values and missingness of the predictor. When associations are identified, the MCAR assumption is violated. We cannot test for MNAR versus MAR.
4. As an extension of point 3, it is especially important to assess whether missingness was associated with the outcome. This can easily be assessed by examining the outcome, e.g., the percentage mortality, by missingness of the predictor (value available/missing). Often, we may note a poorer outcome in those with missing values. The first question is whether this association can be explained by observed predictors. Hereto, logistic regression analysis can be helpful, with missingness as the dependent variable, and the outcome y and other predictors as covariables. If the study was truly prospective, a missing X–y association can only occur through other characteristics; it is logically impossible to have selective missingness on the outcome when the data were collected before the outcome was known. The other characteristics that mediate the observed missingness—outcome association may be known; this is a MAR on x situation. If some of the mediating predictors are not known, or measured imprecisely (measurement error), some kind of residual confounding occurs, leading to an MNAR situation. Imputation with y may at least partly resolve this situation.
5. Subject matter knowledge should be used to judge plausible mechanisms for the missing values, for example, whether MNAR is plausible. The MCAR assumption can be tested, and may often be rejected in medical research. The MAR assumption cannot be tested, and MNAR, hence, always remains a possibility.

7.6.2   *Simple Approaches*

A historically popular method in epidemiological research was to create a category "missing" for missing values in the regression analysis. Such a "missing indicator method" is especially straightforward for categorical predictors. For example, we can recode a predictor that was incompletely recorded as "absent", "present", and "missing". Such a procedure ignores the correlation of the values of predictors among each other. Simulations have shown that the procedure may lead to severe bias in estimated regression coefficients [207, 385]. The missing indicator should hence generally not be used. An alternative in such a situation might be to change the definition of the predictor, i.e., by assuming that if no value is available from a patient chart, the characteristic is absent rather than missing. This approach is followed in many analyses of observational data with electronic health records: if something is not recorded, it is assumed to be absent [452].

7.6.3   More Advanced Approaches

Systematic missingness of a predictor may occur in some situations:

- a new test or biomarker is only available in a more recent series of patients. Simulations found that imputation works as well as other regression types or Bayesian approaches [405].
- data from several studies are combined in a meta-analysis, while some predictors are systematically missing in some studies. A multilevel structure is then needed in the imputation model to respect the principle of congeniality and appropriately acknowledge between study differences in predictor effects [19]. MI methods have been proposed that use random effects for the study variable, and can provide imputations for continuous and binary predictors. Some methods allow for different variances in predictors per study, which can however only be estimated reliably in large studies [453]. If small clusters are analyzed, it may be better to assume identical variances across clusters (homoscedasticity) [282].

7.6.4   Maximum Fraction of Missing Values Before Omitting a Predictor

When we are interested in the specific effect of a predictor, the validity of an analysis is higher with fewer missing values. If a substantial number of missing values occur specifically in one predictor, it may be convenient to omit this predictor from the analysis. Especially when the predictor is of primary interest, it would not be natural to impute the missing values. For example, when we had missing treatment allocation for some patients in a randomized controlled trial (RCT), we would never impute these missing values.

It is difficult to provide a guide to what is still an acceptable number of missing values. Evidence for selective missingness (e.g., MAR on y) may already make a CC analysis of a predictor with 10% missings suspect; in other cases 20% missingness may be quite acceptable (e.g., MCAR assumed).

Theoretically, MI solves any missing data problem, as long as we correctly model the missing data mechanism. So, the effect of a predictor with 90% missing values could still be estimated, but with relatively large uncertainty.

In practice, we can only approximate the missing data mechanism. Effects of predictors with more than 50% missings in a specific data set may generally be distrusted. Such predictors might hence be discarded from a predictive analysis, because of too many missings. Other considerations may include the reasons for missingness. If missings occur because of the study design, we may be less worried in interpreting findings based on a relatively limited set of known values. For example, in the TBI case study (Chap. 8), missing values occurred especially because some studies included in the meta-analysis did simply not record the predictor.

7.6.5   Single or Multiple Imputation for Predictor Effects?

In prediction research, we may generally think of studying effects of predictors that are of specific interest (in univariate and in adjusted analyses); and of studying predictions (deriving prognostic equations, with the evaluation of model performance). We usually start a prognostic analysis with a univariate analysis of predictor effects, e.g., a cross-tabulation of a predictor with a binary outcome or with time-to-event in a Kaplan–Meier survival analysis. Equivalently, we can calculate the regression coefficients in a univariate logistic or Cox regression to obtain estimates of predictor effects. A complete case analysis is the most obvious approach as long as we do not have a MAR on y or MNAR in y situation (Table 7.5). In Table 7.9 this is indicated as ignoring incomplete records for variable $x1$. An example may be that we are interested in the prognostic effect of the Motor score from the Glasgow Outcome Scale in TBI (see Chap. 8).

Next, we are often interested in adjusted effects, i.e., the effect of $x1$ corrected for correlation with other variables ($x2$ to x_i). The variables $x2$ to x_i are considered as confounders, since they may be associated with the outcome and with $x1$. Such an adjusted analysis may well be done with the imputation of missing data for the confounders ($x2$ to x_i), but without imputation of $x1$. This ensures comparability with the univariate analysis, because numbers will be the same in univariate and adjusted analyses. MI is preferable, although SI will only slightly underestimate the variability in the adjusted regression coefficient for $x1$. MI for the confounding

Table 7.9 Dealing with missing values to estimate predictor effects

Analysis	Predictor of interest $x1$ (e.g. motor score)	Confounders $x2$–x_i (other predictors)
Univariate analysis	Complete case	–
Adjusted analysis	Complete case	SI/MI

variables results in better estimates of the variability in the adjusted regression coefficient. This will be illustrated for traumatic brain injury (see Chap. 8).

An alternative is to perform univariate and adjusted analyses with imputed data, both for the predictor of interest $x1$ and the confounders $x2$ to x_i. Many medical researchers will, however, appreciate univariate analyses that stay closer to the observed data, at least as an initial analysis.

7.6.6 Single or Multiple Imputation for Deriving Predictions?

If we focus on the derivation of predictions from a model, again MI may be the preferred approach. However, given that having multiple completed data sets complicates various analyses, some next best strategies can be envisioned, especially for situations with relatively few missings. Then single imputation may be a reasonable alternative: a stochastic SI data set can easily be created as the first of a series of MI data sets. Every investigator can easily work with such an SI data set, and does not have to bother with the combination of results over different MI data sets. More experienced data analysts may consider this advantage trivial. The GUSTO-I data set, which is used as an example throughout this book, is a CM dataset, with at most 8% imputed values for some of the predictors [329].

The primary disadvantage of stochastic SI is the underestimation of the uncertainty associated with imputed values. A second disadvantage is less stability in the point estimates, because of the random element in stochastic SI. These disadvantages are less relevant with relatively few missing values, and in large data sets. MI may be preferable with relatively small data sets (for example, with less than 100 events), since imputations will vary considerably from imputation to imputation. In addition to the size of the data set, the fraction of missings may guide the number of imputations. For example, we might use the average percentage of missings for the number of imputations: 5 imputations for 5% missingness on average, 20 for 20%, 50 for 50% [600].

To derive predictions for individual subjects in our development data set, it is often advisable to impute missing data for all predictors. An exception is a situation that we know that we cannot obtain complete data in future applications. It may then be reasonable to develop the full prediction model in a selection of subjects where the data will be available in the future.

Finally, we may want to present the prognostic model in a simple form for practical application (Chap. 18). A score chart based on rounded coefficients is easy to obtain with SI. MI will provide better estimates of the variability of the scores, but variability is only of secondary interest, if presented at all. MI may, therefore, have only a minor advantage over SI for model presentation. In summary, multivariable analysis, performance estimation and model presentation can all be done both with SI or MI approaches.

7.6.7   Missings and Predictions for New Patients

If a model is applied in a new setting, predictor values may be missing. Several approaches are possible, including the imputation of missing values with an imputation model derived from the development sample. A straightforward solution is to provide predictions for submodels of a prediction model, i.e., models that only use the available predictors [167].

7.6.8   *Performance Across Multiple Imputed Data Sets

Various performance measures can be estimated for prediction models (Chaps. 15 and 16). Normally distributed measures can readily be combined with Rubin's rules across imputed data sets, for example, an estimate for calibration-in-the-large with a model intercept, and the calibration slope with a regression coefficient for the linear predictor. The area under the ROC curve, or concordance statistic (c), ranges between 0 and 1. A logit transformation makes that we can better combine estimates, either from multiple imputed data sets, or in the context of a meta-analysis (Table 7.10) [521].

A specific challenge lies in the estimation of optimism in performance when missing values have been imputed. We will discuss various techniques for internal and external validation in Chap. 17, including cross-validation and bootstrap resampling. For example, bootstrapping might be performed within each imputed data set. This is a common and straightforward approach: we determine measures of model performance within imputed datasets and subsequently pool these for overall measures of model performance [677]. Alternatively, we might impute within each bootstrap sample. Such multiple imputation after bootstrapping is computationally intensive. Any differences will especially arise in small data sets with many missing values, where we would need a substantial number of imputations.

Table 7.10 Parameter of interest in prediction modeling studies and ways to combine estimates after MI [521, 677]

Parameter	Rubin's rules on
Regression coefficients	original
Tests of coefficients	Wald tests
Linear predictor per patient	original
Calibration in the large	model intercept/log(baseline hazard)
Calibration slope	original
AUC or c-statistic	logit(c)

7.6.9   Reporting of Missing Values in Prediction Research

Suggested reporting guidelines [84] emphasize 3 major issues:

1. Quantification of the completeness of predictor data;
2. Approaches to dealing with missing predictor data (including imputation methods), and
3. Exploration of the missing data (including results for complete case and completed case analysis, Table 7.11).

Some examples of dealing with missing values are in Table 7.12. Methods include single imputation (simple, conditional mean, stochastic regression), or multiple imputation. More details of these studies are provided at the book's website www.clinicalpredictionmodels.org.

Table 7.11 Guidelines for reporting of prognostic studies with missing predictor data [84]

Issue	Aspect
Quantification of completeness	If completeness of data is an inclusion criterion, specify numbers excluded
	Provide total n and n with complete data
	Report frequency of missingness for every predictor
Approach to dealing with missing data	Provide sufficient details on the methods used, including references if imputation was done
	Specify the n of patients and number of events for all analyses
Exploration of missing data	Discuss reasons for missingness
	Present comparisons of characteristics between cases with and without missing data

Table 7.12 Imputation methods as applied in some examples

Method	Characteristics	Example
Simple imputation	Mean or most frequent category	Guillain-Barré: few missings [631]
Conditional mean imputation	Estimate predicted value based on correlations between predictors	Historical examples: GUSTO-I [329], ReHiT study [551]
Stochastic regression imputation	Draw imputed value from distribution of predicted values	Adjusted analysis in the IMPACT study [398]
Multiple imputation	Develop imputation model and draw imputed value from the distribution of predicted values; combine estimates over m imputed data sets	Ovarian cancer [99], testicular cancer [617], prostate cancer marker missing in historic patients [405]

7.7 Concluding Remarks

Missing values pose important challenges in prediction research. Straightforward methods such as complete case analysis are often oversimplistic from a methodological point of view. Most simulations that have been performed on imputation conclude that imputation methods are superior to complete case analysis [275]. Indeed, multiple imputation is gaining rapidly in acceptance in medical research.

The best solution for missing values is to ensure that no data are missing. It may sometimes be possible to retrieve missing data by going back to medical charts. In some settings, it may be reasonable to define missing as "No" [452]. If characteristics are measured multiple times, we may sometimes use a measurement from another time point, as will be illustrated for the Motor score component of the Glasgow Coma Scale in a case study (Chap. 8). If missing values do occur, they have to be dealt with in a reasonable way, i.e., such that the research questions are addressed efficiently.

The research question is not to estimate the missing values correctly. We aim to estimate model parameters (univariate effects, adjusted effects, multivariable effects) and make predictions (derive predictive equations, assess performance). These parameters should be valid for the population where the model will be applied in the future. The sample serves to learn for this future application, and we should use all available information. Imputation of some missing values prevents that we throw away useful information recorded for other predictors. The primary benefit of imputation is hence an increase in power to detect prognostic effects, and in deriving better predictions. A second benefit of imputation is comparability of results over analyses. The price we pay for these benefits is making the MAR assumption, which can be addressed with an appropriate imputation model. We hence need to include all variables (predictors, outcome, and auxiliary variables) that are potentially correlated with the missingness of the predictor in the imputation model.

As in any statistical analysis, the sensible judgment of the analyst is important, based on subject knowledge and the research question. Comparing results of the complete case and completed case analyses may be informative, and together with a judgment about the plausibility of assumptions in a particular situation, we can decide on which is the primary analysis.

7.7.1 Summary Statements

- Missing values in predictors are common, and lead to inefficiency, difficulties in comparing results between analyses with different numbers, and potentially biased regression coefficients and predictions

- Theoretical analyses and simulations conclude that imputation methods, especially multiple imputation, are often superior to complete case analyses
- Advanced stochastic single imputation methods, based on the first data set of a multiple imputation sequence, may be a reasonable start to address a number of prognostic research questions
- Imputation methods make the assumption of MAR; more specifically, MAR given the information used in the imputation process
- The MAR assumption is not testable, but becomes more reasonable with imputation models that include a wide range of characteristics, including predictors, the outcome, and auxiliary variables.

7.7.2 *Available Software and Challenges*

Multiple imputation software is widely available nowadays, and further improvements may be expected during the coming years. For R, the `mice` library is freely available (developed by Van Buuren et al.) [599]. It includes state of the art functions, has flexible settings, but the computation time can be substantial. An alternative is the `aregImpute` function developed by Harrell, which performed well in a number of assessments. Stata has sophisticated functions. With any imputation procedures, we should check distributions of the observed and imputed values, e.g., by histograms.

Several methodological challenges may require further study:

- In what circumstances is MI needed, and is SI not sufficient, in prognostic research?
- What are the main risks when incorrectly specifying the imputation model?
- How should we deal with missing values in a meta-analysis context? [19] (Chap. 8).
- If some sort of selection process is done, e.g., stepwise selection, how can this be combined with imputation? [678] (Chap. 11).
- How should we perform internal validation, e.g., bootstrapping, when missing values are imputed? Is it sufficient to validate the modeling process within each imputed data set? [401, 677] (Chaps. 17 and 23).

Questions

7.1. Missing values versus incomplete cases

(a) How many values are missing from the required values for a model with 3 predictors $x1 - x3$, estimated in 1000 subjects, where $x1$ has 100, $x2$ 200, and $x3$ 400 missing values?

(b) If the missing values occur completely at random, how many subjects would approximately be discarded in a complete case (CC) analysis?

7.2. MCAR, MAR or MNAR?

Consider a prognostic study among patients undergoing heart valve surgery aiming to quantify the predictive value of intraoperative characteristics (e.g., intraoperative blood pressure and complications) for mortality after 30 days (outcome). What type of missingness pattern do we have in the following two situations?

(a) Among patients who actually developed an intraoperative complication, the intraoperative data are often missing?

(b) Among patients with a less severe indication for surgery based on presurgical data, the intraoperative data are missing?

Suppose that clinicians do not perform a diagnostic test if their impression is that the patient does not have the diagnosis of interest. This impression may partly be captured by clinical variables that are observed, but also depend on some predictors that are not registered in the data.

(c) Is this a MAR or MNAR situation?

7.3. MAR on y in Fig. 7.1

Why does a missing value mechanism of $x1$ MAR on y result in bias both for $b1$ and $b2$ in Fig. 7.1?

7.4. Problems of overall mean imputation

What is the effect of performing overall mean imputation (i.e., imputing the mean of the observed values for the missing values) on estimated regression coefficients and standard errors?

7.5. Imputation with outcome

Consider 90% missingness for a predictor $x1$ which is not related to other predictors. It is recommended to perform SI or MI with the outcome as one of the variables in the imputation model (Table 7.7). What would happen to the univariate regression coefficient of $x1$ if a completed data set were analyzed, where values were imputed without using y?

7.6. Complete case analysis or imputation?

    (a) For what missingness patterns is complete case analysis a reasonable solution?

    (b) In what respects is multiple imputation preferable above single imputation.

Chapter 8
Case Study on Dealing with Missing Values

Background A case study is presented on prognostic modeling in patients with moderate and severe traumatic brain injury (TBI). Individual patient data from several studies were available to: (a) quantify predictor effects; (b) develop and validate prognostic models. Missing values were a key issue. Some values were systematically missing per study, since few studies recorded all predictors of interest. The use of single and multiple imputation methods is illustrated with a detailed description of the analyses in R software.

8.1 Introduction

8.1.1 Aim of the IMPACT Study

The overall aim of the IMPACT study was to optimize the methodology of randomized clinical trials in the field of TBI, such that chances of demonstrating benefit with an effective new therapy or therapeutic agent would be maximized [357]. Randomized controlled trials (RCTs) in TBI are complex due to the heterogeneity of the population. None of the multicenter RCTs conducted in this field over the past decades have convincingly shown the benefit of new therapies in the overall population [374]. The project was labeled IMPACT: International Mission on Prognosis and Analysis of Clinical Trials in TBI: http://www.tbi-impact.org/ [357]. Individual patient data (IPD) from trials and surveys were made available for methodological research.

Prognosis was central to the aims of the project. Prognostic models can be used for the efficient selection of patients (excluding those with an extreme prognosis, either very poor or very good) and for covariate adjustment of the treatment effect (with several advantages as described in Chap. 2) [242]. In TBI, the outcome is commonly assessed with the Glasgow Outcome Scale (GOS), which is an ordinal

© Springer Nature Switzerland AG 2019

E. W. Steyerberg, *Clinical Prediction Models*, Statistics for Biology
and Health, https://doi.org/10.1007/978-3-030-16399-0_8

scale (Table 8.1) [281]. The scale ranges from dead, vegetative state, severe disability to moderate disability and good recovery. In trial analyses, the GOS is often dichotomized as mortality versus survival (category 1 vs. 2–5), or as unfavorable versus favorable (category 1–3 vs. category 4, 5), although it is preferable to exploit the ordinal nature of this scale [464]. One approach is the "sliding dichotomy" analysis, in which the split for dichotomization of the GOS is differentiated according to the baseline prognosis established prior to randomization [397]. Another approach is to use a proportional odds model for the GOS as an ordered outcome (see Chap. 4).

We aimed to predict the dichotomized 6-month GOS. Missing data were a key problem in the prognostic analysis [371]. We focus on approaches for dealing with missing data for two types of research questions: predictor effects and prediction of 6-month outcome.

8.1.2 Patient Selection

Our focus was on patients with severe TBI (Glasgow Coma Score, GCS 3–8), but cohorts that included patients with moderate TBI (GCS 9–12) were also considered. The GCS is a measure for the level of consciousness. Essentially, an individual patient data meta-analysis (IPD-MA) of 11 studies was performed, including 8 RCTs, and 3 relatively unselected prospective surveys, with the potential for analyzing data on 9205 patients. Complete outcome data were available for 8719 of the 9205 patients (95%). We further excluded children, leaving 8530 patients for analysis. The studies are arbitrarily designated as 1–11 in Table 8.2. The meta-analysis was a continuation of analyses of 2 related RCTs (Tirilazad, Table 8.2: study ID 1 and 2) [259].

8.1.3 Potential Predictors

Extensive univariate analyses were performed within the IMPACT study to assess potential predictors. In combination with a review of the literature, we identified 16 predictors for further multivariable analyses [398]. These predictors included

Table 8.1 Definition of the Glasgow Outcome Scale [281]

Category	Label	Definition
1	Dead	–
2	Vegetative	Unable to interact with the environment; unresponsive
3	Severe disability	Conscious but dependent
4	Moderate disability	Independent, but disabled
5	Good recovery	Return to normal occupational and social activities; may have minor residual deficits

Table 8.2 Availability of predictor values by study, as included in the IMPACT database ($n = 8530$, completely missing in bold) [357]

Study	1	2	3	4	5	6	7	8	9	10	11	Total
n	1118	1041	409	919	1510	350	812	604	126	822	819	8530
Core predictors												
Age (%)	100	100	100	100	100	100	100	100	100	100	100	100
Motor score (%)	100	100	100	100	100	100	100	100	100	100	100	100
Pupils (%)	93	95	97	**0**	98	100	92	100	**0**	96	99	85
Secondary insults												
Hypoxia (%)	88	89	100	93	**0**	**0**	98	100	67	99	**0**	64
Hypotension (%)	97	97	**0**	93	**0**	98	99	100	83	99	100	75
CT												
CT class (%)	99	99	100	99	**0**	**0**	**0**	**0**	100	98	99	61
tSAH (%)	97	95	99	99	100	73	**0**	87	100	95	100	87
EDH (%)	98	99	**0**	99	100	100	95	**0**	100	100	100	87
Cisterns (%)	89	87	99	99	**0**	**0**	**0**	86	100	**0**	**0**	45
Shift (%)	89	88	99	99	100	**0**	**0**	89	100	**0**	100	73
Laboratory values												
Glucose (%)	96	99	**0**	95	96	85	**0**	**0**	98	**0**	**0**	57
pH (%)	76	82	**0**	68	**0**	**0**	**0**	90	100	**0**	**0**	40
Sodium (%)	98	96	**0**	96	96	95	**0**	64	98	**0**	**0**	62
Hb (%)	99	98	**0**	90	30	97	**0**	**0**	93	**0**	**0**	45
Platelets (%)	**0**	**0**	**0**	90	29	**0**	**0**	40	93	**0**	**0**	19
Prothrombin time (%)	**0**	**0**	**0**	**0**	29	**0**	**0**	48	91	**0**	**0**	10

demographic characteristics (age) [399], injury details (cause of injury) [85], secondary insults (hypoxia and hypotension) [372], clinical measures of injury severity
(Glasgow Coma scale and pupillary reactivity) [364], characteristics of the admission
CT scan [359], and laboratory values [595]. For prognostic modeling, a core set of 3
strong predictors emerges from the literature since the 1970s, consisting of age, motor
score, and pupillary reactivity [400]. We subsequently expanded this core model to a
7-predictor model by including secondary insults and CT characteristics (CT classification, traumatic subarachnoid hemorrhage) [559]. Further modeling studies were
performed with the inclusion of more predictors, but are omitted here.

8.1.4   Coding and Time Dependency of Predictors

An important issue was the definition of predictors across the 11 studies.
Definitions varied between data sets. The data extraction was guided by a data
dictionary and original study documentation, which standardized the format of
variables entered into the pooled data set. A consistent set of categories for coding
was sought for each variable by collapsing more extensive coding into a simpler
format. For example, the presence of hypoxia on admission was collapsed into a
binary coding present/absent, although some datasets contained a more detailed
coding as "No/Suspect/Definite".

A further issue was related to the time of measurement of a predictor. We aimed
to consider predictors that would be available when patients were to be enrolled in a
RCT, in line with the overall aim of the project. An interesting example is the motor
score, which is the prognostically most important element of the GCS among those
with moderate or severe injuries. Four time points for assessment were defined:
pre-hospital, first hospital (in case of secondary referral), admission, and post stabilization. Most data sets had data for at least 2 of these time points. For prognostic
analysis, we aimed to select the latest reliable assessment on admission to correspond with a baseline assessment prior to randomization, i.e., the post-stabilization
score. If this was missing we used the next reliable value going back in time
(admission, first in-hospital, pre-hospital). However, sometimes the Motor score is
not clinically obtainable because of early sedation or paralysis, required for artificial
ventilation. The motor score was then coded as a separate category ("9", untestable), rather than considered as a missing value. This approach made the motor
score available for all patients.

It can be debated whether a more formal analysis should have been used for
defining the baseline Motor score; e.g., a multiple imputation procedure might have
considered all four time points, providing a formally imputed post-stabilization
Motor score. MI might also have provided estimates for the untestable patients
("category 9"). However, the necessity for sedation and paralysis is related to the
severity of injuries. In this specific case missingness in the sense of "untestable"
may possibly be of prognostic relevance, and imputation of a virtual motor score for
"untestable" patients was hence not considered appropriate.

8.2   Missing Values in the IMPACT Study

Missing values were present in the outcome and in predictors. We discuss dealing with both below.

8.2.1   Missing Values in Outcome

Data on 6-month outcome were available for 10 of the 11 studies. For one study, only the 3-month GOS was measured (study 5). Since the GOS is assumed to be relatively stable between 3 and 6 months, we simply carried the 3-month GOS forward to 6-month GOS. This approach is consistent with the way in which missing outcome had been imputed in a small number of patients in the individual studies (Last Value Carried Forward approach, LVCF). We note that LVCF generally is a quite poor approach to missing outcomes, since any changes in time are missed [668]. We chose not to further attempt imputation of the 6-month GOS in the 5% of patients in whom outcome remained missing, as not to compromise the interpretation of our outcome measure. A more formal MI procedure could have been followed, incorporating the GOS patterns over time as available in some of the studies (e.g., 1, 3, 6, 12 months), and correlations of outcomes with predictors and study.

8.2.2   Quantification of Missingness of Predictors

Table 8.2 summarizes the availability of predictors within the 11 studies of the IMPACT database. The main reason for missingness was the systematic absence of a predictor within a given dataset. If the dataset included a predictor, availability was generally high, with only sporadic missingness. Data for age and motor score (including the untestable category) were complete, but some studies had no data for pupils (studies 4 and 9, Table 8.2). If pupils were recorded, data were complete in >90% of the patients within most of the studies. Secondary insults (hypoxia and hypotension) had not been recorded in some studies, but if recorded, data were again quite complete. CT scans are usually performed within hours after admission, after stabilization of the patient. CT scans provide important diagnostic information, and are often classified according to the Marshall classification [368]. This classification was available in 7 of the 11 studies, for 61% of the 8530 patients. Other important CT characteristics, such as traumatic subarachnoid hemorrhage (tSAH) and the presence of an epidural hematoma (EDH, Fig. 8.1) were available in slightly higher numbers of patients.

Laboratory values were available for only a few studies (Table 8.2). Glucose, pH, sodium and Hb levels were available for around 50% of the patients, but

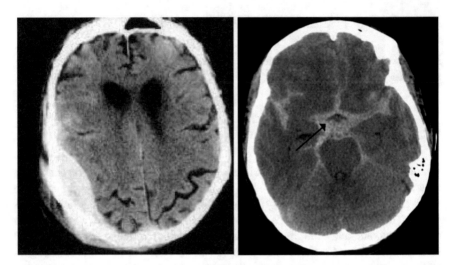

Fig. 8.1 Example of an epidural hematoma (EDH, left) and traumatic subarachnoid hemorrhage (tSAH, right). An EDH is located directly under the skull and mainly causes brain damage due to compression. Consequently, the prognosis is favorable if it can be evacuated rapidly. A developing EDH is one of the greatest emergencies in neurosurgery. Subarachnoid hemorrhage is bleeding into the subarachnoid space—the area between the arachnoid membrane and the pia mater surrounding the brain, implying a poor prognosis

platelets and prothrombin time (which are related to blood clotting), were available for less than 20% (Table 8.2). The latter percentages were that low that we did not consider these predictors for a prediction model; admittedly this judgment is arbitrary. A series of models was developed, with different selections of studies, based on the availability of predictors per study.

8.2.3   Patterns of Missingness

We further examined patterns of missingness, following the steps discussed in Chap. 7.

a. *How many missings occur for each potential predictor?*

We can use the naclus and naplot functions to further visualize missing value patterns. As was also noted in Table 8.2, missing values were most frequent for laboratory parameters and some CT characteristics (Fig. 8.2, left panel). Many patients had multiple missing values, e.g., 2277 of 8530 patients had 4 missing values, and 4 patients even had 10 missing values among 10 key predictors (Fig. 8.2, right panel).

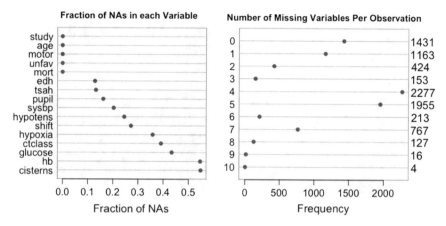

Fig. 8.2 Fraction of missing values per potential predictor (left panel), and number of missing values per subject (right panel)

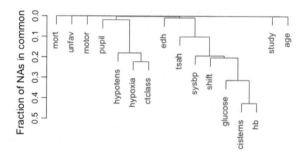

Fig. 8.3 Combinations of missing values in predictors ("NAs"), based on a hierarchical cluster analysis of missingness combinations in 8530 patients with TBI

b. *Missing value mechanisms*

For analysis of the mechanism of missingness, we examine combinations of missing predictors, associations between predictors and missingness, and associations between outcome and missingness. As proposed by Harrell, we used the `naclus` function to visualize missing value patterns (Fig. 8.3) [225]. Characteristics of CT scans, such as shift and cisterns are often missing in combination, while also laboratory values are missing in such patients (glucose and hb). Key insights in missing value frequency and patterns of missingness can also be obtained with the `aggr` function (Fig. 8.4).

c. *Associations between predictors and missingness*

Table 8.2 shows that missingness of most predictors strongly depends on the study. We explored in detail whether there were other determinants of missingness for CT characteristics, some key laboratory variables and presenting characteristics. No clear associations were found in relation to age (Fig. 8.5). The main determinant of

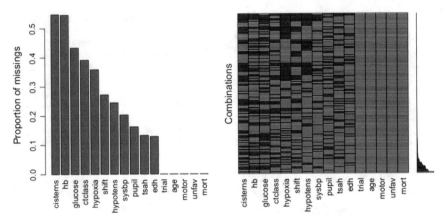

Fig. 8.4 Proportion of missings and combinations of missing values in predictors (aggr function in VIM)

missingness was the study: some studies did not register a particular predictor. No "MAR on *X*" patterns were evident.

d. *Associations between outcome and missingness*

Figure 8.5 further demonstrates no clear associations between missingness and an unfavorable 6-month Glasgow Outcome Scale (GOS) outcome. To explore the relation between missingness and outcome in more detail, logistic regression models for missingness of a predictor were constructed, but again no clear patterns were noted. Hence, there were no indications of a "MAR on *y*" mechanism.

e. *Plausible mechanisms for missingness*

The most plausible mechanism for missingness was that a predictor was simply not recorded for some studies. Within studies, a mechanism close to MCAR had occurred. We conclude that missingness was essentially MCAR, conditional on the study. Hence, we would like to stratify on study when making imputations. We imputed values conditional on values of the other predictors, and with the study as the main effect. We excluded some studies from analyses if we judged that too many predictors were 100% missing in a study [559].

8.3   Imputation of Missing Predictor Values

8.3.1   Correlations Between Predictors

Table 8.3 shows that the correlations between variables were generally modest. Some more substantial correlations ($r > 0.4$) were noted among CT scan characteristics and between some laboratory values. The associations between cisterns/

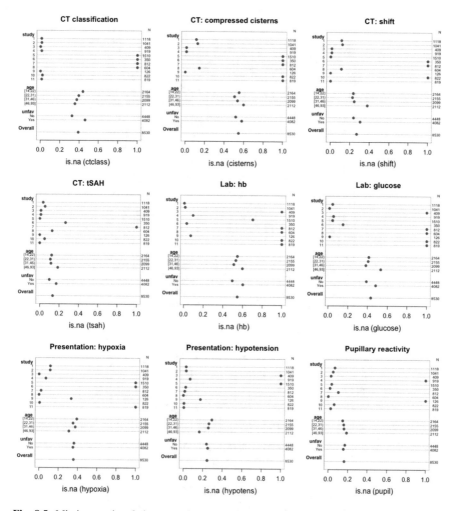

Fig. 8.5 Missingness in relation to study, age, and outcome (unfavorable status according to the Glasgow Outcome Scale at 6 months). The study was the main determinant of missingness. Only weak associations were observed with age and the 6-month outcome ("unfav")

shift and the CT classification are to be expected, as these characteristics are used in the definition of the CT classification. Hb and platelets are correlated, as both will decrease following blood loss.

Table 8.3 Rank correlations between predictors, with correlations > 0.4 in **bold**

	Study	Age	Motor	Pupil	Hypoxia	Hypotens	CTclass	tSAH	EDH	Cisterns	Shift	Glucose	Sodium	Hb	Platelet
Study[a]	1	0.17	0.28	0.22	0.19	0.16	0.08	0.22	0.12	0.34	0.26	0.24	0.08	0.31	**0.52**
Age	0.17	1	-0.01	0.03	0.00	0.05	0.20	0.14	0.01	0.03	0.14	0.06	-0.07	-0.05	-0.17
Motor	0.28	-0.01	1	0.37	0.15	0.14	0.11	0.05	-0.02	0.21	0.11	0.11	-0.03	-0.06	-0.01
Pupil	0.22	0.03	0.37	1	0.14	0.17	0.22	0.11	-0.02	0.23	0.16	0.18	-0.06	-0.05	-0.03
Hypoxia	0.19	0.00	0.15	0.14	1	0.29	0.02	0.01	-0.05	0.02	-0.02	0.12	-0.01	-0.03	0.02
Hypotens	0.16	0.05	0.14	0.17	0.29	1	-0.02	0.05	-0.06	0.02	-0.03	0.15	0.02	-0.23	-0.14
CTclass	0.08	0.20	0.11	0.22	0.02	-0.02	1	0.14	0.31	**0.44**	**0.48**	0.15	-0.06	-0.04	-0.01
tSAH	0.22	0.14	0.05	0.11	0.01	0.05	0.14	1	-0.04	0.13	0.07	0.10	-0.02	0.01	-0.04
EDH	0.12	0.01	-0.02	-0.02	-0.05	-0.06	0.31	-0.04	1	0.06	0.15	0.00	0.01	-0.05	-0.05
Cisterns	0.34	0.03	0.21	0.23	0.02	0.02	**0.44**	0.13	0.06	1	**0.51**	0.09	-0.03	-0.08	0.07
Shift	0.26	0.14	0.11	0.16	-0.02	-0.03	**0.48**	0.07	0.15	**0.51**	1	0.03	-0.01	-0.11	-0.10
Glucose	0.24	0.06	0.11	0.18	0.12	0.15	0.15	0.10	0.00	0.09	0.03	1	-0.13	-0.04	0.21
Sodium	0.08	-0.07	-0.03	-0.06	-0.01	0.02	-0.06	-0.02	0.01	-0.03	-0.01	-0.13	1	0.04	-0.08
hb	0.31	-0.05	-0.06	-0.05	-0.03	-0.23	-0.04	0.01	-0.05	-0.08	-0.11	-0.04	0.04	1	**0.46**
Platelet	**0.52**	-0.17	-0.01	-0.03	0.02	-0.14	-0.01	-0.04	-0.05	0.07	-0.10	0.21	-0.08	**0.46**	1

[a]Based on Generalized Spearman Rank Correlation as calculated with the spearman2 function; other correlations based on standard Spearman rank correlation. All correlations were calculated with pairwise available patients

8.3.2 Imputation Model

An initial imputation model included all relevant potential predictors and the outcome (6-month GOS, in 5 categories). No auxiliary variables were used. A relatively simple imputation model was fitted using the `mice` library. We show the commands below for illustration, with more details at www.clinicalpredictionmodels.org.

```
# mice imputation model for pmat as predictor matrix, with default settings
names(TBI1)
 [1] "study" "age" "hypoxia" "hypotens" "cisterns" "shift" "tsah" "edh" "pupil"
[10] "motor" "ctclass" "sysbp" "hb" "glucose" "unfav" "mort"
p <- 16
pmat   <- matrix(rep(1,p*p),nrow=p,ncol=p)
diag(pmat)   <- rep(0,p)
pmat[,c(1:2, 10, 15:16)]  <- 0 # set some columns to zero
pmat[ c(1:2, 10, 15:16),] <- 0 # set the rows for the same variables to zero

# define data to be used and the imputation method for each column, seed =1
gm <-mice(TBI1, m=10, imputationMethod=c("polyreg","pmm","logreg","logreg",
"logreg","logreg","logreg","logreg","polyreg","polyreg","polyreg","pmm","pmm",
"pmm", "logreg","logreg"), predictorMatrix = pmat, seed=1)
```

The printed result includes a summary of the procedure:

```
Number of multiple imputations:   10
Missing cells per column:
study age hypoxia hypotens cisterns shift tsah   edh pupil
  0    0    3057     2090     4673  2321 1137  1105  1387
motor ctclass sysbp   hb glucose unfav mort
  0    3338  1733 4659    3700     0    0
```

The `gm` object has 10 imputed data sets of the IMPACT database. In total, 16 variables were considered in the imputation model, corresponding to Table 8.3. Data were complete for the outcome (`unfav` and `mort`), `study`, `age`, and Motor score (`motor`).

8.3.3 Distributions of Imputed Values

The distributions of imputed values can be checked for the plausibility of imputations (e.g., within a plausible range, no strange peaks, Fig. 8.6). We note rather stable distributions of imputed values, with similarity to the complete data. The last graph shows imputations for glucose, with values truncated at 2 and 20, as in the original predictor definition.

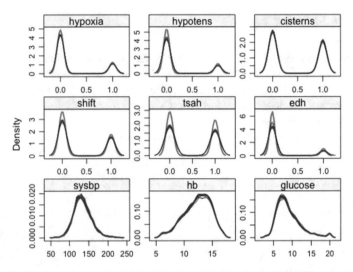

Fig. 8.6 Distribution of imputed and original values with `mice` in the IMPACT study (n = 8530)

8.3.4 *Multilevel Imputation*

Our `mice` imputation model did stratify by the study as the main effect, since the study was a strong determinant of missingness, and predictor values may depend on the specific study. This is a typical situation for a meta-analysis context, where results from several studies are combined. Sporadic and systematic missing values may occur by the study. MI methods have been proposed that use random effects for the study variable, and can provide imputations for continuous and binary predictors [19]. Some methods allow for different variances in predictors per the study, which can, however, only be estimated reliably in large studies [453]. If small clusters are analyzed, it may be better to assume identical variances across clusters (homoscedasticity) [282].

8.4 Predictor Effect: Adjusted Analyses

After imputation, we can estimate the adjusted effects of each predictor of interest in turn, using imputed versions of other predictors. These other predictors are hence considered as potential confounders. We present all results with `mice` for adjusted analyses. As confounders, we considered 7 predictors that had also shown convincing effects in previous TBI studies. These include the 3 core predictors (age, Motor score, pupils), 2 secondary insults (hypoxia, hypotension), and 2 CT characteristics (CT classification and tSAH). The outcome was GOS at 6 months, dichotomized as unfavorable versus favorable in logistic regression models. For

Table 8.4 Logistic regression coefficients of predictors in univariate and adjusted analyses. Numbers are estimated coefficients (estimated SE)

		Univar	Adjusted		
	n	$n = 5192 - 8530$	CC $n = 2428$	SI $n = 5192 - 8530$	MI $n = 5192 - 8530$
Age (per decade)	8530	0.32 (0.015)	0.36 (0.033)	0.35 (0.017)	0.35 (0.018)
Motor score	8530				
1 or 2		1.87 (0.065)	1.65 (0.16)	1.61 (0.073)	1.61 (0.074)
3		1.38 (0.077)	1.36 (0.16)	1.25 (0.085)	1.24 (0.086)
4		0.69 (0.065)	0.71 (0.13)	0.62 (0.070)	0.61 (0.071)
5 or 6		zero (ref)	zero (ref)	zero (ref)	zero (ref)
9 (untestable)		0.91 (0.112)	1.06 (0.26)	0.90 (0.125)	0.87 (0.127)
Pupillary reactivity	7143				
Both pupils reactive		zero (ref)	zero (ref)	zero (ref)	zero (ref)
One nonreactive		0.97 (0.076)	0.51 (0.15)	0.58 (0.085)	0.57 (0.085)
Both nonreactive		1.77 (0.067)	0.94 (0.14)	1.15 (0.076)	1.15 (0.077)
Hypoxia	5473	0.80 (0.072)	0.49 (0.12)	0.42 (0.085)	0.41 (0.085)
Hypotension	6440	0.99 (0.070)	0.68 (0.13)	0.43 (0.077)	0.37 (0.082)
CT class	5192				
1 or 2		zero (ref)	zero (ref)	zero (ref)	zero (ref)
3 or 4		1.08 (0.079)	0.77 (0.13)	0.77 (0.089)	0.77 (0.090)
5 or 6		0.96 (0.066)	0.67 (0.11)	0.56 (0.075)	0.54 (0.077)
Traumatic SAH	7393	0.99 (0.050)	0.84 (0.10)	0.72 (0.057)	0.73 (0.057)

illustration, we show the adjusted logistic regression coefficients of each of these predictors in turn (Table 8.4). We estimate adjusted effects in the complete cases (CC), as well as in completed data sets with single (SI) or multiple imputation (MI). SI and MI contain a random element for the imputed values.

Numbers of patients differ dramatically across the univariate and CC analyses, since only 2428 patients had complete values for all 7 predictors. Per predictor, values were complete for some (age, Motor score). Values were frequently incomplete for CT class, leaving $n = 5192$ for analysis. The coefficients for most of the predictors were largest in univariate analyses, and smaller in adjusted analyses. This reflects the positive correlations between predictors as noted in Table 8.3. The adjusted estimates were largely similar for SI or MI. The SEs in the CC analyses are higher than in the imputed analyses, reflecting smaller numbers. As expected, the MI analyses showed larger SEs than SI analyses, but differences were minor (third decimal).

Technical details of the model fitting are further discussed below with detailed code for R programs. We first describe the modeling for complete predictors (age, motor, 8.4.1), followed by the approach followed for predictors with missing values, such as pupils (Sect. 8.4.2).

8.4.1 Adjusted Analysis for Complete Predictors: Age and Motor Score

age and motor were completely available ($n = 8530$). Univariate effects can easily be estimated with logistic models (Table 8.4):

```
lrm(unfav ~ study + age, data = TBI1)
lrm(unfav ~ study + motor, data = TBI1)
```

Here, unfav refers to unfavorable GOS at 6 months, study is the study indicator, such that analyses are stratified by study, while assuming a common effect of the predictor across the studies.

A CC model with adjustment for confounders included only 2428 patients, due to exclusion of patients with any missing value for the other predictors (pupil, hypoxia, hypotens, CTclass, tsah). Only patients from studies 1, 2, and 10 are included:

```
## CC, n = 2428
lrm(unfav~study+age+motor+pupil+hypoxia+hypotens+ctclass+tsah, data = TBI1)
```

```
Frequencies of Missing Values Due to Each Variable
unfav study age motor pupil hypoxia hypotens ctclass tsah
    0     0   0     0  1387    3057     2090    3338 1137
  Obs Model L.R. d.f. P     C    R2 Brier
 2428         840   14 0 0.823 0.393 0.168

            Coef    S.E.    Wald Z Pr(>|Z|)
Intercept -1.9537 0.2060   -9.48 <0.0001
study=2   -0.1482 0.1211   -1.22 0.2212
study=10   0.0717 0.1372    0.52 0.6012
age        0.0357 0.0033   10.67 <0.0001
motor=3   -0.2876 0.1801   -1.60 0.1104
motor=4   -0.9308 0.1621   -5.74 <0.0001
motor=5/6 -1.6454 0.1597  -10.30 <0.0001
motor=9   -0.5833 0.2682   -2.17 0.0296
pupil=2    0.5143 0.1489    3.45 0.0006
pupil=3    0.9437 0.1437    6.57 <0.0001
hypoxia    0.4911 0.1248    3.94 <0.0001
hypotens   0.6786 0.1332    5.10 <0.0001
ctclass=2  0.7678 0.1343    5.72 <0.0001
ctclass=3  0.6749 0.1148    5.88 <0.0001
tsah       0.8409 0.1014    8.29 <0.0001
```

For SI, we create a completed data set from the first cycle of the MI object:

```
## SI, n = 8530
lrm(unfav~study+age+motor+pupil+hypoxia+hypotens+ctclass+tsah,
    data = complete(gm, action=1))
```

The MI model for age and motor score is fitted using the fit.mult.impute function, which automatically combines results over imputed data sets.

```
## MI, n = 8530
fit.mult.impute(unfav~study+age+motor+pupil+hypoxia+hypotens+ctclass+tsah,
           lrm, xtrans = gm, data = TBI1)
```

```
Variance Inflation Factors Due to Imputation:
Intercept study=2 study=3 study=4 study=5 study=6 study=7 study=8 study=9 study=10
     1.03    1.01    1.02    1.03    1.01    1.03    1.03    1.02    1.03    1.01
  study=11 age motor=3 motor=4 motor=5/6 motor=9 pupil=2 pupil=3 hypoxia hypotens
     1.01 1.02    1.02    1.04       1.02    1.04    1.22    1.42    1.59    1.28
 ctclass=2 ctclass=3 tsah
      1.09       1.45 1.11
  Obs  Model L.R. d.f.    C   R2  Brier¹
 8530       2529   22 0.80 0.34  0.183

              Coef    S.E.    Wald Z Pr(>|Z|)
Intercept  -1.5490 0.1139  -13.60 <0.0001
study=2    -0.1249 0.1023   -1.22 0.2220
     ...
study=11   -0.2572 0.1096   -2.35 0.0190
age         0.0348 0.0018   19.73 <0.0001
motor=3    -0.3662 0.0859   -4.26 <0.0001
motor=4    -0.9941 0.0738  -13.46 <0.0001
motor=5/6  -1.6050 0.0735  -21.82 <0.0001
motor=9    -0.7389 0.1284   -5.75 <0.0001
pupil=2     0.4997 0.0845    5.92 <0.0001
pupil=3     0.9777 0.0802   12.19 <0.0001
hypoxia     0.2945 0.0837    3.52 0.0004
hypotens    0.4976 0.0795    6.26 <0.0001
ctclass=2   0.5022 0.0730    6.88 <0.0001
ctclass=3   0.3656 0.0706    5.18 <0.0001
tsah        0.6325 0.0557   11.36 <0.0001
```

For the two complete[1] predictors (age and motor), we note very similar effects in SI or MI analyses (Table 8.4). Indeed, all results were similar for SI and MI (Table 8.5): model statistics (LR statistic, c statistic, R^2 estimate), as well as regression coefficients and standard errors.

8.4.2   Adjusted Analysis for Incomplete Predictors: Pupils

Pupillary reactivity was recorded for 7143 patients. This selection of patients was used in univariate and adjusted analyses, for fair comparability of univariate and adjusted effects.

```
# pupils
TBIc    < complete(gm, action = "long", include=TRUE) # completed data set
TBI2   <- TBIc[!TBIc$.id %in% TBIc$.id[is.na(TBIc$pupil)], ] # magic
gm2    <- as.mids(TBI2) # make this an MI object
fit.CC <- lrm(unfav ~ study + pupil, data = TBI2[TBI2$.imp==0,]) # orig data
fit.SI <- lrm(unfav ~ study+age+motor+pupil+hypoxia+hypotens+ctclass+tsah,
              data = TBI2[TBI2$.imp==1,]) # first imputed data
fit.MI <- fit.mult.impute(unfav ~ study+age+motor+pupil+ ... + tsah,
               lrm, xtrans = gm2) # 10 imputed sets
```

---

[1]These statistics are averaged over the 10 model fits.

Table 8.5 Multivariable regression coefficients and rounded prognostic scores for a 7 predictor model in the IMPACT study. Most scores are similar to complete case (CC), single imputation (SI) or multiple imputation (MI). Some differences in scores are noted for the effects of CT class (>2 points differences in **bold**)

	CC, $n = 2428$		SI, $n = 8530$		MI, $n = 8530$	
			mice		mice	
	Coef	Score	Coef	Score	Coef	Score
Age (per decade)	0.36	1[a]	0.35	1[a]	0.35	1[a]
Motor score[b]						
1 or 2	1.64	16	1.61	16	1.61	16
3	1.36	14	1.25	13	1.24	12
4	0.71	7	0.62	6	0.61	6
5 or 6	zero (ref)		zero (ref)		zero (ref)	
9	1.06	11	0.90	9	0.87	9
Pupillary reactivity						
Both pupil reactive	zero (ref)		zero (ref)		zero (ref)	
One nonreactive	0.51	5	0.46	5	0.50	5
Both nonreactive	0.94	9	0.91	9	0.98	10
Hypoxia	0.49	5	0.37	4	0.29	3
Hypotension	0.68	7	0.47	5	0.50	5
CT class						
1 or 2	zero (ref)		zero (ref)		zero (ref)	
3 or 4	0.77	**8**	0.51	5	0.50	5
5 or 6	0.67	**7**	0.37	4	0.37	4
Traumatic SAH[c]	0.84	8	0.62	6	0.63	6

[a]Age effect per 3 years
[b]Coded with 5/6 as the reference category for better interpretability
[c]SAH: subarachnoid hemorrhage

The results were as follows for the estimates of pupil coefficients and SE.

	2: One nonreactive pupil			3: Both pupils nonreactive		
	Uni	Adj, SI	Adj, MI	Uni	Adj, SI	Adj, MI
Coefficient	0.97	0.58	0.57	1.77	1.15	1.15
SE	0.076	0.085	0.085	0.067	0.076	0.077

Again, the results obtained with single or multiple imputation procedures were very similar. Analyses for the other predictors with missing values were performed in a similar way. A series of papers presents further results for the other predictors with missing values [85, 359, 364, 372, 595].

8.5 Predictions: Multivariable Analyses

After studying the adjusted effects per predictor, we were interested in the multi-variable effects of all predictors combined. We aimed to estimate a *global* prediction model: predictor effects are the same in each study, although the baseline risk can vary per study. So the intercept is study dependent, and the predictor effects are constant across studies.

We here focus on a model including the 7 predictors that were also used for adjustment before: 3 core predictors plus secondary insults plus CT characteristics. A CC analysis was possible with only 2428 patients, representing a loss of $8530 - 2428 = 6102$ patients (72%), while only 18% of the required values were missing ($11,009/(7 * 8530)$).

The multivariable coefficients are shown in Table 8.5, together with rounded prognostic scores. Scores were based on multiplying coefficients by 10, and rounding to whole numbers ("round(10*fit$coef)"). We note that the SI and MI coefficients and prognostic scores were largely similar. Scores never differed by more than 2 points. The CC analysis gave somewhat different estimates compared to SI or MI, demonstrating the limitation of CC analysis.

8.5.1 *Multilevel Analyses

The analyses for adjusted effects (Sect. 8.4) and the prediction models (Sect. 8.5) assumed global effects, i.e. that the effect of predictors was similar across studies. We adjusted for study as the main effect, as would be done in any meta-analysis. A richer model allows predictor effects to vary by study [30, 31]. Imputation should then also allow for differential imputation by study, as described in Sect. 8.3.4 [19]. We can quantify the between-study heterogeneity with random effect models, such as available in the glmer function in the lme4 package (see Chap. 21).

8.6 Concluding Remarks

This case study illustrates how we may deal with missing values in assessing predictor effects (univariate and adjusted effects, Sect. 8.4), and in multivariable modeling to derive a prediction model (Sect. 8.5), after inspection of missing value patterns (Sect. 8.2) and constructing an imputation model (Sect. 8.3). The difference in numbers of patients was dramatic between complete case (CC) and single or multiple imputed (SI and MI) data sets. A simple imputation model could easily be constructed, which is consistent with assuming global effects of predictors across studies. More advanced imputation is needed if we allow the effects of predictors to differ across studies in a meta-analysis context.

Questions

8.1 Missingness mechanisms

We state that most predictors were missing completely at random (MCAR), conditional on study (Sect. 8.2.3 e).

   (a) Does Table 8.2 support a MCAR mechanism?

   (b) What do we learn from Fig. 8.5 with respect to MAR on x, or MAR on y mechanisms?

   (c) Can we exclude a MNAR mechanism from the presented Tables and Figures?

8.2 Imputation results (Sect. 8.4.1).

   (a) For the MI model, the fit.mult.impute function lists "Variance Inflation Factors Due to Imputation". What do these factors refer to? When are they larger than 1? Which predictor has the largest VIF?

   (b) Compare the predictor effects of age between the CC, SI and MI models. When is the standard error estimated as the smallest?

   (c) Why is the standard error of a regression coefficient in a MI model slightly larger than that of a SI model?

Chapter 9
Coding of Categorical and Continuous Predictors

Summary When developing a prediction model, an important consideration is how we code the predictors. Raw data from a study are often not in a form appropriate for entering in regression models and must first be inspected and managed before the statistical analysis starts. As in any data analysis, we will usually start with obtaining an impression of the data under study, such as the occurrence of missing values and the distribution of predictors and outcome. Descriptive analyses, such as frequency tables and graphical displays, are useful to this aim. We will consider various issues in coding of unordered and ordered categorical predictors. For continuous predictors, we specifically discuss how we can limit the influence of outliers and interpret regression coefficients.

9.1 Categorical Predictors

Categorical predictors can be unordered, for example, a diagnostic category, or a type of hospital. Categorical predictors are usually coded as "factor" variables, with coding as dummy variables. For example, smoking was coded originally as "1" for never, "2" for past, and "3" for the current smoker in the GUSTO-I study. For analysis as a factor, we might create two dummy variables for category 2 versus 1 and 3 versus 1. Logistic regression coefficients for these dummy variables refer to the comparison of past vs never smokers and current vs never smokers. Dummy coding may often be convenient in prediction research. Specific attention should be paid to the choice of reference category (here: never smokers). By default, the lowest or highest numbered category is used as a reference in many statistical packages. If this category is relatively small, comparisons with this reference category may show statistically nonsignificant and unstable results, while the factor has an important predictive effect overall and is statistically significant. The predictions from a model are usually not affected by the choice of reference category.

© Springer Nature Switzerland AG 2019

E. W. Steyerberg, *Clinical Prediction Models*, Statistics for Biology and Health, https://doi.org/10.1007/978-3-030-16399-0_9

It may be convenient to combine categories if these are relatively small. For example, a cancer study might list a very large number of stages (e.g., T1a, T1b, T1c, T2a, T2x, etc.) that might be converted into a smaller number of groups (e.g., T1, T2, T3, and T4). In other situations, some categories might be very small and thus combined in an "other" category. If small categories are kept, some sort of penalized estimation or shrinkage is required to obtain reliable estimates (Chap. 13) [646]. When this combination of categories is based on the similarity of the relation with the outcome, overfitting may occur and the apparent model performance will be optimistic. In practice, a balance has to be sought between combining categories blinded to the outcome (e.g., based on frequency distributions) and adequately capturing patterns of the outcome by category. Using the coding from previous studies may often be helpful in smaller sized data sets.

Ordered categorical predictors are also common in prediction research. They pose a challenge to the analyst. Options include

- ignore the ordering, treat as an unordered categorical variable, with dummy variable coding;
- simplify to a dichotomous predictor;
- assume linearity of effect, as if we model a continuous predictor, perhaps with nonlinear extensions, such as adding a square term [225];
- enforce monotonicity of effect by some specific coding and penalized estimation; this is more flexible than coding as a continuous predictors [179, 646].

Table 9.1 illustrates that a dramatic loss of information may occur by dichotomization of an ordered predictor such as Killip class [472]. Simply assuming linearity of ordered predictor may sometimes work well.

Table 9.1 Impact of various coding schemes for categorical predictors in GUSTO-I ($n = 40,830$)

Predictor	Coding	df	LR statistic[a]
Unordered			
Location of infarct	Anterior versus other	1	343
	Ant/Inf/Other	2	361
Ordered			
Killip class (indicating left ventricular function)	Shock (3/4 versus 1/2)	1	861
	Linear (1–4)	1	1388
	Linear + square	2	1388
	Factor	3	1389
Smoking	Never/past/current	2	483
	Linear (1–3)	1	482

[a]LR statistic calculated as the difference between a model with and without the predictor on the -2 log likelihood scale

9.1.1 Examples of Categorical Coding

In patients with an acute MI, location of infarction is an important predictor of 30-day mortality. In GUSTO-I, the categorization was as anterior versus inferior versus others. The "other" location category contained only 3% of the patients [329]. A refined coding with "other" is only possible in large studies; in smaller sized studies we might combine the inferior and other categories, such that we compare Anterior location versus other location of the MI. Table 9.1 shows that the refined coding with 3 categories led to a slightly better predictive performance than the combined coding with 2 categories. The LR statistics were 361 versus 343, calculated as the differences between a model with and without the location of infarction on the -2 log likelihood scale (Table 9.1), at the expense of 1 df extra.

An example of an ordered predictor is Killip class, a measure for left ventricular function ranging from I to IV. It can be recoded as shock (Killip 3/4 versus 1/2) [395]. Alternatively, we can analyze ordered predictors as continuous variables. An easy relaxation of the linearity assumption is possible by adding a square term: y ~ Killip + Killip^2. A simple linear coding captures much of the predictive information (χ^2 1388). Adding a square term, or considering all categories as a factor variables with 3 dummy variables, did not add much (χ^2 1388 and 1389, respectively), while dichotomization would lose a substantial amount of predictive ability (χ^2 861). For a less clearly ordered variable such as smoking (never/past/ current), linear coding had the same performance as a factor variable, using 1 instead of 2 df (Table 9.1).

9.2 Continuous Predictors

Continuous variables formally should be measured at an interval or ratio scale, and should be able to take any value in a range. We noted in Table 9.1 that treating ordered variables as linear was sometimes reasonable for prediction.

9.2.1 *Examples of Continuous Predictors

Age is a good example of a continuous predictor variable that is relevant in many medical prediction problems. We already found that the age effect could often quite well be captured with a linear term (Chap. 6). Remarkably, age has often been considered as a dichotomized variable in prognostic studies, for example in traumatic brain injury [260]. Even worse than dichotomization as such is the search for optimal cut-points [12]. In GUSTO-I, a dichotomy at 65 years leads to a χ^2 of 1463

Table 9.2 Impact of various coding schemes for continuous predictors in GUSTO-I ($n = 40{,}830$)

Predictor	Coding	df	Model χ^2
Age	<=65 versus >65 years	1	1463
	<=60, 61–70, >=70	2	1814
	Linear	1	2099
	Linear + square	2	2112
	RCS, 5 knots[a]	4	2122
ST elevation	>4 versus <=4	1	256
	Linear (0–10)	1	281
	Linear + square	2	306
	RCS, 5 knots[a]	4	350
	Factor	10	364

[a]RCS denotes restricted cubic spline function; 5 knots lead to 4 df for the transformation of the predictor (see Sect. 9.3) [228]

instead of 2099 for age as a linear variable (Table 9.2). Considering 3 categories limits the loss in information somewhat (χ^2 1814, 86% of the information of age as a linear variable).

The predictor "number of leads with ST elevation" ranges from 0 to 10 in the GUSTO-I data (Chap. 22). The number of categories is large for consideration as a factor variable, but this can technically still be done. Simple linear coding leads to a slightly better performance than a dichotomy at 4 or more leads (χ^2 281 versus 259). Adding a square term led to further improvement in fit, exceeded by a restricted cubic spline function with 4 df (χ^2 350) [225].

9.2.2   Categorization of Continuous Predictors

Dichotomization of a continuous predictor has many disadvantages [472]. The first unnatural aspect is the step in predictions, as illustrated for age <=65 versus >65 years in Fig. 9.1. Would risks be really very different for patients who had their 65th birthday yesterday compared to patients who had their 65th birthday today? Similarly, the assumption of a constant risk below or above a threshold is unnatural. A patient of age 40 likely has lower risks of mortality than a patient of age 64; and a patient of age 90 is different from a patient of age 66. There are only 2 points where the dichotomized version of age may be considered adequate, i.e., around the intersections of predicted risks with the predicted risks according to the continuous variable (either linear or transformed). Moreover, if there had been a different distribution of ages, e.g., no patients older than 70 years old, the step function in Fig. 9.1 would have been much different. The continuous model, which conditions on all values of age, would remain relatively unchanged.

In contrast, the analysis of ST elevations as a predictor of mortality is more complex. A reasonable fit is achieved with a linear + square coding (Table 9.2,

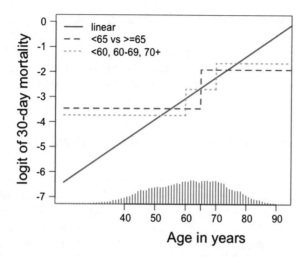

Fig. 9.1 Relation between age and 30-day mortality in GUSTO-I ($n = 40,830$). Age is modeled as a linear variable, dichotomized at age 65, or categorized in 3 groups (Table 9.2). The distribution of ages is shown at the bottom of the graph

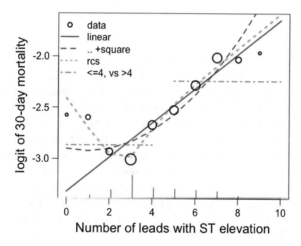

Fig. 9.2 Relation between the number of leads with ST elevation and 30-day mortality in GUSTO-I ($n = 40,830$). ST elevation is modeled as a linear variable, with extension with a square term, as a restricted cubic spline with 4 *df* (5 knots), and a dichotomized version of ST elevation (>4 leads, see Table 9.2). The observed risk for each number of leads with ST elevation is shown with circles (o), with size proportional to the square root of the number of events

Fig. 9.2). The risk associated with a low number of elevated leads (0–3) could also be well captured with a dichotomous categorization as >4 versus <=4 elevated leads. This example illustrates the importance of visual inspection of transformations. It is exceptional in leading to some credit for dichotomization, which is only rarely defendable over continuous coding [472].

In epidemiological research, continuous variables are often divided into 4 or 5 categories. This may be attractive as an exploratory step for predictor—outcome relations, but should not be used in a final prediction model [391]. Jumps in predictions are unnatural, and smooth relations are biologically far more plausible. Smooth functions can be coded with a limited number of degrees of freedom.

9.3   Nonlinear Functions for Continuous Predictors

When we consider a continuous predictor as a linear term in a prediction model, we assume that the effect is the same at each part of the range of the predictor. For example, in Fig. 9.1 we assume that the effect of being 10 years older is the same at age 30 (40 versus 30 years) and 70 years (80 versus 70 years) for patients with an acute MI. If a nonlinear function is expected, various options can readily be considered in regression models. Below we discuss nonlinear modeling of continuous predictors with (1) polynomials; (2) fractional polynomials, and (3) spline functions.

9.3.1   Polynomials

A classic approach to continuous predictors in regression analysis is to add polynomial terms as extensions to a model with a linear term. Commonly, square and cubic terms are considered [197]. For example, we can examine models with x, $x + x^2$, and $x + x^2 + x^3$, where x is a continuous predictor. This results in nested models, and we can statistically test each extension. From a pragmatic point of view, there is no objection to considering a model such as $x + x^3$, but it is more common to consider sequential extensions with terms of an increasingly higher order. Other common transformations to consider are the inverse (x^{-1}) and square root ($x^{0.5}$), and logarithmic ($\log(x)$ or $\ln(x)$, $\exp(x)$). We may use these terms as replacement of the linear term x, or an extension to a model with x as a linear term included. Polynomials are limited in the shapes they can take. We, therefore, consider wider families of models.

9.3.2   Fractional Polynomials (FP)

Fractional polynomials (FPs) have been advocated as a flexible approach to modeling continuous predictors [477]. FPs are an extension of earlier proposals on the transformation of predictors [69]. FPs allow for smooth and flexible transformation of continuous predictors by combining polynomials. FPs extend ordinary polynomials by including nonpositive and fractional powers from the set $-2, -1, -0.5, 0, 0.5, 1, 2, 3$. This defines 8 transformations, including inverse (x^{-1}), log (x^0), square root $(x^{0.5})$, linear (x^1), squared (x^2) and cubic transformations (x^3). In addition to these 8 "FP1" functions, 28 "FP2" functions can be considered of the form $x^{p1} + x^{p2}$; if $p1 = p2$ we define another 8 FP2 functions as $x^p + x^p \log(x)$, for a total of 36 FP2 functions [486]. These functions are assumed to use 2 and 4 *df*, respectively: 1 *df* for searching the transformation, and 1 *df* for estimation of the regression coefficient.

For medical problems, two terms (FP2 transformations) have been suggested as sufficient to describe nonlinear relations, e.g., *age^2 + age^0.5*. Such parametric combinations can be written down easily. Procedures have been proposed to select FP transformations in multivariable models [15, 477].

A disadvantage of FPs is a distortion of the global shape by values at the tails of the predictor distribution. The influence of extreme values can be prevented by a type of truncation ("winsorizing"), but the global shape of fractional polynomials remains influenced by the values at the tails. Furthermore, fractional polynomial functions depend on a change of origin of the covariate, and negative values cannot be handled. A pragmatic approach to these issues has been proposed to improve the robustness of FP models [476].

9.3.3 Splines

Quite flexible transformations are provided by spline functions. Various types of spline functions can be considered, such as natural splines. These can be fitted with a generalized additive model (gam) [230]. GAMs are also often used for non-parametric regression functions, such as lowess or loess. The extreme flexibility leads sometimes to wiggly patterns of predictions, which are unlikely to be reproduced in new data. Smoothness can be enforced by parameters in the model fitting process, e.g., penalty terms in the likelihood function (see Chap. 13) [231]. Without such penalty, splines may easily overfit patterns in the data.

Restricted cubic spline (RCS) functions have been proposed for a more stable approach to continuous predictor modeling [228]. RCSs are cubic splines (containing x^3 terms) that are restricted to be linear in the tails. These splines are still very flexible. They can take more forms than a parametric transformation with the same *df* in the model. For example, adding x^2 restricts the relation to be parabolic, while a RCS with 2 *df* (3 knots) incorporates a wider family of functions. See Harrell for many illustrations of the form that a RCS can take [225].

A spline function requires the specification of knots. The spline will bend around these knots. The exact position of the knots is not critical to the shape that the spline will take. It is common to specify the location from the distribution of the predictor variable [225]. More challenging is the choice of the number of knots. Empirical illustrations have shown that using 5 knots (4 df) is sufficient to capture many nonlinear patterns. In smaller data sets, it may often be reasonable to use linear terms or splines with 3 knots (2 df), especially if no strong prior information suggests that a nonlinear function is necessary [225]. If a large data set is available, 4 or 5 knots may be reasonable, especially if we anticipate a nonlinear function for an important predictor.

RCS of increasing complexity are not nested functions, so testing of higher order transformations to simplify a complex nonlinear model in a stepwise manner is not formally correct. It is, however, possible to study the increase in model Likelihood Ratio (LR) while taking the extra degrees of freedom into account, e.g.,as Chi-square—2 * df (a rephrasing of Akaike's Information Criterion) [225].

9.3.4   *Example: Functional Forms with RCS or FP

We examined the transformations for continuous predictors in the GUSTO-I study; both in a large subsample ($n = 785$) and the full data set ($n = 40,830$, Fig. 9.3). In the subsample, we first fit a second order fractional polynomial (FP2); the optimal model is $age^{-2}+age^{3}$. We compare the shape to a restricted cubic spline (RCS) function. An FP2 function uses 4 df, but the shape cannot have more than 2 bendings. An RCS with 5 knots also uses 4 df. For age, weight, and height, FP2 functions were explored in univariate and multivariable logistic regression analysis; no statistically significant nonlinearity was identified in the subsample of 785 patients. In the full GUSTO-I data set, age^{2} was chosen as the optimal transformation. For weight and height nonlinearity was not statistically significant. Overall, the use of RCS or FP functions led to very similar patterns in Fig. 9.3. This was also found in a case study of prostate cancer patients [406].

9.3.5   Extrapolation and Robustness

Extrapolation beyond the range of observed data is always dangerous, but is readily possible with RCS and FP functions. An interesting intermediate approach is to aim for a parametric transformation that captures most of the nonlinearity of a predictor. Adequacy of the fit can be tested by adding RCS functions based on the transformed variable [228]. For example, in a prostate cancer prediction problem, PSA values were linearly related to outcome after a log transformation [562], while the original model in this prediction problem was constructed with RCS functions with 5 knots [295]. The log transformation often performs well for laboratory

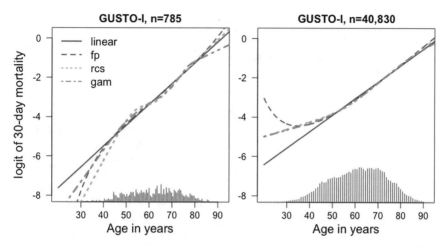

Fig. 9.3 Comparison of 3 nonlinear fits in a sample from the GUSTO-I data (left, $n = 785$) and the full data set (right, $n = 40,830$). Fractional polynomials (fp), restricted cubic splines (rcs), and general additive models (gam) each had 4 degrees of freedom ($df = 4$). In the full data set, rcs and gam follow very similar shapes, while the fp function behaves differently at young ages. Deviations from linearity occur at the extremes of the distributions, where limited data are available

measurements. Restricting a continuous predictor to a parametric transformation may seem to harm the apparent performance somewhat. But it may limit optimism in performance and increase a model's robustness. Care should always be given to predictions at the tails of a distribution [470].

9.3.6   Preference for FP or RCS?

Various empirical comparisons between FPs and RCSs have been made [51, 572]. The main differences are expected to occur at the tails of the distribution, where the RCS was restricted to have linear behavior, which contributes to robustness (see Fig. 9.3). If we have a predictor where a true curvature occurs at the tails, this will be captured by the FP and less so by the RCS. If such curvatures are spurious, RCS will do better. In practice, both approaches may perform similarly in fitting a nonlinear relation given the same number of df, especially with winsorizing to limit the impact of extreme values (see below). Sample size is also crucial: "From limited information, a suitable explanatory model cannot be obtained. Prediction performance from all types of nonlinear models is similar" [51]. A number of options for dealing with continuous predictors in prediction models are summarized in Table 9.3.

Table 9.3 Options for dealing with continuous predictors in prediction models

Procedure	Characteristics	Recommendation
Dichotomization	Simple, easy interpretation	Bad idea
More categories	3, 4, or 5 categories capture more prognostic information, but are not smooth, sensitive to the choice of cut-points and unstable	Only for illustration
Linear	Simple	Often reasonable as a start
Polynomials	Square, cubic terms added; tails may behave unstably	Reasonable as checks for nonlinearity
Transformations	Log, square root, inverse, …	May provide robust summaries of nonlinearity
Fractional polynomials (FP)	Flexible combinations of polynomials; tails may behave unstably	Flexible descriptions of nonlinearity
Restricted cubic splines (RCS)	Flexible functions with robust behavior at the tails of predictor distributions	Flexible descriptions of nonlinearity
Splines in gam	Flexible functions with smoothness set by penalty terms	Highly flexible descriptions of nonlinearity

9.4   Outliers and Winsorizing

Outliers are an important concern in many statistical analyses. Outliers are values that are outside the typical range for a variable. In Box plots, a box is usually shown with the median and the interquartile range (IQR, 25–75 percentile). Outliers are defined by Tukey as values at least 3 times the IQR above the third quartile or at least 3 times the IQR below the first quartile [251]. We consider outliers as any values that potentially have a large influence in a regression model.

The first question to address for an outlier is whether the value is perhaps a data entry error. The records of a patient could be checked for the plausibility of a value, e.g., the hospital chart or the case report form when the patient participated in a trial.

Another check is on biological plausibility. This judgment requires expert opinion and depends on the clinical setting. For example, a systolic blood pressure of 250 mmHg is biologically plausible in the acute care situation for traumatic brain injury patients, but may not be plausible in an ambulatory care situation. Implausible values may best be considered as errors and hence set to missing.

For biologically possible values, various statistical approaches are subsequently possible. To reduce the influence on the regression coefficients ("leverage") we may consider transforming the variable by "winsorizing" (Table 9.4). Winsorizing means replacement of extreme values with a certain percentile value from each end, while trimming or truncation formally means the removal of outliers. With winsorizing, very high and very low values are shifted to the center:

Table 9.4 Dealing with outliers and extreme values of continuous predictors in prognostic research

Procedure	Method	Recommendation
Outlier detection	Box plot	Verify correctness (data entry error?) and biological plausibility (missing if implausible value)
Winsorizing	Shift low and high values to the center of a distribution	Shift approximately 1% of very low and 1% of very high values to lower and upper ends of a range

$$\text{If } x > x_{max} \text{ then } x = x_{max};$$
$$\text{If } x < x_{min} \text{ then } x = x_{min};$$
$$\text{else } x = x$$

Here, x_{max} and x_{min} may be defined as upper and lower percentile points, or by clinical input. A reasonable choice may be to use the 1 and 99 percentiles for winsorizing [476].

9.4.1   Example: Glucose Values and Outcome of TBI

As an example, we consider glucose values measured at admission to predict 6-month outcome of patients with traumatic brain injury (TBI, Chap. 8). We consider 2159 patients from the Tirilazad trials, who had both glucose values and outcome available in $n = 2095$.

1. The upper threshold for biologically possible glucose values was set at 100 mmol/l. Only 3 patients had values above this threshold, which were set to missing.
2. We winsorize glucose values to the interval [3–20 mmol/l] to limit the influence of extreme values (Fig. 9.4). The glucose–outcome relation becomes slightly more linear after winsorizing (Fig. 9.5).

9.5   Interpretation of Effects of Continuous Predictors

Effects of predictors can be interpreted through various presentations. A general way is to examine the predictions by predictor values, for example, as the predicted probabilities from a logistic model. A graph is often very useful, especially for

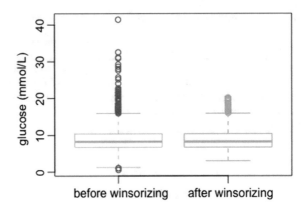

Fig. 9.4 Distribution of glucose for 2095 TBI patients before and after winsorizing of values close to the 1 and 99% percentiles

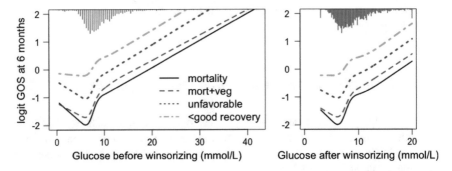

Fig. 9.5 Relation of glucose to Glasgow Outcome Scale (GOS) at 6 months after TBI before (left) and after (right panel) winsorizing to the interval [3–20 mmol/l]. The lowest line (solid) indicates the probability of mortality (GOS 1), the second the combination of mortality and vegetative state (GOS 1 or 2), the third unfavorable outcome (GOS 1, 2, or 3), and the fourth line the probability of less than good outcome (GOS < 5). Relations were analyzed with restricted cubic spline functions (5 knots, 4 *df*) in logistic regression models. The glucose–outcome relation becomes slightly more linear after winsorizing. The distribution of glucose values is indicated at the top of each graph

nonlinear effects of predictors. For binary outcomes, the choice of scale is critical. Linear transformations from logistic regression models are straight lines at the log odds (or logit) scale, but nonlinear at the probability scale. Similarly, we can plot the effects of continuous predictors of survival outcomes at the log hazard scale or as survival probabilities.

We can interpret the coefficients from a regression model by converting them to odds ratios (logistic regression) or hazard ratios (survival models, e.g., Cox regression). For binary variables such as gender, scaling is straightforward: the odds ratio (OR) will refer to the comparison of females versus males if females are coded one unit higher than males (e.g., 1/0).

For continuous variables, the scaling is important for interpretability and comparability of effects. For example, the predictive effect is usually small if age is coded in years. In GUSTO-I, the univariate logistic regression coefficient is 0.084, or an OR of 1.088 per year older, in the analysis of 30-day mortality. A simple improvement is to divide the age variable by 10 before estimating the model, such that the age effect is interpreted by decade. We can also multiply the coefficient that was estimated by year: In GUSTO-I, the univariate logistic regression coefficient becomes $10 * 0.084$, and the OR $1.088^{10} = 2.32$. Similarly, for other variables with a wide range in units, e.g., laboratory measurements, division by 10, 100, or 1000 may help. Comparability of effects of different continuous variables is still difficult then.

Another approach is to standardize linear, continuous predictors by dividing them by their standard deviation.[1] A variant on this approach was proposed by Harrell, i.e., to compare the effects of predictors at the 75 versus 25 percentiles [225]. For linear, continuous variables, this can be achieved by dividing the values by the interquartile range. Note that such rescaling does not affect *p*-values or predictions in any way. The interpretation becomes dependent on the distribution of the predictor in the data set as analyzed; this is a disadvantage when comparing effects across studies.

For nonlinear coding of continuous variables, we can again compare the predicted outcomes at specific points of the distribution, e.g., the 75 versus 25 percentile [225]. Interpretability is most difficult for parabolic relations (e.g., a quadratic form); an OR near 1 may be found when comparing the 75 versus 25 percentile predictions. A somewhat related, simple alternative is to code a nonlinear variable with 2 dummy variables: one indicating values below the 25 percentile and 1 indicating values above the 75 percentile. The middle category is defined by the 25–75 percentile and serves as a reference category for both dummy variables. Admittedly, such categorized coding implies a loss of information. Moreover, the effects in the dummy coding depend on the distribution of the predictor. Such coding is, therefore, more useful for illustration of a predictor effect than for making predictions.

9.5.1   *Example: Predictor Effects in TBI*

Various continuous predictors were measured at admission to predict 6-month outcome of patients with traumatic brain injury (TBI). The relation of age and

---

[1]Note that standardization does not work well for categorical variables or nonlinear transformations such as polynomials.

Table 9.5 Examples of coding of continuous predictors in predicting the outcome of TBI

Predictor	Procedure	Interpretation
Age (linear)	Compare predictions at age 40 to 30 years	Age by decade
	Coding: divide by 10	Age by decade
	Compare predictions at age 45 to 21 years	Age by IQR
	Coding: divide by 24 (24 is IQR)	Age by IQR
Systolic blood pressure (quadratic relation)	Illustrate nonlinear effect by making 3 categories, with dummy variables for <120 mmHg, >150 mmHg	Effects for relatively low and high blood pressure

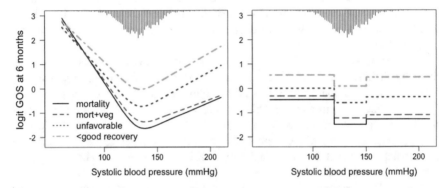

Fig. 9.6 Relation of systolic blood pressure to Glasgow Outcome Scale (GOS) at 6 months after TBI before (left) and after (right panel) categorization as <120, 120–150, and >150 mmHg. The lowest line (solid) indicates the probability of mortality (GOS 1), the second the combination of mortality and vegetative state (GOS 1 or 2), the third unfavorable outcome (GOS 1, 2, or 3), and the fourth line the probability of less than good outcome (GOS < 5). The coding with continuous values had a higher R^2 than the categorized coding (8.1% versus 5.2% for mortality)

glucose to outcome were reasonably linear. Effects were presented for the interquartile range (IQR, Table 9.5).

The relation of systolic blood pressure with outcome was nonlinear: low blood pressure was especially associated with a poor GOS, and GOS was also poorer at higher blood pressure values. This relation was modeled with a restricted cubic spline with 3 knots (2 *df*, Fig. 9.6).

The 75 percentile is a pressure of 142; the 25 percentile 121 mmHg. The OR for the comparison of predictions at these points is 1.6 [1.4–1.9] for mortality. For illustration, we categorize blood pressure at 120 and 150 mmHg. This leads to ORs of 2.8 and 1.2 for blood pressure <120 and >150 versus 120–150 mmHg respectively. So, the 6-month mortality was more than twice as high with relatively low blood pressure, and 1.2 times worse with a relatively high pressure compared to an intermediate pressure level. This categorized coding has a R^2 of 5.2%. compared to 8.1% for the continuous coding, arguing against the use of dummy coding for predictive purposes. Hence, such categorized coding may only be reasonable to illustrate effects rather than to replace the nonlinear continuous variable in a prediction model.

9.6 Concluding Remarks

We have seen that some decisions on coding can be made while we are blinded to the relation of the predictor to the outcome in our sample. Such blinding limits overfitting. Another general strategy is to use the coding of predictors as used in other studies.

Special attention is required for continuous predictors. Most natural processes have a more or less smooth association with an outcome. Simple extensions of linear terms, such as the square and square root, can be useful, as well as more flexible functions such as restricted cubic splines (RCS) and fractional polynomials (FP).

We focused on the effects of single predictors, which are usually first considered in a univariate analysis. The effects may also be studied with adjustment for other predictors ("confounders", multivariable analysis). If the aim is to derive a prediction model, we are less interest in the specific forms of the relation of each predictor with the outcome. A detailed modeling strategy has been proposed for the simultaneous selection of predictors for a model and their FP transformations ("multivariable fractional polynomial (MFP) modeling" [477].). Harrell has suggested to determine the number of degrees of freedom with RCS in univariate analyses, and use the chosen level of complexity in further multivariable analyses, irrespective of statistical significance of higher order terms [225]. Another reasonable strategy might be to fit a model with all continuous predictors in flexible forms, e.g.,with 4 *df*, and then decide on reducing *df* per predictor based on their contribution to the model, e.g., according to partial R^2. Stronger predictors are then given more flexibility than weaker predictors, without considering the degree of nonlinearity. Approaches to nonlinearity in the multivariable analysis are discussed in more depth in Chap. 12.

9.6.1 Software

RCS and FP functions can be used with any statistical program, but may require some programming. RCS functions are very easy to use with R (rcs function in Harrell's rms library) and Stata. Algorithms for fractional polynomials are available for R (mfp), Stata, and SAS [485]. Examples are available at www.clinicalpredictionmodels.org.

Questions

9.1. Dichotomization: a bad idea [472]

   (a) What are the problems of dichotomization when focusing on the effect of one specific predictor, such as age?
   (b) What are the problems of dichotomization when studying the effect of gender (male versus female) and potential confounders, such as age, are dichotomized in an adjusted analysis?
   (c) What are the problems of dichotomization of predictors, such as age, when we aim to make individualized predictions?

9.2. Categorization of continuous predictors
   In an analysis of BNP, the authors of a paper state: "To produce odds ratios, cut-points were used for age (65 years) and BNP (62 pg/mL) to reduce them to nominal variables [352]."

   (a) Why should continuous predictors not be categorized?
   (b) For be useful?
   (c) What suggestion would you have for the authors if they want to calculate interpretable odds ratios for continuous predictors?

9.3. Winsorizing extreme values

   (a) Why are extreme values a problem in regression analysis?
   (b) How could you define winsorizing in one simple statement in R software for a continuous predictor x?

9.4. Flexible continuous functions
   What are the advantages and disadvantages of flexible modeling of continuous predictors, e.g., using restricted cubic spline functions?

Chapter 10
Restrictions on Candidate Predictors

Summary A major challenge in prediction modeling is that we may have more candidate predictors available for the analysis than we would like to include for further analysis, in particular if our data set is relatively small. A small sample size leads to problems as discussed in Chap. 5, such as limited power to test effects of potential predictors, and too extreme predictions when predictions are based on the standard regression coefficients (overfitting). We discuss some procedures to increase the robustness and validity of a prediction model, including restriction of the number of candidate predictors based on subject knowledge, considering distributions of predictors, combining similar variables, and averaging the effects of similar variables. We provide a detailed description of a case study of modeling similar effects of aspects of family history for robust prediction of the presence of a genetic mutation.

10.1 Selection Before Studying the Predictor–Outcome Relation

From a statistical modeling perspective, it would be ideal to prespecify a prediction model completely. This implies that candidate predictors are selected without studying the predictor–outcome relation in the data under study. Potential approaches are to use subject knowledge, external to the study; and to study the distribution of predictors in the data under study.

© Springer Nature Switzerland AG 2019
E. W. Steyerberg, *Clinical Prediction Models*, Statistics for Biology and Health, https://doi.org/10.1007/978-3-030-16399-0_10

10.1.1   Selection Based on Subject Knowledge

The list of candidate predictors can often be reduced based on a review of the literature on the specific topic, combined with consulting experts in the field. The development of a prognostic model in situations without such subject knowledge on at least some predictors is nearly impossible, unless huge sample sizes are available. In many medical problems, a list in the order of 5–20 potential predictors is reasonable to develop an adequate prediction model. Even in genetic research, it has been suggested that at most 20 genes should be included in a prediction model (although many more are usually considered, necessitating very large sample sizes) [336]. On the other hand, simulations show that many genes are needed for adequate predictive power if effects per gene are small [278].

10.1.2   *Examples: Too Many Candidate Predictors

In predicting the underlying diagnosis in children presenting with fever without an obvious cause, models were developed that considered 57 candidate predictors [57]. The sample size was relatively small, with 231 patients including 58 with the diagnosis of interest (severe bacterial infection). The model was developed with stepwise methods after a univariate screening for statistically significant predictors. The model seemed to perform reasonable, but external validation showed poor results [55]. On further analysis, bootstrapping of the full modeling process indicated a substantial decrease in expected model performance. A large part of the poor performance in new patients could be attributed to the modeling strategy with too many candidate predictors [535].

Similarly, a prediction model for diagnosing Lynch syndrome was published in *NEJM*, considering over 37 candidate predictors (with dichotomization of continuous predictors) in a cohort where 38 mutations were found among 870 participants. Simulations showed over 50% bias for 5 of 6 originally selected predictors, unstable model specification, and poor performance at validation [563]. Indeed, the proposed model performed poorly in a comparative international validation study of 3 prediction models [290].

10.1.3   Meta-Analysis for Candidate Predictors

We may consider to perform a systematic literature review or even a formal meta-analysis to identify candidate predictors. Some objections can be made against meta-analysis of univariate effects of predictors. Correlations between variables make that their effects are different in multivariable analyses. In the case of negative correlations, the univariate effects are suppressed. This results in no relation between the predictor and outcome in univariate analysis, while multivariable analysis does show a relation. This situation may be relatively rare, but if this is suspected, the univariate effect of the predictor from previous studies should not be used as guidance to whether the candidate predictor is considered. In medical applications, most correlations between variables are positive, making univariate effects larger than multivariable effects.

Another question is whether we should only count the number of times that a predictor was identified as "important", or perform a formal meta-analysis, which summarizes effect estimates. Counting may be sufficient for identification of the key predictors in a prediction problem. Meta-analysis is desired if we want to use the univariate effects of previous studies as a kind of prior estimate in our model (see Chap. 15). Publication bias is an important objection to such a formal meta-analysis of predictors. Many studies will not report the effect of a predictor if not statistically significant; this biases the reported effects to more extreme values (Winner's curse [267], see Chaps. 5 and 11). One approach is to consider only studies that report the results for all predictors considered, but this may severely limit the numbers of studies in the meta-analysis.

10.1.4   Example: Predictors in Testicular Cancer

We reviewed the prognostic value of a core set of prognostic factors for the histology of residual masses in testicular cancer [554]. The predictors that emerged as most relevant in the review were subsequently used in a prediction model. Some further fine-tuning was done [566]. This fine-tuning included searching for good transformations of continuous variables, and choosing between 3 variables related to mass size: pre-chemotherapy mass size, post-chemotherapy mass size, and reduction in mass size (calculated as [presize–postsize]/presize).

10.1.5   Selection Based on Distributions

After restricting the list of potential predictors, we should consider the distributions of predictors for missing values and width of the distribution. We may choose to eliminate variables that have a large number of missing values, especially if

- the predictor is relatively important in the problem, such that imputation of missing values will be suspect to many readers;
- the predictor will be missing in applications of the model;

Also, we may choose to eliminate variables that have a narrow distribution. Especially if the variable is not expected to be important, this may be reasonable.

The situation is more difficult when a predictor has a very skewed distribution but is known to be highly predictive. For example, in GUSTO-I, shock occurred in 2% of the patients but had a large effect (univariate OR 11). Several options are available to deal with such a variable, such as

1. include the variable as a predictor, since the effect is substantial;
2. omit the variable from the model, since the effect cannot be estimated reliably; the model might be presented with a warning that specific conditions, such as shock, are not included in the model;
3. omit patients with shock, making the model applicable only to patients without shock.

As a default strategy we might prefer option 1, i.e., to include important variables, even though they are infrequent. The second option, in fact, holds for all potential predictor variables that are not included in a model: predictions only consider information on variables that were included. The third option may only be defendable when we postulate that patients with shock are different with respect to predictor–outcome relations of other variables, i.e., we assume interaction with shock for other predictors.

10.2   Combining Similar Variables

Sometimes variables can be grouped such that less degrees of freedom (*df*) are used for modeling their effects. Such combination is a trade-off between greater robustness against missing details of the effects of individual predictors.

10.2.1   Subject Knowledge for Grouping

Grouping can often be based on subject knowledge. As an example, we consider the coding of "atherosclerosis", which is a systemic disease that is reflected in many symptoms. These symptoms can hence be considered as one group reflecting the underlying concept of "presence of atherosclerotic disease" (Table 10.1) [314]. We could code "presence of atherosclerotic disease" as 0 or 1, depending on the presence of any symptom. We could also make a simple unweighted sum, by counting the number of symptoms. For 6 symptoms, the sum ranges from 0 to 6. We could winsorize such an unweighted sum as 0, 1, 2, 3+ , depending on the distribution, and start modeling with this sum as a linear, continuous predictor.

Another example is the coding of comorbidity. The presence of concomitant diseases ("comorbidity") is important in many prediction problems. Various systems have been proposed to quantify comorbidity. Weighted sumscores can be used such as proposed in the Charlson score [93] or ACE-27 [439] Note that these scores

Table 10.1 Illustrations of simple summary variables based on combinations of different predictors

Concept	Variables	Range
Atherosclerotic disease in predicting renal artery stenosis [314]	Any femoral or carotid bruit, angina pectoris, claudication, myocardial infarction, CVA, or had vascular surgery	0–1
Comorbidity in predicting surgical mortality in esophageal cancer [560]	Count of chronic pulmonary disease, cardiovascular disease, diabetes, liver disease, renal disease	0–5
Comorbidity in predicting mortality in various cancers [287, 439]	Count of ACE-27 elements	0–27
Family history in predicting a genetic mutation [40]	Sum of # affected 1st degree family members plus 0.5 * # affected 2nd degree family members	0–3

were derived for specific populations. Subject matter knowledge hence needs to support that it is reasonable to apply such as a predefined weighted score in another setting.

Alternative codings may be considered, depending on sample size. In very large data sets, e.g., using >100,000 subjects, a detailed coding can be imagined, which considers study-specific regression coefficients for each comorbidity. Also, a simple score can be attractive, for example, the sum of a number of comorbidities [158, 287]. Such an unweighted sum may be rather robust and may generalize well to new settings. Such a simple sum was applied in a prediction model for surgical mortality after esophagectomy (Table 10.1) [560].

10.2.2   Assessing the Equal Weights Assumption

Simple sums of predictors make the assumption of equal weights for each predictor. This assumption can be assessed by adding the conditions one by one in a regression model that already contains the sumscore. The coefficient of the condition added in a model indicates the deviation from the common effect based on the other conditions. We can use an overall test for the decision whether a simple sum is reasonable, or that a more refined coding is required. In the example of comorbidity, we may consider the sum of 5 comorbidity conditions (Table 10.2). We may assess the effect of each of the 5 conditions by fitting 5 logistic regression models, with a separate coefficient for the deviation from the common effect for each of the 5 conditions in turn. We note that the deviations from the common effect are relatively small, except for liver disease and renal disease. Renal disease even seemed to have a protective effect. Both effects were based on small numbers. The standard errors of the estimates were large, and the effects were statistically nonsignificant. The overall test for deviations from the simple sum had a χ^2 statistic of only 3.6, 4 df, and a p-value of 0.46, in a model with the simple sum and 4 comorbidities added (chronic pulmonary disease,

Table 10.2 Illustration of testing deviations for each condition in a sum score. Data from esophageal cancer patients who underwent surgery (2041 patients from SEER-Medicare data, 221 died by 30 days [560]). The overall test for deviations from a simple sum score had a p-value of 0.46 (overall test, 4 *df*)

Model	Logistic regression coefficient	*p*-value
Comorbidity sumscore	0.44 (± 0.13)	<0.001
. + chronic pulmonary disease	–0.22 (± 0.31)	0.48
. + cardiovascular disease	–0.13 (± 0.33)	0.69
. + diabetes	+0.32 (± 0.29)	0.27
. + liver disease	+1.31 (± 1.03)	0.20
. + renal disease	–1.09 (± 1.11)	0.33

cardiovascular disease, diabetes, renal disease). We hence may stick to our assumption of a similar effect for liver disease as for the other 4 comorbidities, and a similar effect for renal disease as for the other 4 comorbidities.

10.2.3   Biologically Motivated Weighting Schemes

Instead of equal weights, we can sometimes base weights on a biological relation. For example, when we model family history, we know that the genetic distance between family members is 0.5 between 2nd and 1st degree relatives, and 0.25 between 3rd and 1st degree relatives. This relation can be used to define a variable for family history (Table 10.1).

Such a coding was used in a model to predict the likelihood of a genetic mutation in patients suspected for Lynch syndrome [40, 534]. A proband with 1 affected 1st degree family member receives a similar score for family history (1) as a proband with 2 affected 2nd degree family members. An implicit assumption here is that the numbers at risk are similar for 1st and 2nd degree family members, e.g., with similar numbers and similar age distributions.

10.2.4   Statistical Combination

Harrell proposed to use principal component analysis (PCA) to summarize the information from all candidate predictors [226]. This clustering technique does not use the information on the predictor–outcome relation. An objection to such clustering is that the interpretability of regression coefficients is lost. Moreover, all predictor values have to be filled to calculate predictions. There is some similarity with the clustering analysis applied in some studies of genetic markers [511]. The machine learning community seems to embrace principal components analysis [283].

10.3   Averaging Effects

In regression modeling, we usually start with modeling main effects of variables. We subsequently may assess interaction effects as tests for additivity of effects. Conceptually, the main effects average over underlying subgroup effects. This averaging may be reasonable as long as no strong interactions exist, and adds to the robustness of the model. This issue has a parallel with how we study treatment effects in RCTs, where we should focus on the main effect rather than subgroup effects [298−300]. Subgroup effects should be considered as secondary analyses, and may often be misleading [18, 240, 658].

10.3.1   Chlamydia Trachomatis Infection Risks

The starting point for modeling determines how our final model may look. For example, prediction of Chlamydia trachomatis infections has traditionally focused on infection prevalences in women. However, when we have a data set which contains infection status for both men and women, we may debate how to view model development. On the one hand, we may develop a male model fully independent from the female model. This is equivalent to assuming interactions between all predictors and sex. The models for males and females may adequately fit risk patterns for both sexes separately, but the predictions will be less reliable because of the reduced sample size. The obvious alternative is to start with a model in the combined data, and assuming similar effects in males and females. This assumption can specifically be tested by interaction terms of sex * predictor. In a case study, only the effect of urogenital symptoms clearly differed between the sexes [191].

10.3.2   *Example: Acute Surgery Risk Relevant for Elective Patients?

In the Chlamydia trachomatis example, we were interested in prediction for both males and females. In another case, we were specifically interested in patients undergoing elective replacement of a heart valve [619]. In our data set, we also had information on patients undergoing acute valve replacement. Should these patients be excluded? We decided to include these patients in our modeling process, with inclusion of the main effect for acute versus elective surgery. We tested whether predictive effects were different between these types of patients, and found no such indication for any predictor separately nor in an overall test for interaction. Hence, it might be reasonable to assume that increasing the sample size by adding these high-risk acute surgery patients helped to improve our predictions for elective patients. More precisely stated, we assume that the relevance of any bias is smaller than the increase in precision by increasing sample size. This assumption seems reasonable from the data, but paradoxically a small sample size limits the power to detect differential effects. Therefore, subject matter knowledge is the main guidance to when effects would be so different that the bias in the predictions for the patients of interest harms the modeling in the total group.

10.4 *Case Study: Family History for Prediction of a Genetic Mutation

We consider the case study of diagnosing mutations in patients suspected of Lynch syndrome, or "hereditary nonpolyposis colorectal cancer" (HNPCC) [40]. Mutations can be diagnosed with a genetic test, which is costly. Therefore, some selection of patients for testing is required. Family history has traditionally been used for such selection, with simple rules. These rules include young age at diagnosis of colorectal cancer (CRC) as an important predictor, e.g., "2 family members with CRC <50 years". Also, the number of 1st and 2nd degree relatives is important, with more family members making a mutation as the cause of the cancer more likely.

10.4.1 Clinical Background and Patient Data

Lynch syndrome is the most common hereditary colorectal cancer (CRC) syndrome in Western countries, accounting for 2–5% of all CRCs [356]. Lynch syndrome is associated with underlying mutations in the mismatch repair system, most commonly in the *MLH1* and *MSH2* genes. Empirically derived prediction models have been developed for the likelihood of mutations in individual patients or families, enabling a more refined selection of subjects compared to simple rules. Some models use logistic regression [40, 42, 345, 672], while others use Bayesian methods [96]. Several aspects of family history are considered in these models, related to the presence and age at diagnosis of cancer in the proband (the index person who is first being tested in a family), and the presence and age at diagnosis of cancer in his/her relatives. Modeling family history is complex, since the spectrum of cancers associated with *MLH1* and *MSH2* mutations is diverse. Mutation carriers are mainly at risk of developing colorectal and endometrial cancer [356]. Young age at diagnosis is suspect for being a mutation carrier, and family members with various degrees of genetic relation to the proband need to be considered.

We consider a development sample of 898 patients, who were tested for the presence of mutations (130 with mutation). Patients usually had one or more of various cancer diagnoses, including colorectal cancer (CRC, $n = 536$), women with endometrial cancer ($n = 91$), and other HNPCC-related cancer ($n = 100$). Of the

898 patients, 118 had multiple cancers. Details on predictor and outcome definitions and modeling issues are described elsewhere [40, 534].

10.4.2   Similarity of Effects

Colorectal cancer (CRC) at a young age is a well-known predictor of a mutation. Especially if multiple CRCs occur in the same patients, this is very suspect for an underlying genetic cause. Further, CRC in the family history points at HNPCC. We illustrate the modeling of CRC effects for the prediction of the presence of a mutation:

(1) What are the effects of a CRC diagnosis below age 50?
(2) How can we estimate the effect of age of CRC diagnosis as a continuous predictor?
(3) How can we estimate a single effect of CRC diagnosis as a continuous predictor for those with one or multiple CRCs diagnoses?
(4) Is there need for a nonlinear transformation in the age effect?

(1) We first study the effect of CRC below 50.

We make 2 dummy variables: 1 for having 1 CRC below age 50 years (CRC1 < 50) and another for having 2 CRC diagnoses with the first diagnosis made below age 50 years (CRC2 < 50). The model is

$$\text{Mutation} \sim \text{CRC1} < 50 + \text{CRC2} < 50,$$

where Mutation indicates the presence of a mutation (0/1), and $\sim$ indicates the logistic regression link.

We can also use 2 terms for each, reflecting probabilities of mutation below and over 50 years: Mutation $\sim$ CRC1 < 50 + CRC1 >= 50 + CRC2 < 50 + CRC2 >= 50.

In the first formula, 2 coefficients are estimated for those with CRC at age <50 years ("CRC < 50"). All other patients form the reference category. Estimated coefficients were 0.58 and 1.86. In the second formula, 4 coefficients are estimated for those with CRC, and patients without CRC are the reference (Fig. 10.1). Coefficients for CRC1 were 0.54 and −0.50, and for CRC2 2.09 and 1.82 (age <50 and age >=50 years, respectively). Therefore, patients with 1 CRC, diagnosed after age 50, had a lower estimated probability of mutation compared to patients without a CRC.

(2) We now turn to the age of CRC diagnosis as a continuous predictor.

We need to insert an age for those without CRC. A simple strategy would be to impute "0" for patients without CRC. An indicator variable would then be used for "CRC", referring to the difference in probability of mutation at age zero between those with and without CRC. To obtain a more interpretable effect of the indicator variable for CRC, we set age at 45 years, since 45 years is around the average age

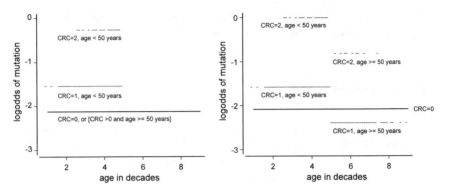

Fig. 10.1 Mutation prevalence in relation to the presence of a single or multiple CRCs diagnosed before age 50 in the proband (left), or before or after age 50 (right)

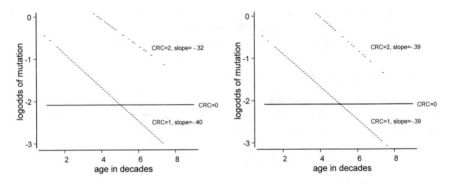

Fig. 10.2 Mutation prevalence in relation to the presence of a single or multiple CRCs, with age at diagnosis as a linear term (left, assuming separate age effects; right, assuming identical age effects)

of patients with CRC diagnoses. Further, we scaled the age per decade ($CRCage10 = CRCage/10$). The interpretation of the indicator variables CRC1 and CRC2 is as the presence of one or two CRCs versus no CRC at the age of 45 years. For calculation of the linear predictor and graphical display (Fig. 10.2), the specific coding is irrelevant. We may analyze the effect of the age at diagnosis of CRC with separate coefficients for CRC1 and CRC2 patients:

$$Mutation \sim CRC1 + CRC2 + CRC1age + CRC2age,$$

where CR1age and CRC2age indicate the age of CRC diagnosis; in those without CRC, the age is arbitrarily set close to the mean age of diagnosis (45 years). The main effects CRC1 and CRC2 are interpretable as the effect at age 45 of having a CRC diagnosis (one or multiple CRCs).

(3) We may also assume a single CRCage effect for both CRC1 and CRC2 patients.

Table 10.3 Performance of alternative modes for the effect of CRC and its age of diagnosis in patients tested for mutations in HNPCC (898 patients, 130 mutations). The third coding is preferred (3 *df*), with age as a single linear term ("CRCage")

Model	*df*	R^2 (%)	*c* statistic
CRC1 < 50 + CRC2 < 50	2	4.6	0.602
CRC1 < 50 + CRC2 < 50 + CRC1 >= 50 + CRC2 >= 50	4	6.9	0.634
CRC1 + CRC2 + CRCage	3	7.6	0.651
CRC1 + CRC2 + CRC1age + CRC2age	4	7.6	0.649

We consider the simpler model: Mutation $\sim$ CRC1 + CRC2 + CRCage, where CRCage is a single variable for those with one or multiple CRC diagnoses. A test of whether the more complex model is better than the simpler one is provided by a likelihood ratio test (comparison of the χ^2 statistics, 1 *df*). The age effects were very similar in both groups (CRC1age -0.40, CRC2age -0.32), and the difference in effects was far from significant ($p = 0.80$). Hence, it is reasonable to assume a single age effect for patients with one or two CRCs; performance remained identical (Table 10.3).

(4) We may subsequently test for nonlinearity in the age effect.

Nonlinearity can be tested in a number of ways, including adding a square term, or coding with a restricted cubic spline (Chap. 9). A linear coding was found reasonable, since we found no improvement in the fit by adding a square term ($p = 0.50$) or considering restricted cubic splines (3 knots, nonlinearity $p = 0.76$; 4 knots, nonlinearity $p = 0.94$).

10.4.3   CRC and Adenoma in a Proband

Adenoma polyps can be considered as precursors of CRC. They, hence, occur on average before the age of diagnosis of CRC. But the predictive effect for a, e.g., 10 years younger diagnosis of adenoma is a priori expected to be similar to the age–outcome relation for CRC. Let us first consider the CRC and adenoma effects plus their age effects:

$$\text{Mutation} \sim \text{CRC1} + \text{CRC2} + \text{CRCage} + \text{Adenoma} + \text{AdenomaAge}$$

The coefficients for the age effects are -0.38 for CRC and -0.36 for adenoma. It is tempting to estimate only 1 coefficient for these 2 effects. However, among a total of 141 patients with adenomas, only 100 had *only* adenomas as their diagnosis. CRC and adenoma are hence not mutually exclusive. How can we force the CRCage and AdenomaAge effects to be identical? In other words, we want to estimate one $\beta_{\text{CRCAdenoma}}$ instead of β_{CRC} and β_{Adenoma} in a regression equation as

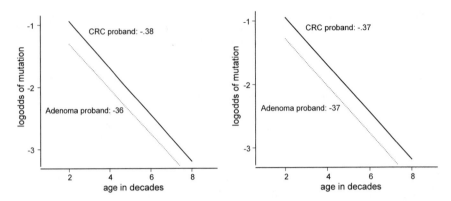

Fig. 10.3 Mutation prevalence in relation to age at diagnosis of CRC and age at diagnosis of adenoma as a linear term (left, assuming separate age effects; right, assuming identical age effects)

$$\text{Mutation} \sim \beta_{\text{CRC}} * \text{CRCage} + \beta_{\text{Adenoma}} * \text{AdenomaAge} + \ldots .$$

The requirement is that $\beta_{\text{CRC}} = \beta_{\text{Adenoma}}$. This is achieved quite simply:

$$\text{Mutation} \sim \beta_{\text{CRCAdenoma}} * (\text{CRCage} + \text{AdenomaAge}) + \ldots .$$

Again, we include the indicator variables CRC1, CRC2, and adenoma in such a model. CRCage and AdenomaAge are set to 45 years for those with missing diagnoses, and recorded per decade for better interpretability of effects. The value of $\beta_{\text{CRCAdenoma}}$ was -0.37: in between the effects for the 2 separate coefficients β_{CRC} and β_{Adenoma} (Fig. 10.3).

10.4.4 Age of CRC in Family History

A further extension is to consider the effects of age at CRC diagnosis in 1st and 2nd degree relatives (Fig. 10.4). A CRC diagnosis at a young age in a relative is more suspect for HNPCC than a CRC diagnosis at a more advanced age. We can again assume that the age effects should be similar, and add indicator variables for the presence of 1st or 2nd degree relatives. Four separate age effects are fitted with the formula:

$$\text{Mutation} \sim \text{CRC1} + \text{CRC2} + \text{CRCage} + \text{Adenoma} + \text{AdenomaAge}$$
$$+ \text{CRC1st} + \text{CRCage1st} + \text{CRC2nd} + \text{CRCage2nd},$$

where CRCage and AdenomaAge indicate age at diagnosis of CRC and adenoma in the proband, respectively, and CRCage1st and CRCage2nd indicate the age at diagnosis of CRC in 1st and 2nd degree relatives respectively. CRC1 and CRC2

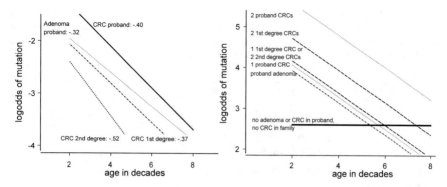

Fig. 10.4 Mutation prevalence in relation to age at diagnosis of CRC in the proband, 1st or 2nd degree relatives, and age at diagnosis of adenoma. Separate logistic regression coefficients were estimated for the four age effects in model 5a (left). In the right panel, one single age effect is estimated by considering the sum of all four ages, and family history is summarized in a single weighted score instead of 4 separate family history effects (1 or 2 1st degree relatives with CRC, 1 or 2 2nd degree relatives with CRC, model 5c). The predictive performance of model 5c was similar to that of model 5a while using 5 instead of 11 degrees of freedom (Table 10.4)

refer to 1 or 2 CRCs in the proband, Adenoma to adenoma in the proband, CRC1st and CRC2nd to the number of CRC affected 1st and 2nd degree relatives.

A single effect for the 4 age variables is estimated by calculating the sum of all four ages, to force the 4 age coefficients to be the same:

$$\text{sumCRC.Adenoma.CRC1st.CRC2nd.age}$$
$$= \text{CRCage} + \text{AdenomaAge} + \text{CRCage1st} + \text{CRCage2nd}$$

We reduce a model with 4 age effects to a model with a single common age effect for CRC and adenoma.

Moreover, we can combine the family history of 1st and 2nd degree relatives as CRCfam = CRC1st + 0.5 * CRC2nd, instead of considering indicator variables for having 1 or 2 1st degree relatives, and 1 or 2 2nd degree relatives with CRC. Therefore, we reduce a concept with 4 to 1 *df*.

The chosen coding for CRC and adenoma effects, hence, is as

$$\text{Mutation} \sim \text{CRC1} + \text{CRC2} + \text{adenoma} + \text{CRCfam} + \text{CRC.Adenoma.CRC1st.CRC2nd.age}$$

In total, we reduce a model with 11 to 5 *df*. We find that the performance of both model variants is similar (Table 10.4). Importantly, more stability is expected, and better generalizability to other patients.

Table 10.4 Performance of alternative modes for the predictive effect of age of diagnosis for CRC and adenoma in the proband, and CRC in 1st and 2nd degree relatives. Models created with data from patients tested for mutations in HNPCC (898 patients, 130 mutations). The fourth coding is preferred, with a single, linear term for a continuous age effect

Model	df	R^2 (%)	c statistic
CRCage + AdenomaAge; adenoma; CRC1 + CRC2;	5	8.4	0.662
CRCAdenomaAge; adenoma; CRC1 + CRC2	4	8.4	0.662
CRCage + AdenomaAge + CRC1stAge + CRC2ndAge + adenoma; CRC1 + CRC2; CRC1st (0, 1, 2), CRC2nd (0, 1, 2)	11	19.4	0.767
1 age effect[a]; adenoma; CRC1 + CRC2; CRCfam	5	18.3	0.757

[a]The age effect was labelled: CRC.Adenoma.CRC1st.CRC2nd.age reflecting 4 age effects in 1 summary variable

10.4.5   Full Prediction Model for Mutations

A final predictive model was constructed where other diagnoses were treated in a similar way. For endometrial cancer, we create an indicator variable with as reference category females without endometrial cancer and all males ("endo"). Age at diagnosis in the proband was combined with age at diagnosis in 1st and 2nd degree relatives, and family history was coded as for CRC: # affected 1st degree relatives + 0.5 # affected 2nd degree relatives.

For other HNPCC-related cancers, indicator variables were created for the proband ("other") and relatives ("rother", scored as for CRC and endo). No age effect was identified. The final model hence was

$$Mutation \sim CRC1 + CRC2 + Adenoma + CRCfam + CRC.Adenoma.CRC1st.CRC2nd.age$$
$$+ \quad Endo + EndoFam + EndoAge + Other + OtherFam$$

This model incorporates information on CRC, adenoma, endometrial cancer, and other cancer diagnoses from the proband and from 1st to 2nd degree relatives with only 10 df. The R^2 was 24.9%, and the c statistic 0.81. External validation was performed with 1016 new patients from the same setting [40]. The R^2 was 24.0% and c statistic 0.80.

This case study illustrates how predictors related to the same underlying phenomenon can be combined for parsimonious and robust modeling. Such a strategy may especially be useful in relatively small data sets, where the specification of complex models would not be reasonable, and lead to unstable estimation of regression coefficients. Further statistical detail is provided elsewhere [534]. Model updates have been developed [291], and an extensive validation study compared various prediction models for Lynch syndrome [290].

10.5 Concluding Remarks

Model specification is the most difficult step in prediction modeling. We considered several steps to develop more robust models for prediction purposes by reducing the effective degrees of freedom considered in the modeling process.

1. The first step obviously is to match the number of candidate predictors with the available effective sample size, which is mainly determined by the number of events for binary outcomes. If we have a small sample for modeling, a more restricted set of candidate predictors is necessary compared to the situation of a large sample. Subject matter knowledge may assist in limiting the selection, such as literature review and consultation of subject experts.
2. Second, we may consider distributions of predictors. We may exclude candidate predictors based on the number of missing values and skewness of distributions, for example, binary predictors with less than 5% being positive.
3. Related predictors can sometimes be combined in summary scores, such as illustrated for comorbidity.
4. Finally, we may want to average effects of predictors across groups for more stability, exploit biological relations, and estimate single effects for combinations of predictors. As illustrated for the case study on mutation prevalence in Lynch syndrome, this may lead to a parsimonious, robust model, which still captures most of the prognostic information.

The risk of such restrictions is that we may exclude certain predictors and miss specific predictor effects from a model; the specific circumstances should guide us in what strategy is most reasonable in balancing external information to what information is available in the data set under study.

Questions

10.1 Data reduction
   (a) What is meant with candidate predictors, in contrast to included predictors in a model?
   (b) Which problems can occur when considering many candidate predictors for inclusion in a prediction model (see also Chap. 4)?
   (c) What kind of strategies do not use the predictor–outcome relation in reducing the number and degrees of freedom of the candidate predictors?
   (d) What kind of strategies use the predictor–outcome relation while attempting to reduce the number and degrees of freedom of the candidate predictors (see also Chap. 11)?

10.2 Combining similar variables
   What objections can be made against the combination of similar variables in summary predictors (e.g., comorbidity scores), or the combination of effects of similar predictors (e.g. age effects in family history)?

10.3 Interpretation of case study (Sect. 10.4)
   The case study illustrates robust coding of family history for prediction of an underlying mutation in Lynch syndrome patients.
   (a) CRCage may be coded as (45–years)/10. How can we then interpret the coefficients for CRCage, CRC1, and CRC2 in the following regression formula:

$$\text{Mutation} \sim \text{CRC1} + \text{CRC2} + \text{CRCage}$$

   (b) The model for aspects of CRC in the family was

$$\text{Mutation} \sim \text{CRC1} + \text{CRC2} + \text{adenoma} + \text{CRCfam} +$$
$$\text{CRC.Adenoma.CRC1st.CRC2nd.age}$$

   What would the values of the predictors be for someone with no CRC or adenoma, and no CRC in the family?
   (c) How can we test for deviations of the age effects in 1st and 2nd degree relatives in the variable CRC.Adenoma.CRC1st.CRC2nd.age (2 age effects versus 1 age effect for relatives)?
   (d) Endometrial cancer can only occur in females. How do we code the predictors Endo and EndoFam to obtain interpretable coefficients?

10.4 Splitting analyses
   A researcher considers to analyze males and females separately, and proposes to split the files for such analyses. A colleague says there is no need to do so. How can the effects of predictors for males and females be analyzed in one dataset? Write down the regression formula with predictors p and sex for outcome y.

Chapter 11
Selection of Main Effects

Background Model specification is the most difficult part of prediction modeling. Especially in smaller data sets, it is virtually impossible to obtain a reliable answer to the question: which predictors are important and which are not? In this chapter, we focus on the problems that are associated with model reduction techniques such as stepwise selection, including overfitting and the quality of predictions from a model. Specific issues include instability of selection, biased estimation of coefficients and exaggeration of p-values. We explore the influence of including noise variables as predictors in a model, and find that their influence is not as detrimental to legitimize widespread use of selection methods. Alternative approaches are discussed, such as limiting the number of candidate predictors, e.g. based on a meta-analysis of available literature, and some modern selection methods, such as the LASSO and elastic net.

11.1 Predictor Selection

11.1.1 Reduction Before Modeling

In the previous chapters, we have discussed several approaches to limit the degrees of freedom that are considered in the modeling process. Use of subject matter knowledge is essential to preselect candidate predictors, e.g., from a systematic review of the literature, and from discussions with experts in the field. We should also consider strategies for robust coding of predictors (Chap. 10). These steps may reduce the chance that there are noise variables among the candidate predictors. Prediction modeling then turns into an estimation problem rather than a testing problem [529]. Ideally, we end up with a limited list of say 5–10 candidate predictors, which can all be entered in a "full model", which contains the main effects of all candidate predictors [225]. Model specification is then restricted to

© Springer Nature Switzerland AG 2019
E. W. Steyerberg, *Clinical Prediction Models*, Statistics for Biology and Health, https://doi.org/10.1007/978-3-030-16399-0_11

consideration of model assumptions such as additivity (with interaction terms) and nonlinearity (with nonlinear terms, see Chap. 12) [14].

11.1.2 Reduction While Modeling

In many prediction problems, we may end up with a list of over 10 candidate predictors, and we may consider to reduce this set of predictors for various reasons [236].

- One reason is that it is not practical to use a large set of predictors in medical practice. Formally, this is only an argument if variables are not all available in future patients, or have a cost associated with their collection.
- Some predictors may have very small or implausible effects, which makes it questionable why they are included in a model. In some circumstances, we may also have a list of new predictors, where some are expected to have no true relation to the outcome at all. For example, when predicting valve fracture with production characteristics, it was unclear which specific aspects would be important [58].
- In genetic and proteomic research, identification of which characteristics are predictive from a very large set of candidate predictors is the main goal. Such explanatory model building may make such analyses quite exploratory in nature, more aimed at biological knowledge discovery than prediction.

11.1.3 Collinearity

Another argument in favor of model reduction includes collinearity, which refers to the issue that predictors may be strongly correlated with each other. Collinearity is reflected in "variance inflation factors" (VIF) , which measure the degree to which collinearity among the predictors degrades the precision of estimate coefficients. Collinearity may hamper reliable and stable estimation of regression coefficients of the correlated variables, especially if correlations are very strong (say correlation coefficient $r > 0.8$, or VIF > 10) [653].

Is collinearity relevant for prediction models?

- Correlations do of course exist between predictors. We can perform multivariable analysis to consider the joint effects of predictors which cannot be inferred from univariate analysis.
- In many practical examples, correlations are relatively modest, with $r < 0.5$. For example, the strongest correlation in the GUSTO-I study is between height and weight with $r = 0.54$. All other correlations are weaker, typically with r around 0.1–0.2.
- Sometimes, we create highly correlated variables, e.g., age and age^2 ($r > 0.95$), but we can estimate their coefficients.

If predictors are relatively strongly correlated, it may be wiser to combine them in a single combined variable. For example, a strong correlation generally exists between diastolic blood pressure (DBP) and systolic blood pressure (SBP), with r of 0.62 in one study [14]. When choosing between DBP and SBP, "mean blood pressure" may be a better choice ((2xDBP + 1xSBP)/3) than choosing either one of them [5]. But again, subject matter knowledge is important. For example, systolic pressure may be the more relevant predictor for cardiovascular risk [571].

11.1.4 Parsimony

Another argument in favor of smaller models is made by referring to the principle of parsimony ("Occam's razor"). This principle states that simpler explanations are preferred over more complex explanations. This is an appealing philosophical principle when judging 2 alternative theories. It is, however, not obvious how this principle translates to prediction models [134]. Better predictive abilities cannot necessarily be expected from a simpler model, especially if we try to identify the simpler model from a richer model.

The traditional reasoning is that a model where some less significant variables are eliminated is more parsimonious than a full model with more predictors, and is hence to be preferred. When we consider how predictive regression models are created we, however, come to the opposite conclusion:

- a fully prespecified model does not ask more from the data than: what are the estimated regression coefficients?
- a reduced model asks two questions:
  (a) which variables can be eliminated?
  (b) what are the coefficients of the remaining predictors, given that the other variables are eliminated?

So, a reduced model reflects the answer to 2 questions rather than the answer to 1, which is arguably more complex.

A practical issue may be that smaller models are easier to interpret and use in practice. For example, prediction rules with a few, simple predictors may be easy to remember for clinicians. Hence "parsimony" comes at a price: such smaller models are conditional on selecting the right predictors from the candidate predictors.

11.1.5 Nonsignificant Candidate Predictors

Many may argue that statistically nonsignificant variables should not be included as predictors in a model, since their effects are not proven. This belief may result from mixing the fundamental statistical concepts of hypothesis testing and estimation. Prediction is about estimation; hence it is quite reasonable to include a predictor with a p-value higher than the magical value of 5%. Especially, this is reasonable if the data set is relatively small, the predictor uncommon (a rare but strong predictor such as "shock" in GUSTO-I), or when the predictor is well known from previous research to be predictive. Non-significance does not mean that there is evidence for a zero effect of a predictor; as always the absence of evidence is not evidence of absence [11]. Finally, simulation studies with true noise variables in a model show only a limited decrease in predictive ability [543] (see www.clin-icalpredictionmodels.org for additional material).

11.1.6   Summary Points on Predictor Selection

In sum, some arguments can be put forward in favor of predictor selection based on findings in our data:

- Larger models are less practical to work with;
- Some predictors may have very small or implausible effects.

False arguments include

- Statistically nonsignificant variables should be excluded: for estimation, significance testing is not relevant, especially if estimated effects are supported by subject knowledge;
- Collinearity precludes obtaining reliable predictions: although collinearity makes estimates of individual coefficients unstable, reliable predictions can still be obtained;
- Referring to the parsimony principle: this principle may hold when prespecified models are compared, not when models are selected by studying patterns in the data.

11.2   Stepwise Selection

We will first consider traditional approaches such as stepwise selection of predictors in a model, followed by some promising alternative approaches to model specification.

11.2.1   Stepwise Selection Variants

Currently, stepwise selection methods are probably the most widely used in medical applications. These automated methods aim to include only the most significant predictors in a model. Significance is determined with a selection criterion: the F test in linear regression; a likelihood ratio (LR), Wald, or score statistic, in logistic or Cox regression models. Forward selection starts with the inclusion of the most significant candidate predictor to a model that does not contain any predictor. Backward selection starts with elimination of the least significant candidate predictor from a full model including all candidate predictors. Forward and backward selection may also be combined, such that an iterative procedure is followed [236].

A backward selection approach is generally preferred if stepwise selection is attempted. First, the modeler is forced to consider the full model with a backward approach, and can judge the effects of all candidate predictors simultaneously [225]. Second, correlated variables may remain in the model, while none of them might enter the model with a forward approach [133].

An extension of stepwise selection strategies is "all possible subsets regression". Here, every possible combination of predictors is examined to find the best fitting model. All possible subsets regression can identify combinations of predictors not found by the more standard forward or backward procedures. This comes at a price: we examine many models, with multiple testing, easily resulting in overfitted models [133].

11.2.2 Stopping Rules in Stepwise Selection

The stopping rule for inclusion or exclusion of predictors is a central issue in stepwise selection methods. It is far more important than the specific variant of the stepwise selection method (e.g., forward, backward, combined, all possible subsets). Usually, one applies the standard significance level for testing of hypotheses ($\alpha = 0.05$), but the Akaike Information Criterion (AIC) or Bayesian Information Criterion (BIC) are also often used. In all possible subset selection, the stopping criterion often is to maximize Mallow's C_p, which is similar to optimizing AIC. Stopping rules are usually applied for testing contributions of individual predictors, but may also be applied to the pooled degrees of freedom of unselected predictors [225].

AIC and BIC compare models based on their fit to the data, but penalize for the complexity of the model. With AIC, we require that the increase in model chi-square (χ^2) has to be larger than 2 times the degrees of freedom: $\chi^2 > 2\ df$. When considering a predictor with 1 df, such as gender, this implies $\chi^2 > 2$, equivalent to $p < 0.157$. With 2 df, $\chi^2 > 4$, or $p < 0.135$, and with 4 df, $p < 0.092$ (Table 11.1).

Table 11.1 *P*-value associated with Akaike's Information Criterion (AIC) for selection of candidate predictors with different degrees of freedom (*df*)	*df*	Minimum χ^2	Critical *p*-value
	1	2	0.157
	2	4	0.135
	3	6	0.112
	4	8	0.092
	5	10	0.075

Table 11.2 *P*-value
associated with Bayesian
Information Criterion (BIC)
for selection of candidate
predictors

N	Minimum χ^2	Critical *p*-value
20	3.0	0.083
50	3.9	0.048
100	4.6	0.032
200	5.3	0.021
500	6.2	0.013
1000	6.9	0.009
2000	7.6	0.006

With BIC, we penalize the model fit such that χ has to exceed $\log(n)$. The effective sample size should be used for n, e.g., the number of events in Cox regression for survival data [655]. With small sample size, e.g., $n = 20$, BIC is equivalent to $p < 0.083$ for selection. With larger sample sizes, the critical *p*-value is much lower (Table 11.2). Hence, selection with BIC will generally lead to smaller models than selection with AIC. The theory behind AIC and BIC criteria can be found elsewhere in detail [231]; for the applied researcher, the *p*-value that is effectively used as a stopping criterion is most relevant.

There is no specific reason to stick to a critical *p*-value of 0.05, or lower, as implied by applying BIC. Using AIC has been recommended [14]. The use of higher *p*-values ($p < 0.20$ or $p < 0.50$) has been found to provide more power for the selection of predictors with relatively weak effects [327], and to provide better predictions in small data sets with a set of established candidate predictors [542].

11.3   Advantages of Stepwise Methods

Stepwise selection methods have a number of advantages. They are usually relatively straightforward to apply in any statistical package [236]. Some care should be taken with missing values; if we start with a full model, the number of available cases is restricted by the combination of missing values in any of the candidate predictors. It is therefore important to use imputed data set to deal with missing values. Multiple imputation (MI) poses some complexities if we would select predictors per imputed data set, where predictor may be selected in some replicates of the data set and not in other replicates. The preferable approach is to perform selection based on the results from the combined data sets [678]. For example, with a backward procedure, we first obtain *p*-values for each predictor in a full model, fitted on MI data sets. We then eliminate the least significant predictor, provided that the *p*-value is higher than our stopping criterion. We refit the model in the MI data, and eliminate the next predictor. We stop when all predictors have *p*-values less than the stopping criterion.

Stepwise methods are also relatively objective. When another analyst is provided with the same data set and the same list of candidate predictors, the resulting selection should be very similar. The objectivity of stepwise selection makes it possible to replay this model reduction strategy in the validation procedures such as the bootstrap (Chap. 16). Optimism can hence be estimated including model uncertainty [94, 535].

Stepwise methods usually reach their goal of making a model smaller. In larger data sets, such as GUSTO-I, all variables that are important for prediction will have small p-values. Sometimes $p < 0.01$ is therefore chosen in large samples. In small data sets, only a few variables may have such small p-values, resulting in small models (sometimes referred to as "underfitting"). This argues for the use of a higher p-value in smaller data sets.

11.4   Disadvantages of Stepwise Methods

Stepwise methods have severe disadvantages, including

(1) instability of the selection;
(2) biased estimation of coefficients;
(3) misspecification of variability and exaggeration of p-values;
(4) provision of predictions of worse quality than from a full model.

These issues are explained and illustrated below.

11.4.1   Instability of Selection

Stepwise selection considers a high number of combinations of predictors. Some of these combinations may actually be rather similar in how they fit the data. This instability may be illustrated by the observation that the selection of predictors may change when we consider a somewhat different selection of patients for a model [27, 563].

The instability of selection can well be illustrated with subsamples of our GUSTO-I case study; very different selections arise (Table 11.3). For example, the selected predictors were age (dichotomized at 65 years, "a65" [395]), hypotension ("hyp") and shock ("sho") in sample number 5 ($n = 429$ patients). We also considered the selection in the other 110 small subsamples where a logistic regression model could technically be fitted. The predictors a65, hyp, and sho were among the predictors most often selected (80%, 47%, 53%, respectively). The specific selection of these 3 predictors was, however, replicated in only 7 of the 110 other small subsamples.

The conclusion from this case study is similar to what was found in other studies: the specific selection of predictors is unstable and should be interpreted with much caution [27, 563]. Statements such as "the only independent predictors

Table 11.3 Illustration of variability in selection with backward selection with $p < 0.05$ in 20 small subsamples from GUSTO-I [541]. The full 8-predictor model could technically be fitted in 111 of the 121 subsamples

	a65	sex	dia	hyp	hrt	hig	sho	ttr
1	7.9					2.5		
3	4.0	3.9				3.9	5.3	
4	11.7			10.9			10.3	
5	3.9			3.3			39.3	
6	4.1	4.1						
7					3.6	3.9	12.0	
8	14.5	3.6			6.4			
9		3.8				44.3	45.5	
11	4.1						6.0	
13	14.5				3.3			
14	5.7						20.8	
...								
116	11.8					7.7		
117	5.5				2.8			3.9
118	4.2		4.0			9.9		
119	3.6				2.8		4.4	
120	3.2			5.0			15.0	
121	7.6	2.8		8.2			24.9	
Selected (%)	80	22	13	47	23	29	53	11

Table 11.4 Summary of the number of predictors selected with different selection strategies in subsamples from the GUSTO-I data set. Numbers are mean ± SD

Samples	Full	$p < 0.05$	AIC	$p < 0.5$
Small subsamples	8	2.8 ± 1.1	4.2 ± 1.1	6.3 ± 1.2
Large subsamples	8	4.8 ± 1.1	6.0 ± 1.0	7.0 ± 0.9
Regions	8	6.6 ± 1.0	7.1 ± 0.8	7.8 ± 0.4

in this prediction problem were age, hypotension, and shock" are overinterpretations unless the sample size was huge [236]. Even worse overinterpretations are related to the order of entry of a predictor in a forward stepwise procedure, or rank order of the p-value in the selected model [133].

The instability of selection depends on a number of factors. One crucial aspect is the sample size. In a large sample, more stability is to be expected, since we have more power to detect truly important effects. Table 11.4 illustrates that more predictors were selected in larger subsamples than in smaller subsamples. When considering 16 large regions in GUSTO-I of at least 2000 patients (178 events on average), around 6 to 7 predictors had statistically significant effects, eliminating predictors such as *ttr* and *dia* which had minor prognostic effects.

Although a larger sample size helps in many ways, we are usually tempted to study more candidate predictors in such situations. This introduces instability again: having more candidate predictors implies having more potential combinations of predictors. So, a crucial aspect is the ratio between the number of candidate predictors and the effective sample size. Sometimes, a ratio of 1 predictor per 10 events is advocated; this is, however, only a reasonable lower bound for prespecified models. For reliable selection among candidate predictors, a 1 in 25 [236], or a 1 in 50 rule [543] has been suggested. So, if we consider 8 candidate predictors, at least 200–400 events should preferably be analyzed in a logistic regression model when we want to make statements on which predictors are important and which are not. The total GUSTO-I model easily fulfills the 1 in 50 criterion with 2851 events in 40,830 patients, but this is exceptional.

The instability of selection procedures can well be studied for one specific data set with bootstrapping procedures (Chaps. 5 and 16). For larger data sets, the instability will not show up as extreme as with the small subsamples in Table 11.3. Also, when a few predictors have strong effects, and others have weak effects, this should be apparent from the selection pattern over bootstrap samples.

11.4.2   Testimation: Biased in Selected Coefficients

The problem of estimation after testing (*testimation*) was already introduced in Chap. 5. This bias is a key problem if the selection is based on observed patterns in the data (*Winner's curse* [267]). It clearly shows up in stepwise selected coefficients: the distributions of selected coefficients are biased away from zero.

We illustrate the theoretically expected patterns with different critical p-values for selection: $p < 0.50$ (liberal selection for prediction [543], AIC [14] or $p < 0.157$ for estimates with 1 df, $p < 0.05$ (the default in many statistical packages), $p < 0.01$, and $p < 0.001$ (a more stringent selection criterion, as sometimes applied in very large data sets). We assume that a true effect has mean value $\mu = 1$ and a sample size such that $SE = 0.5$ (Fig. 11.1). For logistic regression, a coefficient with value 1 implies a true odds ratio of 2.7; a SE of 0.5 corresponds to a study of a binary predictor with 50:50 distribution, in a sample with 35 events and 35 non-events. Equivalently we can think of a study with true odds ratio 1.65 with 140 events and 140 nonevents (coefficient 0.5 and SE 0.25). If no selection is applied, we expect no bias in estimates such as regression coefficients. With a liberal p-value of 0.50, we would keep 91% of estimates, which causes a small bias (+9%). The bias increases to 39% for $p < 0.05$ selection, +60% for $p < 0.01$ and +88% for $p < 0.001$ selection, given a true effect of 1 and a SE of 0.5.

The bias in selected estimates depends on a number of characteristics, including the true effect size and the statistical power for selection of an estimate (Fig. 11.2). The stringency of the stopping rule is also important, with more bias for selection with lower p-values. Biases over 100% can arise if true effects are small, and when estimates are from small studies with low statistical power. We further illustrate these theoretically expected patterns with empirical data from GUSTO-I.

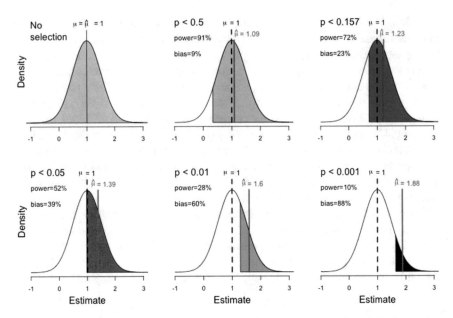

Fig. 11.1 Illustration of testimation bias for a true effect of $\mu = 1$ and SE $= 0.5$. If we select estimates based on increasingly stringent *p*-values, the bias increases from 9% for $p < 0.50$ to 88% for $p < 0.001$

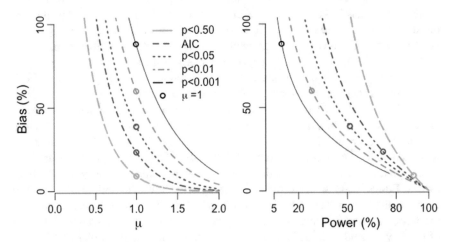

Fig. 11.2 Illustration of testimation bias in relation to the size of the true effect while SE $= 0.5$, and in relation to the statistical power for selection of the estimate. Results for $\mu = 1$ correspond to Fig. 11.1. Estimates are expected to have a large bias if selected in small sample sizes with low statistical power, while the true effect was small

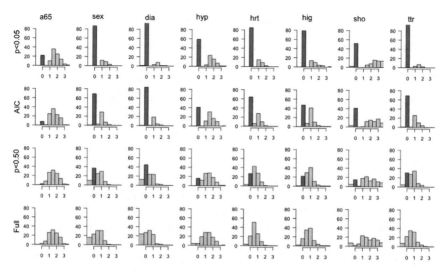

Fig. 11.3 Distribution of logistic regression coefficients in 111 small subsamples within GUSTO-I. First row: $p < 0.05$ selection; second row: AIC selection; third row: $p < 0.5$ selection; fourth row: full model with all 8 predictors included. a65: age > 65; dia: diabetes; hyp: hypotension; hrt; heart rate > 80; hig: high risk (anterior infarction or previous MI); sho: shock; ttr: time to relief > 1 h. Note that the coefficients in the stepwise selected models should be interpreted with caution: they are based on different sets of selected predictors. The general pattern is that the coefficients in the stepwise selected models are either zero (marked in red), or a value clearly above zero, since predictors with small effects are not selected. The coefficients follow an approximately normal distribution in the full models (last row)

11.4.3 *Testimation: Empirical Illustrations

We further illustrate the bias that is induced by stepwise selection in 111 small subsamples in GUSTO-I. Predictors such as diabetes (*dia*) and time to relief (*ttr*) were often not selected for the model with the default criterion of $p < 0.05$ (Table 11.3, first row in Fig. 11.3). We set the coefficients to zero for such nonselected predictors. From zero there is a gap; only larger estimated coefficients were statistically significant. The gap is smaller when we select with a higher *p*-value (AIC or $p < 0.50$). The higher statistical power for selection implies that more coefficients are included with a more relaxed stopping rule, and that fewer coefficients are set to zero. The testimation problem is smaller in larger samples (see www.clinicalpredictionmodels.org for graphs). Similar bias has been observed in a case study of Lynch syndrome patients [563].

11.4.4 Misspecification of Variability and p-Values

As noted in Figs. 11.1 and 11.3, the distribution of coefficients from stepwise selected models has a strange shape. From an unconditional perspective,

Table 11.5 Standard errors of estimated coefficients in logistic regression models after backward selection with $p < 0.05$, calculated from an unconditional or conditional perspective (standard deviation in Fig. 11.3), and as asymptotically estimated in the models (average SE)

SE estimation	a65	sex	dia	hyp	hrt	hig	sho	ttr
Empirical unconditional	0.87	0.55	0.53	0.98	0.55	0.77	1.51	0.46
Conditional	0.52	0.27	0.36	0.47	0.29	0.62	0.75	0.27
Asymptotic conditional	0.57	0.48	0.55	0.61	0.48	0.59	0.88	0.62

coefficients are set to zero when the predictor was not selected. From a conditional perspective, only the values of coefficients of selected predictors are considered. The asymptotic standard error (SE) of the selected coefficient is estimated as if the model was prespecified. The means of these asymptotic SEs were somewhat larger than the empirical SEs of the conditional coefficients for each of the 8 predictors, but smaller than the unconditional SEs (Table 11.5). The latter SEs reflect that the coefficient might have been set to zero, but the interpretation of this SE is difficult, if not impossible. In sum, the distribution of coefficients is less straightforward to interpret or quantify when a stepwise selection procedure has been followed. Some may hence consider reporting of 95% confidence intervals for coefficients in a stepwise model rather meaningless.

Another consideration is the variability of predictions (rather than predictor effects), given covariate patterns. This variability has been studied with bootstrapping techniques. Predictions were far more variable than expected from estimates which were made as if the model was prespecified [10, 21].

Furthermore, the testimation bias in coefficients and misspecification of variability leads to an exaggeration of p-values. The p-value of predictors in a stepwise model should generally not be trusted; the p-value is calculated as if the model was prespecified. This interpretation of p-values is only valid for a full model, without selection.

11.4.5   Predictions of Worse Quality Than from a Full Model

Apparent performance usually does not suffer much from stepwise selection procedures. The eliminated variables have by definition relatively weak effects, otherwise, they would have been omitted.

Of more interest is the validity of the predictions outside the studied sample. We can assess the validity with internal validation techniques such as bootstrapping, and with external validation, i.e., evaluation in completely new patients. Both types of validation have shown that the performance of stepwise selected models is usually worse than that of a full model, without selection [226]. Table 11.6 provides an illustration of bootstrap validation in a small sample from the GUSTO-I

Table 11.6 Illustration of bootstrap validation of model performance, as indicated by R^2 in subsample #5 of the GUSTO-I database ($n = 429$, see also Table 5.4)

Method	Apparent	Bootstrap	Test	Optimism	Optimism-corrected
Full 8-predictor model (%)	22.7	24.7	17.2	7.6	15.1
Stepwise, 3 predictors $p < 0.05$ (%)	17.6	18.7	12.7	5.9	11.7

study. This same pattern was found in a simulation study considering all small subsamples within the training part of GUSTO-I, and evaluating them on an independent validation part of GUSTO-I [542].

11.5   Influence of Noise Variables

An argument for stepwise methods is that it helps to eliminate variables that have no true relation to the outcome (noise variables, with true regression coefficient of zero). As discussed before, the likelihood of having such noise variables in our model can be reduced by considering only predictors with external knowledge on their relevance (from the literature, expert opinion). Various simulation studies have considered the behavior of stepwise selection in the presence of noise variables. In one simulation, stepwise selection produced models in which 30–70% of the selected predictors were not related to the outcome, i.e., were pure noise, when candidate predictors consisted of a mix of noise and true predictors [133]. The frequency of inclusion of noise and true predictors depended on the number of noise variables among the candidate predictors and on the correlations between candidate predictors. Stepwise methods were, hence, far from a guarantee for exclusion of noise variables.

A simulation study in 2 data sets with a mix of true and noise predictors focused on the predictive performance of the models. Stepwise selection with AIC was optimal in that study [14].

In GUSTO-I, we added 9 noise variables to the 8 predictors considered thus far for some further simulations [542, 543]. The performance was evaluated in independent test patients (see Chap. 24). As expected, we noted that discriminative ability (c statistics) for the full model was worse by adding noise variables, compared to a model including 17 true predictors (Table 11.7: c 0.78 with true predictors, 0.75 with 8 true and 9 noise predictors). The stepwise models succeeded in removing noise variables: with $p < 0.05$ selection only 1 in 20 was retained in the model, which is approximately 1 in every 2 models (since 9 noise variables were considered per model). The exclusion of noise variables comes at the price of at the same time excluding some true predictors. For example, the $p < 0.05$ selected models contained on average 0.5 of the 9 noise predictors and 4.8 of the 8 true predictors (Table 11.7). The performance of stepwise models was worse when only true predictors were considered, but also when more than half of the candidate

Table 11.7 Selected predictors and performance of models with 17 true predictors or 9 noise variables and 8 true predictors in 23 large subsamples from GUSTO-I [543]. Models were created in a large subsample (#4, n = 795, 52 events) and evaluated in the independent test part of GUSTO-I (part B, n = 20,318)

	True predictors		Noise variables added	
	17-predictor model	$p < 0.05$	8 + 9 noise model	$p < 0.05$
#Predictors				
Noise	0	0	9	0.5
True	17	5.9	8	4.8
Validated c statistic	0.784	0.762	0.753	0.746

predictors were in fact noise (Table 11.7). Apparently, the $p < 0.05$ stopping rule led to a suboptimal balance between the elimination of noise variables and the inclusion of a sufficient number of true predictors in this case study. This suggests that the omission of a true predictor may be far worse than the inclusion of a noise variable [543].

11.6   Univariate Analyses and Model Specification

A common way to select predictor variables for a regression model is to first study the univariate relation between each variable and the outcome. When a variable meets a univariate criterion, e.g., $p < 0.2$, the variable is considered further for multivariable modeling (Table 11.8). This strategy may seem advantageous to reduce problems of overfitting and stepwise selection. However, univariate preselection is just a variant of stepwise selection. All candidate predictors are considered in the first step, but only those meeting the univariate criterion are considered in the following steps. This is in contrast to the standard forward (or backward) selection, where all candidate predictors are considered in each step as long as they have not been removed from the model. The difference between univariate prescreening and standard backward selection is shown in Tables 11.8 and 11.9 for a hypothetical example.

11.6.1   Pros and Cons of Univariate Preselection

Univariate preselection has some practical advantages, which include:

- Predictors are eliminated at an early stage if no regression coefficient can be estimated with standard fitting algorithms, e.g., for "shock" in the small GUSTO-I subsamples. A model can be developed with the remaining predictors;

Table 11.8 Hypothetical example of univariate screening of candidate predictors, followed by stepwise backward selection. Candidate predictors are marked in gray, omitted predictors as red, and the finally selected predictors are in green. We note that 3 candidate predictors are omitted from further consideration based on univariate insignificance (#6, #7, #8), and 2 because of multivariable insignificance (#4, #5). The final model includes 3 predictors (#1, #2, #3)

	1	2	3	4	5	6	7	8
Univariate screening								
Multivariable modeling								
Omitted #5								
Omitted #4								
Selected model								

Table 11.9 Hypothetical example of backward stepwise selection of candidate predictors #1–#8. We note that the hypothetical final model might include 1 of the 3 candidate predictors which were insignificant in univariate analysis (#6). The model also includes the 3 predictors selected after univariate screening (#1, #2, #3)

	1	2	3	4	5	6	7	8
Multivariable modeling								
Omitted #8								
Omitted #7								
Omitted #5								
Omitted #4								
Selected model								

- In a large data set, with many predictors, the computational burden is lower when starting with a smaller set of predictors in a "reduced full model".

On the other hand, univariate screening of candidate predictors does not reduce the problems as noted for stepwise methods (Sect. 11.4). Other variants of univariate preselection are eye-balling relations between continuous predictors and outcome, and inspection of exploratory cross-tables. In these informal inspections, the relation between a predictor and the outcome is used. Such informal data inspections may hence contribute to overfitting.

11.6.2   *Testing of Predictors within a Domain

A variant of univariate screening is to test the relevance of predictors within a cluster of related variables, representing a disease domain. For example, we may consider preselection of 1 or more predictors from variables related to hypertension: diastolic blood pressure, systolic blood pressure, treatment for high blood pressure. Such an approach has some attractiveness, but problems of stepwise selection apply here too. Some increase in power can be obtained by requiring that all domains have to be included in the final model, even when not statistically significant after the preselection. Alternative approaches are to combine variables within such a cluster, e.g., as mean blood pressure, or preselection based on prior information, e.g., evidence from other studies (see Chap. 10).

11.7   Modern Selection Methods

A number of more modern selection methods have emerged over the past decades. Some methods use resampling methods such as the bootstrap to identify important variables. Others have proposed principles of Bayesian analysis, such as Bayesian model averaging [252]. Some methods use shrinkage of regression coefficients to zero as a method of selection. Finally, many methods are under consideration by computer scientists and statisticians that may prove valuable in the future but are not discussed here [231].

11.7.1   *Bootstrapping for Selection

Several authors have proposed to define prediction models based on the selection in bootstrap samples [28, 95, 487]. For example, one may apply backward stepwise selection in bootstrap samples drawn from the original sample. Candidate predictors are ranked according to their frequency of selection in the bootstrap samples. A cut-off is then applied for selection of predictors in the model that is fitted in the original sample, e.g., all predictors selected in >50% of bootstrap samples. Evidence for the advantages of this method is still unconvincing. Models constructed with this procedure will generally be very similar to the stepwise model in the original sample, provided that the stopping rule is similar (selection >50% of bootstraps). Predictors with low p-values in the original sample tend to be selected with high frequency in bootstrap samples.

11.7.2   *Bagging and Boosting

Bagging (for "bootstrap aggregating") is a method for generating multiple versions of a linear predictor and using these to obtain an aggregated linear predictor [78]. Multiple versions are formed by making bootstrap replicates of the sample and using these as new model development sets. The aggregation averages over multiple versions of a predictor to make predictions. If perturbing the development set can cause clear changes in the predictor constructed, then bagging can improve accuracy [78].

Bagging is somewhat related to "boosting", which is a general method for improving the performance of any learning algorithm [490]. Bagging works by taking a bootstrap sample from the training set. Boosting works by changing the weights on the training set. Greater weights are given to observations that were difficult to classify, and lower weights to those that were easy to classify.

11.7.3 *Bayesian Model Averaging (BMA)

Researchers usually ignore the uncertainty associated with modeling procedures such as stepwise selection. Bayesian model averaging (BMA) aims to appropriately consider this uncertainty [252]. This method selects a subset of all possible models (up to $K = 2^p$, where p is the number of predictors, ignoring interactions) and uses the posterior probabilities of the models to perform hypothesis testing and prediction. Equations relating to the problem of optimal model selection have been developed [252]. Here, $M = \{M_1, M_2 ..., M_k\}$ is used to denote the set of all possible models to be considered and Δ is used to identify the quantity of interest. For example, Δ can indicate the regression coefficient in a logistic regression model. Then the posterior distribution of Δ, given the data D is

$$\Pr(\Delta|D) = \sum_{k=1}^{K} \Pr(\Delta/M_k, D) \Pr(M_k|D)$$

This is an average of the posterior distributions under each model M_k ($\Pr(\Delta |M_k, D)$), weighted by the corresponding posterior model probabilities given the data ($\Pr(M_k | D)$, with $k = 1, 2, ..., K$). Hereto, we need to estimate how likely each coefficient is given a particular model and how likely each model is. This estimation requires two prior probabilities: one for the coefficient values and one for the likelihood of each model M_k. For the coefficients, a multivariate normal prior with mean at the maximum likelihood estimate and variance equal to the expected information matrix for one observation has been suggested. This can be thought of a prior distribution that contains the same amount of information as a single, typical observation. Essentially, this prior distribution is non-informative. When there is little information about the relative plausibility of the models considered, taking them all to be equally likely a priori is believed by many to be a reasonable choice.

For an analysis with p potential predictors, the number of models K can be enormous. To get around this problem, we may exclude models that are far less probable than the best model. This strategy is also known as "Occam's window" approach [448]. For example, we may choose to discard models that are 20 times less likely as posterior models based on the data than the most likely model. This approach makes the BMA procedure computationally better feasible.

Software is increasingly available that calculates a posterior model probability, parameter estimates, and standard errors of those estimates. This enables the testing of hypotheses, such as that the effect of a predictor is zero. Also, the regression coefficient can be estimated (as the posterior mean) with a standard error (based on the posterior standard deviation). Essentially, each estimated regression coefficient

from a potential model is weighted with the posterior likelihood that this model is
the final model:

$$E(\beta_j|D) = \sum_{M_k \in A} \hat{\beta}_j \Pr(M_k/D)$$

Similarly, we can make predictions for future patients with all models with a
posterior likelihood larger than zero, and then weight each prediction with the
posterior likelihood that this model is the final model.

11.7.4   Shrinkage of Regression Coefficients to Zero

Shrinkage is the principle of reducing the regression coefficients to improve the
quality of predictions. Several variants of shrinkage will be discussed in Chap. 13.
Some variants of shrinkage methods lead to regression coefficients which are set to
zero. Hence, model reduction is achieved, since variables with zero coefficients can
be dropped. Examples of these methods include the "Garotte" [77], elastic net
[689], and the "least absolute shrinkage and selection operator" (LASSO) [581].
The LASSO minimizes the log likelihood subject to a restriction on the sum of the
absolute values of the parameters. This restriction shrinks some coefficients to zero.
The LASSO showed promising results in simulation studies and in predicting
30-day mortality in subsamples from GUSTO-I (see Chaps. 13, 22–24).

11.8   Concluding Remarks

The problem of overfitting starts with considering too many candidate predictors in
a data set. This problem is difficult to solve with standard statistical techniques
which are still widely used by default in medical research nowadays, such as
stepwise selection [563]. Faraway has labeled the issues discussed here as "the cost
of data analysis" [157]. We can estimate the "effective degrees of freedom" of a
multistep modeling procedure [685].

   Improvements in model selection can be sought in various directions. This first is
to limit the necessity for selection by using subject matter knowledge, especially in
relatively small data sets. Another strategy is to use better algorithms to discover
patterns in the data, including better fitting algorithms (such as the "LASSO"),
bootstrapping, or following Bayesian estimation methods [206, 252]. The uncertainty
of model selection is an important source of overfitting, which needs to be prevented if
possible, e.g., by analyzing larger data sets, and by limiting the use of stepwise or
related methods. The LASSO and variants of such a method are promising techniques
when prediction and parsimony are goals of prediction modeling.

Questions

11.1 Stepwise selection methods
Stepwise methods are abundant in the medical literature, both in the context of addressing epidemiological questions on predictor effects and in the context of deriving prediction models.

(a) What decisions need to be made when one wants to use stepwise selection methods?
(b) What are the major advantages and disadvantages of stepwise selection?

11.2 Models considered in all subset regression
Suppose we consider 10 candidate predictors, and use a variant of stepwise selection that considers all combinations of predictors in selecting a model ("all possible subset regression", Sect. 11.2.1).

(a) How many models do we consider?
(b) And how many if we pre-specify that 4 predictors have to be included?

11.3 Bias by stepwise methods (Fig. 11.1)
What bias can we expect by stepwise selection with $p < 0.05$, if predictors are studied with SE = 0.5:

(a) if the true regression coefficient = 0.5 (Odds ratio 1.6)?
(b) if the true regression coefficient = 2 (Odds Ratio 7.4)?

11.4 Application of stepwise methods
Consider the paper by Sanada et al. published in 2007 [482].

(a) How many subjects were studied?
(b) How many candidate predictors were considered?
(c) How many predictors were selected by stepwise selection?
(d) What alternatives might have been used for model specification?
(e) Consider the Letter to the editor from Malek et al., who is very critical with respect to stepwise selection [362]. They propose an alternative selection strategy, called "hierarchical analysis". What is your opinion on this strategy?

Chapter 12
Assumptions in Regression Models: Additivity and Linearity

Background In this chapter, we discuss assessment of assumptions in multivariable regression models. Specifically, we consider the additivity assumption, which can be assessed with interaction terms. We also consider the linearity assumption of continuous predictors in a multivariable regression model, where multiple nonlinear terms can be included to allow for nonlinear relations between predictors and outcome. Throughout we stress parsimony in strategies to extend a prediction model with interactions and nonlinear terms, since better fulfillment of assumptions in a particular sample does not necessarily imply better predictive performance for future subjects. We consider several case studies for illustration of strategies to deal with additivity and linearity.

12.1 Additivity and Interaction Terms

The generalized linear regression models discussed in this book all have a linear predictor at their core: $lp = b1 * x1 + b2 * x2 + \ldots + b_i * x_i$, for models with i predictors.

The regression coefficients $b1$ to b_i refer to the main effects of predictors $x1$ to x_i. This formulation implies additivity of effects at the linear predictor scale. We leave out the intercept a for simplicity; this is a constant that needs to be used to make predictions with the model. For a logistic regression model, we can calculate odds ratios as exp(b); the odds ratios are multiplied to obtain the odds of the outcome. Hence, the effects of predictors are assumed to be multiplicative at the odds scale. For a Cox regression model, exp(b) is the hazard ratio; the assumption is that these hazard ratios can be multiplied at the hazard scale.

The scale is essential for consideration of additivity. If a treatment reduces risk as 20 to 10% in one risk stratum, and 10 to 5% in another risk stratum, the relative risk is 0.5 in both. The odds ratios are also quite similar (0.44 and 0.47,

© Springer Nature Switzerland AG 2019
E. W. Steyerberg, *Clinical Prediction Models*, Statistics for Biology
and Health, https://doi.org/10.1007/978-3-030-16399-0_12

respectively). Hence, we could say that there is a consistent halving of the risk. But on an absolute scale, the benefit is clearly dependent on the risk (10 vs. 5% reduction).

The most common regression modeling procedure is to start model specification with main effects of predictors only. Some epidemiological textbooks advice to consider interactions early in the modeling process, with main effects included for all variables that have a relevant interaction term [306]. Interactions between predictors can be considered by multiplicative terms of the form x1 * x2 (two-way or first-order interactions), and x1 *x2 * x3 (three-way, or second-order interactions); higher order interactions are uncommon to consider for regression models. As mentioned in Chap. 4, tree models assume higher order interactions to be present. The interpretation of a two-way interaction is that the effect of one predictor depends on that of another predictor. The effect is different, depending on the value of another predictor. The effect of a predictor cannot be interpreted alone; we need to know the value of another predictor to interpret its effect.

12.1.1 Potential Interaction Terms to Consider

Prior subject knowledge may help to guide us to select interaction terms. For example, interaction terms that were identified in previous studies could be assessed. Some types of interactions have been suggested that warrant consideration in prediction models (Table 12.1) [225].

On the other hand, clinical insight, e.g., on pathophysiology, is difficult to use. This is because using main effects in a model assumes already that predictors act in a multiplicative way on the risk scale (e.g., odds ratios and hazard ratios are multiplied). Reasoning why a certain combination of predictors would not act in an additive way

Table 12.1 Examples of interactions to potentially consider in clinical prediction models (based on Harrell [225])

Interaction	Example
Severity of disease * treatment	Less benefit with less severe disease
Place * treatment	Benefit varies by the treatment center
Place * predictors	Predictor effects vary by center/region
Calender time * treatment	Learning curves for some treatments
Calender time * predictors	Increasing or decreasing impact of predictors over the years
Age * predictors	Older subjects less affected by risk factors; or more affected by certain types of disease
Follow-up time * predictors	Non-proportionality of survival effects, often a decreasing effect over the follow-up time
Season * predictors	Seasonal effect of predictors

on, e.g., the log(odds) scale is quite difficult to imagine. Similarly, non-additivity at the log(hazard) scale is difficult to picture for survival models. Some researchers are motivated to study an interaction term when 2 predictors are correlated. But correlation does not imply anything on the effects of predictors conditional on each other. Two predictors may not have any correlation and still, have interacting effects.

12.1.2 Interactions with Treatment

Various interactions with treatment can be considered. The benefit of treatment may depend on the severity of the disease, with less relative benefit for those with less severe disease. The reverse may also be true, especially in oncology, where less relative benefit occurs for those with more severe disease. For example, surgery in esophageal cancer can be curative, but only for patients without distant metastases. Note that absolute benefit will anyway depend on the severity of the disease, even when the relative benefit is constant [299, 300, 333]. For example, the absolute benefit of tPA treatment depended strongly on the risk profile of patients with an acute MI, while it might be assumed that the relative effect of treatment was constant [86]. In addition to the severity of the disease, a treatment effect may depend on the setting, e.g., the center where a patient was treated. This is especially the case when specific skills and facilities are required for the treatment. For example, surgical mortality is known to vary widely between centers for some procedures, such as resection of esophageal cancer. Similarly, some treatments have a learning curve, which can be modeled by including a treatment * calendar time interaction term, with calendar time reflecting cumulative experience.

In randomized controlled trials, subgroup effects for treatment effects are often performed, e.g., whether the treatment works better for older than younger patients. Such subgroup effects should be supported by an interaction test for difference in effect; not with one p-value for older and one p-value for younger patients [441]. Even when subgroup analyses are prespecified, results should be interpreted cautiously because of multiple testing of the treatment effect [333]. Multiple testing inflates the risk of false positive conclusions. Indeed, we found not more statistically significant interactions than expected by chance if no differences between subgroups existed for cardiovascular trials [240] and for male–female differences in relative effect estimates [659]. Subgroup analyses are, therefore, best interpreted as secondary analyses which motivate further study rather than as conclusive analyses for a more patient-centered treatment effect estimate.

12.1.3 Other Potential Interactions

Predictor effects may differ by place and time, which would limit their generalizability (see part III). Basic issues to consider are whether predictor definitions were consistent across centers and during time. Measurement error may affect performance negatively [355]. In some individual patient data analyses, predictor effects were, however, surprisingly consistent, even when definitions varied over studies (e.g., studies in traumatic brain injury [357].). As might be expected, interactions of predictors by place of treatment were small within the GUSTO-I trial, where data were collected in a highly standardized and controlled way [539].

Various aspects of "time" can interact with predictor effects: calendar time (e.g., patients treated during the years 2000–2015), age (e.g., 30–90 years), follow-up time (e.g., 0–10 years), and season (months January–December). For example, the effects of predictors may change over the years because of improvements in treatment or changing definitions. The effects of risk factors for developing a cardiovascular disease are known to decrease with aging. Predictors having less effect in the elderly might be explained as that older subjects have proven to survive with the risk factors. For survival analysis, predictors are usually assumed to have proportional effects during follow-up, e.g., in the Cox proportional hazards model, but also in a Weibull model. Such proportionality of effects may not be tenable in the follow-up of oncological patients, where relative risks of predictors for early events decrease with time, while others may increase. For example, nonproportional effects have been noted in breast cancer survival, with no effect of stage of disease after 10 years of follow-up [402]. The proportionality assumption is equivalent to assuming no interactions between predictors and follow-up time.

Furthermore, some predictors may have a different impact during the season, e.g., for infectious and respiratory diseases (Table 12.1). Other interactions may be relevant in specific prediction problems. For example, the sex-specific effects of predictors are commonly modeled separately for cardiovascular disease risks.

12.1.4 *Example: Time and Survival After Valve Replacement

A follow-up study was done spanning over 25 years for the survival of patients after aortic valve replacement [254]. Various changes had taken place in case-mix between the first valve replacement (in 1967) and the latest replacement analyzed (in 1994). During the 25+ years period, 1449 mechanical valves were implanted. Overall early mortality (<30 days) was 5%, and was analyzed with logistic regression. Survival rates at 5, 10, and 15 years were 80%, 63%, and 49%, respectively. Poisson regression analysis was used to disentangle the effects of calendar time, age, and follow-up. All three aspects of time appeared to be important. A substantial drop in both early and late mortality was identified around the introduction of a new treatment (cardioplegia; in 1997), but no strong interactions with calendar time were found. A changing, nonproportional effect was observed for several prognostic factors during follow-up. For example, increasing effects during follow-up were found for older age ($p < 0.05$), urgency (urgent operations and acute endocarditis) ($p < 0.05$), and ascending aorta surgery ($p = 0.12$). Early year of operation, male gender and previous cardiac surgery (all $p < 0.05$) were more important during the early years of follow-up. The effects of concomitant coronary bypass surgery and concomitant mitral valve surgery were more or less constant during follow-up. This study illustrated that a Poisson regression model could be used to disentangle different aspects of time in survival analysis, including interaction effects. This model was easier to work with compared to the Cox regression model.

12.2   Selection, Estimation, and Performance with Interaction Terms

In clinical prediction models with a typical number of predictors, say 5–10, the number of potential interactions is substantial. If interactions are considered, it has been suggested to first perform an overall test for all interactions [225]. We can also obtain partial overall p-values, e.g., for all interactions with age. If this p-value is low, we may consider proceeding with studying specific interactions for inclusion in the model. This approach limits the multiple testing problem, at the price of lower power for including specific interactions. An alternative is to perform tests for individual interaction terms with a rather stringent p-value, such as 0.01 for inclusion, at the cost of more testimation bias. We illustrate the problems with the selection of interaction terms with a small subsample from the GUSTO-I study.

12.2.1   Example: Age Interactions in GUSTO-I

We study interaction with age in the relatively large subsample from GUSTO-I (sample5, $n = 785$, 52 deaths). We first fit all interactions, and then perform and overall test based on the Wald statistics. The overall test has a p-value of 0.14; but the interaction AGE * HRT is statistically significant ($p = 0.03$, not adjusted for multiple testing). Some might be tempted to include this interaction in the model. It appears that HRT (a fast heart rate, tachycardia) has a stronger effect at higher age (a positive interaction). Equivalently, we can state that age has a stronger effect in those with tachycardia (Fig. 12.1).

12.2.2   Estimation of Interaction Terms

A first distinction that some epidemiologists like to make is between "qualitative" and "quantitative" interactions. A qualitative interaction means that a predictor has

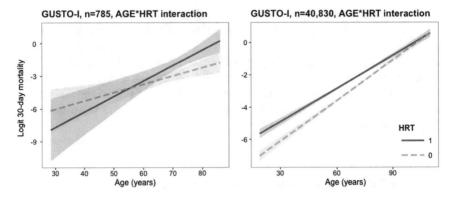

Fig. 12.1 Age by HRT interaction in GUSTO-I. In a subsample ($n = 785$, 52 deaths), a positive interaction was noted, in contrast to a slightly negative interaction in the full data set ($n = 40,830$, 2850 deaths)

an opposite effect in one group versus another group of patients. Quantitative interaction means that the effect of a predictor is in the same direction, but different in size in one group than another group of patients (see e.g., Fig. 12.1, $n = 785$). This distinction is especially important when we aim to interpret the effects of predictors; we will more be tempted to include a qualitative interaction than a quantitative interaction.

Another issue is that we can have somewhat counterintuitive effects of interactions. For example, Fig. 12.1 suggests that the presence of a fast heart rate (HRT = 1, tachycardia) is protective for 30-day mortality at ages younger than 55. If we consider this implausible, we can code the interaction such that no effect of HRT is present below age 55 (Fig. 12.2). Admittedly, the age cut-point of 55 years is data-driven. The general idea is that we incorporate subject-specific knowledge to prevent the incorporation of random noise in the model.

```
# No interaction
full8 <- glm(DAY30~AGE+KILLIP+HIG+DIA+HYP+HRT+TTR+SEX,
data=gustos,family="binomial")
# Linear interaction, 3 df
update(full8,.~.+AGE*HRT) # full.int model
# Interaction over age 50, 3 df
update(full8,.~.-HRT + ifelse(AGE>55,(AGE-55)*HRT,0)+ifelse(AGE>55,(AGE-55)*(1-
HRT),0))
# Interaction over age 50, 2 df
update(full8,.~.-HRT + ifelse(AGE>55,(AGE-55)*HRT,0))
interact_plot(full.int, pred = AGE, modx = HRT, interval=T, ...) # Fig 12.1 and
12.2
```

More generally, we can use a smart coding for interaction terms once we decide to include such a term in a model. This is especially useful when we want to readily obtain standard errors and confidence intervals for predictors in interaction with other predictors [161]. The approach is to test for interactions in models with

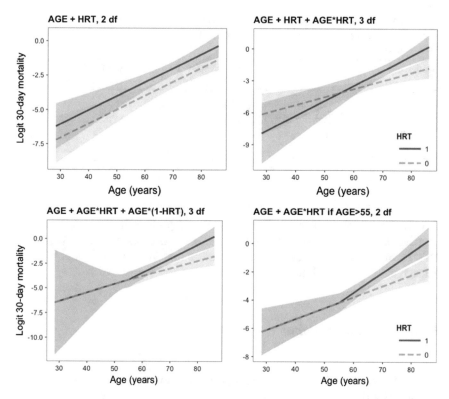

Fig. 12.2 Age by HRT relations to 30-day mortality in a subsample of GUSTO-I ($n = 785$, 52 deaths). Panel *a*: main effects only; panel *b*: simple interaction; panel *c*: separate effects for "HRT over age 55 and "no HRT over age 55"; panel *d*: one age effect and an additional effect of "HRT over age 55 years". The predictions for panel *c* and *d* are very similar; in panel *c*, 3 age effects are estimated, while in panel *d* 2 age effects are estimated

standard multiplicative terms of the form $x1 * x2$. We can estimate effects with a smarter coding of the form $x1+(1 - x1)*x2+ x1 * x2$ instead of $x1 + x2 + x1 * x2$. More details are at www.clinicalpredictionmodels.org.

12.2.3   Better Prediction with Interaction Terms?

We may wonder whether we predict better with the AGE * HRT interaction (Table 12.2). We hereto test the models as shown in Fig. 12.2 in a large, independent part of GUSTO-I ($n = 20,318$). Surprisingly, we find that a model with the AGE*HRT interaction (Fig. 12.2, panel *b*), performs worse in this external data set than a model without this interaction term. The models without the counterintuitive effect of tachycardia below age 55 perform similar, both at apparent validation and

Table 12.2 Performance (c statistics) of models developed in a subsample of GUSTO-I ($n = 785$) in an independent part of GUSTO-I ($n = 20,318$). The model with main effects contained 8 dichotomized predictors

Model	df	Apparent ($n = 785$)	Validation ($n = 20,318$)
Main effects	8	0.828	0.805
Main effects + AGE * HRT interaction	9	0.831	0.796
One age effect < 55, 2 age effects > = 55	9	0.832	0.798
HRT effect only for age > 55 years	8	0.832	0.798

at external validation in $n = 20,318$. The explanation for this remarkable finding is that the interaction between AGE and HRT was positive in the subsample, but negative in the full GUSTO-I data set (less effect of HRT at older ages, Fig. 12.1). This example illustrates that considering interaction in an unstructured way can damage the predictive ability of a model.

12.2.4 Summary Points

- Interaction depends on the scale; logistic and Cox regression models assume additivity at a logarithmic scale;
- Interaction terms to consider in a prediction model depend on the context, but some types of interactions may warrant specific consideration;
- For better interpretation, we may use a smart coding of interactions, and eliminate counterintuitive effects, e.g.. that a predictor becomes protective for some patients;
- The performance of a prediction model does not necessarily increase by including an interaction term;
- Prespecifying that interaction terms will not be included in a model may be preferable to the exploratory determination of which terms to include.

12.3 Nonlinearity in Multivariable Analysis

We discussed the assessment of continuous predictor variables in Chap. 9 for the univariate situation, where each predictor is considered separately. Harrell advocates to use restricted cubic spline functions to define transformations of continuous variables [225, 228]. An RCS function consists of pieced-together cubic splines (containing x^3 terms) that are restricted to be linear in the tails. These functions have many favorable properties, such as appropriate flexibility combined with

Table 12.3 Approaches to non-linearity in multivariable clinical prediction models

Approach	Characteristic	Multivariable strategy	R implementation
Restricted cubic splines	Cubic splines, with restriction in shape at the ends of the predictor distribution	Keep complexity as defined a priori or based on findings in univariate/multivariable analysis	rcs in Design package
Fractional polynomials	Combine one or two polynomials	Search iteratively for optimal transformations	mfp package
Splines in GAM	Spline functions with smoothing depending on effective degrees of freedom	Degrees of freedom set by the analyst or from a generalized cross-validation (GCV) procedure	gam and mgcv package

stability at the tails of the function. We can also consider multivariable modeling with fractional polynomials [477, 486], or with smoothing spline transformations (in multivariable generalized additive models, "GAM", Table 12.3). The flexibility of a smoothing spline transformation in a GAM is determined by penalty terms, which relate to the effective degrees of freedom (df). One variant is that the effective df are set by the analyst [230]. Alternatively, a generalized cross-validation (GCV) procedure can be used to define statistically optimal transformations for multiple continuous predictors in a GAM [680]. We discuss these approaches in more detail below in the context of multivariable model development.

12.3.1 Multivariable Restricted Cubic Splines (RCS)

A RCS requires the specification of knots, which can be based on the distribution of the predictor variable [225]. The key issue is the choice of the number of knots: 5 knots implies a function with 4 df, 4 knots 3 df, and 3 knots 2 df (Chap. 9). Although 5 knots are sufficient to capture many non-linear patterns, it may not be wise to include 5 knots for each continuous predictor in a multivariable model. Too much flexibility would lead to overfitting (Chap. 5). One strategy defines a priori how much flexibility will be allowed for each predictor, i.e. how many df will be spent. In smaller data sets, we may choose to use only linear terms. Or we may use splines with at most 3 knots (2 df), especially if no strong prior information suggests that a non-linear function is necessary [225]. Alternatively, we might examine different RCS transformations (5, 4, 3 knots) in univariate and/or multivariable analysis, and choose an appropriate number of knots for each predictor based on the findings in the data. Formally, the transformations with 5, 4, or 3 knots are not nested models, however. Alternatively, we might choose the complexity of non-linear functions based on the χ^2 statistic of each predictor, with more flexibility for stronger predictors.

12.3.2   *Multivariable Fractional Polynomials (FP)*

As discussed in Chap. 9, fractional polynomials are formulated as a power trans-formation of a predictor x: x^p, where p is chosen from the set $-2, -1, -0.5, 0, 0.5, 1, 2, 3$. This defines 8 transformations, including inverse (x^{-1}), log (x^0), square root ($x^{0.5}$), linear (x^1), squared (x^2), and cubic transformations (x^3). In addition to these 8 FP1 functions, 28 FP2 functions can be considered of the form $x^{p1} + x^{p2}$; when $p1 = p2$ one defines another 8 FP2 functions as $x^p + x^p \log(x)$, for a total of 36 FP2 functions [477, 486]. FP1 and FP2 transformations are considered with 2 *df* and 4 *df*, respectively.

Estimation algorithms have been developed for various software packages, including R [485]. The `mfp` algorithm applies a special type of backward stepwise selection procedure for the determination of reasonable functional forms for each continuous predictor. The algorithm starts with a full model including all predictors, with all continuous predictors in linear form. The predictors are considered in order of decreasing statistical significance, such that relatively important predictors are considered before unimportant ones [477].

For a certain continuous predictor, we may search within the 44 FP2 transfor-mations for the best fitting function. The best transformation is compared to deleting the predictor. This procedure uses 4 *df* to test for inclusion of the continuous pre-dictor, as having "any effect". If this test is significant, we may continue with a test for nonlinearity: FP2 versus linear, using 3 *df*. Finally, we test an FP2 versus FP1 transformation as a test of a more complex function against a simpler one (2 *df* test for model simplification). The functional form for this predictor is kept, and the process is repeated for each other predictor. The first iteration stops when all the variables have been processed. The next cycle is similar, except that the functional forms from the initial cycle are retained for all variables excepting the one currently being processed. Updating of FP functions and selection of variables continues until the functions and variables included in the model do not change [477, 486].

This test procedure aims to preserve the overall type I error (a "closed test" [363]). The price is that we are slightly conservative if the true predictor—outcome relation is linear, i.e., a straight line. This is because, in step 1, we test for overall effect with 4 *df*, leading to lower statistical significance in case of a truly linear relation which would, in fact, need only 1 *df*.

12.3.3   *Multivariable Splines in GAM*

In a generalized additive model (GAM), flexible, smooth functions are defined for continuous predictors. The smooth functions can be defined by splines or other "basis functions" [680]. To avoid overfitting, we statistically penalize "wiggliness" using a smoothing parameter. The penalization reduces the effective degrees of freedom used by each continuous predictor. The optimal smoothness can be determined with prediction error criteria, e.g. in generalized cross-validation (GCV) procedure. Further details are provided elsewhere [231, 680].

In multivariable modeling, splines in a GAM may serve as a reference standard for comparison of simpler, parametric transformations, such as FP (or RCS) functions [470]. We compare several approaches in a case study below. In practice, the analyst would not have to perform all of these transformations but choose one approach that he/she is familiar with.

12.4 Example: Nonlinearity in Testicular Cancer Case Study

We aim to predict the presence of tumor tissue in patients treated with chemotherapy for testicular cancer. We consider 6 predictors, of which 3 are coded as binary (Teratoma, prechemotherapy elevated AFP, prechemotherapy elevated HCG), and 3 continuous (prechemotherapy LDH, reduction in mass size during chemotherapy, postchemotherapy size). The LDH values were standardized by dividing by the upper limit of the local upper normal value ("LDHst" variable).

In initial analyses, we used restricted cubic spline (RCS) functions to study nonlinearity in the effects of the continuous predictors [551]. Subsequently, we used simple parametric transformations, mainly based on visual assessment of the univariate RCS functions [566]. The chosen transformations were logarithmic for LDHst; linear for the reduction in size; and square root postchemotherapy size (Fig. 12.3). We now explore the transformations that would be chosen with other modeling strategies, including fractional polynomials (FP) and smoothing splines in generalized additive models (GAM).

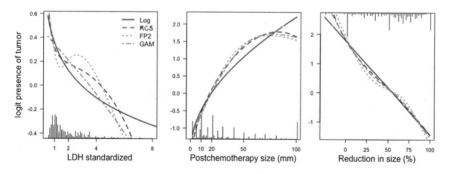

Fig. 12.3 Non-linearity in univariate analysis of LDH, postchemotherapy size and reduction in mass size. Curves are shown for a parametric approximation (log, sqrt, linear), restricted cubic spline (RCS) functions with 4 knots (3 *df*), a fractional polynomial (FP, 4 *df*), and a generalized additive model (GAM) with spline smoother. The distributions of predictor values are shown at the bottom of the graphs

We compare RCS, FP, and GAM functions. We use FP2 transformations, RCS with 4 knots (3 *df*), and GAM splines with optimized effective *df*.

1. For LDH, the transformations lead to different results. The relation of LDH to the tumor is rather different for a logarithmic transformation compared to other transformations. A simple linear term might also have been reasonable. This is supported by the FP procedure (Table 12.4). LDH has an effect (p value for "any effect" = 0.02), but nonlinearity was nonsignificant in the closed test procedure ($p = 0.48$).
2. For postchemotherapy size, the RCS, FP2, and GAM transformations agree visually (Fig. 12.3), and the square root transformation looks somewhat reasonable. The FP procedure indicates significant nonlinearity ($p = 0.0002$), and non-significant improvement by an FP2 function over an FP1 function ($p = 0.46$). The chosen FP1 function is logarithmic rather than the square root.
3. Finally, the reduction in mass size seems to be fit adequately with a linear term. The RCS, FP2, and GAM transformations fluctuate around the straight line, with the most wiggly pattern for the GAM. The FP procedure confirms that there is no reason to include non-linear terms ($p = 0.64$). The R code for these analyses is available at www.clinicalpredictionmodels.org.

The key R commands are shown below.

```
lrm(Tum~rcs(LDHst,4),data=n544) # 4 knots, 3 df
mfp(Tum~fp(LDHst,df=4), alpha=1,data=n544,family=binomial) # FP2, 4 df
gam(Tum~s(LDHst),data=n544, family=binomial) # optimal smoothing
```

12.4.1   *Details of Multivariable FP and GAM Analyses

Multivariable fractional polynomials were fitted without selection ("full model", 3 *df* for dichotomous + 3 * 4 = 12 *df* for continuous predictors, in total 15 *df*), and with a variant of a backward stepwise selection algorithm (Table 12.4). We found that winsorizing each of the three continuous predictors at their 1 and 99% quantiles before for the FP analyses led to slightly different choices of FP transformations than using the original variables.

The FP2 transformations in the full model were log(LDHst) +LDHst^3; sqrt (postsize) + sqrt(postsize)*log(postsize); and 1/reduction + 1/sqrt(reduction). A multivariable FP procedure with $p < 0.05$ for selection led to a model with linear terms for the 3 continuous predictors and 3 binary predictors (each of the 6 predictors $p < 0.01$). All tests for non-linearity were non-significant (Table 12.4). Selection with $p < 0.20$ led to a linear term for LDHst, log(postsize), and 1/reduction in FP1 transformations. Postchemotherapy size and Reduction in size had p-values for non-linearity of 0.03 and 0.08, but FP2 transformations were not much better than FP1 transformations (p-values 0.46 and 0.27, respectively, Table 12.4).

Table 12.4 Fractional polynomial analysis of 3 continuous predictors in the testicular cancer data set ($n = 544$)*

Predictor	Analysis	P value "any effect" (FP2 vs. no effect, 4 df)	P value "non-linearity" (FP2 vs. linear, 3 df)	P value "FP2" (FP2 vs. FP1, 2 df)	FP1	FP2
LDH (standardized)	Univariate	0.021	0.48	0.59	2	$-2, 3$
	Full model	<0.0001	0.18	0.73	0 (= log)	**0 (= log), 3**
	Stepwise $p < 0.05$	0.0003	0.46	0.62	0.5	0 (= log), 3
	Stepwise $p < 0.20$	<0.0001	0.28	0.66	0 (= log)	0 (= log), 3
Postchemotherapy size (mm)	Univariate	<0.0001	0.0002	0.46	0 (= log)	0.5, 1
	Full model	0.0004	0.004	0.45	0 (= log)	**0.5, 0.5**
	Stepwise $p < 0.05$	0.012	0.086	0.30	0 (= log)	$-0.5, -0.5$
	Stepwise $p < 0.20$	0.0005	0.034	0.46	**0 (= log)**	$-0.5, -0.5$
Reduction in size (%)	Univariate	<0.0001	0.64	0.63	0 (= log)	$-1, 3$
	Full model	0.0005	0.06	0.16	-1	**$-1, -0.5$**
	Stepwise $p < 0.05$	0.0002	0.64	0.78	-1	$-1, 3$
	Stepwise $p < 0.20$	0.0009	0.08	0.27	-1	$-1, -0.5$

* Fractional polynomials were considered in univariate logistic regression analysis, and in 3 multivariable logistic regression models. A full model included 3 binary predictors (Teratoma (yes/no, 1 df), Elevated AFP (yes/no, 1 df), Elevated HCG (yes/no, 1 df)), and 3 continuous predictors to handle with FP2 functions (LDH standardized, Reduction in size, Postchemotherapy size). Values in bold are the selected polynomial transformations

12.4.2   *GAM in Univariate and Multivariable Analysis*

For comparison, we examine the smooth functions selected as optimal with a generalized cross-validation procedure (GCV, Fig. 12.4). In univariate analysis, a (near) linear term is found optimal for LDH (1.2 effective *df*). Postchemotherapy size and reduction are modeled with a nonlinear function using 2.5 and 2.9 effective *df*, respectively. In multivariable analyses, nonlinear functions are used for all 3 continuous predictors, using 2.9, 3 and 4.5 effective *df* for LDHst, postchemotherapy size and reduction, respectively (Fig. 12.4). Hence, more complex transformations were chosen in multivariable than in univariate analyses. The multivariable functions for LDH looks much like a log transformation, as chosen previously. For postchemotherapy size, we see no surprises, in contrast to "Reduction", where we note an implausible wiggly shape between 20 and 100% reduction in size. Hence, the smooth functions might not be smooth enough from a pathophysiological perspective. Further external validation might indicate whether the chosen "optimal" transformations are merely examples of overfitting.

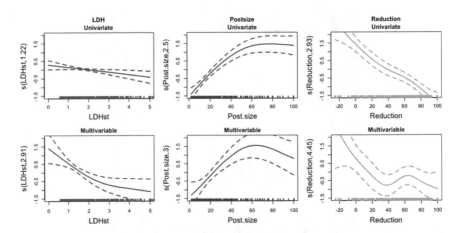

Fig. 12.4 Generalized additive models (GAMs) with optimal smoothing spline transformations and 95% confidence intervals for prediction of tumor tissue in testicular cancer (*n* = 544). Top row: optimal transformation in univariate logistic regression analysis according to a generalized cross-validation procedure; bottom row: multivariable logistic regression analysis with 6 predictors, smoothing based on generalized cross-validation. The degrees of freedom of the optimal smoothing spline transformation are shown in each y-axis label. The distribution of predictor values if shown at the bottom of the graphs

Table 12.5 Predictive performance of logistic regression models with alternative codings of 3 continuous predictors. Apparent performance is based on the original data set ($n = 544$); optimism-corrected performance is based on bootstrap validation (500 repetitions). bw: backward selection; GCV: Generalized cross-validation

Strategy	Apparent df	Model LR (χ^2)	R^2_{app} (%)	$R^2_{opt\text{-}corr}$ (%)	c_{app}	$c_{opt\text{-}corr}$
Simple bad idea: dichotomize	3 + 3	182	38.1	36.2	0.814	0.807
Assume linearity	3 + 3	205	41.8	39.6	0.831	0.824
FP2 no selection	3 + 12	227	45.6	41.6	0.849	0.835
bw $p < 0.20$ selection	3 +>3	221	44.7	40.6	0.841	0.827
RCS no selection	3 + 9	234	46.8	43.4	0.852	0.838
GAM, GCV	3 + (2.9 + 3 + 4.5)	238	47.3	39.1	0.854	0.829

12.4.3   *Predictive Performance

Finally, we study the predictive performance of the alternative nonlinear transformations (Table 12.5). As a reference, we show results for dichotomization of the three predictors LDH, postchemotherapy size, and reduction in size. Any approach to using continuous predictors performs better than this bad idea [472]. With linear terms only, we use 6 df, and achieve a model LR of 205 (apparent R^2 41.8%, internally validated R^2 39.6%). If we fit a full FP2 model without selection, we use 15 df, and achieve a model LR of 227. The increase by 22 (from 205 to 227) with 9 df is statistically significant (overall LR test, $p = 0.009$). If we apply a liberal p-value for model selection ($p < 0.20$), the model LR increases to 221. Using RCS functions with each 4 knots leads to a slightly better fit than the FP2 functions (LR 234 vs. 227). Smoothing splines were similar in fit to the RCS model.

All model LR statistics and R^2 estimates indicate apparent performance. Internal validation, including all modeling selection steps, may provide a fair indication of the expected increase in performance, after correction for optimism (see Chap. 17). Using a bootstrap resampling procedure, we find that the largest optimism was in the GAM model, which performs not better than FP2 or RCS modeling (Table 12.5). The optimism-corrected R^2 and c statistics were similar with FP2 or RCS transformations, both used without selection.

12.4.4 *R Code for Nonlinear Modeling in Testicular Cancer Example

```
# RCS: multivariable logistic regression with 3 rcs functions, each 4 knots
library(rms)
lrm(Tum ~    Teratoma+Pre.AFP+Pre.HCG+
             rcs(LDHst,4)+rcs(Post.size,4)+rcs(Reduction,4), data=n544,...)

# FP: multivariable fractional polynomial
library(mfp)
mfp(Tum ~    Teratoma+Pre.AFP+Pre.HCG+fp(LDHst)+fp(Post.size)+fp(Reduction),
             alpha=1,data=n544,family=binomial)
mfp(Tum ~    Teratoma+Pre.AFP+Pre.HCG+fp(LDHst)+fp(Post.size)+fp(Reduction),
             alpha=0.2, select=0.2,data=n544,family=binomial) #p<0.20 selection

# GAM: multivariable gam
library(mgcv)
gam(NEC ~ Teratoma+Pre.AFP+Pre.HCG+s(LDHst)+s(Post.size)+s(Reduction),
    data=n544, family=binomial)

# Validate performance by bootstrapping, key code
for (i in 1:B) { # B repetitions
  n544B <- n544[sample(nrow(n544), replace=T),] # bootstrap sample created
  full.gam.gcv.B  <- gam(Tum ~ Teratoma+Pre.AFP+Pre.HCG+
                         s(LDHst)+s(Post.size)+s(Reduction),data=n544B,...)
  val.prob(y=n544B$Tum, logit=predict(full.gam.gcv.B)) # validate at B
  val.prob(y=n544$Tum, logit=predict(full.gam.gcv.B, n544)) # val at orig
  # optimism is decrease in performance; storage of results omitted here
  ...          } # end B repetitions
```

12.5   Concluding Remarks

On the one hand, one may see the additivity and linearity assumptions as essential components of a generalized linear model. Hence, one might argue that we should assess these assumptions thoroughly. When we want to describe and interpret the effect of a specific predictor, this may make sense. In contrast, a thorough assessment of assumptions increases the risk of overfitting if we are primarily interested in obtaining predictions from a model. We will be tempted to adopt the model specification based on findings in the data, i.e., extend the model with interaction terms and/or nonlinear terms. The price of striving for such perfection is that we may end up with a model that performs worse for future patients than a parsimonious model without interaction terms or nonlinear terms. Instead, we might strive for a "wrong, but useful" model [68]. Such a model should provide well-calibrated and discriminating predictions, despite possibly violating some underlying model assumptions.

In the examples in this chapter, model performance did not increase impressively. Differences were small between models with fractional polynomials (FP), restricted cubic splines (RCS), or GAM. Of course, results may be different in other situations, but strong qualitative interaction or *U*-shaped nonlinearity may be relatively rare. In general, it may be sobering to assess the increase in predictive performance by the inclusion of interaction terms and non-linear terms with bootstrap or other internal validation procedures.

Note that prediction modeling techniques deal with interactions differently. A procedure such as Naïve Bayes estimation uses univariate effects of predictors in a multivariable prediction context; additivity is assumed, and interactions are not studied. In contrast, tree models assume high-order interaction by default. Similarly, neural networks and other machine learning algorithms assume high-order interactions, allowing for their flexibility to fit a model to a data set. Shrinkage or penalized estimation may be particularly valuable to reduce interaction effects that were identified among a large set of potential interactions (see Chap. 13).

12.5.1 Recommendations

Several measures can be taken to prevent overfitting by considering additivity and linearity assumptions.

(1) We should balance the number of interaction and non-linear terms to be considered with the effective sample size in the analysis (Table 12.6). We might only consider interactions in studies with relatively large sample sizes, i.e., many events compared to the number of terms considered. In smaller data sets, we may simply have to rely on the additivity assumption to be reasonable. We can also say that we estimate average (or "marginal") effects of predictors across subgroups; we know that we will never be able to exclude that we missed a relevant high order interaction.

Table 12.6 Approaches to limit overfitting by assessing additivity and linearity assumptions

Approach	Description
Limited number of interaction/nonlinear terms	Only consider interaction term that is a priori plausible (Table 12.1); Consider non-linear terms only for predictors with a presumed strong, and likely nonlinear, effect
Overall testing	Perform overall tests per interacting predictor (e.g., all age interactions)
Compare flexible vs. simple model	Compare the validated performance of a flexible model (e.g., including interactions and nonlinearities) with a simple model without interaction and assuming linearity; use internal validation approaches (Chap. 17)
Extra shrinkage of interaction/nonlinear terms	Use a stronger shrinkage factor or more penalty in a penalized estimation procedure for interaction and nonlinear terms (Chap. 13)

For the linearity assumption we might consider nonlinear terms only for predictors with a presumed strong, and likely nonlinear, effect. If previous studies have used a nonlinear transformation for a predictor, we could also consider this transformation. Subject knowledge should also support the choice for a transformation; plotting the effect of a transformed predictor is essential (see Figs. 12.1, 12.2, 12.3 and 12.4).

(2) We should use overall tests, rather than focus on separate tests for interaction and nonlinear terms. Note that based on an overall test, we would not have continued estimation of the interaction of age and a fast heart rate (HRT, tachycardia) in the GUSTO-I subsample (Sects. 12.2–12.4). Interaction terms make life a bit more difficult for model presentation, arguing against their inclusion in a model unless their relevance is substantial for the specific prediction problem.

(3) As an extension of this overall testing approach we might compare the performance of a flexible model to a simple model without interaction and nonlinear effects (e.g., Table 12.5). The flexible model may, for example, be a neural network, or a GAM. Both the simple model and the flexible model should be validated, e.g., with bootstrapping, to assess the validated rather than apparent improvement that might be achieved with the inclusion of interaction and nonlinear terms.

(4) Finally, we may use shrinkage techniques to reduce the regression coefficients of selected interaction or nonlinear terms. Some extra shrinkage may compensate for the "testimation bias" (see Chaps. 5 and 11), which is expected when terms were included in a model because they were relatively large [225]. The search for interactions and nonlinear terms makes that the effective degrees of freedom of a flexible model is larger than the final degrees of freedom of a fitted model. This is recognized by FP transformations, where FP1 is tested with 2 *df*, and FP2 with 4 *df*.

Questions

12.1. Additivity and interaction

(a) Explain the additivity assumption in your own words, and the relevance of the scale for assessing additivity?

(b) Explain the interaction terms in your own words?

(c) How many interaction terms can be assessed in a model with 10 binary predictors?

(d) What is the probability that at least one of these is statistically significant at the $p < 0.05$ level, if the underlying model has main effects only?

12.2. Assumptions and model performance

(a) Why would you consider testing of the additivity assumption with interaction terms?

(b) Which key problem can occur when interactions and non-linearities are included in the model? How can this be prevented?

(c) Model performance increases with more flexible non-linear functions. In Table 12.5 the maximum Model LR is 238. Is this model hence to be preferred for predicting the outcome, or do you think other considerations are also relevant?

Chapter 13
Modern Estimation Methods

Background In this chapter, we discuss methods to estimate regression coefficients which lead to better predictions than obtained with traditional estimation methods. These modern estimation methods include uniform shrinkage methods (heuristic or bootstrap based) and penalized maximum likelihood methods (with various forms of penalty, including ridge regression and the LASSO). We illustrate the application of these methods with a data set of 785 patients from the GUSTO-I study.

13.1   Predictions from Regression and Other Models

In linear regression, we aim to minimize the mean squared error, which is calculated as the square distance between observed outcome Y and prediction $\hat{Y}$. The prediction $\hat{Y}$ can be based on a multivariable combination of predictors, e.g., age, sex, smoking, and salt intake are used to predict blood pressure. As discussed in previous chapters, we can improve predictions from multivariable models for future subjects if the predictions are shrunk towards the average. We can reduce the mean squared error for future subjects by using slightly biased regression coefficients [109, 627]. This is because the slightly biased predictions have lower variance. The challenge is to find the optimal balance between increasing bias and decreasing variance. This "bias-variance" trade-off underlies the problem of overfitting (Chap. 5).

In generalized linear regression models, such as logistic or Cox models, maximum likelihood methods are the classical methods for estimation of regression coefficients. Similar to linear regression, the estimated coefficients can be

© Springer Nature Switzerland AG 2019
E. W. Steyerberg, *Clinical Prediction Models*, Statistics for Biology
and Health, https://doi.org/10.1007/978-3-030-16399-0_13

considered as optimal for the sample under study. But again, introducing some bias in the coefficients may lead to better predictions for future subjects.

13.1.1   *Estimation with Other Modeling Approaches

Neural networks are examples of generalized nonlinear models (see Chap. 4). One popular estimation technique is minimizing the Kullback–Leibler divergence, which can be considered as a distance between two probability densities [318]. One density is provided by the observed outcomes, another by the estimates from the model. Minimizing the Kullback–Leibler divergence is similar to maximizing the likelihood in a generalized linear regression model. Neural networks are quite flexible and will hence be severely overfitted when they are fully optimized to fit the data. Therefore, a common procedure is "early stopping": the model is not fully trained for maximum fit to the data, but training is stopped at the point where predictive ability is expected to be best. Commonly, the optimal number of iterations to train the model is determined from a cross-validation procedure, where the model is trained on part of the data and tested on an independent part [140]. The optimal number of iterations is then used in the full training part to develop the neural network. This procedure is a form of shrinkage: parameters are used with suboptimal fit to the data but best predictive ability.

13.2   Shrinkage

Shrinkage of regression coefficients towards zero is a classic approach to improve predictions from a regression model [109, 627]. We label this method *shrinkage after estimation*, since the shrinkage is applied to regression coefficients after the model has been fitted initially with traditional methods (Table 13.1).

Table 13.1 Characteristics of some shrinkage methods

Name	Label	Characteristic
Uniform shrinkage	Shrinkage after estimation	Application of a shrinkage factor to regression coefficients. The shrinkage factor is determined with a heuristic formula or by bootstrapping
Penalized maximum likelihood	Shrinkage during estimation	Regression coefficients are estimated with penalized maximum likelihood and a restriction on the sum of squared coefficients ("Ridge", $L2$ penalty)
LASSO	Shrinkage for selection	Regression coefficients are estimated with penalized maximum likelihood with a restriction on the sum of the coefficients ("LASSO", $L1$ penalty)
Elastic net	Shrinkage and selection	Regression coefficients are estimated with a combination of $L1$ penalty and $L2$ penalty

Penalized estimation is an alternative method, which uses a penalty factor in the estimation of the regression coefficients: larger values of standardized regression coefficients are penalized in the fitting procedure, leading to smaller values being preferred. We refer to this method as *shrinkage during estimation*. Although one single penalty factor is used, the degree of shrinkage varies by predictor. A variant of penalized estimation was proposed by Firth [165]. This method estimates regression coefficients even in situations where separation occurs, and traditional maximum likelihood estimates would go to infinity [209]. Another variant of penalized estimation is the LASSO ("least absolute shrinkage and selection operator") [581]. This approach penalizes the sum of the absolute values of the regression coefficients. This leads to some coefficients becoming zero. A predictor with a coefficient of zero can be excluded from the model, which means that the LASSO implies *shrinkage for selection*. The penalized and LASSO variants of penalization are combined in the "Elastic Net" [689]. Penalized regression, shrinkage, or regularization methods are used as synonyms here, and discussed in more detail below.

13.2.1 Uniform Shrinkage

A simple and straightforward approach is to apply a uniform (or *linear*) shrinkage factor for the regression coefficients. Shrunk regression coefficients are calculated as $s * b_i$, where s is a uniform shrinkage factor and b_i are the estimated regression coefficients. The shrinkage factor s may be based on a heuristic formula [109, 627]:

$$s = \left(\text{model } \chi^2 - df\right)/\text{model } \chi^2,$$

where model χ^2 is the likelihood ratio χ^2 of the fitted model (i.e., the difference in log likelihood between the model with and without predictors) and df indicates the effective degrees of freedom. The effective df may be best estimated by the df of all candidate predictors considered for the model, rather than the df of the selected predictors for the model. The required shrinkage increases when larger numbers of predictors are considered (more df), or when the sample size is smaller (smaller model χ^2).

We can also calculate the shrinkage factor s with bootstrapping [225, 627].

1. Take a random bootstrap sample of the same size as the original sample, drawn with replacement.
2. Select the predictors according to the selection procedure (if used) and estimate the logistic regression coefficients in the bootstrap sample.
3. Calculate the value of the linear predictor for each patient in the original sample. The linear predictor is the linear combination of the regression coefficients as estimated in the bootstrap sample with the values of the predictors in the original sample.

4. Estimate the slope of the linear predictor, using the outcomes of the patients in the original sample.

Steps 1–4 need to be repeated many times to obtain a stable estimate of the shrinkage factor as the mean of the slopes in step 4. For example, we may use 200 bootstrap samples, although a fully stable estimate of the shrinkage factor may require 500 bootstrap repetitions [535]. The shrinkage factor may take values between 0 and 1.

13.2.2 Uniform Shrinkage: Illustration

As an example, we consider a subsample from the GUSTO-I study of patients with an acute myocardial infarction (see Chap. 24). The data set ("sample4") consists of 785 patients, of whom 52 had died by 30 days. We consider two models for prediction of 30-day mortality after an acute MI: an 8-predictor model and a 17-predictor model. For estimation of the heuristic shrinkage factor, we need the model χ^2 statistics of each model. These were 62.6 and 73.5. The heuristic shrinkage estimate s was hence $(62.6 - 8)/62.6 = 0.87$. The 17-predictor model required more shrinkage, with $s = (73.5 - 17)/73.5 = 0.77$.

A bootstrap procedure was performed with 500 replications. This resulted in identical estimates of the slope of the linear predictor (0.87 and 0.77, respectively). The regression coefficients are shown in Table 13.2.

Table 13.2 Logistic regression coefficients estimated with standard maximum likelihood ("original"), uniform shrinkage, penalized maximum likelihood, Firth regression, and the LASSO for sample4 (795 patients with acute MI, 52 deaths by 30 days)

Predictor	Original	Shrunk	Penalized[a]	Firth	LASSO
SHO	1.12	0.97	1.17	1.10	1.10
A65	1.49	1.30	1.21	1.44	1.38
HIG	0.84	0.74	0.72	0.81	0.74
DIA	0.43	0.38	0.36	0.46	0.32
HYP	0.99	0.86	0.83	1.03	0.82
HRT	0.96	0.84	0.84	0.94	0.88
TTR	0.59	0.51	0.49	0.57	0.47
SEX	0.07	0.06	0.11	0.08	0.00
Effective shrinkage	1	0.87	0.87 0.81–1.49	0.98 0.96–1.14	0.91 0–0.97

[a]Penalized maximum likelihood or ridge regression (L2 penalty from `pentrace` in `rms`). Elastic Net regression identified the ridge regression model as optimal

13.3   Penalized Estimation

Penalized maximum likelihood estimation is a generalization of the ridge regression method, which can be used to obtain more stable parameters for linear regression models [139]. Instead of maximizing the log likelihood in generalized linear models, a penalized version of the log likelihood is maximized, in which a penalty factor λ is used with squared values of the estimated coefficients b_i:

$$\text{PML} = \log L - 0.5 \, \lambda \, \Sigma (s_i b_i)^2,$$

where PML is penalized maximum likelihood, L is the maximum likelihood of the fitted model, λ is a penalty factor, b_i is the estimated regression coefficient for each predictor i in the model, and s_i is a scaling factor for each b_i to make $s_i b_i$ unitless [225, 646]. It is convenient to use the standard deviation of each predictor for the scaling factor s_i [225]. Shrinkage of the coefficients is achieved by penalizing the regression model with a penalty term called $L2$-norm, which is the sum of the squared coefficients.

13.3.1   *Penalized Maximum Likelihood Estimation

The PML can also be formulated as PML $= \log L - 0.5 \, \lambda \, b' \, P \, b$, where λ is a penalty factor, b' denotes the transpose of the vector of estimated regression coefficients b_i (excluding the intercept), and P is a nonnegative, symmetric penalty matrix. For penalized estimation, the diagonal of P consists of the variances of the predictors and all other values of P are set to 0 [225]. If P is defined as $\text{cov}(b)^{-1}$ (i.e., the inverse of the covariance matrix of the estimated regression coefficients b), shrinkage of the regression coefficients is achieved which is identical to the use of a uniform shrinkage factor as determined by leave-one-out cross-validation [646]. If P is equal to the matrix of second derivatives of the likelihood function, PML is similar to applying a uniform shrinkage factor $s = 1/(1 + \lambda)$.

The main question in penalized estimation is how to choose the optimal penalty factor λ_{opt}. Maximizing a modified Akaike's Information Criterion (AIC) is an efficient method [198]. Traditionally, the AIC is defined as $-2 \log L + 2p$, where L is the maximum likelihood of the fitted model and p is the degrees of freedom equal to the number of fitted predictors. A more convenient formulation is as

$$\text{AIC}_{\text{model}} = \text{model } \chi^2 - 2p,$$

where model χ^2 is the likelihood ratio χ^2 of the fitted model (i.e., the difference in $-2 \log$ likelihood between the model with and without predictors). For penalized maximum likelihood estimation, we use a modified AIC, defined as

$$\text{AIC}_{\text{penalized}} = \text{model } \chi^2_{\text{penalized}} - 2 * df_{\text{effective}},$$

where model $\chi^2_{\text{penalized}}$ refers to likelihood ratio χ^2 of the penalized model and $df_{\text{effective}}$ is the degrees of freedom after penalizing the coefficients. In standard logistic regression, the df are equal to the number of predictors in the model; the higher the number of predictors, the higher the df and the more likely the model is overfitted. Due to the penalization, the $df_{\text{effective}}$ used in penalized estimation is lower than the actual number of predictors. More technically, $df_{\text{effective}}$ is derived from the reduction in variance of penalized estimates in comparison to the variance of standard estimates of b_i:

$$df_{\text{effective}} = \text{trace}[I(b)\text{cov}(b)],$$

where $I(b)$ is the information matrix as computed without the penalty function and $\text{cov}(b)$ is the covariance matrix as computed by inverting the information matrix calculated with the penalty function. If both $I(b)$ and $\text{cov}(b)$ are estimated without penalty, $I(b)\text{cov}(b)$ is the identity matrix and trace $[I(b)\text{cov}(b)]$ is equal to the number of estimated coefficients b_i in the model [198]. With a positive penalty function, the $\text{cov}(b)$ becomes smaller and $df_{\text{effective}}$ decreases. With higher penalty values, the model $\chi^2_{\text{penalized}}$ decreases (poorer fit to the data), but so does the $df_{\text{effective}}$. The maximum of $\text{AIC}_{\text{penalized}}$ (model $\chi^2_{\text{penalized}} - 2 * df_{\text{effective}}$) is sought by varying the values of λ. For example, we may vary λ over a grid such as 0, 1, 2, 4, 6, 8, 12, 16, 24, 32, 48. Larger values of λ are required for more complex models and larger data sets. The optimal penalty factor λ_{opt} is the value of λ that maximizes $\text{AIC}_{\text{penalized}}$. With this optimal λ, the final model is estimated. An alternative is to use cross-validation or bootstrapping to find λ_{opt}, which is more computer intensive compared to finding the maximum of $\text{AIC}_{\text{penalized}}$.

13.3.2   Penalized ML: Illustration

We may search for a penalty factor λ_{opt} over a grid using the `pentrace` function in the `rms` package. The fitting procedure for the 8-predictor model is as follows:

```
# logistic regression model with 8-predictors
full8        <- lrm(DAY30~SHO+A65+HIG+DIA+HYP+HRT+TTR+SEX, data=gustos)
# determine performance over range of penalties
p8     <- pentrace(full8, c(0,2,4,6,8,10,12,14,16,18,20,22, 24, 28, 32,40))
# fit penalized model
full8.pen    <- update(full8, penalty=p8$penalty)
```

The $\text{AIC}_{\text{penalized}}$ is calculated with the effective degrees of freedom ($df_{\text{effective}}$) and is plotted in Fig. 13.1. The optimum penalty factors λ_{opt} was estimated as 8 for the 8-predictor model and 24 for the 17-predictor model. So λ_{opt} was larger for the more complex mode, as expected. The effective degrees of freedom were 6.9

Fig. 13.1 AIC$_{penalized}$ in relation to the penalty factor. Optimum values are 8 and 24 for the 8- and 17-predictor models, respectively. The more complex model with 17-predictors needs more penalization

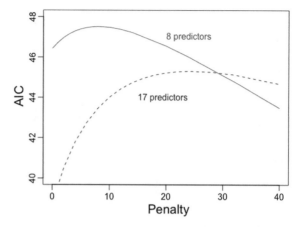

(instead of 8) and 10.8 (instead of 17). Note that the AIC$_{penalized}$ was worse for the 17-predictor model compared to the 8-predictor model. This reflects that the 17-predictor model was overfitted with only 52 events in the data set. The effective shrinkage was 0.87 (Table 13.1).

13.3.3 *Optimal Penalty by Bootstrapping

For comparison, we also performed a bootstrap procedure to find the optimal penalty factor λ_{opt}. We created logistic regression models with a range of penalty factors in bootstrap samples drawn with replacement. The models were tested in the original sample. A linear predictor was calculated with the penalized coefficients from the bootstrap sample and the predictor values in the original sample: lp = $X_{original}$ %*% $b_{penalized,bootstrap}$. Various performance measures can be calculated. We focus on the slope of the linear predictor, since the primary objective of shrinkage methods is to improve calibration. As expected, the slope is below 1 when no shrinkage is applied (Fig. 13.2). It appears that the slope is 1 if we apply a penalty factor of 7 for the 8-predictor model and 12 for the 17-predictor model. These values are slightly lower than obtained from maximizing the AIC$_{penalized}$. This could be explained by the fact that AIC considers the model χ^2 as criterion rather than the slope of the linear predictor. The model χ^2 is also influenced by the discriminative ability, which was higher with a larger penalty value for the 17-predictor model (Fig. 13.2).

13.3.4 Firth Regression

Firth regression was proposed as a method to reduce bias in maximum likelihood estimates [165]. Bias occurs especially in sparse data, where either the event is rare or some categorized predictor has few subjects. An example in GUSTO-I is the

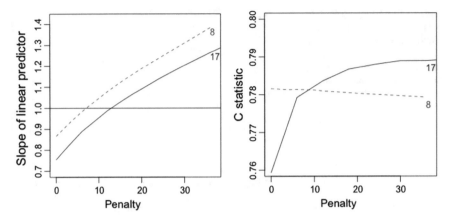

Fig. 13.2 Slope of the linear predictor (left panel) and C statistic (right panel) in relation to the penalty factor according to a bootstrap procedure. For slope, the optimum values are 7 and 12 for the 8- and 17-predictor models, respectively, while penalties of 0 and around 42 would optimize the *c* statistic

occurrence of Shock (<5% of subjects). With sparse data, all the subjects may have the same event status (0 or 1). This phenomenon is known as separation. It causes severe problems fitting the model with standard maximum likelihood. A symptom of separation, or near separation, is that we note large standard errors. Software may report an error ("non-convergence") or a warning, while very small or very large regression coefficient estimates are still returned with huge SE. One solution for this situation is to apply exact logistic regression [235]. Firth regression is computationally less demanding.

13.3.5   *Firth Regression: Illustration*

We use the package `brglm` ("Bias Reduction in Binomial-Response Generalized Linear Models") because of convenience in fitting and making predictions over the `logistf` package. The model can be fitted using maximum penalized likelihood, where the penalization is done using Jeffreys invariant prior or using bias-reducing modified scores. These methods gave identical results in the example of the 8-predictor model in a subsample from GUSTO-I. No cross-validation is needed:

```
# logistic regression model with 8-predictors
model8.Firth <- brglm(DAY30~SHO+A65+HIG+DIA+HYP+HRT+TTR+SEX, data=gustos)
```

The estimated coefficients are very close to the maximum likelihood estimates (Table 13.2). The effective shrinkage was only 0.98, which is insufficient for prediction purposes, although the stability of Firth estimation is an advantage over other shrinkage approaches.

13.4 LASSO

A method to achieve model selection through shrinkage is the LASSO (least absolute shrinkage and selection operator) [232, 581]. The LASSO can also be used for generalized linear models such as the logistic or Cox model [582]. The LASSO preferentially shrinks some predictor coefficients to zero by penalizing the absolute values of the regression coefficients.

13.4.1   *Estimation of a LASSO Model

The LASSO estimates the regression coefficients of standardized predictors by minimizing the log likelihood subject to $\Sigma|b| \leq t$, where t determines the shrinkage in the model. We estimate the final set b_i with the value of t that gives the lowest mean squared error in a cross-validation procedure [582].

We may use the glmnet package for R to perform LASSO analyses [232]. The logistic regression coefficients were estimated given a bound ("L1 Norm") to the sum of absolute standardized regression coefficients, $|b|$. This is implemented as setting alpha = 1. For ridge regression (Sect. 13.3), we may specify alpha = 0. The predictors are standardized such that sum $|b|$ does not depend on coding of predictors.

```
# Fit LASSO for a range of penalties
glmmod <- glmnet(full8$x, y=full8$y, alpha=1, family="binomial")
plot(glmmod, xvar="norm", ...) # Fig 13.3 upper left
# Find the best lambda using cross-validation for the full8 model
set.seed(123)
cv <- cv.glmnet(x=full8$x, y=full8$y, alpha = 1, family=c("binomial"))
plot(cv,...) # Fig 13.3 upper right
model8.L1 <- glmnet(x=full8$x, y=full8$y, alpha=1, lambda=cv$lambda.min,
family=c("binomial"))
coef(model8.L1) # Coefficients in Table 13.2
```

We find that with a strong penalty, quite small coefficients are estimated for the predictors A65 (Age > 65 years), SHO (Shock), and HRT (Heart rate). This occurred both in the 8- and 17-predictor models (Fig. 13.3). The other predictors had coefficients set to zero. With larger bounds, nonzero coefficients were estimated for these predictors as well. With high L1 norm values (low penalty λ) all predictors were selected with the original, unshrunk coefficients.

The optimum penalty can be estimated by a cross-validation procedure (Fig. 13.3). This suggests an optimal selection of 7 predictors in the 8-predictor

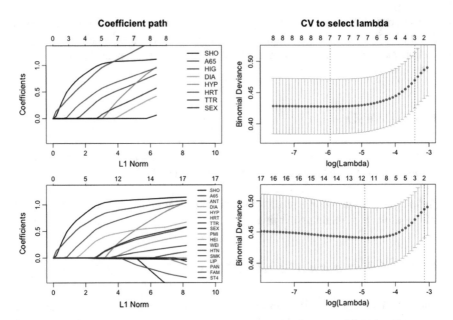

Fig. 13.3 Coefficients and cross-validated performance for the 8- and 17-predictor models (top and bottom graphs, respectively), according to the sum of the absolute values of the estimated regression coefficients (L1 Norm = |standardized betas|) in sample 4 from GUSTO-I (n = 785, 52 deaths). We note that larger coefficients are estimated in the 8-predictor model for SHO and A65 (left graphs), with an expected better performance according to cross-validation (right graphs)

model ($\log(\min(\lambda))$ = -5.9), and a selection of 14 predictors for the 17-predictor model ($\log(\min(\lambda))$ = -4.9). The coefficients for the final model can be chosen at the lowest cross-validated λ value, or more conservatively, at a 1 standard error larger value of λ [232]. For the 8-predictor model, the effect of SEX was set to zero, and the coefficient of DIA was small (coefficient 0.32) with the optimal penalty. The effective shrinkage was 0.91 (Table 13.2). For the 17-predictor model, the predictors LIP, PAN, and ST4 were dropped. Note that the penalty for the 17-predictor model is larger than for the 8-predictor model, and that the cross-validated performance was worse (binomial deviance, equivalent to the model likelihood ratio scale, Fig. 13.3).

13.5   Elastic Net

A combination of LASSO-type selection and ridge-type penalization is possible with the Elastic Net [232, 689]. Elastic Net produces a regression model that is penalized with both the *L1* and *L2* norms. The Elastic Net selects a limited number of predictors, similar to the LASSO, while it may predict slightly better than the

LASSO, depending on the specific setting. In addition, the Elastic Net shows a grouping effect, where strongly correlated predictors tend to be in or out of the model together [689].

13.5.1   *Estimation of Elastic Net Model*

The Elastic Net requires two parameters labeled alpha and lambda. The mixing parameter alpha lies between 0 and 1 ($0 \leq \alpha \leq 1$). Setting $\alpha = 1$ is the LASSO penalty *L1* and $\alpha = 0$ the ridge penalty *L2*, with the penalty is defined as $(1 - \alpha)/2$ $|\beta|_2^2 + \alpha|\beta|_1$. We may consider a range of possible α and L1/L2 values for the Elastic Net model, with the optimum combination based on their performance in a cross-validation procedure. This can be achieved with the `cva.glmnet` function from the `glmnetUtils` package. In the subsample of GUSTO-I, the optimal alpha value was 0, equivalent to ridge regression. An R script is available at www. clinicalpredictionmodels.org.

13.6   Performance After Shrinkage

Shrinkage leads to less extreme distributions of predictions. The linear predictor is shrunk towards the average compared with standard maximum likelihood, either with uniform shrinkage, penalized maximum likelihood estimation (PMLE), or the LASSO (Fig. 13.4). Shrinkage hence prevents that too extreme predictions are derived from the development data set. Indeed Table 13.3 illustrates that the calibration slope is closer to 1 in independent test data when shrinkage was applied in small samples drawn from the GUSTO-I data set (see Chaps. 22 and 24).

Fig. 13.4 Distribution of the linear predictor in sample 4 from GUSTO-I with standard maximum likelihood, uniform shrinkage, Ridge and Firth regression, and the LASSO. The penalized fits were obtained with the `cv.glmnet` function in `glmnet` and Firth regression with `brglm`

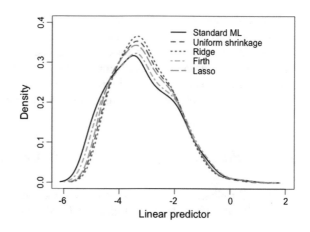

Table 13.3 Discrimination (*c* statistic) and calibration (calibration slope) of the 8- and 17-predictor models based on small and large subsamples (average *n* = 336 and *n* = 892, respectively), and based on the total training part (*n* = 20,512), as evaluated in the independent test part (*n* = 20,318). Mean values are shown for several estimation methods with a fixed selection of predictors

Training data		8 predictors	17 predictors
		C statistic	C statistic
Total training (*n* = 20,512, 1423 deaths)	Standard ML	0.789	0.802
61 small subsamples (*n* = 336, 23 deaths on average)	Standard ML	0.75	
	Uniform	0.75	
	shrinkage	0.76	
	Penalized ML	0.75	
	LASSO		
23 large subsamples (*n* = 892, 62 deaths on average)	Standard ML	0.78	0.78
	Uniform	0.78	0.78
	shrinkage	0.78	0.79
	Penalized ML	0.78	0.78
	LASSO		
		Calibration slope	Calibration slope
Total training (*n* = 20,512, 1423 deaths)	Standard ML	0.944	0.959
61 small subsamples (*n* = 336, 23 deaths on average)	Standard ML	0.66	
	Uniform	1.01	
	shrinkage	0.93	
	Penalized ML	0.83	
	LASSO		
23 large subsamples (*n* = 892, 62 deaths on average)	Standard ML	0.86	0.76
	Uniform	0.97	0.95
	shrinkage	0.96	0.98
	Penalized ML	1.01	0.93
	LASSO		

Discrimination was similar with or without shrinkage. Generally, LASSO is expected to perform better in situations of some predictors with large effects, and the remaining predictors with small coefficients. Ridge regression will perform somewhat better when many predictors have coefficients of roughly equal size. The Elastic Net is expected to perform well for in-between situations; it preserves some of the advantages of LASSO in reducing the number of predictors in the model.

13.6.1   Shrinkage, Penalization, and Model Selection

Uniform shrinkage and penalized estimation methods are defined for prespecified models. If we apply a selection strategy such as stepwise selection, fewer predictors are included in the selected model, and we might expect less need for shrinkage of coefficients. However, we know that a "testimation" problem arises, i.e., coefficients of selected predictors are overestimated (Chaps. 5 and 11). This selection bias should be taken into account when calculating a shrinkage factor. This may be achieved by considering the *df* of the candidate predictors in the heuristic formula (instead of the number of selected predictors) [627]. In a bootstrap procedure, we can include the selection process in step 2 [225]. Empirical research suggests that the required shrinkage is more or less similar in prespecified or selected models [542]. For penalized estimates of the regression coefficients after selection, we can apply the penalty factor that was identified as optimal for the full model, before selection took place. A more refined option is to fit a LASSO or Elastic Net model, where selection is achieved through shrinkage of coefficients to zero [232].

A specific situation is that a substantial number of interaction terms are tested, and one or more are included in the final model. For shrinkage, we could still use the original *df* of the model with main effects and all interactions considered. A more elegant solution was suggested by Harrell for penalized ML estimation, i.e., to penalize the interaction terms more than the main effects, for example, with twice the penalty of the main effects [225]. This approach may be used to limit the impact of treatment by predictor interactions if we develop a prediction model for individualized treatment effect in an RCT [300]. Similarly, nonlinear effects and nonlinear interaction terms might be penalized by twice and four times the penalty of the main effects, respectively [225].

13.7 Concluding Remarks

Shrinkage of regression coefficients is an important way to battle overfitting; on average, too extreme predictions are prevented. Note that having a larger data set, considering fewer predictors, and incorporating external knowledge are better ways to prevent overfitting. Shrinkage is especially needed in small data sets, and/or situations with large numbers of candidate predictors. Using advanced shrinkage procedures is readily possible with modern software, implemented in, e.g., R. The glmnet package may be the most versatile, while rms has easy options for *L2* penalized estimation. Penalty factors are a general concept in smooth estimation of model parameters; they are important in curve fitting (e.g., with splines) and generalized additive models [231]. The LASSO currently receives interest for prediction analysis in Big Data and other situations with large numbers of potential predictors [452].

Questions

13.1 Shrinkage and model performance
Explain how shrinkage can influence
(a) the predictions from a model, (b) calibration, and (c) discrimination?

13.2 Penalized maximum likelihood

(a) Why might we label PML "shrinkage during estimation" (Table 13.1)
(b) How is it possible that one penalty term leads to differential shrinkage in Table 13.2?
(c) In the prediction of abnormalities at CT scans [519], we can assess the effect of PML on the various coefficients. Which coefficients are penalized most?

13.3 Shrinkage methods and stepwise selection (Sect. 13.3.3)
How can shrinkage and penalization be used when the model is developed with stepwise selection:

(a) Uniform shrinkage with Van Houwelingen's formula or bootstrapping?
(b) Penalized maximum likelihood?

Chapter 14
Estimation with External Information

Background In this chapter, we discuss methods that estimate regression coefficients based on the combination of findings in the sample under study with external information from published studies. The aim is to develop a global model, which has broad applicability. Such a model might be informed by a meta-analysis based on individual patient data (IPD) from multiple studies. We illustrate this approach with a meta-analysis of 15 studies of traumatic brain injury. Another aim is to obtain a better model for a specific, local setting. This aim may be addressed by a simple "adaptation" method for univariate regression coefficients, which are obtained from a meta-analysis. We illustrate this method in a case study of operative mortality of abdominal aneurysm surgery. We discuss some further approaches to estimation of regression coefficients, including stacked regressions and Bayesian estimation with explicit prior information.

14.1 Combining Literature and Individual Patient Data (IPD)

Let's consider the common situation that several studies have been published for a particular clinical prediction problem, in which the relation between patient characteristics and the outcome of interest is described. Obviously, some of that knowledge should be useful in model building, beyond using individual patient data (IPD)? If the published papers describe findings from comparable patient series, we may try to combine the available evidence quantitatively in a meta-analysis. The reported findings in these papers may vary substantially, however, for example:

© Springer Nature Switzerland AG 2019
E. W. Steyerberg, *Clinical Prediction Models*, Statistics for Biology
and Health, https://doi.org/10.1007/978-3-030-16399-0_14

Table 14.1 Characteristics of model development with a focus on a locally applicable model versus a globally applicable model. We assume we have a data set with individual patient data (IPD) and literature data, i.e., published prediction studies

Modeling aspect	Local model	Global model
Model specification	Mixture of IPD and literature	Focus on consensus in literature
Model coefficients	IPD with literature as background	Meta-analysis of literature
Baseline risk	IPD	Literature

(a) Only univariate results can be obtained for the effects of potential predictors;
(b) Some multivariable models have been proposed, with different sets of predictors;
(c) A common multivariable model is found in some studies, with identical predictors.

In practice, situations (a) and (b) may be most common. Situation (c) might be ideal but rare. For each situation, we may want to focus on a model with local or global applicability (Table 14.1).

14.1.1   A Global Prediction Model

A global model may readily be aimed for if multiple studies have published the same prediction model. We may then perform a meta-analysis, with the aim to produce a single, global model. Pooling of published regression coefficients might use multivariate meta-analysis techniques (e.g., the mvmeta function) for the combined set of predictors, although a naïve pooling of each multivariable regression coefficient may work reasonably well [129]. Ignoring stratification by study is overly naïve in any meta-analysis, and should be avoided [6]. A more relevant situation is that we have access to individual patient data (IPD) from different cohorts. We can then directly model the predictor effects, although some predictors may be systematically missing per study (see Chaps. 7 and 8).

The baseline risk for the global model poses specific challenges, both when the model is based on reported regression coefficients or based on IPD analyses. We may use a random effect model for the model intercept in logistic regression or a frailty model in survival analysis (see Chap. 21). A random effect model may provide estimates of a global average plus the between-study heterogeneity in baseline risk. If this between-study heterogeneity is small, the average risk may apply broadly.

Similarly, we can assess the heterogeneity in regression coefficients between studies [31]. If this heterogeneity is small, the global model is supported. If substantial differences are noted, we may search for explanations. Are some studies from specific settings where the measurement of predictors was different, or a different selection process had occurred [355]? Outlier studies might be excluded to define the global model more precisely.

The general philosophy for a global model is that we may except some bias by pooling heterogeneous data sources, if compensated by lower variance because of higher numbers. The global model has a single set of coefficients that is assumed to apply broadly. We illustrate the estimation of a global model for a case study.

14.1.2 *A Global Model for Traumatic Brain Injury

For illustrative purposes, we consider 15 cohort studies of patients suffering from traumatic brain injury (TBI, see Chap. 8). These studies were included in the IMPACT project, where a total of 25 prognostic factors were considered for prediction of 6-month outcome [343].

We develop a "global model" by considering individual patient data (IPD) from the 15 studies, with stratification by study (Table 14.2). We may estimate the following simple global model:

$$p(\text{Mortality}) = -1.35 + 0.28 * \text{age} - 0.38 \\ * \text{motor score} + 0.61 \text{ irresponsive pupils},$$

Table 14.2 Multivariable logistic regression models to predict mortality 6 months after TBI in 15 studies. We show estimated regression coefficients with associated standard errors per study, and results from a two-stage meta-analysis. We also show the between-study variance parameter τ and prediction intervals for the regression coefficients

Study	Intercept	Age	Motor score	Pupillary reactivity
1	−1.22 (0.09)	0.20 (0.05)	−0.39 (0.08)	0.41 (0.11)
2	−1.40 (0.10)	0.21 (0.07)	−0.40 (0.08)	0.36 (0.11)
3	−1.35 (0.22)	0.28 (0.09)	−0.28 (0.12)	0.71 (0.23)
4	−1.34 (0.09)	0.20 (0.06)	−0.14 (0.07)	0.74 (0.11)
5	−1.73 (0.10)	0.21 (0.05)	−0.52 (0.06)	0.52 (0.08)
6	−1.41 (0.19)	0.30 (0.09)	−0.45 (0.13)	0.82 (0.17)
7	−0.93 (0.11)	0.43 (0.05)	−0.30 (0.09)	1.01 (0.12)
8	−0.73 (0.12)	0.47 (0.07)	−0.42 (0.10)	0.57 (0.12)
9	−1.28 (0.35)	0.38 (0.16)	−0.23 (0.22)	0.34 (0.26)
10	−1.41 (0.12)	0.40 (0.05)	−0.45 (0.09)	0.80 (0.12)
11	−1.44 (0.11)	0.22 (0.06)	−0.40 (0.09)	0.43 (0.11)
12	−1.49 (0.17)	0.24 (0.10)	−0.39 (0.11)	0.68 (0.14)
13	−1.43 (0.14)	0.22 (0.09)	−0.42 (0.11)	0.68 (0.14)
14	−1.61 (0.11)	0.17 (0.07)	−0.34 (0.09)	0.29 (0.16)
15	−2.07 (0.18)	0.52 (0.07)	−0.59 (0.15)	0.91 (0.16)
Two-stage pooled estimated coefficient	−1.35 (0.07)	0.28 (0.03)	−0.38 (0.03)	0.61 (0.06)
Estimated τ	0.25	0.09	0.07	0.17
95% Prediction interval	[−1.92, −0.78]	[0.08, 0.48]	[−0.55, −0.20]	[0.21, 1.01]

where age is coded per 10 years, motor score ranges from 1 to 6, and 1 or 2 pupils may be irresponsive. The between-study variance parameter τ was checked for each predictor and was reasonably small for each.

Rather than the average intercept (-1.35), we might also consider the baseline risk from a single, representative study. For example, we might estimate the intercept for study #14, which was an RCT that enrolled patients between 2001 and 2004, with the global model coefficients in an offset variable:

$$\text{Mortality}|\text{Study 14} \sim \alpha_{14} + \text{offset}(\text{global linear predictor}),$$

where the global linear predictor is the linear combination of global coefficients with the covariate values in Study 14. Further explorations of heterogeneity are possible, as discussed elsewhere [127].

14.1.3 Developing a Local Prediction Model

We now assume that we have access to individual patient data (IPD) from only one specific setting. We may focus on obtaining a better model for that setting by using information from the published literature. If the IPD are representative for other settings, we may still hope for global applicability of the model. No checks for heterogeneity can be performed with limited data however.

At least, a literature review may reveal which predictors have been studied frequently, suggesting a set of candidate predictors. Some predictors may stand out as being studied relatively often, with relatively substantial effect. Model specification may hence be informed by findings from outside the data set under study (Chap. 11).

The model coefficients may be estimated with external information as well. We focus on the situation that only univariate regression coefficients are available from the literature. How might we utilize such external information?

14.1.4 Adaptation of Univariate Coefficients

An "adaptation method" has been proposed to take advantage of the univariate literature data in the estimation of the multivariable regression coefficients in a prediction model [129, 544]. The aim is better prediction of the outcome in individual patients from a specific setting. This adaptation method is closely related to an earlier proposal by Greenland for meta-analysis [201]. For example, when studying the relation between coffee consumption and acute myocardial infarction, one study may have corrected the regression coefficient for a confounder (for example, alcohol consumption), while other studies have not. Greenland proposed to use the change from unadjusted to adjusted regression coefficient to adapt the unadjusted coefficients in the latter studies. We discuss two variants of an adaptation method for the regression model as estimated in the single IPD data set.

14.1.5 *Adaptation Method 1

We aim to perform a regression analysis that combines information from literature and individual patient data. The regression coefficients can be formulated as

$$\beta_{m \mid I+L} = \beta_{u \mid L} + \left(\beta_{m \mid I} - \beta_{m \mid I} \right),$$

where $\beta_{m \mid I+L}$ refers to the multivariable coefficient based on the combination of individual patient data and literature data (the "adapted coefficient"), $\beta_{u \mid L}$ is the univariate coefficient from a meta-analysis of the literature, and $\beta_{m \mid I} - \beta_{u \mid I}$ is the difference between multivariable and univariate coefficient in the IPD data set (the "adaptation factor"). Hence, we simply use the change from univariate to multivariable coefficient in our IPD data to adapt the meta-analysis coefficient.

For the variance of the adapted coefficient ($\mathrm{var}(\beta_{m \mid I+L})$), we may add the difference between variances of the multivariable and univariate coefficient to the variance of the univariate coefficient from the literature, ignoring all covariances [544]:

$$\mathrm{var}(\beta_{m \mid I+L}) = \mathrm{var}(\beta_{u \mid L}) + \mathrm{var}(\beta_{m \mid I}) - \mathrm{var}(\beta_{u \mid I}).$$

14.1.6 *Adaptation Method 2

A more general way to formulate the adaptation formula is

$$\beta_{m \mid I+L} = \beta_{u \mid L} + c \,(\beta_{m \mid I} - \beta_{u \mid I}), \quad \text{where } c \text{ is a factor between 0 and 1.}$$

If $c = 1$, the same formula as proposed by Greenland arises. If c equals 0, the literature data is effectively discarded. The estimate of $\beta_{m \mid I+L}$ is unbiased for any choice of c, if the expectation of $\beta_{u \mid L} - \beta_{u \mid I} = 0$, that is, the individual patient data form a random part from the studies included in the meta-analysis. Actually, this implies that the method may provide global model estimates. We found that we can derive a formula for c such as to minimize the variance of $\beta_{m \mid I+L}$:

$$c_{\mathrm{opt}} = r(\beta_{m \mid I} - \beta_{u \mid I}) * \mathrm{SE}(\beta_{m \mid I}) * \mathrm{SE}(\beta_{u \mid I}) / [\mathrm{var}(\beta_{u \mid L}) + \mathrm{var}(\beta_{u \mid I})],$$

where $r\,(\beta_{m \mid I} - \beta_{u \mid I})$ refers to the correlation between multivariable and univariate coefficient in the individual patient data.

This variant of the adaptation method indicates that adaptation will be especially advantageous if the literature data set is larger (resulting in a smaller var($\beta_{u \mid L}$)), or when the correlation r ($\beta_{m \mid I} - \beta_{u \mid I}$) is larger. The latter correlation is expected to be large if the collinearity between covariables is small [544]. The adaptation factor will then be close to 1 and method 1 may yield good results too.

14.1.7 *Estimation of Adaptation Factors*

Meta-analysis techniques may be used to estimate the univariate coefficients from the literature data. The literature data may include the individual patient data for maximal efficiency. The meta-analysis may assume fixed effects (for example, Mantel–Haenszel method, or conditional logistic regression), or random effects (for example, DerSimonian Laird method or likelihood-based methods) [83]. The calculations for method 1 use estimates that are readily available. For example, logistic regression analysis with standard maximum likelihood (ML) provides estimates of the univariate and multivariable coefficients in the individual patient data.

For the second method, the estimation of the optimal adaptation factor requires estimates of the variances of the regression coefficients, and an estimate of the correlation between univariate and multivariable coefficients. The latter correlation cannot easily be estimated with logistic regression methods. We therefore used bootstrap re-sampling to estimate the coefficients $\beta_{m \mid I}$ and $\beta_{u \mid I}$ repeatedly, and their correlation.

14.1.8 *Simulation Results*

The adaptation methods were applied in the GUSTO-I data [544]. First, we assessed the correlation between multivariable and univariate coefficients across 121 small subsamples. We observed a strong correlation for the combination of age and sex in a two-predictor model (Fig. 14.1). Results were somewhat less favorable for predictors with stronger collinearity. For example, weight and height had a Pearson correlation coefficient of 0.54, and the correlation between their univariate and multivariable coefficients was 0.80 and 0.83, respectively. The strong r ($\beta_{m \mid I} - \beta_{u \mid I}$) supports the use of the adaptation method.

Next, the values of c_{opt} were quite close to 1 (0.98 ± 0.015 and 0.99 ± 0.020 for age and sex (mean $\pm$ SD) in the 121 small subsamples). Hence, Greenland's method ($c = 1$) and adaptation method 2 (c_{opt} estimated with bootstrapping) resulted in very similar estimates of the adapted coefficients (Fig. 14.2). Both methods lead to much better estimates of the multivariable regression coefficients in the small subsamples. These very favorable results were obtained by using univariate results from approximately half of the GUSTO-I data ($n = 20{,}000$). When using univariate results from a neighboring, small subsample, the sample size was

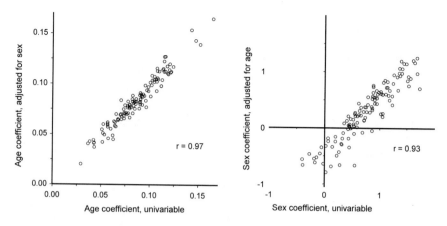

Fig. 14.1 Correlations between univariate and multivariable regression coefficients in a two-predictor model consisting of age and sex estimated in 121 small subsamples of the GUSTO-I data set [544]

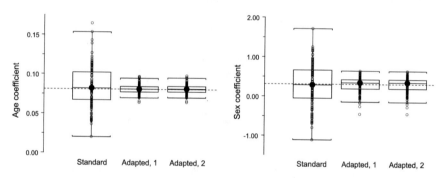

Fig. 14.2 Regression coefficients in the two-predictor model consisting of age and sex. Box plots show the standard ML, and adapted estimates (methods 1 and 2) for 121 small subsamples with $n = 20,000$ as literature data; - - - - indicates the coefficient observed in the total GUSTO-I data set ($n = 40,830$) [544]

effectively doubled. This pattern was also reflected in the values of the adaptation factor from method 2; close to 1 with $n = 20,000$ as literature data, ± 0.50 with a neighbor subsample as literature data [544].

14.1.9   Performance of the Adapted Model

Finally, we compared the predictive performance of the adaptation method to the performance obtained with uniform shrinkage, penalized ML, or the LASSO in 23 large subsamples from GUSTO-I (Table 14.3). The discriminative ability improved

Table 14.3 Discrimination (c statistic) and calibration (calibration slope) of the 8- and 17-predictor models based on large subsamples (average $n = 892$), and based on the total training part ($n = 20,512$), as evaluated in the independent test part of GUSTO-I ($n = 20,318$). Mean shown for two variants of the adaptation method and several other modern estimation methods

Training data		8 predictors	17 predictors
		c statistic	c statistic
Total training ($n = 20512$, 1423 deaths)	Standard ML	0.789	0.802
23 large subsamples ($n = 892$, 62 deaths on average)	Standard ML	0.78	0.78
	Uniform shrinkage	0.78	0.78
	Penalized ML	0.78	0.79
	LASSO	0.78	0.79
	Adapted 1	0.79	0.78
	Adapted 2	0.79	0.79
		Slope	Slope
Total training ($n = 20512$, 1423 deaths)	Standard ML	0.944	0.959
23 large subsamples ($n = 892$, 62 deaths on average)	Standard ML	0.86	0.76
	Uniform shrinkage	0.97	0.95
	Penalized ML	0.96	0.98
	LASSO	1.01	0.93
	Adapted 1	0.92	0.86
	Adapted 2	0.92	0.86

slightly (+0.01), but some problems were noted in calibration. Miscalibration was better than for the standard ML estimates, but some form of shrinkage should actually have been built into the adaptation method (see www.clinicalpredictionmodels.org for some possibilities).

14.2   Case Study: Prediction Model for AAA Surgical Mortality

In our examples with GUSTO-I, no relevant differences were noted between adaptation methods 1 and 2. Since method 1 is much simpler to apply, we only consider this method further. We applied adaptation method 1 in the prediction of perioperative mortality (in-hospital or within 30 days) after elective abdominal aortic aneurysm surgery [555]. Individual patient data were available on a relatively small sample (246 patients, 18 deaths). Patients were operated on at the University Hospital Leiden between 1977 and 1988. Univariate literature data were available

Table 14.4 Meta-analysis results for operative mortality of elective aortic aneurysm surgery: coefficient (SE) per predictor

Predictor	Fixed effect	Random effect
Age (per decade)	0.79 (0.06)	0.79 (0.11)
Female sex	0.36 (0.08)	0.36 (0.18)
History of MI	1.03 (0.27)	1.03 (0.32)
Congestive heart failure	1.59 (0.33)	1.59 (0.41)
ECG: Ischemia	1.52 (0.31)	1.51 (0.38)
Impaired renal function	1.32 (0.25)	1.30 (0.26)
Impaired pulmonary function	0.89 (0.23)	0.85 (0.24)

from 15 published series with 15,821 patients (1153 deaths) in total. Predictors were age and sex, cardiac comorbidity (history of myocardial infarction (MI), congestive heart failure (CHF), and ischemia on the ECG), pulmonary comorbidity (COPD, emphysema, or dyspnea), and renal comorbidity (elevated preoperative creatinine level). These predictors were chosen since they were reported in at least two studies and were also available in the Leiden data set.

14.2.1   Meta-Analysis

Univariate logistic regression coefficients were estimated both with fixed and random effects methods from the literature data. As expected, the estimates of the coefficients were very similar, but the SEs were somewhat larger with the random effect method (Table 14.4).

A number of practical issues merit discussion with respect to the meta-analysis of the literature data. First, definitions of predictors varied, especially for pulmonary and renal comorbidity. Despite these differences, it was considered reasonable to assume one single effect for each predictor across the studies (nonsignificant tests for heterogeneity of odds ratios; nonsignificant interaction terms between study and effect estimates in logistic regression).

Second, the number of studies that described a predictor varied. The effect of age was reported in 15 studies, sex and renal function in six, pulmonary function in five, MI in three, and CHF and ECG findings in only two. This somewhat limits the value of the adaptation method in this case study.

Third, the analysis of age as a continuous variable was hampered by the fact that mortalities were described in relatively large age intervals, for example, younger or older than 70 years. For logistic regression analysis, we estimated the mean ages in these age intervals using study-specific descriptions as far as available (mean and SE) [208]. The effect of age would have been estimated more accurately if smaller age intervals had been reported.

Table 14.5 Individual patient data results ($n = 246$) for operative mortality of elective aortic aneurysm surgery: coefficient (SE) for Standard ML, and coefficient estimates for Shrunk and Penalized models

Predictor	Univariate	Standard ML	Shrunk	Penalized	$r(\beta_{m|l}, \beta_{u|l})$
Age (per decade)	0.98 (0.38)	0.58 (0.39)	0.48	0.34	0.91
Female sex	0.28 (0.79)	0.30 (0.86)	0.25	0.17	0.81
History of MI	1.50 (0.50)	0.74 (0.57)	0.61	0.57	0.88
Congestive heart failure	1.78 (0.55)	1.04 (0.59)	0.86	0.67	0.92
ECG: Ischaemia	1.72 (0.55)	0.99 (0.62)	0.83	0.63	0.87
Impaired renal function	1.24 (0.70)	1.12 (0.77)	0.93	0.74	0.85
Impaired pulmonary function	0.84 (0.53)	0.61 (0.59)	0.51	0.39	0.90

14.2.2   Individual Patient Data Analysis

In the individual patient data, multivariable logistic regression coefficients were usually smaller than the univariate coefficients, reflecting a predominantly positive correlation between predictors (Table 14.5). Correlations were strongest between the three cardiac comorbidity factors (r 0.26, 0.32, and 0.45). We note that the number of predictors (7) was large relative to the number of events (18 deaths). Bootstrapping estimated a shrinkage factor of 0.83 (200 replications, convergence in only 119), and penalized ML was performed with 14 as the penalty factor. The correlation between univariate and multivariable coefficients was estimated between 0.81 and 0.91 (Table 14.5).

14.2.3   Adaptation and Clinical Presentation

The literature and individual patient data were combined with the adaptation method, using the random effect estimates from the literature data. The adaptation factor was always set to 1 (Table 14.6; for method 2, c_{opt} was estimated between 0.63 and 0.86, results not shown). Compared to shrunk or penalized coefficients, the adapted estimates for sex, renal, and pulmonary function were somewhat higher and lower for a history of MI.

For application in clinical practice, scores were created by rounding each adapted coefficient after multiplication by 10 and shrinkage of 90% ((1 + bootstrap shrinkage factor)/2 $\approx$ 0.90). The intercept was calculated with the linear predictor as an offset variable in a logistic regression model. The offset was the linear combination of the scores (divided by 10) and the values of the covariables in the individual patient data.

Table 14.6 Individual patient data results ($n = 246$) for operative mortality of elective aortic aneurysm surgery. Numbers are logistic regression coefficients (SE)

Predictor	$\beta_{m\,|\,I} - \beta_{u\,|\,I}$	Adapted	Score
Age (per decade)	−0.40	0.38 (0.14)	3
Female sex	+0.02	0.38 (0.40)	3
History of MI	−0.76	0.27 (0.41)	2
Congestive heart failure	−0.74	0.85 (0.47)	8
ECG: Ischaemia	−0.73	0.79 (0.48)	7
Impaired renal function	−0.12	1.18 (0.41)	11
Impaired pulmonary function	−0.23	0.62 (0.34)	6

Score: rounded value of 10 * 90% * Adapted

$$\text{Mortality} \sim a + \text{offset}(\text{score}/10).$$

The intercept a was estimated as −3.48. Note that offset with score divided by 10 preserves the shrinkage. If we had estimated a model with the linear predictor as the single predictor, the slope b would be 1/90% = 1.1:

$$\text{Mortality} \sim a + b * (\text{score}/10).$$

The intercept was further adjusted for a presumably lower mortality in current surgical practice (5%) than that observed in the individual patient data (7.6%). This adjustment can be considered as a form of recalibration to contemporary circumstances. It was achieved by subtracting ln(odds(5%)/odds(7.6%)) = −0.44 from the previous intercept estimate: −3.48 − 0.44 = −3.92. This results in a final formula to estimate the risk of perioperative mortality in current elective abdominal aortic aneurysm surgery:

$$\text{p(Mortality)} = 1 / \left[1 + e^{(-(\text{score}/10 - 3.92))} \right].$$

The c statistic was 0.83 in the individual patient data with standard, shrunk, or penalized estimation. The optimism-corrected estimates were 0.80 for standard or shrunk estimation, and 0.81 for penalized estimation (bootstrapping with 200 replications). For the final model with adapted coefficients, we expect a performance at least as good as these methods, but this needs to be confirmed in further validation studies. The main limitation in this case study is the limited sample size in the IPD (only 18 events).

14.3   Alternative Approaches

Several alternative approaches are possible to include published regression results in a multivariable model. We discuss three approaches below: using an overall calibration factor for the univariate literature coefficients, stacked regression, and Bayesian methods.

14.3.1 Overall Calibration

One variant of naïve Bayes was already suggested in Chap. 4, i.e., use of a uniform, overall calibration factor for all univariate coefficients. In the case study of aortic aneurysm mortality, the calibration factor is 0.69 for a linear predictor based on the univariate coefficients from the literature multiplied with the predictor values in the IPD. The multivariable coefficients are reasonably close to those estimated with our adaptation method, except for cardiac comorbidity factors (scores 7, 11, and 10 for MI, CHF, and ISCHEMIA, versus 2, 8, and 7 with the adaptation method, respectively). This is explained by the relatively strong correlations among these factors, while the overall calibration only reflects an average correlation between the seven predictors.

14.3.2 Stacked Regressions

Rather than a set of univariate regression coefficients, we may often find that some prediction models have been published with different sets of predictors. If some look promising we might analyze these models with "stacked regression", i.e., we include the linear predictor of each literature model in our analysis. Each linear predictor is given a weight to create a linear combination of the included models. If the weight is close to zero, the model has no relevant contribution, and the model might be dropped [128]. With this approach, we may obtain a weighted sum of predictor effects which respects the relative weights as proposed in the publications, while we use a low number of degrees of freedom.

14.3.3 Bayesian Methods: Using Data Priors to Regression Modeling

Some have argued that a Bayesian perspective needs to be incorporated into basic biostatistical and epidemiological training [202]. In small data sets with many predictors, Bayesian approaches may offer advantages over conventional frequentist methods. Specifically, estimation of regression coefficients is difficult for data with few or no subjects at crucial combinations of predictor values.

Bayesian estimation consists of setting prior values for the regression coefficients, which are combined with the estimates in the data to produce posterior estimates of the coefficients. When the prior values are all zero, the coefficients are pulled towards zero. This is similar to shrinkage, as discussed in Chap. 13. Setting a prior to zero may be reasonable for a variable with very doubtful value as a predictor. A negative or positive effect is then equally likely, making zero the best prior guess. We may allow for the possibility that the effect is nonzero, while we consider large values unlikely. The degree of shrinkage is then determined by the width of the prior distribution. The narrower the prior distribution, the more the prior shrinks the coefficient towards zero [209]. The other factor that determines the effective shrinkage is the information in our data set. With many events, we will obtain limited shrinkage. The final estimate is an average of the prior expectation and the conventional estimate.

An even more interesting role for Bayesian approaches in regression is in using informative priors. For example, we may hypothesize a priori that a predictor has an odds ratio of 2, with values smaller than 0.5 and larger than 8 being highly unlikely. Setting a reasonable informative prior is the most difficult task for any Bayesian analysis. Expert judgment can be used, or literature review [209]. When using informative priors, the source of these priors should be well documented, and sufficient variability allowed in the prior distribution. Presentation of prior information can be presented as "informationally equivalent", e.g., assuming knowledge of 100 patients with a certain outcome [204]. This kind of reasoning may be increasingly acceptable to many in the medical field [209].

14.3.4 Example: Predicting Neonatal Death

Greenland describes a case study of predicting neonatal-death risk in a cohort of 2992 births with 17 deaths [202]. He estimates logistic regression models with 14 predictors, assuming small to large effects for most predictors. He finds that the predictive ability of the Bayesian model is better than a model based on standard maximum likelihood. He also illustrates how Bayesian estimation can be achieved relatively easily with data augmentation: records are added to a data set, reflecting predictive effects of predictors [204]. In the case of a multivariable model, the prior distributions refer to the multivariable effects of predictors, which may be more complicated to elicit from experts or from literature than univariate effects (Sect. 14.2).

14.3.5 *Example: Aneurysm Study

In the prediction of perioperative mortality of aortic aneurysms, we might try to use informative priors based on the literature. The meta-analysis, however, provides univariate effects, and we need to translate these to priors for multivariable effects. The difference between univariate and multivariable coefficients is directly related to the correlation between predictors. If we have some guesses for these correlations, this may give some hints on how the multivariable coefficients compare to the univariate coefficients. For example, with substantial correlations, we might halve all univariate coefficients; with no correlation, we keep the multivariable effect at the univariate estimate. Being on the conservative side with informative priors may be sensible to make Bayesian analysis more acceptable.

14.4   Concluding Remarks

The methods in this chapter emphasize the central role of subject knowledge in developing prediction models in small data sets. Literature data may guide the selection of predictors (Chap. 11), as well as improve the estimates of the regression coefficients. Especially when the data set is relatively small, this strategy will result in more reliable regression models than using a strategy that considers a data set with individual patient data as the sole source of information.

A potential problem of meta-analyses is that publication bias may have led to overestimation of the regression coefficients. Also, performing a meta-analysis may not be realistic if definitions of risk factors vary substantially in the literature.

Bayesian methods provide another perspective on estimation of regression coefficients. As with any Bayesian method, the main criticism will be on the choice of prior distribution. Many papers have been written about Bayesian approaches, but Bayesian methods have not yet made it to mainstream predictive modeling, other than as computational tools with non-informative priors. Bayesian approaches may be used in the context of model updating (Chap. 20) [514, 573]. A variant is empirical Bayes estimation (Chap. 21). Empirical Bayes methods have an important role in, e.g., estimating between center effects and provider profiling. With this variant, the distribution of center effects is determined empirically from the data, and the effect for a particular center can be estimated in the context of this distribution.

Note that the field of machine learning may be seen as in contrast with Bayesian approaches, in that machine learning generally downplays the role of context and prior knowledge by relying strongly on the data alone. On the other hand, machine learning modelers are aware of risks of overfitting and employ penalization methods which often behave similar to Bayesian approaches [209].

Questions

14.1 We examine the effect of the adaptation method with a different set of univariate literature estimates in the aneurysm case study

- What would happen to the adapted effects when larger univariate coefficients were found in the literature?
- What would happen to the adapted effects when the univariate coefficients were identical in the literature and in the individual patient data?
- What would happen to the adapted effects when there was virtually no correlation between predictors?

14.2 What is the relation between shrinkage and Bayesian methods according to Greenland [209] (https://www.bmj.com/content/352/bmj.i1981)?

Chapter 15
Evaluation of Performance

Background When we develop or validate a prediction model, we want to quantify the quality of the predictions from the model ("model performance"). Predictions are absolute risks, which go beyond assessments of relative risks, such as regression coefficients, odds ratios, or hazard ratios. We can distinguish apparent, internally validated, and externally validated model performance (Chap. 5). For all types of validation, we need performance criteria in line with the research questions, and different perspectives can be chosen. We first take the perspective that we want to quantify how close our predictions are to the actual outcome. Next, more specific questions can be asked about calibration and discrimination properties of the model, which are especially relevant for prediction of binary outcomes in individual patients. We illustrate the use of performance measures in the testicular cancer case study.

15.1 Overall Performance Measures

The distance between the predicted outcome $\hat{y}$ and actual outcome y is a central to quantify overall model performance from a statistical perspective [231]. The distance, or residual, is $y - \hat{y}$ for continuous outcomes. For binary outcomes, $\hat{y}$ is equal to the predicted probability p, and for survival outcomes, it is the predicted time to an event. These distances between observed and predicted outcomes are related to the concept of "goodness-of-fit" of a model, and the amount of variability that is explained. Better models have smaller distances between predicted and observed outcomes $(y - \hat{y})$.

© Springer Nature Switzerland AG 2019
E. W. Steyerberg, *Clinical Prediction Models*, Statistics for Biology
and Health, https://doi.org/10.1007/978-3-030-16399-0_15

15.1.1   *Explained Variation:* R^2

The explained variation (R^2) is an overall measure to quantify the amount of information in a model in a given data set. R^2 is useful to guide various model development steps for all types of regression models commonly used in prognostic research, including linear and generalized linear models (e.g., logistic, Cox). With R^2, we can readily compare the impact of different encoding of predictors, different shapes of the relations of continuous predictors to the outcome, different selections of predictors, and the impact of including interaction terms (see previous chapters).

R^2 is the most commonly used performance measure for continuous outcomes. For generalized linear models, Nagelkerke's R^2 can well be used [403], although many alternatives are available, and some may prefer other definitions [7]. As discussed in Chap. 4, this R^2 is based on a logarithmic scoring rule: $(y - 1) *$ $(\log(1 - p)) + y * \log(p)$. The logarithm of predictions p is compared to the actual outcome Y. For binary outcomes, the log likelihood for a patient with the outcome is $\log(p)$; without the outcome $\log(1 - p)$. When a very low prediction is made for a patient who actually had the outcome, this prediction has a severe score (Fig. 15.1). This gives an infinite disadvantage for a prediction model that gives a prediction of 0 or 1 while the outcome is discordant.

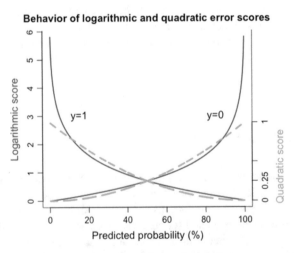

Fig. 15.1 Logarithmic and quadratic error scores of a subject with ($y = 1$) or without ($y = 0$) the outcome in relation to predicted probability (p). The logarithmic score was calculated as $y *$ log $(p) + (1 - y) * (1 - p)$, as in Nagelkerke's R^2 (solid line ——). The quadratic score was calculated as $(y - p)^2$, as in the Brier score (dashed line - - -). Lines were scaled such that they crossed at $p = 50\%$. We note that the logarithmic score severely penalizes false predictions close to 0 or 100%

15.1.2 Brier Score

An alternative for binary outcomes is to use a quadratic scoring rule, where the squared differences between actual outcomes y and predictions p are calculated. This calculation is done in the Brier score, which is simply defined as $(y - p)^2$. We can also write this similar as the logarithmic score: $y * (1 - p)^2 + (1 - y) * p^2$, with y the outcome and p the prediction for each subject. For a subject, the score can range from 0 (prediction and outcome equal) to 1 (discordant prediction); a prediction of 50% has a score of 0.25 both when the outcome is 0 or 1. The Brier score is hence less severe than Nagelkerke's R^2 in penalizing false predictions close to 0% or 100% (Fig. 15.1). The Brier score for a model can range from 0% for a perfect model to 0.25 for a non-informative model with a 50% incidence of the outcome. When the incidence is lower, the maximum score for a model is lower, e.g., for 10%: $0.1 * (1 - 0.1)^2 + (1 - 0.1) * 0.1^2 = 0.090$. A disadvantage of the Brier score is hence that the interpretation depends on the incidence of the outcome.

Similar to Nagelkerke's approach to the LR statistic, we should scale Brier by its maximum score: $\text{Brier}_{scaled} = 1 - \text{Brier} / \text{Brier}_{max}$, where $\text{Brier}_{max} = \text{mean}(p) * (1 - \text{mean}(p))^2 + (1 - \text{mean}(p)) * \text{mean}(p)^2$, with mean($p$) indicating the average probability of the outcome. Brier_{scaled} ranges between 0 and 100%, and hence has better interpretability [568].

15.1.3 Performance of Testicular Cancer Prediction Model

We consider a development sample containing 544 patients [551], and a validation sample 273 patients treated at Indiana University Medical Center [644]. We developed a logistic regression model with five predictors: teratoma elements in the primary tumor, prechemotherapy levels of AFP and HCG, postchemotherapy mass size, and reduction in mass size.

Internal validation of performance was estimated with bootstrapping (500 replications). Bootstrap samples were created by drawing random samples with replacement from the development sample. The prediction model was fitted in each bootstrap sample and tested on the original sample.

The R code is

```
# 5 predictors in data set n544; develop testicular cancer model
full          <- full <- lrm(tum ~
ter+preafp+prehcg+sqpost+reduc10,data=n544)
val.prob(logit=full$linear.predictor, y=full$y) # apparent
validate(full, B=500)   # Internal validation with 500 bootstraps
# External validation; refit model for matrix x and comparison of coefs
val.prob(y=val$tum, logit=predict(full, val)) # external validation in val
```

Nagelkerke's R^2 was 38.9% in the development sample, and slightly lower at internal validation (Table 15.1). At external validation, the R^2 was estimated

Table 15.1 Overall performance of testicular cancer prediction model[a]

	Development	Internal validation	External validation
R^2 (%)	38.9	37.4	26.7
Brier	0.174	0.178	0.161
$Brier_{max}$	0.248	0.248	0.201
$Brier_{scaled}$ (%)	29.8	28.2	20.0

[a]Development and internal validation with n = 544 patients, external validation in n = 273 patients. Internal validation with 500 bootstrap resamples using Harrell's `validate.lrm` function. $Brier_{scaled} = 1 - Brier/Brier_{max}$

considerably lower, as 26.7%. Note that R^2 is based on the difference between a Null model ("intercept only") and a model with recalibrated predictions (intercept + calibration slope * logit of predictions) [225]. So, the R^2 is estimated after recalibration of the predictions.

The Brier score was 0.174 and 0.178 at development and internal validation, respectively. Remarkably, the Brier score was better at external validation (0.161). The external Brier score was simply calculated by comparing predictions with actual outcome, without recalibration as was done for R^2. The interpretation of the Brier score is easier with the scaled version, which compensates for the fact that the maximum Brier score was lower in the external validation set (necrosis in 76 of 273 (28%), $Brier_{max}$ 0.20) than in the development set (necrosis in 245 of 544 (45%), $Brier_{max}$ 0.248). The scaled Brier score was clearly lower at external validation than at internal validation (20% versus 28%, Table 15.1).

15.1.4   Overall Performance Measures in Survival

Nagelkerke's R^2 can readily be calculated for survival outcomes, based on the difference in –2 log likelihood of a model without and a model with the linear predictor. Calculation of the Brier score is not directly possible because of censoring: not all subjects are followed long enough for the outcome to occur. To address the censoring issue, we can define a weight function, which considers the conditional probability of being uncensored during time [194, 494, 495]. The assumption is that the censoring mechanism is independent of survival and the subject's history. We can hence calculate the Brier score at fixed time points. For example, we can compare predicted survival versus observed survival at 1, 2, and 5 years of follow-up. Choosing many consecutive time points leads to a time-dependent graph. This is useful as a benchmark curve, based on the Brier score for the overall Kaplan–Meier estimator, which does not consider any predictive information. The survival estimates of the overall Kaplan–Meier curve only depend on time of follow-up. An interesting example is provided by a case study on the disappointing contribution of microarray data to prediction of survival for patients with diffuse large-B-cell lymphoma [494].

15.1.5 Decomposition in Discrimination and Calibration

Overall statistical performance measures incorporate both calibration and discrimination aspects. For example, the Brier score can formally be decomposed into indicators of calibration and discrimination [54, 396]. Discrimination relates to how well a prediction model can discriminate those with the outcome from those without the outcome. Calibration relates to the agreement between observed outcomes and predictions and is especially relevant at external validation. Studying discriminative ability and calibration is then more meaningful than an overall measure such as R^2 or Brier score when we want to appreciate the quality of model predictions for individuals. We therefore discuss these aspects in detail.

15.1.6 Summary Points

- R^2 is a common measure to express the amount of variability in outcomes that is explained by the prediction model; commonly, it is a logarithmic scoring rule.
- The Brier score is another commonly reported performance measure for the squared distance between observed and predicted outcomes; it can be seen as a quadratic scoring rule and needs scaling to be interpretable between settings with different event rates.

15.2 Discriminative Ability

Model predictions for binary outcomes need to discriminate between those with and those without the outcome ("Event" versus "No event"). Several measures can be used to indicate how good we classify patients in such a binary prediction problem. The concordance (c) statistic is the most commonly used performance measure to indicate the discriminative ability of generalized linear regression models. For a binary outcome, c is identical to the area under the receiver operating characteristic (ROC) curve (AUC). The ROC curve is a plot of the sensitivity (true positive rate) against 1—specificity (false-positive rate) for consecutive cutoffs for the probability of an outcome. We therefore consider sensitivity and specificity first.

15.2.1 Sensitivity and Specificity of Prediction Models

Sensitivity is defined as the fraction of true positive (TP) classifications among the total number of patients with the outcome (TP/N_{Event}), and the specificity as the fraction of true negative classifications among the total number of patients without

Table 15.2 Classification of subjects according to a cutoff for the probability of an outcome (Event or No event)

	Event	No event
Predicted probability >= cutoff	TP	FP
Predicted probability < cutoff	FN	TN
	N_{Event}	$N_{No\ event}$

TP and FP: numbers of True- and False-Positive classifications; FN and TN: numbers of False and True Negative classifications, respectively. N_{Event} = TP + FN; $N_{No\ event}$ = FP + TN

the outcome (TN/$N_{No\ event}$, Table 15.2). To classify a patient as positive or negative, we need to apply a cutoff to the predicted probability. If the prediction is higher than the cutoff, the patient is classified as positive, otherwise, as negative. It is common to use a cutoff of 50% for classification. This cutoff is often not defendable in a medical context, as we will discuss in detail in Chap. 16. We can examine sensitivity and specificity over the whole range of cutoffs from 0 to 100%. The results can be plotted in a receiver operating characteristic (ROC) curve [223].

15.2.2   Example: Sensitivity and Specificity of Testicular Cancer Prediction Model

For the 544 patients with testicular cancer, we might classify patients as having tumor when the probability is over 50%. With this threshold, we find a sensitivity of 77% and a specificity of 32% (FP rate 68%). With a lower cutoff, for example, 30%, these numbers are 92% and 42%, respectively. This illustrates that a lower cutoff leads to better sensitivity, at the price of a lower specificity. This trade-off is visualized in a ROC curve (Fig. 15.2).

15.2.3   ROC Curve

A plot of a ROC curve has often been used in diagnostic research to quantify the diagnostic value of a test over its whole range of possible cutoffs for classifying patients as positive versus negative [223]. We can also make a ROC curve with consecutive cutoffs for the predicted probability of a binary outcome. We start with a cutoff of 0%, which implies that all subjects are classified as positive. The sensitivity is 100%, and the specificity 0% (upper right point in Fig. 15.2). There are no false-negative classifications, and 100% false-positive classifications, since all subjects without the outcome are classified as positive. We then shift to a slightly higher cutoff, e.g., 1%, where sensitivity may still be 100%, but specificity above 0%. We follow all possible cutoffs till 100%, where all subjects are classified as

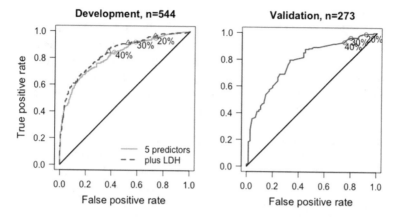

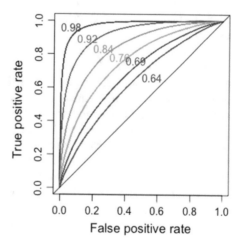

Fig. 15.2 Receiver operating characteristics (ROC) curve for the testicular cancer model in the development data set of 544 patients and validation set with 273 patients. Using cutoffs for the predicted probability of tumor results in specific combinations of true positive rate (sensitivity) and false-positive rate (1 − specificity). The area under the curve (AUC) is 0.82 [0.78–0.85]

Fig. 15.3 ROC plot for five hypothetical prediction models. The AUC values (or *c* statistics) were 0.5, 0.64, 0.69, 0.76, 0.84, 0.92, and 0.98

negative. This is the lower left point in Fig. 15.2. Here, the sensitivity is 0% and specificity 100%.

The curves are more to the upper left corner when the distributions of predictions are more separate between those with and without the outcome (Fig. 15.3). We can draw a diagonal line for a non-informative model, where the sum of TP and TN is 1 at every cutoff. This sum (also known as Youden's index, sensitivity + specificity - 1) is larger than 1 for sensible prediction models. Youden index is maximized in the upper left corner of the ROC plot [564]. We will discuss the choice of an optimal cutoff for classification in the next chapter (Chap. 16).

The area under the curve (AUC) can be interpreted as the probability that a patient with the outcome is given a higher probability of the outcome by the model than a randomly chosen patient without the outcome [223]. An uninformative model, such as a coin flip, will hence have an area of 0.5. A perfect model has an area of 1. The AUC is usually the most important number from a ROC plot; the plot itself suffers from instability and is rather meaningless if no thresholds are indicated (Fig. 15.3, no thresholds, only the area is relevant versus Fig. 15.2, thresholds added).

Some may consider the interpretation of AUC as straightforward. Others may object that we consider a pair of subjects, one with and one without the outcome, and that such conditioning is a rather artificial situation. Statistically, this conditioning on a pair of patients is attractive, since it makes the area independent of the incidence of the outcome (or event rate), in contrast to R^2 or the Brier score, for example. Another objection is that the AUC is thought to be insensitive to improvements in prediction by adding predictors such as biomarkers. Indeed, the AUC is a rank order statistic; on the other hand, improvements in model fit go hand in hand with improvements in AUC, if the underlying statistical model is correct [434]. So, measures such as R^2, Brier score, and AUC should all show an improvement if a true predictor is added to a model. Finally, the AUC is bounded by 1.0; with higher AUC values such as 0.90, only small increments can be expected [425].

A generalization of the area under the ROC curve is provided by the concordance statistic (c) [226]. The c statistic is a rank order statistic for predictions against true outcomes, related to Somers' D statistic. As a rank order statistic, it is insensitive to errors in calibration such as differences in average outcome. For binary outcomes, c is identical to AUC.

Confidence intervals for the AUC (or c statistic) can be calculated with various methods. Standard asymptotic methods may be problematic, especially when sensitivity or specificity is close to 0% or 100% [9]. Bootstrap resampling is a good choice for many situations. For example, a difference in c between a reference and a more complex model is hard to evaluate fairly when the models are developed on the same data [434]. Bootstrapping can be used for comparison of optimism-corrected estimates of the difference in performance (see Chap. 17).

15.2.4 R^2 Versus c

We compare the behavior of Nagelkerke's R^2 and the c statistic for hypothetical prediction models in settings of 50 and 10% event rates (Fig. 15.4). At 50% incidence, a high c statistic such as 0.98 is associated with a R^2 value of 87%. With lower incidence, R^2 is somewhat lower. Prediction models with c between 0.7 and 0.8 typically have R^2 values between 10 and 20%; $R^2 > 50\%$ matches with $c > 0.9$.

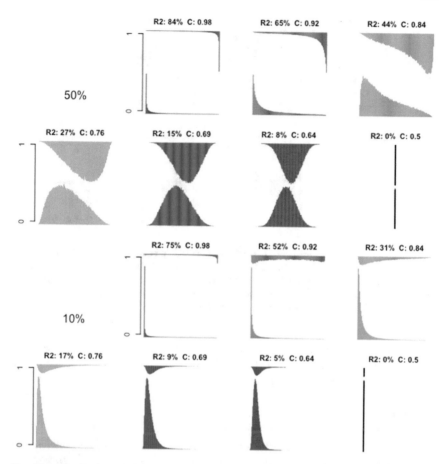

Fig. 15.4 Distribution of observed binary outcomes in relation to predicted probabilities from hypothetical logistic models. The top seven graphs relate to an incidence (event rate) of 50%. The next sets relate to a 10% incidence. For each hypothetical model, Nagelkerke's R^2 and c statistics are shown. If $c = 0.5$ (and $R^2 = 0\%$), predictions are at the incidence of the outcome for all subjects, with or without the outcome, indicated with a single spike. If c is close to 1 (R^2 close to 100%), predictions are close to 0% for those without the outcome, and close to 100% for those with the outcome

15.2.5   Box Plots and Discrimination Slope

The discrimination slope is a simple measure for how well subjects with and without the outcome are separated. Its use as a measure for discrimination is attributed to Yates [684]. It is easily calculated as the absolute difference in average predictions for those with and without the outcome.

Visualization is readily possible with a box plot (Fig. 15.5). The box plot may be a simple and intuitive way to communicate the extent of risk differentiation achieved by the model. The same information can be shown by histograms, which

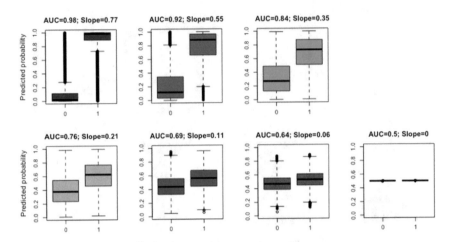

Fig. 15.5 Box plots for predictions from hypothetical prediction models with different discriminative abilities (AUC or *c* statistic, see Fig. 15.4). The discrimination slopes are calculated as the difference in means of predictions for those with and those without the outcome (mean incidence 50%). The standardized differences at the log odds scale were 8, 4, 2, 1, 0.5, 0.25, and 0; for AUC = 0.98, 0.92, 0.84, 0.76, 0.69, 0.64, and 0.5, respectively

will show less overlap between those with and those without the outcome for a better discriminating model (Fig. 15.4). Similar to Fig. 15.4, the incidence of the outcome (event rate) determines the visual impression that a box plot makes, and the magnitude of Yates discrimination slope. With low incidence, the slope is somewhat lower, for the same AUC (or *c* statistic).

The difference in mean predictions is related to the calculation of AUC from the comparison of two standard normal distributions; one for those with events ($y = 1$) and one for those without an event ($y = 0$): AUC = $\Phi((\mu_{y=1} - \mu_{y=0})/\sqrt{2})$, where Φ indicates the cumulative normal distribution. With ($\mu_{y=1} - \mu_{y=0}$) = 1, the AUC is 0.76; with a standardized difference of 0.25, AUC = 0.64; with a difference of 8, AUC = 0.98. So, the calculations of AUC can be thought of as comparing $y = 1$ versus $y = 0$ at the log(odds) scale, while Yates's discrimination slope compares $y = 1$ versus $y = 0$ at the probability scale.

Indeed, the interesting connection is that Pearson R^2 is asymptotically equal to the Yates slope. Improvements in Pearson R^2 or in Yates slope are equivalent to the integrated discrimination index (IDI) [426, 428, 568].

15.2.6   *Lorenz Curve*

An alternative way to judge discriminative ability is by the Lorenz curve (Fig. 15.6). The Lorenz curve has been used in economics to characterize the distribution of wealth in a population [351]. This curve has been used to plot the

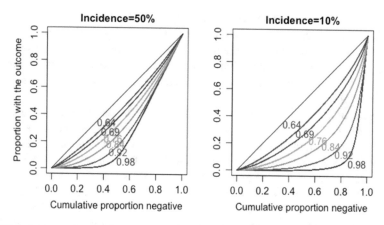

Fig. 15.6 Lorenz curve showing proportion with the outcome versus the cumulative proportion of patients classified as negative, according to rank order of predictions. The outcome incidence is 50% in the left panel and 10% in the right panel. We note that a near-perfect model (c = 0.98) follows a horizontal line and then rises steeply to 100% false-negative rate from the points of 50% and 90% cumulative proportions, respectively

cumulative distribution of wealth against the cumulative distribution of the population, ranked on the basis of individual wealth.

For prediction models, we can plot the cumulative proportion of the population on the x-axis, ranked by predicted probability. On the y-axis, we plot the cumulative proportion of subjects with the outcome. For example, we can show the proportion of subjects developing cancer against the cumulative proportion of the population ranked by cancer risk [46]. In terms of ROC curves, we plot the cumulative rate of false-negative classifications against the cumulative rate of negative predictions. The ROC and Lorenz curves look somewhat similar, except that the Lorenz curve is flipped vertically and horizontally. In case of a non-informative model, a straight line arises, since every rate of the population classified as negative corresponds to the same rate classified as negative among those with the outcome. A good model has a curve under this straight line, with a relatively large proportion of the population classified as negative having only a small part of the outcomes (low false-negative rate). On the upper end of the x-axis, a small part of the population should contain many subjects with the outcome. In the ideal case, a cutoff is used that classifies the fraction as positive equal to the prevalence, and all these have the outcome. Indeed, we note that a c statistic of 0.98 leads to a nearly horizontal line till the 50% cumulative proportion point on the x-axis and increases more or less linearly to 100% after that.

The Gini index is sometimes calculated as a summary measure for the Lorenz curve. The Gini index is the ratio between the area A between the Lorenz curve of the prediction model and the line for a non-informative model and the area under the line for a non-informative model (0.5). Hence, G = 2 * A.

Other summaries are related to quantiles of the cumulative distribution. For example, we can consider the number of missed outcomes when 25% of the population is classified as negative. If we want to be sure not to miss the outcome, usually only few can be classified as negative, unless a model is used with very good discriminative ability. At the upper end of the range, we can consider how many outcomes are concentrated in the upper quarter (above the 75th percentile). We illustrate these principles for the testicular cancer prediction case study (Table 15.4).

An advantage of the Lorenz concentration curve is that the trade-off is clearly visualized between how many subjects can be classified as negative without missing many with the outcome. A disadvantage may be that the appearance of the Lorenz curve depends strongly on the incidence of the outcome. With low incidence, such as screening, the graph looks more impressive (Fig. 15.6, right panel). With 10% incidence, only few cases with disease are missed at 25% classified negative when we use a model with a c statistic of 0.84. The top 25% then easily contains most cases. With a more frequent outcome, more cases are missed at the 25% point, and fewer of the cases are in the top 75 percentile.

15.2.7 Comparing Risk Quantiles

The ROC curve, box plots, and Lorenz curve consider the full distribution of predicted risk. Researchers sometimes express the risks between extreme parts of the risk distribution as summary measures [586]. For example, we may compare the risk among those above the top 90% percentile to the risk in the lowest 10% of the risk distribution. With c statistic of 0.64, this implies we compare a subgroup with 65% risk to a group with 35% risk, if the average risk is 50%. This difference can be expressed as an odds ratio of 3.7 (Table 15.3). The odds ratio is as high as 26 for a c statistic of 0.84. With a lower incidence of 10%, these odds ratios are 3.2 and 13, so still quite impressive (Table 15.3). By comparing those over the 99% percentile to the lowest 1%, we obtain even larger differences in risks, for example, 74% versus 26% for a c statistic of 0.64, odds ratio 7.4 (Table 15.3).

Table 15.3 Comparison of risk among those at high versus low risk according to prediction models with different AUC values

AUC	Incidence 50%			Incidence 10%		
	<1 versus >99%	<10 versus >90%	50–50%	<1 versus >99%	<10 versus >90%	50–50%
0.98	>1M	>1M	135	>1M	>100k	342
0.92	60	53	10	60	23	5.1
0.84	50	26	5.4	40	13	3.8
0.76	30	13	3.3	17	8.0	2.8
0.69	15	6.5	2.4	8.4	4.6	2.1
0.64	7.4	3.7	1.8	5.8	3.2	1.7
0.5	1	1	1	1	1	1

These impressive numbers may be considered statistical cheating, since we focus on extremes and ignore the large middle group of subjects in between the extremes. A fairer comparison might be to split in the middle: at the 50% risk percentile (the median). This is similar to the approach for Royston's D statistic, which was focused on discrimination in survival analysis [475]. The D statistic quantifies the risk difference among two equal-sized groups: those above versus those below the median risk. If we apply this approach to binary outcomes, we find lower odds ratios as a quantification of the separation between those at high versus low risk, e.g., 1.8 and 1.7 for a c statistic of 0.64 with incidence 50% and 10%, respectively (Table 15.3).

15.2.8 *Example: Discrimination of Testicular Cancer Prediction Model

We continue the example of predicting a benign histology in testicular cancer patients after chemotherapy. The c statistic was 0.818 at model development, with small optimism according to bootstrap validation (decrease by 0.006 to 0.812). At external validation, the c statistic was 0.785, with a relatively wide 95% confidence interval of 0.73–0.84 (Table 15.4).

The discrimination slope was 0.30 at model development, with small optimism according to bootstrap validation (decrease to 0.29). At external validation, the slope was much smaller (0.24). Part of this decrease is attributable to the lower average prevalence of necrosis (76 of 273, 28%; versus 245 of 544, 45%). This higher prevalence of residual tumor is also evident from the box plots (Fig. 15.7).

Lorenz curves were created with as x-axis the cumulative fraction at risk of having residual tumor, and hence classified as not undergoing surgical resection (Fig. 15.8). The y-axis was the fraction of missed tumors, i.e., tumor masses left

Table 15.4 Discriminative ability of testicular cancer prediction model developed in $n = 544$ and externally validated in $n = 273$

		Development n = 544, 245 necrosis	Internal validation[a]	External validation n = 273, 76 necrosis
c statistic [95% CI]		0.818 [0.78–0.85]	0.811 [0.78–0.85][b]	0.79 [0.73–0.84]
Yates' slope [95% CI]		0.301 [0.27–0.34][c]	0.295 [0.26–0.33][b]	0.24 [0.18–0.30][c]
Lorenz curve	p25, tumors missed	9%	–	13%
	p75, tumors missed	58%	–	65%

[a]Internal validation with 500 bootstrap samples
[b]Assuming the same SE applies as estimated for model development
[c]Based on bootstrap resampling

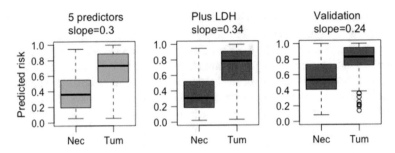

Fig. 15.7 Box plot showing predictions of residual tumor by actual outcome (tumor vs. necrosis) for testicular cancer patients ($n = 544$ and $n = 273$, respectively). The difference between means is Yates' discrimination slope (slope = 0.30, 0.34 and 0.24, respectively)

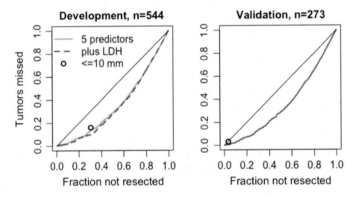

Fig. 15.8 Lorenz curves for prediction of residual tumor. Patients classified as low risk for tumor would not undergo surgical resection (x-axis). With increasing fractions not undergoing resection, the fraction with unresected tumor increases ("Tumors missed")

unresected. The point of 25% classified as necrosis corresponds to using a cutoff of 68% for the probability of necrosis, and only patients with a probability over 68% are not resected. We miss 9% of the tumors with that cutoff. Hence, sparing surgery in 25% leads to missing 9% of the tumors. The point of 75% classified as necrosis corresponds to using a low cutoff (21%), and missing 58% of the tumors. Hence, 42% of the tumors are concentrated in the upper quarter of the distribution.

At external validation, the curve looks similar, which is related to a lower discriminative ability compensated by a higher average prevalence of tumor (72% versus 55%). The 25% and 75% cumulative fractions correspond to cutoffs of 60% and 92% for the probability of tumor, and lead to 13% and 65% missed tumors, respectively.

As a reference, we consider the current widely used policy of resection if the residual mass size exceeds 10 mm [552]. This policy uses only one of the five predictors in the model ("postchemotherapy mass size"), and hence has less discriminative ability (the point is closer to the 45° line in Fig. 15.8). In the development sample, 165 of the 544 patients (20%) had residual masses <= 10 mm, but among them 48 with tumor (fraction tumor missed 48/299, 16%). In the validation sample, only 9 of the 273 patients (3.3%) had residual masses <= 10 mm, but among them 6 with tumor (fraction tumor missed 6/197, 3%). Hence, the reference policy did not perform well in the validation sample.

15.2.9   *Verification Bias and Discriminative Ability

In the testicular cancer validation sample, only 9 of 273 patients had very small residual masses. This reflects the policy for resection in the specific center, where patients with such small masses were not considered candidates for resection [644]. This leads to verification bias [670]: we do not know the histology of these masses, since they were not resected, and cannot evaluate predictions for these patients. We know that the estimation of regression coefficients is not biased by this selection, if we include the selection criterion (residual mass size) in the prediction model. Hence, model predictions are valid even with verification bias [688]. But performance measures such as sensitivity and specificity are biased [45]. The c statistic may not be affected too much because verification bias makes that we merely shift on the ROC curve to a different combination of sensitivity and specificity. As a sensitivity analysis, we might evaluate the model performance after imputing outcome for unresected patients [122, 645].

15.2.10   *R Code for Discriminative Ability

The box plot is created simply with `boxplot`, based on a "full model" including five predictors in the development data:

```
lp    <- full$linear.predictors
boxplot(plogis(lp)~full$y, ...)        # Fig 15.7
```

The discrimination slope is the difference between the mean predicted probabilities by outcome:

```
mean(plogis(lp[full$y==1])) - mean(plogis(lp[full$y==0]))
```

Lorenz concentration curves are created easily with the ROCR package:

```
library(ROCR)
pred.full <- prediction(full$linear.predictor, full$y)
perf.full <- performance(pred.full,"fnr","rnp") # Lorenz curve data+plot
plot(perf.full, xlab="Fraction not resected", ylab="Tumors missed", ...)
abline(a=0,b=1)                  # Fig 15.8 with reference line
```

15.2.11   Discriminative Ability in Survival

Similar to overall performance measures, we can focus on summarizing performance for the full follow-up, or focus on some specific time points. A classic implementation of the c statistic for survival is by Harrell, which considers pairs of risk subject at any time during follow-up [226]. Harrell's overall c statistic indicates the proportion of all pairs of subjects who can be ordered such that the subject with the higher predicted survival is the one who survived longer. Ordering is possible if both subjects have an observed survival time, or when one has the outcome and a shorter survival time than the censored survival time of the other subject. Ordering is not possible if both subjects are censored, or if one has the outcome with a survival time longer than the censored survival time of the other subject. Hence, a censored subject is only considered as a nonevent for the time points where events occurred and the subject was at risk. Harrell's c is sensitive to the censoring pattern. An potential improvement is Uno's c statistic, which uses a weight function to compensate for the censoring [591]. Time-dependent c statistics, or AUC_t, were proposed by Heagerty with various variants [234, 592]. The overall and time-specific discrimination measures usually do not agree numerically [53].

Box plots or Lorenz curves have no easy translation to the survival context, while splitting at the median risk was proposed for the D statistic [475]. Such splitting is also common in oncology, where prognostic groups are often created after constructing a prognostic model. A common procedure is to base these groups on quarters of predicted survival; the lower 25% should have the worst survival, the highest 25% the best survival. This approach can well illustrate the discriminative ability of a model. An example is shown in Chap. 23 (Fig. 23.8).

15.2.12   Summary on Measures for Discrimination

As discussed above, various measures can be used to indicate discrimination (Table 15.5). These all relate to the spread in predictions: how well can we separate low risk from high-risk subjects? The c statistic, or AUC, is the most commonly reported measure [390]. It is a rank order statistic, and hence not sensitive to miscalibration. It is usually not so informative to plot the ROC curve, unless specific thresholds are indicated as in Fig. 15.2. The discrimination slope and Gini index are influenced by calibration. Hence, the preferred measure for discrimination is the c statistic or AUC for binary outcomes.

Further quantitative insight is obtained from realizing how the risk distributions for those with and without events are shifted (see distributions in Fig. 15.4 and box plots in Figs. 15.5 and 15.7). The risk distributions were created from normal distributions for those with and without the event at the linear predictor scale (logodds or logit scale, Table 15.6). A mean difference of 1 leads to a c statistic of 0.76. So, $logit(p)$ is distributed as $N(-0.5, 1)$ and $N(0.5, 1)$ for $y = 0$ and $y = 1$,

Table 15.5 Summary of some measures for discriminative ability of a prediction model for binary outcomes

Measure	Calculation	Visualization	Characteristics
Concordance statistic	Rank order statistic	ROC curve	Insensitive to outcome incidence Readily interpretable as probability of higher predictions among events versus nonevents, by conditioning on pairs
Discrimination slope	Difference in mean of predictions between outcomes	Box plot	Easy interpretation, attractive visualization
Gini index	Shows concentration of outcomes missed by cumulative proportion of negative classifications	Lorenz concentration curve	Shows balance between finding true positive subjects versus total classified as positive

Table 15.6 Quantitative comparison of measures related to discrimination. Prediction models with high to low AUC were based on normal distributions at the log odds scale, with standardized differences between 0 and 8, for a 50% incidence

Standardized difference: $logit|y = 1 - logit|y = 0$	AUC	R^2 (%)	Discrimination slope: $risk|y = 1 - risk|y = 0$	D: odds ratio with median split
8	0.98	84	0.77	135
4	0.92	65	0.55	10
2	0.84	44	0.35	5.4
1	0.76	27	0.20	3.3
0.5	0.69	15	0.11	2.4
0.25	0.64	8	0.05	1.8
0	0.5	0	0	1

respectively. A smaller standardized difference such as 0.25 times the standard deviation leads to $c = 0.64$. With $c = 0.76$, Nagelkerke R^2 was 27%, the discrimination slope was 0.20, and the odds ratio with a split at the median of the risk distribution was 3.3.

15.2.13 Incremental Value of Markers and Discrimination

The incremental value of biomarkers and other predictors is an important study question in many medical fields. The incremental value can be statistically tested by adding the marker to a reference model [425, 558, 561]. The reference model needs

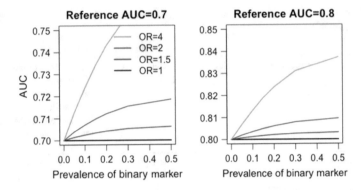

Fig. 15.9 Discriminative ability (AUC) for adding a marker to a reference prediction model with AUC = 0.7 (left panel) or AUC = 0.8 (right panel). Marker effects of OR 1.5, 2, and 4 were simulated over prevalence of the binary marker from 0 to 50%. The increase in AUC is less with a better reference model since AUC is bounded by 1.0

to be refitted to the data for a fair comparison of incremental value [682]. For example, examining promising biomarkers for cardiovascular disease might consider a specific version of the Framingham model as a reference. The predictors in the Framingham model would be entered to estimate coefficients that are optimal to the data at hand. Next, the marker would be added, with a likelihood ratio test to assess statistical significance [425, 434, 647].

The AUC has been considered as insensitive to such addition of predictors to the model [107, 426]. We may examine this perceived insensitivity by adding a binary marker to a model with a reference AUC of 0.7 or 0.8 (Fig. 15.9) [425]. The increase in AUC depends on the effect of the marker (odds ratio 1.5, 2, 4 for illustration), and on the prevalence (range 0–50% considered). It does not depend on the event rate. With a rare characteristic, say with prevalence <5%, we would need a large effect such as OR = 4 to reach an improvement in AUC of approximately 0.01 [433]. Such an improvement is achieved with a weak effect such as OR = 1.5 if the prevalence is 50:50, and not if the reference model already has an AUC of 0.8. If we add a well-distributed marker (prevalence around 50:50) with a strong effect (OR = 4), the AUC reaches 0.83 even if the reference model has AUC = 0.8. So, the AUC will not increase with notable quantity if the ordering of risk predictions changes to a minor extent for a small group of subjects. But large effects for frequent characteristics will correspond to substantial increases in AUC.

15.2.14 Incremental Value of Markers and Reclassification

Another way to assess incremental value of a marker is by reclassification. This approach has received attention as being more meaningful to communicate to medical researchers [107], perhaps also out of frustration that "promising markers"

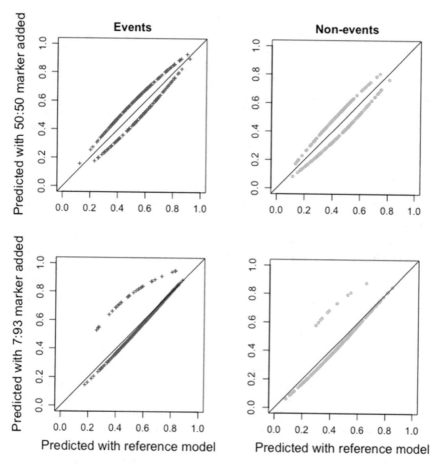

Fig. 15.10 Reclassification plots for a binary marker with 50% prevalence (top row) or 7% prevalence (lower row). Both markers increased AUC by 0.019 from AUC = 0.7. In the 50:50 case, the Net Reclassification Index (NRI) is positive for those with events (+15%) as well as for those without events (+15%). In the 7% prevalence case, the Net Reclassification Index is negative for those with events (−79%) but positive for those without events (+93%)

showed limited increase in AUC [426]. We may compare predictions with the marker to predictions without the marker, separate for those with and without events. The net reclassification improvement (NRI) has been proposed to summarize such reclassification. For binary classification (Table 15.2), the NRI for events is the change in sensitivity, and the NRI for nonevents is the change in specificity. Note that an increase in AUC does not necessarily correspond to an increase in both sensitivity and specificity; one may increase while the other decreases [603].

The change in the full risk distribution can be studied with reclassification graphs for those with and without events (Fig. 15.10). If the marker has a 50:50 distribution, with OR = 2, we find that the increase in AUC is +0.019. We would hope to see higher risk predictions for those with events, and lower for those without events. Indeed, among those with events, 57.6% had higher predictions with the model with the marker compared to the predictions with the reference model without the marker. On the downside, 42.4% had lower predictions, for an NRI of +15%. Identical numerical results are found for those without events: 57.6% had lower predictions, for an NRI of +15%.

A similar improvement of +0.019 in AUC is achieved with a marker with 7% prevalence and OR = 4 (Fig. 15.9). For such a marker, the NRI for events is negative: 11% are reclassified to higher predictions, while 89% are reclassified to lower predictions (NRI −79%). On the other hand, 97% among the nonevents are reclassified to lower predictions, for an NRI of +93%.

The sum of the NRI for events and the NRI for nonevents is referred to as the overall NRI, and sometimes simply as "NRI" [331]. For the first situation, NRI = NRI for events + NRI for nonevents = 0.15 + 0.15 = 0.30. For the second situation, NRI = 0.932 − 0.786 = 0.15. So, the same increase in AUC leads to very different NRI values. The NRI needs careful interpretation as "the sum of the net reclassification improvements for those with events and those without events." It is not correct to interpret the total NRI as "the fraction correctly reclassified", and interpret this number as a percentage. With a 50% event rate, the fraction of the sample that is correctly reclassified is 0.5 * 0.15 + 0.5 * 0.15 = 15% in the first example, and 0.5 * 0.932 − 0.5 * 0.786 = 7.3% in the second [331]. The overall NRI provides for a higher number than the change in AUC, but otherwise may be more confusing than providing meaning on the incremental value of a marker [650]. More meaningful interpretations of the value of marker may come from evaluations of the distributions of predicted values ("predictiveness curves") [432] and especially from decision-analytic measures (see Chap. 16) [648]. In line with decision analysis, a weighted NRI can be calculated ("wNRI") [427]. The wNRI is consistent with improvements in Net Benefit and Relative Utility [607]. These measures provide a weighted sum of changes in sensitivity and specificity and have a strong scientific basis [424].

15.2.15   *R Code for Assessment of Incremental Value

Reclassification statistics can be calculated with the improveProb function

```
fit0   <- lrm(y~x1)
fit1   <- lrm(y~x1+x2)
improveProb(x1=plogis(predict(fit0)),x2=plogis(predict(fit1)), y=y)
```

Tests for model improvement can simply be obtained from the model fit

```
anova(fit1)
```

Table 15.7 A hierarchy of calibration levels for risk prediction models for binary outcomes [602]

Strength of calibration	Definition	Assessment
Mean	Observed event rate equals average predicted risk	Compare event rate with average predicted risk; Evaluate calibration-in-the-large as $a\|b = 1 = 0$, 1 df test
Weak	No systematic overfitting or underfitting and/or overestimation or underestimation of risks	Calibration analysis for calibration-in-the-large and calibration slope; evaluate with Cox recalibration test: 2 df test of the null hypothesis that $a = 0$ and $b = 1$ [114]
Moderate	Predicted risks correspond to observed event rates	Calibration plot with smooth curve, and/ or inspection by grouped predictions
Strong	Predicted risks correspond to observed event rates for each and every covariate pattern	Scatter plot of predicted risk and observed event rate per covariate pattern, impossible with continuous predictors

15.3   Calibration

Another key property of a prediction model is calibration, i.e., the agreement between observed outcomes and predictions. The most common definition of calibration is that if we observe $p\%$ risk among patients with a predicted risk of $p\%$. So, if we predict 70% probability of residual tumor tissue for a testicular cancer patient, the observed frequency of tumor should be approximately 70 out of 100 patients with such a predicted probability. Weaker forms of calibration only require the average predicted risk (mean calibration) or the average prediction effects (weak calibration) to be correct. Strong calibration requires that the event rate equals the predicted risk for every covariate pattern [602]. This implies that the model is fully correct for the validation setting (Table 15.7). Graphical inspection is very useful (a calibration plot) [26, 225].

15.3.1   Calibration Plot

A calibration plot has predictions on the x-axis, and the outcome on the y-axis. A line of identity helps for orientation: perfect predictions should be at the 45° line. For linear regression, the calibration plot results in a simple scatter plot. For binary outcomes, the plot contains only 0 and 1 values for the y-axis. Such probabilities are not observed directly. Smoothing techniques can be used to estimate the observed probabilities of the outcome ($p(y = 1)$) in relation to the predicted probabilities. The observed 0/1 outcomes are replaced by values between 0 and 1 by combining outcome values of subjects with similar predicted probabilities, e.g.,

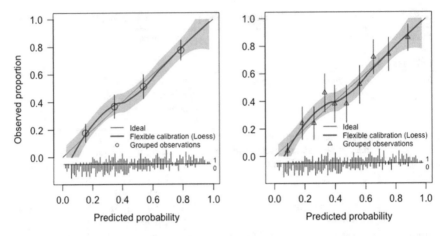

Fig. 15.11 Calibration plots of actual outcome versus predictions for a hypothetical model with *c* statistic 0.76, *n* = 500. Left and right panels only differ in the number of groups (4 vs 10). The distributions of actual 0 and 1 values are shown at the bottom of the graph; the *loess* smoother (with 95% confidence band) is close to the ideal 45 degree line; actual outcomes according to risk groups are shown by circles and triangles (each circle: *n* = 125; triangle: *n* = 50)

using the *loess* algorithm [26]. Confidence intervals can be calculated for such a smooth curve (Fig. 15.11).

The plot visualizes mean calibration (are observed outcome systematically lower or higher than predicted?), weak calibration (is there a general trend in predictions being too extreme, a sign of overfitting at model development?). Moreover, we can plot results for subjects grouped by similar probabilities. This allows us to assess a moderate level of calibration by comparing mean observed proportions per group to the mean predicted outcome. For example, we can plot observed outcome in groups defined by quintile or by decile of predictions (Fig. 15.11). This makes the plot a graphical illustration of the Hosmer–Lemeshow goodness-of-fit test. Note that we also learn about discrimination from a calibration plot: A better discriminating model has more spread between observed proportions per group than a poorly discriminating model. The choice of groups is important for the visual impression of calibration; if small groups are plotted, the variability will be larger (right panel in Fig. 15.11).

15.3.2   Mean and Weak Calibration at Internal and External Validation

The mean calibration will usually be perfect when we compare observed outcomes to the mean predictions in the data set used to develop a model. Such apparent calibration is hence not informative. Similarly, the mean calibration remains uninformative with internal validation techniques such as cross-validation or bootstrapping (see Chap. 17). In contrast, when we validate the model in external data, the calibration of the mean risk is often far from perfect ("poor calibration-in-the-large").

The concept of weak calibration is related to the average strength of the predictor effects. For linear regression, we can write $y_{new} = a + b_{overall} * \hat{y}$, and for generalized linear models $f(y_{new}) = a + b_{overall} *$ linear predictor, where the linear predictor is the combination of regression coefficients from the model and the predictor values in the new data. A link function f is used for y_{new}, e.g., log odds (or logit) in logistic regression. The $b_{overall}$ is named the calibration slope [114]. Ideally, the calibration slope $b_{overall} = 1$. With apparent validation, $b_{overall} = 1$, since this yields the best fit on the data under study with either least squares or maximum likelihood methods. At internal validation, the calibration slope reflects the amount of shrinkage that is required for a model ($b_{overall} < 1$) [109, 627]. It indicates how much we need to reduce the effects of predictors on average to make the model well calibrated for new patients from the underlying population. The calibration slope can hence be used as a shrinkage factor to adjust a model for future use (Chap. 14). At external validation, the calibration slope reflects the combined effect of two phenomena: overfitting on the development data and true differences in the effects of predictors.

15.3.3 Assessing Calibration-in-the-Large and Calibration Slope

For continuous outcomes, calibration-in-the-large can be assessed easily by comparing the mean($\hat{y}$) and mean(y_{new}), and testing the differences $y_{new} - \hat{y}$, e.g., with a one-sample t-test. This test indicates the statistical significance of the mean under- or overestimation of the observed outcome: mean($y_{new} - \hat{y}$). In a linear regression model, we can estimate an intercept a in a model with the residual $y_{new} - \hat{y}$ as the outcome. The recalibration model is simply $y_{new} = a + b_{overall} * \hat{y}$. The deviation of the calibration slope from 1 can be tested in linear regression by a model that studies the residuals: $y_{new} - \hat{y} = a + b_{overall} * \hat{y}$. The significance of $b_{overall}$ is then determined as usual in regression, and indicates on average stronger or weaker effects of the predictors in a model.

For binary outcomes, calibration-in-the-large again refers to the difference between mean($\hat{y}$) and mean(y_{new}). A simple comparison can directly be made, with an odds ratio indicating the average under- or overestimation of the outcome:

$$\text{OR} = \text{odds}(\text{mean}(\hat{y}))/\text{odds}(\text{mean}(y_{new}))$$
$$= [\text{mean}(\hat{y})/(1 - \text{mean}(\hat{y}))]/[\text{mean}(y_{new})/(1 - \text{mean}(y_{new}))].$$

For statistical testing of the difference, we need to be more careful. In logistic regression, the relation between the outcome y and the linear predictor is nonlinear (i.e., logistic). We want to compare $\mathrm{logit}(y_{new} = 1)$ to $\mathrm{logit}(\hat{y})$, where

$$\mathrm{mean}(\mathrm{logit}(y_{new} = 1) - \mathrm{logit}(\hat{y})) \text{ is not equal to } \mathrm{mean}(\mathrm{logit}(y_{new} = 1)) - \mathrm{mean}(\mathrm{logit}(\hat{y})).$$

In a model, we could write

$$\mathrm{logit}(y_{new} = 1) - \mathrm{logit}(\hat{y}) = a; \text{ or}$$
$$\mathrm{logit}(y_{new} = 1) = a + \mathrm{logit}(\hat{y}) = a + \mathrm{offset}(\text{linear predictor}).$$

The intercept a then reflects the difference in log odds between predictions and observed outcome, adjusted for the linear predictor. The offset makes that predictions are taken literally, as in linear regression. We can think of a regression coefficient for the offset variable that is fixed at unity. The statistical significance of intercept a can be tested with standard regression tests, such as the Wald test or the likelihood ratio (LR) test. The alternative hypothesis is $a <> 0 \mid b_{overall} = 1$ (Table 15.8).

Note that $\exp(a)$ can be interpreted as an observed-to-expected (O/E) ratio. This ratio can also be calculated directly by comparing the sum of observed events (O) with the sum of the predictions (E). These ratios will differ, with $\exp(a)$ larger than the simple O/E ratio [210]. This is because the estimation of a was conditional on the linear predictor (as an offset variable), which makes for an adjusted estimate rather than an unadjusted estimate as for O/E. So, $\exp(a)$ can be interpreted as the odds ratios for individuals, given their covariate pattern (a conditional estimate), while O/E reflects the overall average miscalibration (a marginal estimate).

The calibration slope can be estimated from the recalibration model $\mathrm{logit}(y_{new} = 1) = a + b_{overall} * \mathrm{logit}(\hat{y}) = a + b_{overall} * $ linear predictor. The deviation of the calibration slope from 1 ("miscalibration") can be tested by a model that includes an offset variable:

$$\mathrm{logit}(y_{new} = 1) = a + b_{miscalibration} * \text{linear predictor} + \mathrm{offset}(\text{linear predictor}).$$

The slope coefficient $b_{overall}$ reflects the deviations from the ideal slope of 1, and can be tested with Wald or LR statistics (Table 15.8).

For a survival outcome, the calibration slope $b_{overall}$ can be assessed as

Table 15.8 Calibration tests for prediction model $y \sim a + b_{overall} * \hat{y}$. H_0 and H_1 indicate the null and alternative hypothesis, respectively

	H_0	H_1	df
Calibration-in-the-large	$a = 0 \mid b_{overall} = 1$	$a <> 0 \mid b_{overall} = 1$	1
Calibration slope	$b_{overall} = 1$	$b_{overall} <> 1$	1
Recalibration	$a = 0$ and $b_{overall} = 1$	$a <> 0$ or $b_{overall} <> 1$	2

$$\log(\text{hazard}(y_{new} = 1)) = h_0 + b_{overall} * \text{linear predictor}.$$

The model for deviation from a slope of 1 is

$$\log(\text{hazard}(y_{new} = 1)) = h_0 + b_{miscalibration}$$
$$* \text{ linear predictor} + \text{offset(linear predictor)}.$$

Testing of coefficient $b_{miscalibration}$ is as usual, i.e., with a Wald test or LR test. This recalibration test for $a = 0$ and $b = 1$ has several advantages. It can pick up common patterns of miscalibration, i.e., systematic differences between the new data and the model development data, and overfitting of the effects of predictors. Moreover, the test parameters a and $b_{overall}$ are well interpretable, provided that $a \mid b_{overall} = 1$ is reported (rather than a with $b_{overall}$ left free). The slope $b_{overall}$ can directly be taken from the re-calibration model (where a is left free).

With a parametric survival model, we can specify parameters which reflect differences in average survival, after adjustment for predictor effects. Van Houwelingen transformed the baseline hazard from a Cox model to a Weibull model [623]. The Weibull model has two parameters to describe the baseline hazard parametrically (Chap. 4). These two parameters can be refitted for external validation data, together with a single coefficient for the linear predictor, to estimate a recalibrated model.

15.3.4   Assessment of Moderate Calibration

Moderate calibration can best be assessed graphically as discussed above with the calibration plot (Sect. 15.3.1). Smooth curves can be constructed with the *loess* smoother, which may be considered nonparametric, or with a spline smoother such as a restricted cubic spline [26, 602]. A formal test might be done for nonlinearity: compare the fit with an *rcs* versus a linear offset term. In addition to graphical inspection of grouped predictions, we may perform a chi-square test for observed versus expected numbers by group. This test is the often used Hosmer–Lemeshow (HL) test [257].

For the HL test, patients are grouped typically by decile of predicted probability. The sum of predicted probabilities is the number of expected outcomes; this expected number is compared to the observed number in the 10 groups with a chi-square test. At model development, this chi-square test has eight degrees of freedom; at external validation the degrees of freedom are nine. There are many drawbacks to the H-L test [225, 256]. First, there flexibility in the grouping: should we always use deciles to group predictions in tenths, or make the quantiles dependent on the sample size? Should we group by risk interval, e.g., 0–10%, 11–20%, etc. ("interval grouping")? Second, the test has poor power to detect miscalibration in the common form of systematic differences between outcomes in the new data and the model development data, or to detect overfitting of the effects of predictors. Some proposed that the H-L test should only be used in model development, in addition to more specific tests on model assumptions, such as tests for linearity (adding nonlinear transformations) and additivity (adding interaction terms). Reported H-L tests are usually nonsignificant if they reflect apparent validation on the data that were also used to construct the model. Such nonsignificant results may contribute to the face validity of a model as perceived by some readers, but have no scientific meaning.

Various other measures are available for moderate calibration. An intuitively appealing measure of calibration is the absolute difference between smoothed observed outcomes and predicted probabilities (Harrell's E statistic) [225]. This measure is related to the calibration plot, and depends on the way the 0/1 outcomes are smoothed. The difference between smoothed observed outcomes and predicted probabilities can well be judged visually in a calibration plot such as Fig. 15.11, with the distribution of predictions at the x-axis. We can also summarize the miscalibration in a single index such as the estimated calibration index (ECI) [621], which also summarizes the distance between a smooth calibration curve and the ideal 45° line.

15.3.5   Assessment of Strong Calibration

The concept of strong calibration is related to goodness-of-fit, which relates to the ability of a model to fit a given set of data. Ideally, we would identify a true underlying model, which may be utopic (Chap. 5) [602]. Typically, there is no single goodness-of-fit test which has good power against all kinds of lack of fit of a prediction model. Examples of lack of fit are missed nonlinearities, interactions, or an inappropriate link function between the linear predictor and the outcome. Such deviations are better assessed by adding nonlinear terms to a model, adding interaction terms, and examining alternative link functions, if sample size allows for such flexibility in modeling strategy.

An interesting approach is the Goeman–Le Cessie goodness-of-fit test [187, 324]. It assesses the alternative hypothesis that any nonlinearities or interaction effects have been missed in a logistic regression model. Such neglected effects can be detected by studying patterns in the residuals: observations close to each other in covariate space which deviate from the model in the same direction. The approach is to smooth the regression residuals and to test whether these smoothed residuals have more variance than expected under the null hypothesis. This deviation occurs when residuals that are close together in the covariate space are correlated. The test statistic is a sum of squared smoothed residuals.

Another approach to goodness-of-fit is to study observed versus expected outcomes in subgroups of patients, defined by predictor values. For example, we can assess the difference between observed versus expected outcomes in males and females, or other subgroups of patients. If the effect of the subgroup is not well modeled, e.g., an interaction was missed, this might be reflected in this assessment.

There are, however, more direct ways of assessing the influence of subgroup characteristics, as was discussed in Chap. 13 on model specification. So, this check for calibration is also more for face validity of the model and for convincing potential users than a serious check of calibration. Measures for assessment of calibration are summarized in Table 15.9.

15.3.6   Calibration of Survival Predictions

In a survival context, we can assess calibration-in-the-large with a model-based approach [116]. This involves using a Poisson model which uses the linear predictor as an offset. Additionally, we can fit the linear predictor based on the original prediction model as a predictor to obtain the calibration slope. Furthermore, we can fit a model with the linear predictor as an offset and adjusting for a set of dummy variables created by deciles of the linear predictor from the original prediction model. A score test for the group effect of this set is asymptotically equivalent to the Grønnesby and Borgan, or Nam–D'Agostino tests, which are survival analysis variants of the Hosmer–Lemeshow test [132]. Again, these tests produce a p-value that is difficult to interpret: with small external validation samples, we lack statistical power to detect miscalibration. On the other hand, we will commonly find statistically significant miscalibration with large external validation samples. These tests are therefore not very useful.

A calibration plot can also be produced. The calibration of a model can be studied at fixed time points. We can group patients for calculation of survival rates with the Kaplan–Meier method. Harrell suggests to use at least 50 subjects per group, depending on the hazard of the outcome [225]. This observed survival may be compared to the mean predicted survival from the prediction model. A smoothed calibration curve can be obtained by comparing Cox–Snell residuals on the cumulative probability scale against the right-censored survival times [225]. We can also plot the observed t-year risk of the outcome for each tenth of patients (and 95% confidence intervals) against the predicted risk estimated from the Poisson regression model [116]. This model-based approach can be extended to replace the groups with splines. These approaches depend on the baseline hazard being available either for at least some specific time points [471].

15.3.7   Example: Calibration in Testicular Cancer
           Prediction Model

For the prediction model of residual mass histology, we plot the actual outcome versus predicted for the validation sample (Fig. 15.12). We include the distribution of predicted risks, such that discrimination can also be judged. The results for five

Table 15.9 Summary of measures for calibration of a prediction model for binary outcomes

Performance aspect	Calculation	Visualization	Pros	Cons
Calibration-in-the-large	Compare mean (y) versus mean ($\hat{y}$)	Calibration graph	Key issue in validation; statistical testing possible	By definition OK in model development setting
Calibration slope	Regression slope of linear predictor	Calibration graph	Key issue in validation; statistical testing possible	By definition OK in model development setting
Calibration test	Joint test of calibration-in-the-large and calibration slope	Calibration graph	Efficient test of two key issues in calibration	Insensitive to more subtle miscalibration
Harrell's E statistic	Absolute difference between smoothed y versus $\hat{y}$	Calibration graph	Conceptually easy, summarizes miscalibration over whole curve	Depends on smoothing algorithm
Hosmer–Lemeshow test	Compare observed versus predicted in grouped patients	Calibration graph or table	Conceptually easy	Interpretation difficult; low power in small samples
Goeman–Le Cessie test	Consider correlation between residuals	–	Overall statistical test; supplementary to calibration graph	Very general
Subgroup calibration	Compare observed versus predicted in subgroups	Table	Conceptually easy	Not sensitive to various miscalibration patterns

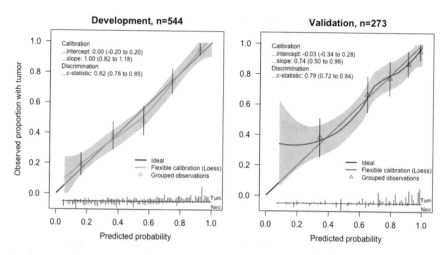

Fig. 15.12   Validity of predictions of tumor in the testicular cancer development sample (n = 544) and in the validation sample (n = 273). The distribution of predicted probabilities is shown at the bottom of the graphs, separately for those with tumor and those with necrosis ("Tum" vs. "Nec"). The triangles indicate the observed frequencies by tenth of predicted probability

Table 15.10   Calibration of testicular cancer prediction model[a]

	Development	External validation
Calibration-in-the-large	0	−0.03
Calibration slope	0.97[a]	0.74
Calibration tests		
Overall miscalibration	$p = 1$	$p = 0.13$
Hosmer–Lemeshow	$p = 0.66$	$p = 0.42$
Goeman–Le Cessie[b]	$p = 0.63$	$p = 0.94$

[a]Internal validation with 500 bootstrap resamples using Harrell's `validate` function
[b]Test statistics of squared smoothed residuals calculated with an R program from Jelle Goeman, available at www.clinicalpredictionmodels.org

risk groups of predicted risk are shown. Tests for miscalibration included the overall test for calibration-in-the-large and calibration slope, and the Goeman–Le Cessie test, which were nonsignificant for model development and external validation (Table 15.10). Note that assessment of calibration makes little sense in the development data, while it is essential at external validation.

15.3.8   *R Code for Assessing Calibration

Calibration plots were made by an extension of Harrell's `val.prob` function called `val.prob.ci.2` [602]. This function also provides assessment of calibration-in-the-large, calibration slope, and the calibration test *p*-value. Goeman developed R code for the functions `mlogit` (for binary of multinomial logistic regression), `smoothU` (for calculation of smoothed residuals), and `testfit` (for the Goeman-Le Cessie goodness-of-fit test).

15.3.9   Calibration and Discrimination

The calibration plot can be extended into a "validation plot" as a central tool to visualize model performance [568]. Moderate calibration is shown by observed outcomes being close to prediction, while discrimination aspects can be indicated with the distribution of the predicted probabilities. The distribution can be shown by a histogram or density distribution. We can also make separate histograms for those with and without the outcome for further insights (see, e.g., Figs. 15.10 and 15.12). It also helps to see the separation according to quantiles of predicted probabilities. For example, when deciles are used to define tenths, these will be relatively far apart for a good discriminating model.

Calibration-in-the-large is a phenomenon that is fully independent of discrimination. For example, we can change the incidence of the outcome in a case–control study, but the discrimination will be unaffected. The calibration slope, however, has a direct mathematical relation with discrimination [629]. If the calibration slope is below unity, the discrimination is also lower at external validation. Hence, over-fitted models will show both poor calibration and poor discrimination when validated in new patients (Chap. 19).

Weak to strong calibration is possible with poor discrimination, for example, when the range of predicted probabilities is small, such as between 9 and 11% for an average incidence of the outcome of 10%. At external validation, such a small range in predictions may arise from a narrow selection of patients (homogeneous case-mix). A drop in discriminative ability compared to the development setting can hence be explained by overfitting (calibration poor), or a more homogeneous case-mix (independent of calibration, see Chap. 19) [629]. On the other hand, a well discriminating model can have poor calibration, which can be corrected with various updating methods (Chap. 20).

15.4   Concluding Remarks

In this chapter, we have discussed a number of performance measures for prediction models; many more can be used, as already systematically discussed in work by Hilden, Bjerregaard, and Habbema in the 1970s [215–217, 247, 248]. Many performance measures are related to each other, e.g., the *c* statistic is related to the Mann–Whitney *U* statistic, which is calculated as a rank order test for the difference between predictions by outcome. The *c* statistic is also linearly related to Somers'

D statistic ($c = D/2 + 0.5$). Recently proposed measures for reclassification have many links to more traditional measures [428, 429].

From a simple statistical perspective, we want a small distance between observed outcome y and predicted outcome $\hat{y}$. Explained variation (R^2) can be used to indicate performance, and quantifies the predictability of the outcome: how much do we know already about the phenomena that lead to the outcome [491]? Diagnostic prediction models would hence be expected to have higher R^2 than prognostic models with long-term outcome. Indeed, prognostic models usually only have R^2 around 20–30%. This indicates that substantial uncertainty remains at the individual level; we can only provide probabilities, and we are far away from providing certainty on the individual outcome [13, 150].

We have focused on measures that are in wide use in medical research nowadays, including the concordance statistic (c, or area under the ROC curve, AUC) for discrimination, and various tests for calibration and goodness-of-fit. We gave some attention to Lorenz curves, although these are not often used; we did not discuss predictiveness curves, which provide useful insight in some applications [432]. The c statistic has been criticized by some, and should not be the only criterion in assessment of model performance. Especially, c is considered to be rather insensitive to inclusion of additional predictors in prediction models, such as novel biomarkers [107, 426]. Our theoretical examples and case study show that the c statistic is a key measure; it is closely related to other performance measures such as R^2 and Brier score [434]. Improvements in model fit will also show improvements in c statistic.

In principle, we might focus our modeling strategy on optimizing performance measures such as the c statistic. Indeed, estimation algorithms have been described that maximize the c statistic rather than the log likelihood [431].

Compared to current practice, calibration should receive more attention, especially when externally validating prediction models [103]. The recalibration test and its components (calibration-in-the-large and calibration slope, with recalibration parameters a and b) should be used routinely in performance assessment at external validation of prediction models.

15.4.1 Bibliographic Notes

The framework of a recalibration model was already proposed by Cox [114], and has been supported by many other researchers for evaluation of model performance [109, 225, 379, 380, 626]. Nice illustrations of diagnostic test evaluation with ROC curves are available at: http://www.anaesthetist.com/mnm/stats/roc/ and illustrations of Lorenz curves and the Gini index are at: http://en.wikipedia.org/wiki/Gini_coefficient.

Questions

15.1 Overall performance measures
Overall performance measures for logistic regression models include Brier score and R^2 type of measures, such as Nagelkerke's R^2.

(a) What values can Brier scores and R^2 take?
(b) What types of scoring rule are Brier and R^2?
(c) What are disadvantages of Brier and R^2?

15.2 Lorenz curve and incidence
In a Lorenz curve, the visual impression of a model with a c statistic of 0.80 depends on the incidence of the outcome.

(a) What happens when a Lorenz curve is made for situation with 1% incidence, such as a screening setting?
(b) And what for 99% incidence?

15.3 Interpretation of validation graphs
The validity of predictions can well be judged graphically. How do you judge

(a) calibration-in-the-large?
(b) calibration slope?
(c) discrimination?

15.4 Relations between calibration, discrimination, and overall performance
Explain the differences and the relation between calibration, discrimination, and overall performance measures.

Chapter 16
Evaluation of Clinical Usefulness

Background Performance measures such as discrimination and calibration consider the full range of risk predictions. We may also want to know whether a prediction model is useful to support medical decision-making: is the model beneficial to guide selection of subjects for screening, for diagnostic work-up, or decision-making on therapy? For such decisions, we need a cutoff for the predicted probability ("decision threshold", or "classification cutoff", see Chap. 2). Patients with predictions above the cutoff are classified as positive; those under the cutoff as negative. We will use the term "clinical usefulness" for a model's ability to make such classifications better than a default policy without the prediction model.

We consider performance measures for classification from a decision-analytic perspective and discuss their relations with performance measures as discussed in the previous chapter. Finally, we discuss study designs for measuring the actual impact of decision rules in clinical practice.

16.1 Clinical Usefulness

In the previous chapter, we saw that the distance between the predicted outcome and actual outcome $(y - \hat{y})$ is central to quantify overall model performance for regression models [231]. For classification, we replace $\hat{y}$ by a binary classifier, such that we classify subjects as positive or negative. The distance $y - \hat{y}$ is 0 for a correct classification and 1 for an incorrect classification. It can be summarized in the error rate (mean(misclassifications)).

A critical issue is the choice of cutoff to classify subjects as positive or negative. The cutoff is set to 50% as a default in some statistical packages. This implies that false-positive and false-negative classifications are equally important, which may be considered "absurd" in medical prediction problems [205]. Missing a patient with the event (a diagnosis or poor prognostic outcome) is usually more important than

E. W. Steyerberg, *Clinical Prediction Models*, Statistics for Biology and Health, https://doi.org/10.1007/978-3-030-16399-0_16

incorrect classification of a patient without the outcome; false-negative errors are more important than false-positive errors. This implies a threshold below 50%. We will consider informal and formal approaches to determining the optimal cutoff below.

The optimal cutoff is defined by the decision context, not by statistical criteria. Once a cutoff is chosen, clinical usefulness measures can be defined. These should consider the relative weight of false-positive and false-negative classifications, e.g., in a kind of weighted error rate [642]. A further approach is to study model performance over the whole range of possible cutoffs, as is done with the receiver operating characteristic (ROC) curve, but now for a "decision curve" [608, 648].

16.1.1   Intuitive Approach to the Cutoff

We consider two situations: treatment for bacterial meningitis and abandoning treatment for patients with traumatic brain injury. Bacterial meningitis is a severe infectious disease, with usually good outcome when treated early with antibiotics, but poor outcome when not treated in time. Several prediction models have been developed to predict the diagnosis "bacterial meningitis" among patients presenting at the emergency ward. If the probabilities from such models are used for decision-making, we should use a rather low cutoff, such as not to miss bacterial meningitis cases.

Several prediction models have been developed for patients with traumatic brain injury. If presenting characteristics are dismal (e.g., high age, severe trauma, poor remaining brain function), the risk of a poor long-term outcome is high. Some researchers have tried to define patients who should not be treated because of very high risk of poor outcome. The cutoff was set close to 100%, since we only want to refrain from treatment in case of near certainty of a poor outcome.

16.1.2   Decision-Analytic Approach: Benefit Versus Harm

The cutoff for treatment against no treatment can formally be defined with a decision-analytic approach (Table 16.1) [648]. The loss (or "costs" in a broad sense) can include patient outcomes (mortality, morbidity, quality of life) as well as economic costs (including diagnostic work-up, therapeutic interventions, admission costs, costs of follow-up, etc.).

Table 16.1 Costs of classification of subjects according to a decision threshold ("cutoff")

	Event	No event
Treatment: Risk >= cutoff	cTP	cFP
No treatment: Risk < cutoff	cFN	cTN

cTP and cFP: costs of True- and False-Positive classifications
cFN and cTN: costs of False- and True-Negative classifications, respectively

We focus on two groups of subjects: those with the event if not treated, and those without the event if not treated. In the first group, the costs relate to undertreatment (false-negative classifications), in the second group to overtreatment (false-positive classifications). In the first group, the costs of these false-negative classifications are referred to as cFN in Table 16.1. These should be compared to the costs of true-positive classifications (cTP); the difference cFN – cTP is the benefit of treatment for those who would have the event without treatment.

In the second group, relevant costs are for those without the event if not treated, who are treated ("overtreated"). The costs of these false-positive classifications (cFP) should be compared to the costs of true-negative classifications (cTN); the difference cFP – cTN is the harm of overtreatment for those who would not have the event anyway.

Specifying a mathematical loss function leads to a simple definition for the optimal decision threshold: the (odds of the) cutoff corresponds to the relative weight of harm versus benefit [172, 420]. Patients with probabilities above the threshold should be treated, those below the threshold not.

Odds(cutoff) = (cFP – cTN)/(cFN – cTP), where cTP and cFP refer to costs of True- and False-Positive classifications, and cFN and cTN to costs of False- and True-Negative classifications, respectively. Equivalently, we can write: Odds (cutoff) = Harm/Benefit.

- Benefit occurs for those with the event when not treated (cFN – cTP); it relates to the correct treatment of those with the event of interest.
- Harm occurs for those without the event when not treated (cFP – cTN); it relates to the unnecessary treatment of those without the event.

So, we note that only the differences between treated and non-treated situations are relevant to decision-making.

16.1.3 Accuracy Measures for Clinical Usefulness

If benefit and harm are weighted equally, the odds of the threshold is 1:1, or a threshold probability of 50%. This cutoff is by default considered in the calculation of the *error rate*, which is defined as (FN + FP)/N (Table 16.2). The complement is the *accuracy rate*: (TN + TP)/N. Often FN classifications are more important than FP classifications, which makes the accuracy rate not a sensible indicator of clinical usefulness [205]. Other disadvantages include that the accuracy rate by definition is high for a frequent or infrequent outcome. For example, if the average mortality is 7% after an acute MI, the accuracy is 93% when we classify all patients as survivors.

The accuracy rate is usually calculated at the simplistic cutoff of 50%, but can also be calculated at clinically defendable thresholds [642]. The harm-to-benefit ratio that underpins the choice of the cutoff should then be used to calculate a

Table 16.2 Classification of
subjects according to a
decision threshold

	Event	No event
Treatment: Risk >= cutoff	TP	FP
No treatment: Risk < cutoff	FN	TN

TP and FP: numbers of True- and False-Positive classifications;
FN and TN: numbers of False- and True-Negative classifications,
respectively

weighted accuracy, or its complement, the *weighted* error rate. We can express the
TN classifications in units of the TP classifications, such that the weighted accuracy
is calculated as (TP + w TN)/n. Similarly, the weighted error rate can be calculated
as (FN + w FP)/n. These rates can also be calculated for a default policy, which
would be followed without using the prediction model. The default policy could be
"treat all" or "treat none". The improvement that is obtained by making decisions
based on predictions from the model is the difference between the weighted
accuracy obtained with the model versus the weighted accuracy of the default
policy [642].

16.1.4   Decision Curve Analysis

In practice, it is often difficult to define the optimal threshold precisely. Difficulties
may lie at the population level, i.e., that we do not have sufficient data to quantify
harms and benefits for the typical threshold in a decision problem. Moreover, the
relative weight of harms and benefits may differ from patient to patient, necessitating individual thresholds [648].

An impression of the order of magnitude of the typical threshold can usually be
obtained from clinical experts. We could consider lower and upper values for the
threshold, with a gray area in between. This approach was, for example, followed in
classifying patients with possibly indolent prostate cancer, where those with
probabilities <30% were advised to undergo surgery, and those with probabilities
>60% to undergo active surveillance [562].

It is attractive to study a range of clinically plausible decision thresholds. This
approach was worked out by Vickers and Elkin [648]. They constructed a "decision
curve", which considers a threshold over the range 0–1. The method starts as
explained above, by noting that the threshold is directly related to the
harm-to-benefit ratio. Next, they create a plot which shows the net benefit of
treating patients according to the prediction model. The formula for net benefit goes
back to work published in 1884:

$$\text{Net Benefit} = \text{NB} = (\text{TP} - w\,\text{FP})/n,$$

where TP is the number of true-positive classifications, FP the number of false-positive
classifications, w is a weight equal to the odds of the threshold ($p_t/(1 - p_t)$), or the ratio
of harm to benefit, and n is the total number of subjects [424]. The crucial issue is the

weight *w*. For example, a threshold of 10% means that $w = 1/9$: the FP classifications are valued at one-ninth of a TP classification. Conversely, $w = 1:4$ implies a threshold of 20%.

The net benefit (NB) of a prediction model should be compared to default policies of "treat none" or "treat all". Treat none means that the NB is zero (since TP and FP are zero). The NB for "treat all" depends on the threshold and the event rate. The NB of a well-calibrated prediction model is at the maximum when the threshold is at the event rate. At this point, the policy "treat all" has a NB of zero, as well as the policy "treat none".

If the prediction model required efforts such as obtaining data from extra medical tests that were invasive, burdensome, or costly, an extended version of the net benefit formula can be used as given below:

$$NB = (TP - w\,FP)/n - \text{test harm},$$

where test harm is expressed per patient in units of the TP result [648]. Alternatively, we can calculate the difference in NB obtained from a test to define the maximum test harm. This is the *test trade-off*: the inverse of the NB indicates the minimum number of patients that we should be willing to undergo the test per positive net benefit [39]. For example, if the NB is 0.01 without considering test harm, we should accept that at least 100 patients are tested per net true positive.

The interpretation of the net benefit is in units of the true positives; how many more patients are correctly treated (TP decisions) at the same rate of not treating those who do not need treatment (TN decisions)? For interpretation of a decision curve, we need to identify a range of plausible threshold probabilities for treatment and study the benefit at all values within this range.

16.1.5 Interpreting Net Benefit in Decision Curves

We present decision curves for prediction models with increasing *c* statistics in Fig. 16.1. With a *c* statistic of 0.5, the net benefit (NB) is identical to the strategy "Treat all" below the decision threshold; no gain is obtained from using such a poor decision model. With a near-perfect model ($c = 0.98$), the NB appears to be substantial over the whole range of thresholds from 0 to 100%. With 50% incidence, the maximum NB is 0.5 at a threshold of 0%. "Treat all" implies 50% correct and 50% incorrect classifications at this threshold. For the 10% incidence, the maximum NB is 0.1. The 0% threshold reflects zero weight for false-positive classifications, which may not be realistic in most medical settings. It would always lead to a "Treat all" strategy: there are no perceived downsides of overtreatment.

For thresholds lower than the incidence (or "event rate"), we would follow a "Treat all" strategy by default, since this strategy provides higher net benefit than "treat none". By basing decisions on a prediction model, we hope to achieve higher net benefit, which implies that some interventions (tests or treatments) are avoided.

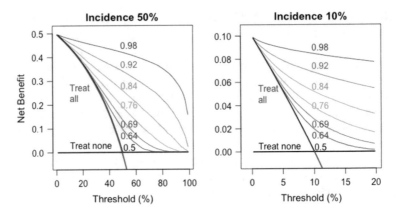

Fig. 16.1 Decision curves for prediction models with increasing c statistics (range: 0.5–0.98), based on the distributions as used in Chap. 15, for incidence (or "event rate") 50 and 10%. We note that the Net Benefit (NB) strongly depends on the c statistic, and that a near-perfect model ($c = 0.98$) is always clinically useful. "Treat all" is associated with a positive NB for thresholds below 50 and 10% (left and right panels, respectively); "Treat none" is dominant to "Treat all" for thresholds above the overall incidence

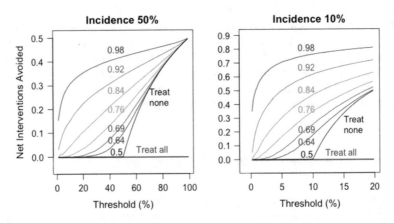

Fig. 16.2 Decision curves for prediction models with increasing c statistics (range: 0.5–0.98), based on the distributions as used in Chap. 15, for incidence 50 and 10%. We note that the fraction of Net Interventions Avoided, or the Net Benefit expressed as true negatives, strongly depends on the c statistic. A near-perfect model ($c = 0.98$) always avoids a substantial number of interventions. The maximum is 50% with an incidence of 50% (left panel) and 90% with an incidence of 10% (right panel). As in Fig. 16.1, "Treat none" is dominant to "Treat all" for thresholds above the overall incidence

This is a reduction in overtreatment (less false positives), at the expense of missing some true positives. We might therefore want to express net benefit in net fractions of interventions avoided, so in terms of net true negatives (Fig. 16.2). We calculate the net fraction of interventions avoided as the difference between net benefit from the prediction model minus the net benefit of "Treat all", since this is the natural reference [38, 39, 608]. We weight this difference by the benefit-to-harm ratio:

Table 16.3 Net benefit of various prediction models at decision thresholds equal to incidences of the outcome. The default policies of treat all or treat none have a net benefit of zero at these points. Net benefit is expressed in units of true-positive decisions (TP)

Prediction model	Incidence	
c statistic	10%	50%
0.5	0	0
0.64	0.020	0.10
0.69	0.028	0.14
0.76	0.039	0.19
0.84	0.052	0.26
0.92	0.068	0.34
0.98	0.085	0.42

$$\text{Net interventions avoided} = (\text{NB} - \text{NB}[\text{``treat all''}]) * \text{B/H}.$$

We use the benefit-to-harm ratio (B/H) rather than the harm-to-benefit ratio, or $1/w$. The fraction interventions avoided has 0% as a reference for "Treat all". So, Fig. 16.2 is a mirror image of Fig. 16.1, with a non-informative model being equivalent to "treat none" above the decision threshold.

The maximum gain from using a prediction model is when the threshold is equal to the incidence of the outcome or event rate [429]. Note that the threshold at the event rate may not be clinically defendable [302, 608]. The default policies of "treat all" or "treat none" both have a net benefit of zero at the event rate. Table 16.3 shows that the maximum gain is less than 0.01 at an incidence of 1%; but increases to over 0.4 for a near-perfect prediction model in the setting of incidence 50%. Net benefit refers here to identifying true-positive cases. If we reverse the coding the outcome, we consider identifying the true negatives, for whom interventions can be avoided.

16.1.6   Example: Clinical Usefulness of Prediction in Testicular Cancer

In the testicular cancer example, the residual mass histology is classified as residual tumor versus benign (necrosis). Malignant histology should surgically be resected, but resection of benign tissue is harmful (risks of surgical complications, hospital admission, costs). A decision analysis suggested a threshold of 70% for the probability of benign histology, or 30% for residual tumor [557]. This implies a ratio of 3:7 for unnecessary versus necessary surgery. The clinical relevance of resection of residual tumor is more than twice as important as unnecessary resection of benign tissue.

At model development, the sensitivity and specificity were 92% and 42%, respectively, at a cutoff of 30% for the probability of tumor (Table 16.4). At external validation, only 23 patients had predictions below 30%. The specificity was

Table 16.4 Classification table for the development ($n = 544$) and validation ($n = 273$) sets of testicular cancer patients at a cutoff for the risk of residual tumor of 30%. Sensitivity to detect tumor, specificity to detect necrosis, and net benefit (NB) in units of tumors detected are calculated for both data sets

	Development ($n = 544$)		Validation ($n = 273$)	
	Necrosis	Tumor	Necrosis	Tumor
Prediction <30%	102	24	16	7
Prediction >= 30%	143	275	60	190
	245	299	76	197
	Spec = 42%	Sens = 92%	Spec = 21%	Sens = 96%
	$NB_{model} = 0.393$		$NB_{model} = 0.602$	
	$NB_{treat\ all} = 0.357$		$NB_{treat\ all} = 0.602$	
	Increase in NB = 0.036		Increase in NB = 0	

lower (21%) and the sensitivity higher (96%) than at model development. The accuracy rate was $(102 + 275)/544 = 69\%$ at development, and, remarkably, slightly better at validation: $(16 + 190)/273 = 75\%$. The error rates are the complements of the accuracy rate (31 and 25%).

Resection of all masses leads to 299 tumor resections, but also to 245 unnecessary resections. This is a better choice than resection in none, since the average probability of tumor tissue was 55%, which is above the threshold of 30%. Using the model with a cutoff of 30% would lead to 275 necessary resections plus 102 correct omissions of resection in patients with necrosis. Missing $299 - 275 = 24$ patients with tumor (FN decisions) is more than compensated by the increase in correct omission of resection from 0 to 102 (TN decisions). The Net Benefit = (TP $- w$ FP)/$n = (275 - 3/7 * 143)/544 = 0.393$, in contrast to $(299 - 3/7 * 245)/544 = 0.357$ for resection in all.

In the validation sample, resection of all masses would lead to 197 tumor resections and 76 unnecessary resections. Using the model with a cutoff of 30% would lead to 190 necessary resections plus 16 correct omissions of resection in patients with necrosis. The Net Benefit = (TP $- w$ FP)/$n = (190-3/7 * 60)/273 = 0.602$, in contrast to $(197 - 3/7 * 76)/273 = 0.602$ for resection in all. Hence, the model is not clinically useful in the validation setting. Put simply: sparing resection in 16 patients with necrosis does not compensate missing tumor in 7, when we weigh tumor as 7/3 of necrosis (Table 16.4).

16.1.7   Decision Curves for Testicular Cancer Example

Thus far, we assumed a constant utility function, i.e., a weight of 3:7 for necrosis:tumor, for the decision to perform surgery on a residual mass in a testicular cancer patient. The corresponding threshold of 30% for the probability of tumor is

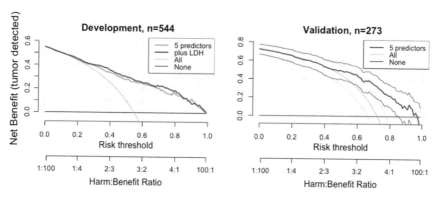

Fig. 16.3 Decision curves of predictions of tumor in patients with testicular cancer in the development sample ($n = 544$) and in the validation sample ($n = 273$). We note that the 5-predictor model can slightly be improved in the development sample by adding the tumor marker LDH. The 5-predictor model is not clinically useful in the validation setting around the relevant risk threshold of 30%. The lines for resection in all and resection in none cross at the frequencies of tumor (55% and 72%, respectively). In the validation sample, 95% confidence intervals are based on bootstrap sampling

an average and may vary for individual patients based on their personal weighing of surgical risks against increased chances of long-term survival [648]. Instead of a single relative weight, we may consider a range of weights in a decision curve for the testicular cancer prediction model (Fig. 16.3). This curve shows that the model is clinically useful for thresholds over 20% risk of tumor in the development sample, or harm-to-benefit ratios over 1:4; equivalent to thresholds for the probability of necrosis below 80%. In the validation sample, the model is only useful in the range of 55–95% for the probability of tumor, confirming that the model is not clinically useful in the validation setting when we assume a decision threshold of 30% [567]. The lines for resection in all and resection in none cross at the prevalence of tumor histology (55% and 72%, respectively). At these points, the model would have maximum gain in net benefit. Uncertainty can be indicated with 95% confidence intervals from a bootstrap procedure if desired [302].

We can correct the estimates of net benefit for statistical optimism by a cross-validation procedure (Fig. 16.4). We can also plot the net benefit in units of net unnecessary resections prevented, where we focus on not resecting patients with benign residual masses (with necrosis, Fig. 16.4). Finally, some may prefer to assess net benefit scaled to the event rate (standardized net benefit, Fig. 16.4) [302].

16.1.8 Verification Bias and Clinical Usefulness

The general policy is to resect residual masses if detected on CT scan. This implies resection if the radiologist considers a lymph node as enlarged, i.e., >10 mm.

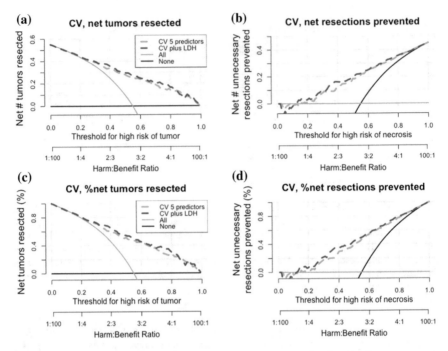

Fig. 16.4 Decision curves for patients with testicular cancer in the development sample ($n = 544$). **a** Cross-validation with 10 folds; **b** Net benefit in terms of unnecessary resections of necrosis prevented; the treat none line crosses at 45% for the probability of necrosis; panels **c** and **d** show results for standardized net benefit, i.e., NB divided by event rate

Patients masses <= 10 mm are generally not considered candidates for resection, and these patients are hence not included in our evaluations of clinical usefulness [644]. Such verification bias affects performance measures such as sensitivity and specificity, and also the clinical usefulness measures. The conclusion from Fig. 16.3 is that the prediction model has limited to no clinical usefulness; hence, we cannot easily reduce resections in those who underwent resection under current policies. There is, however, a large group of patients who are currently not considered for resection. Among the patients with small or "normal" residual masses, some will harbor residual tumor cells. These patients likely would benefit from resection, while they are currently not considered candidates in most centers. An exploratory analysis in 241 patients from a MRC/EORTC trial suggested that 84 (31%) of these might be candidates for resection, using the decision threshold of 30% risk of tumor [645]. For a full evaluation of NB, we might consider imputation of outcomes in those not undergoing resection, if we have access to the distribution of predictor values [122].

*16.1.9   *R Code*

Classification tables can readily be calculated with the `table` command. Andrew Vickers maintains a function `dca` for R and Stata which enables drawing decision curves (https://www.mskcc.org/departments/epidemiology-biostatistics/biostatistics/decision-curve-analysis). The `rmda` package provides many functions for decision curve analysis, with or without standardization to event rate (which makes NB similar to Relative Utility [37, 607]). Options include confidence intervals and perform optimism correction. Examples of decision curve code are at www.clinicalpredictionmodels.org. Key R code is shown below:

```r
library(rmda) # "risk model decision analysis"
# Model development
baseline.model <- decision_curve(tum ~
      ter+preafp+prehcg+sqpost+reduc10, #fitting a logistic model
      data = n544, bootstraps = 500) # bootstrap for 95% CI
set.seed(1)  # for reproducibility of cross-validation in models
      baseline.model.cv   <- cv_decision_curve(tum ~
      ter+preafp+prehcg+sqpost+reduc10, data=n544, folds=10) # CV, 10 folds
LDH.model <- decision_curve(tum ~ ...+lnldhst, ...)
set.seed(1)  # identical folds as above in CV
LDH.model.cv <- cv_decision_curve(tum ~ ... +lnldhst, folds=10) # CV
# Validation
val$pred <- plogis(predict(full, val)) # predict with full model, 5
predictors
val.5pred <- decision_curve(tum ~ pred, data = val,
      fitted.risk =T, bootstraps = 500) # validation with 95% CI based on B
# Plot the curves
par(mfrow=c(1,2), mar=c(4.2,4.2,3,.5), pty="m")
plot_decision_curve(list(baseline.model,LDH.model), # Basic + LDH in Dev
      curve.names=c("5 predictors","plus LDH"), standardize = F, # NB
      confidence.intervals=F, xlab="Risk threshold", # Change labels
      cost.benefit.xlab= "Harm:Benefit Ratio", ...)
plot_decision_curve(val.5pred, curve.names=c("5 predictors"),
      standardize = F, confidence.intervals=T, ...) # Basic in Val
# End plot Figure 16.3 #

# Show results with optimism correction in development setting
plot_decision_curve(list(baseline.model.cv, LDH.model.cv),
      curve.names = c("CV 5 predictors", "CV plus LDH"), ...) # Fig 16.4A
# With opt-out rather than opt-in
set.seed(1)
full.cv.o   <- cv_decision_curve(tum ~ ..., ..., policy="opt-out")
set.seed(1)
LDH.model.cv.o <- cv_decision_curve(tum ~ ..., ..., policy="opt-out
plot_decision_curve(list(full.cv.o, LDH.model.cv.o),
      curve.names = c("CV 5 predictors", "CV plus LDH"),
      cost.benefit.xlab = "Benefit:Harm Ratio") # Fig 16.4B
# Standardized
plot_decision_curve(list(...), standardize = T,...) # Fig 16.4C and D
# End plot Figure 16.4 #
summary(baseline.model, measure="NB") # Summary of analysis
```

16.2   Discrimination, Calibration, and Clinical Usefulness

From a statistical perspective, some may argue that discrimination is the primary criterion of a prediction model, since miscalibration can relatively easily be corrected when we apply a model in a new setting. The debate on recalibration is especially strong on the issue of assessment of incremental value, where recalibration may be desired if we purely focus on the value of the marker [38]. Recalibration would not be appropriate if we focus on real-life decision-making, since we do not know about any miscalibration yet when we apply a model in practice [330, 331]. Hence, clinical usefulness of a model in clinical practice depends at least on the combination of discrimination and calibration. Obviously, some discriminative ability is important for any clinical usefulness, as is clear from the decision curves in Fig. 16.1. Some refer to c statistics over 0.7 as "acceptable" or "modest", over 0.8 as "good", and over 0.9 as "excellent". This is, however, very problematic: it is not possible to indicate a minimum value for the c statistic to make a model clinically useful. In addition to not considering calibration aspects, the consequences of decisions are not considered in the c statistic.

Once the ratio of harms to benefits is used to define a clinically relevant threshold, the distribution of predictions around this threshold is a major determinant of clinical usefulness. The net benefit of a model with well-calibrated predictions is maximum if the decision threshold has the same value as the incidence of the outcome: threshold = event rate [429]. Approximately, half of the predictions are then above and the other half below the threshold. If nearly all predictions are above or below the threshold, the model cannot be clinically useful.

16.2.1   Discrimination, Calibration, and Net Benefit in the Testicular Cancer Case Study

As an example, we review the performance of the testicular cancer prediction model according to various criteria (Table 16.5). We note that overall performance, discrimination, and calibration look quite satisfactory, although predictive effects were slightly weaker than anticipated at external validation (calibration slope 0.74). The external validation data set was relatively small, hence providing limited power for tests of miscalibration. The clinical usefulness measures show a less fortunate pattern. Sensitivity is quite high but specificity is low. Hence, we can spare only few patients with necrosis a resection. Indeed, there was no clinical usefulness at the cutoff of 30% in the external data set. Hence, reasonable calibration and discrimination are necessary but not sufficient for clinical usefulness; it is crucially important where the threshold is located in the risk distribution. If the threshold would be closer to the event rate, the clinical usefulness would be higher. We can illustrate the impact of poor to good discrimination and poor to good calibration on net benefit with a web application (Fig. 16.5).

Table 16.5 Summary of performance measures for the prediction model in testicular cancer case study

Aspect	Measure		Development	Validation
Overall performance	R^2		38%	27%
	Brier$_{scaled}$		28%	20%
Discrimination	c statistic		0.81	0.79
	Discrimination slope		0.29	0.24
	Lorenz curve	p25	9%	13%
		p75	58%	65%
Calibration	Calibration-in-the-large		–	–0.03
	Calibration slope		0.97[*1]	0.74
	Test for miscalibration		p = 1	p = 0.13
Clinical usefulness at threshold p (tumor) = 30%	Sensitivity		92%	96%
	Specificity		42%	21%
	Accuracy		69%	75%
	Net Benefit—resection in all		0.39 – 0.36 = 0.03[*2]	0.60 – 0.60 = 0

[*]Internally validated measure by bootstrapping[1] and cross-validation[2]

16.2.2 Aims of Prediction Models and Performance Measures

Performance measures have different relevance in relation to the aim of the prediction model (see also Chap. 2). As discussed above, clinical usefulness requires considering a decision threshold, which is determined by the relative weight of harms and benefits of a test strategy or treatment. Clinical usefulness then depends on the combination of calibration, discrimination, and the distribution of predictions around the decision threshold.

- One application of a model is in targeting preventive activities to certain "high-risk" groups for efficient use of sparse resources. Discrimination is then the primary requirement; the main issue is to reasonably order subjects according to risk. If sparse resources are not an issue, the targeting should be based on harm to benefit considerations, making clinical usefulness the most relevant aspect of performance.
- If the aim is to inform or make decisions in clinical practice, calibration is an essential requirement. Miscalibration implies that we provide biased information, which can lead to worse decision-making than with a default policy that ignores the model predictions (a loss in net benefit). Of course, discriminative ability is also required, but limited discrimination will lead to a limited, but never a negative, net benefit. Miscalibration can lead to poorer decision-making

DCA and calibration

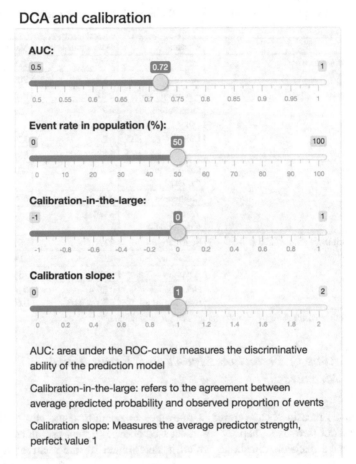

AUC: area under the ROC-curve measures the discriminative ability of the prediction model

Calibration-in-the-large: refers to the agreement between average predicted probability and observed proportion of events

Calibration slope: Measures the average predictor strength, perfect value 1

Fig. 16.5 Screenshot from Daan Nieboer's ShinyApp webpage that interactively shows the fascinating relation between calibration, discrimination, and clinical usefulness https://dcacalibration.shinyapps.io/dcacalibration/

than without the prediction model [606]. Further exploration of this issue is provided in Chap. 19.

- Furthermore, prediction models may have several roles in research. In RCTs, inclusion criteria can be according to a model, e.g., to select high-risk groups for investigation of a new treatment. For such an application, both calibration and discrimination are essential. Vickers et al. have described a method to determine eligibility for an RCT-based on net benefit considerations, including the expected effect of a treatment [649].
- Another use of prediction models is for covariate adjustment in an RCT. Then discrimination is most important. If no strong predictors are known, covariate adjustment has no benefit over unadjusted analysis in an RCT. Calibration is not

an issue when covariate effects are included in a model to estimate adjusted treatment effects.

- When a prediction model is used for confounder adjustment or case-mix adjustment, calibration is also automatically corrected for. Confounder adjustment can be achieved with various approaches, such as traditional regression analyses including the exposure and confounders, and propensity score adjustment. Discrimination of a model with confounders can range from low to high values, which does not make the adjustment less or more valid. With very high discrimination, we may even suspect that we adjust for a predictor that is too close to the outcome that we want to analyze; hence, very high discrimination is suspicious. Similarly, a high c statistic of a propensity score does not imply validity; it merely means that we can predict who gets treatment and who gets not. Most relevant is that all relevant confounders are included in the adjustment, i.e., covariates that are associated with treatment decisions and with outcome. The latter requires subject knowledge rather than statistical criteria.
- Another goal may be to assess the clinical utility of a new marker or test [651]. In Chap. 15, we discussed the net reclassification improvement (NRI) as a summary measure for reclassification by a marker for those with an event (higher risk is desired) and those without an event (lower risk is desired). The NRI can also be used for risk categorization. In the case of a binary classification, the NRI for events is the change in sensitivity, and the NRI for nonevents is the change in specificity. The sum is the change in Youden index, which implicitly weights events versus nonevents by the event rate [426, 564]. It hence falls short as measure for clinical usefulness. A weighted variant of the NRI has been proposed (wNRI), which is consistent with the increase in Net Benefit [427]. Decision curves are increasingly recognized as important tools to show the incremental clinical utility over a range of clinically plausible thresholds [608, 651].

16.2.3 Summary Points

- Discriminative ability is the primary requirement if we want to use the model to identify a high-risk group, or use the model to perform covariate adjustment in a randomized controlled trial.
- For informing patients and medical decision-making, calibration is the primary requirement, which determines clinical usefulness together with discrimination and the distribution of predictions around the decision threshold.

16.3   From Prediction Models to Decision Rules

Prediction models provide diagnostic or prognostic probabilities. They may assist medical decision-making without dictating to clinicians what to do precisely. One motivation for providing probabilities only is that decision thresholds may differ from patient to patient. Some argue, however, that prediction models will more likely have an impact on clinical practice when clear actions are defined in relation to the predictions [451]. They favor presentation as a decision rule rather than as a prediction model.

Few prediction rules have undergone formal analysis to determine whether they improve outcomes when used in clinical practice ("impact analysis") [558]. The clinical impact of most published prediction or decision rules is unknown.

For application as a decision rule, prediction models may require simplification to provide clear advice on actions with high and low predictions. A decision threshold has to be defined, either chosen informally or by formal decision analysis,

Table 16.6 Developing and evaluating clinical prediction models and decision rules [451]

Level of evidence	Definitions and standards of evaluation	Clinical implications
Level 1		
Derivation of prediction model	Identification of predictors for multivariable model; blinded assessment of outcomes	Needs validation and further evaluation before using in actual patient care
Level 2		
Narrow validation of prediction model	Assessment of predictive ability when tested prospectively in one setting; blinded assessment of outcomes	Needs validation in varied settings; may use predictions cautiously in patients similar to sample studied
Level 3		
Broad validation of prediction model	Assessment of predictive ability in varied settings with wide spectrum of patients and physicians	Needs impact analysis; may use predictions with confidence in their accuracy
Level 4		
Narrow impact analysis of prediction model used as decision rule	Prospective demonstration in one setting that use of decision rule improves physicians' decisions (quality or cost-effectiveness of patient care)	May use cautiously to inform decisions in settings similar to that studied
Level 5		
Broad impact analysis of prediction model used as decision rule	Prospective demonstration in varied settings that use of decision rule improves physicians' decisions for wide spectrum of patients	May use in varied settings with confidence that its use will benefit patient care quality or effectiveness

considering the relative weights of false-negative and false-positive decisions. In some diagnostic rules, we may not want to miss any patient with the outcome of interest (e.g., Ottawa Ankle rules [196], CT head rules [519]). This implies that we aim for a sensitivity of 100%, and hope for reasonable specificity. We accept false-positive classifications, since the 100% sensitivity implies an infinite cost of false-negative classifications.

Reilly et al. have proposed a set of criteria for assessing the impact of prediction models as decision rules (Table 16.6) [451]. These progressive evidentiary standards emphasize that a prediction model rises to the level of a decision rule only if clinicians use its predictions to help make decisions for patients ("level 5").

The first level of evidence is at the development of a prediction model. Reilly et al. emphasize the model selection aspects ("Identification of predictors") and blinded assessment of outcomes. We have seen that overfitting and measures to prevent overoptimistic expectations of model performance are important to consider.

Levels 2 and 3 are related to model validation, which indeed is essential before application of a model can be recommended. Validation in multiple settings is required to gain insight in between setting heterogeneity. If such heterogeneity is limited, we may be somewhat confident that we can apply a model for a new setting (see Chap. 21).

Levels 4 and 5 consider impact analysis, where a prediction model is used as a decision rule. We assess whether the rule improves physicians' decisions, and ideally also whether patient outcomes improve. Prediction rules might hence contribute to quality of care and better cost-effectiveness.

16.3.1   Performance of Decision Rules

Sensitivity and specificity are often used as performance criteria for a decision rule. As discussed before, these criteria may also be used for validation of a prediction model at certain cutoffs. Decision rules generally may improve physicians' specificity more than sensitivity; physicians ascribe greater value to true-positive decisions (provide care to patients who need it, benefit) than to true-negative decisions (withhold care from patients who do not need it, preventing harm). This is equivalent to weighing FN more than FP classifications, or a ratio of harm to benefit less than 1. This implies a threshold for treatment below 50%. An important issue is that the sensitivity and specificity of a decision rule in clinical practice is not only influenced by the quality of the prediction model but also by the adherence of clinicians to the rule. Validation of a prediction model may indicate the efficacy of a rule (the maximum that can be attained with 100% adherence), while impact analysis will indicate the effectiveness in practice.

Clinicians may choose to overrule the decision rule, which may improve sensitivity and/or specificity. But overruling may also dilute the effects of the rule [75]. There may be various barriers to the clinical use of decision rules, such as skepticism of guidelines (in general and with respect to the specific rule), questions on the clinical sensibility of the rule, too high confidence in clinical judgment, fear of medicolegal risks, concern that important factors are not addressed by the decision rule, concern on patient safety; and practical issues such as availability of the rule at the time of decision-making, and ease of use.

An impact analysis should ideally be designed as an RCT [289]. Randomization by center is an obvious approach to organizational changes such as using a decision rule in practice. But there is a risk for contaminating intervention and control groups and the logistic and economic challenges of multicenter studies are substantial. Some previous evidence of impact is required, which may come from single center evaluations. Such evaluation quantifies the actual effects of using the rule in clinical practice, which is critical information when planning multicenter ("level 5") studies. The Ottawa Ankle rules provide an excellent case study for model development, validation, and impact assessment [437, 569].

16.3.2   Treatment Benefit in Prognostic Subgroups

Prediction models may indicate subgroups of patients with a poor prognosis, often suggesting that these patients may need more aggressive treatment. Note that this assumes a curative intend. In contrast, in oncology, palliative treatments are generally considered when cure is not possible, and more aggressive treatment may do more harm than good. Prediction models may also define good prognosis groups, where less intensive treatment may be sufficient. For example, the International Germ Cell Classification proposed a distinction in good, intermediate, and poor prognosis groups [4]. In this clinical area, several RCTs have been performed. More aggressive treatment was studied in "poor risk" patients (e.g., high dose instead of standard dose chemotherapy), and less intensive therapy in "good prognosis" patients (e.g., three instead of four cycles of cisplatin-based chemotherapy).

16.3.3   Evaluation of Classification Systems

New classification systems will come up which include genetic profiles or other novel biomarkers. Systematic studies are required to validate these new systems, and provide evidence on any treatment benefits in subgroups as indicated by such new classification systems. For example, the MINDACT [88] and TAILORx [524] trials evaluated a genetic profile to indicate which women with early-stage breast cancer might benefit from chemotherapy. For efficient design, the MINDACT trial focused on the patients whose risk classification was discordant between the genetic profile and the traditional classification with clinical–pathological information only. Women who were determined to be at high risk for relapse of breast cancer by both the genetic profile and traditional clinical pathological criteria received chemotherapy, as is current standard practice. Those who were low risk by both criteria did not receive chemotherapy. However, the women who were determined to be at high risk for distant relapse by one criterion and low risk by the other were randomly assigned to one of two arms. Such as study is important for the evaluation of treatment benefit, but also validates the prognostic model by comparing outcomes between various prognostic groups under standard treatment. The design of trials of markers in oncology is discussed in more detail elsewhere [483].

A limitation of this design is that differences between groups may be small, leading to large sample sizes requirements. Indeed, the MINDACT trial was eventually found to be underpowered to provide reliable answers to regulators on the exclusion of benefit of chemotherapy [88]. Moreover, the prognostic value of a classification can usually well be determined in observational data, e.g., in a prospective validation study. The definition of low- and high-risk groups should relate to the expected benefits and harms. In the case of early breast cancer, the benefits of chemotherapy may be relatively small, casting doubt on the choice of the threshold for what is considered "high risk" [88]. In contrast, the TAILORx trial considered benefit of chemotherapy across a continuous risk score, which allows for a more refined assessment of which women with early breast cancer should be treated with chemotherapy [524].

16.4 Concluding Remarks

In this chapter, we have discussed measures for clinical usefulness of prediction models. We should not naively calculate error rates (or accuracy), with implicit equal weighing of false-positive and false-negative classifications. We noted that the c statistic was not sufficient to indicate clinical usefulness, although a low c statistic made it unlikely that a model was clinically useful. Good calibration was required, and the distribution of predictions had to be on both sides of the decision threshold. Usefulness is high for a perfectly calibrated model, with a substantial c statistic, in a clinical problem where the decision threshold is equal to the event rate [429]. A further discussion follows in Chap. 19.

Note that the determination of the decision threshold is fully independent from developing and validating the prediction model. The threshold is determined by clinical context. It should ideally be based on a formal weighting of harms and benefit of a treatment, compared to the alternatives of no treatment and treatment for all. Clinical usefulness is hence context dependent, and not in the hands of the modeler [302, 608, 651]. Impact of a prediction model as a decision rule is one further step in the evaluation [250, 451].

Compared to current practice, calibration should receive more attention when evaluating prediction models. The recalibration test and its components (calibration-in-the-large and calibration slope) should be used routinely in performance assessment in external data. We note that measures of clinical usefulness are increasingly being considered [608]. Decision curves are promising tools by providing simple graphs to summarize a model's quality for a range of plausible decision thresholds.

Questions

16.1   Calculation of Net Benefit (Sect. 16.1.5).

Net Benefit is defined as: $NB = (TP - w\ FP)/n$, where TP means a true-positive classification, FP false-positive classification, w the harm-to-benefit ratio, and n the sample size.

(a)   What is the NB if we classify all subjects as positive, in a setting of 50% incidence of the outcome, and a relative weight of FP classifications as 1:1?

(b)   And what if the relative weight of FP classifications is 1:2?

(c)   Recalculate the sensitivity, specificity, accuracy, and net benefit for the 273 validation patients in Table 16.4.

16.2   Decision curves (Fig. 16.1).

(a)   Why is the "Treat all" strategy in Fig. 16.1 associated with a negative NB for thresholds over 50%?

(b)   What will happen to the decision curves when a lower incidence than 50% is considered? Or a higher incidence?

16.3   Verification bias (Sect. 16.1.8).

What is verification bias? How does it affect clinical usefulness, e.g., in the right panel of Fig. 16.2?

16.4   Usefulness for decision-making versus research purposes.

When would you consider a model clinically useful? And when useful for research?

16.5.   Critical reflection on an Editorial.

Consider the Editorial in JNCI on discrimination, calibration, and interpretation of risks [150].

(a)   What is wrong in Fig. 2? Compare to Fig. 16.5 (https://dcacalibration. shinyapps.io/dcacalibration/).

(b)   What is the decision threshold for this problem? What is the basis for this threshold?

(c)   How clinically useful is the Gail model with this threshold, according to Net Benefit?

Chapter 17
Validation of Prediction Models

Background A prediction model should provide valid outcome predictions for new patients. Essentially, the data set to develop a model is not of interest other than to learn for the future. Validation, hence, is an important aspect of the process of predictive modeling. An important distinction is between apparent, internal and external validation. In this chapter, we focus on internal and external validation techniques, with illustrations in case studies.

17.1 Internal Versus External Validation, and Validity

A general framework for validation and validity concepts is shown in Fig. 17.1. We develop a model within a sample of patients that is representative for an underlying population. This underlying population has specific characteristics, e.g., a specific hospital with a certain profile of how patients come to this hospital. By necessity, the sample is historic in nature, although we generally will aim for recent data, which are representative of current practice. At least we should determine the internal validity (or "reproducibility" [285]) of our predictive model for this underlying population. We do so by testing the model in our development sample ("internal validation"). Internal validation is the process of determining internal validity. Internal validation assesses validity for the setting where the development data originated from.

A further aspect is the external validity (or "generalizability"/"transportability") of the prediction model to populations that are "plausibly related" [285]. Generalizability is a desired property from both a scientific and practical perspective. Scientifically speaking hypotheses and theories are stronger when their generalizability is larger. Practically, we hope to be able to validly apply a prediction model to our specific setting, that may be different in some respects from the model development setting. To know whether such application is reasonable, external validity needs to have been assessed for a setting similar to that for the intended application and the performance needs to have been found adequate. If no

© Springer Nature Switzerland AG 2019
E. W. Steyerberg, *Clinical Prediction Models*, Statistics for Biology and Health, https://doi.org/10.1007/978-3-030-16399-0_17

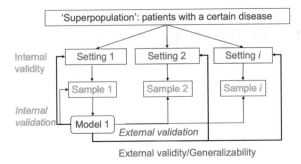

Fig. 17.1 A conceptual framework on internal versus external validation, and validity. We consider a superpopulation, consisting of several subpopulations (referred to as "settings"). We develop a model in sample 1 from setting 1. Internal validation is the process of determining internal validity for setting 1. External validation is the process of determining generalizability to settings 2 to *i*

validation results are available for the setting, or setting similar to where the model will be applied, such application is essentially a leap of faith. Alternatively, validation may have been performed and have suggested ways for model updating (Chaps. 20 and 21).

The definition of "plausibly related" populations is not self-evident. It requires subject knowledge and expert judgment on epidemiological study design aspects [130]. We define "plausibly related" as that populations can be thought of as parts of a "superpopulation" (Fig. 17.1). We could also state that we consider populations that would be reasonable to apply the previously developed model. Populations will be slightly different, e.g., treated at different hospitals or in different time frames. Various aspects may differ between these populations, e.g., the selection of patients (e.g., referral center versus more standard setting, or primary care versus secondary care, severity of disease), and definitions of predictors and outcome. Also, the degree of measurement error may differ between settings [355].

For example, a superpopulation could be formed by "patients with an acute MI". The GUSTO-I trial would represent a subpopulation, defined by the inclusion criteria for this trial, the participating centers, and the time of accrual. We can think of further subpopulations within the trial, defined by regions, countries, and centers [536].

17.1.1 Assessment of Internal and External Validity

We learn about external validity by testing the model in samples from other settings than the model development setting (sample 2 to *i* in Fig. 17.1, "external validation"). These samples are fully independent from the development data. The more often the model is externally validated and the more diverse these settings, the more we learn about the generalizability of the model. This is similar to the approach to assessing any scientific hypothesis [285].

In the case of prediction models, we may often find that the baseline risk differs across settings. One example was the validation of the nomogram for prediction of indolent cancer [562]. This model was developed for a clinical setting, with an overall probability of indolent cancer of 20%. Validation was in a screening setting with 50% probability of indolent cancer. This difference in baseline risk could not be explained by differences in predictors. If we have multiple validation studies, we can better quantify the heterogeneity in baseline risk and in predictor effects between validation settings [457].

17.2   Internal Validation Techniques

Several techniques can be used to assess internal validity. Some of the most common in medical research are discussed here (Table 17.1).

17.2.1   Apparent Validation

With apparent validation, model performance is assessed directly in the sample where it was derived from (Fig. 17.2). Naturally, this leads to an optimistic estimate of performance, since model parameters were optimized for the sample. However,

Table 17.1 Overview of characteristics of some techniques for internal validation

Method	Development	Validation
Apparent	Original 100%	Original 100%
Split-sample	50–67% of original	Independent 50–33%
Cross-validation[a]		
Classical	2 × 50% to 10 × 90% of original	Independent 2 × 50% to 10 × 10%
Jack-knife	$n \times (n - 1$ of original)	Independent $n \times 1$ patient
Bootstrap	Bootstrap sample of size n	Original 100%

[a]More stable cross-validation results are obtained by repeating the cross-validation many times, e.g., 10 times ("multi-fold cross-validation", 10 × 10 fold cross-validation)

Fig. 17.2 Apparent validation refers to assessing model performance in the sample where the model was derived from

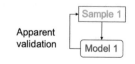

we use 100% of the available data to develop the model, and 100% of the data to test the model. Hence, the procedure gives optimistic but rather stable estimates of performance.

17.2.2   Split-Sample Validation

With split-sample validation, the sample is randomly divided into two groups. This very classical approach is similar to the design of an external validation study, where subjects are fully independent from the development study. However, the split in derivation and test set is at random in split-sample validation. In one group the model is created (e.g., 50% of the data) and in the other, the model performance is evaluated (e.g., the other 50% of the data, Fig. 17.3). Typical splits are as 50:50, or 2:1 [13].

Several aspects need attention with respect to split-sample validation. If samples are split fully at random, substantial imbalances may occur with respect to the distribution of predictors and the outcome. For example, if we perform split-sample validation with a small subsample from GUSTO-I ($n = 429$), the average incidence of 30-day mortality is 5.6% (24/429), but it may easily be 4% in a 50% random part and 7% in another part. Similarly, the distribution of predictors may vary. For predictors with skewed distributions, the consequences may be even worse. For example, a random development sample may not contain any patient with shock which occurred in only 1.6% (7/429). A practical possibility is to stratify the random sampling by outcome and relevant predictors.

The drawbacks of split-sample methods are numerous [225, 382, 533]. One major objection is related to variance. Only part of the data is used for model development, leading to less stable model results compared to development with all development data. Also, the validation part is relatively small, leading to unreliable assessment of model performance. Further, the investigator may be unlucky in the split; the model may show a very poor performance in the random validation part. It is not more than human that the investigator is tempted to repeat the splitting process until more favorable results are found. Another objection is related to bias. We obtain an assessment of the performance when a part of the data is used, while we want to know the performance of a model based on the full sample.

In sum, split-sample validation is a classical but inefficient approach to model validation. It dates from the time before efficient but computer-intensive methods were available, such as bootstrapping [148]. Simulation studies have shown that rather large sample sizes are required to make split-sample validation reasonable [547]. But with large samples, the apparent validity is already a good indicator of model performance. Hence, we may conclude that split-sample validation is a method "that works when we do not need it" [533, 546]. It should be replaced in medical research by more efficient internal validation techniques, and by approaches to assess external validity.

Fig. 17.3 Split-sample validation refers to assessing model performance in a 50% random part of the sample, with model development in the other 50%

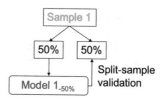

17.2.3 Cross-Validation

Cross-validation is an extension of split-sample validation, aiming for more stability (Fig. 17.4). A prediction model is tested on a random part (a fold) that was left out from the sample. The model is developed in the remaining part of the sample. This process is repeated for consecutive fractions of patients. For example, the data set may be split by deciles to create groups containing 1/10th of the patients each, with model development in 9 of the 10 and testing in 1 of the 10. This is repeated 10 times ("10-fold cross-validation"). In this way, all patients have served once to test the model. The performance may be estimated as the average over all assessments [225]. A more elegant solution is to estimate the performance in one round for all left out folds. The predictions for each fold were then each time based on the remainder of the sample.

Compared to split-sample validation, cross-validation can use a larger part of the sample for model development (e.g., 90%). This is an advantage. However, the whole cross-validation procedure may need to be repeated several times to obtain truly stable results, for example, 10 times 10-fold cross-validation. The most extreme cross-validation is to leave out each patient once, which is equivalent to the jack-knife procedure [148]. With large numbers of patients, this procedure is not very efficient.

A limitation of cross-validation is that the procedure may not properly reflect all sources of model uncertainty, such as the model instability caused by automated variable selection methods. An example is at www.clinicalpredictionmodels.org, where we consider the stability of a backward stepwise selection procedure in the large subsample from GUSTO-I (sample 4, $n = 785$, 52 deaths). A 10-fold cross-validation procedure suggests a quite stable selection of "important predictors": SHO, A65, HIG, and HRT. In contrast, bootstrapping shows a much wider

Fig. 17.4 Cross-validation refers to assessing model performance consecutively in a random part of the sample, with model development in the other parts. With 10-fold cross-validation, 10 parts with 1/10 of the sample serve as validation parts

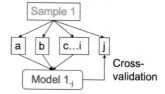

variability. The underestimation of variability is easily recognized for jack-knife cross-validation, where the development sample is identical to the full sample except for 1 patient. Hence, largely the same predictors will generally be selected in each jack-knife sample as in the full sample. Such model uncertainty can better be captured with bootstrap validation.

17.2.4   Bootstrap Validation

As discussed in Chap. 5, bootstrapping reflects the process of sampling from the underlying population (Fig. 17.5). Bootstrap samples are drawn with replacement from the original sample, reflecting the drawing of samples from an underlying population. Bootstrap samples are of the same size as the original sample [148]. In the context of model validation, 200 bootstraps may often be sufficient to obtain stable estimates, but in one simulation study, we reached a plateau only after 500 bootstrap repetitions [535]. With current computer power, bootstrap validation is a feasible technique for most prediction problems with at least 500 repetitions.

For bootstrap validation a prediction model is developed in each bootstrap sample. This model is evaluated both in the bootstrap sample and in the original sample. The first reflects apparent validation, the second reflects validation in new subjects. The difference in performance indicates the optimism. This optimism is subtracted from the apparent performance of the original model in the original sample [148, 225, 542, 547]. The bootstrap was illustrated for estimation of optimism in Chap. 5.

Advantages of bootstrap validation are various. The optimism-corrected performance estimate is rather stable, since samples of size n are used to develop the model as well as to test the model. This is similar to apparent validation, and an advantage over split-sample and cross-validation methods. Compared to apparent validation, some uncertainty is added by having to estimate the optimism. When sufficient bootstraps are taken, say at least 500 repetitions, this additional uncertainty is small beyond the uncertainty that is inherent to analyzing a small sample.

Importantly, simulations have shown that bootstrap validation can appropriately reflect all sources of model uncertainty, especially variable selection [535].

Fig. 17.5 Bootstrap validation refers to assessing model performance in the original sample for a model (Model 1*) that was developed in a bootstrap sample (Sample 1*), drawn with replacement from the original sample

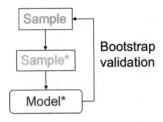

The bootstrap also seems to work reasonably well in high-dimensional settings of genetic markers, where the number of potential predictors is larger than the number of patients ("$p > n$ problems"), although some modifications may need to be considered [494].

Disadvantages of bootstrap validation, and other resampling methods such as cross-validation, include that only automated modeling strategies can be used, such as fitting a full model without selection, or following an automated stepwise selection approach. In many analyses, intermediate steps are made, such as collapsing categories of variables, truncation of outliers or omission of influential observations, assessing linearity visually in a plot, testing some interaction terms, studying both univariate and multivariable p-values, or assessing proportionality of hazards for a Cox regression model. It may be difficult to repeat all these steps in a bootstrap procedure. In such situations, it may be reasonable to at least validate the full model containing all predictors to obtain a first impression of the optimism [225]. For example, when we consider 30 candidate predictors, and build a final model with predictors that have multivariable $p < 0.20$ in a backward stepwise selection procedure, after univariate screening with, e.g., $p < 0.50$, the optimism can be approximated by validating the full 30-predictor model. Another reasonable approximation for the optimism in this example may be to simply perform backward stepwise selection with $p < 0.20$, ignoring the univariate screening. We would definitely be cheating if we validated the finally selected model and ignored all selection steps. In one study, we found an optimism estimate of 0.07 for the c statistic when we replayed all modeling steps (based on univariate and multivariable p-values) in contrast to only 0.01 when we considered the final model as predefined [535].

17.2.5 Internal Validation Combined with Imputation

As discussed in Chaps. 7 and 8, missing values may be imputed multiple times to allow for optimal statistical analysis. It is not immediately clear how internal validation, such as cross-validation or bootstrapping, should be combined with such multiple imputation (MI) [493, 641]. For validation of model performance, it has been proposed to distinguish between ideal model performance and pragmatic model performance [677]. The first refers to the model's performance in a future clinical setting without missing values in predictors. The latter refers to the model's performance in a real-world clinical setting where some individuals have missing predictors. We focus on assessing the ideal model performance. Pragmatic model performance may be assessed for example by a set of partial prediction models constructed for each potential observed pattern of predictors: submodels [167].

We can think of two main approaches when using multiple imputation (MI):

(1) *M* imputed data sets are created and bootstrapping is applied to each of them;
(2) *B* bootstrap samples of the original data set (including missing values) are drawn and in each of these samples the data are (multiply) imputed.

Approach 1 is computationally simpler than approach 2, since imputation takes more computer time than bootstrap cross-validation. An attractive variant of approach 2 might be to do only 1 imputation per bootstrap sample [74]. Approaches 1 and 2 have been applied and compared for issues such as estimation of 95% confidence intervals of predictors and variable selection [244, 669, 678]. It appears that we may well follow approach 1 (bootstrap within imputed sets) to estimate model performance for a future setting with complete data [677]. The optimism-corrected estimates are derived per imputed data set and subsequently pooled to give an overall estimate for the expected model performance. A detailed case study is provided in Chap. 23.

17.3   External Validation Studies

External validation of models is essential to assess general applicability of a prediction model. Where internal validation techniques are all characterized by random splitting of development and test samples, external validation considers patients that differ in some respect from the development patients (Fig. 17.1). External validation studies may address aspects of historic (or temporal), geographical (or spatial), methodological and spectrum transportability [285]. Temporal transportability refers to performance when a model is tested in different historical periods. Especially relevant is a model's validity in more recently treated patients. Geographic transportability refers to testing in patients from other places, e.g., other hospitals or other regions. Methodological transportability refers to testing with data collected by using alternative methods, e.g., when comorbidity data are collected from claims data rather than from patients' charts. Spectrum transportability refers to testing in patients who are, on average, more (or less) advanced in their disease process, or who have a somewhat different disease [285]. Spectrum transportability is relevant when models are developed in secondary care and validated in primary care, or models developed in randomized trials are validated in broader, less selected samples.

In addition to these aspects, we may consider whether external validation was performed by the same investigators who developed the model, or by investigators not involved at the development stage [513]. If model performance is found adequate by fully independent investigators, in their specific setting, this is more convincing than when this result was found by investigators who also developed the model.

A simple distinction in types of external validation studies is shown in Table 17.2: temporal validation (validation in more recent patients), geographic

Table 17.2 Types of external validation studies [285]

Method	Characteristics
Temporal validation	Prospective testing, more recent patients
Geographic validation	Multisite testing
Fully independent validation	Other investigators at other site(s)

validation (validation in other places), and fully independent validation (by other investigators at other sites). Mixed forms of these types can occur in practice. For example, we validated a testicular cancer prediction model in 172 patients: 100 more recently treated patients from hospitals that participated in the model development phase and 72 from a hospital not included among the development centers [545].

17.3.1   Temporal Validation

With temporal validation, we typically validate a model in more recently treated patients. A straightforward approach is to split the development data into two parts: one part containing early treated patients to develop the model and another part containing the most recently treated patients to assess the performance. Note that this is a non-random split.

17.3.2   *Example: Validation of a Model for Lynch Syndrome

We aimed to predict the prevalence of Lynch-syndrome-related genetic defects (*MLH1* or *MSH2* mutations) based in proband and relative characteristics ("family history"). Predictors included type of cancer diagnosis, age, and number of affected relatives. We developed a model with 898 patients who were tested between 2000 and 2003. This model was tested in a validation sample containing 1016 patients who were tested between 2003 and 2004 [40, 534].

In the validation sample, the outcome definition was slightly different, since not only mutations but also deletions of genes were assessed. This may have contributed to the slightly higher prevalence of mutations (15% at validation versus 14% at development), while the case-mix remained similar (mean predicted probability for validation sample 13%). This difference in prevalence may easily be adjusted for by using a slightly higher intercept in the logistic regression model (+0.25). The effects of the predictors were similar in the development and validation samples. Also, the discriminative ability remained at a similar level as at development with c statistic around 0.80.

The good performance at external validation may not be too surprising given that definitions of predictors were exactly the same. For the final model, both data sets were combined, such that 1914 patients were analyzed. This leads to more stable estimation of the effects of the predictors [40]. Later on, more validations were performed, including an international validation across multiple cohorts, including population-based and clinic-based cohorts [290] (Table 17.3).

Table 17.3 Multivariable logistic regression analysis for the PREMM model for Lynch syndrome prediction. Effects of predictors are shown for the development ($n = 898$) and validation ($n = 1016$) patients (OR, odds ratio), as well as in the combined data set ($n = 1914$) used for estimation of the final prediction model. Model performance includes assessment of discrimination and calibration

	Development, $n = 898$	Validation, $n = 1016$	Combined, $n = 1914$
Predictors	OR [95% CI]	OR [95% CI]	OR [95% CI]
Proband			
CRC 1	2.2 [1.9–2.5]	7.0 [6.0–8.1]	3.8 [3.6–4.1]
CRC 2+	8.2 [5.6–12]	37 [25–55]	16 [14–20]
Adenoma	1.8 [1.5–2.2]	1.5 [1.2–1.7]	1.5 [1.4–1.6]
Endometrial cancer	2.5 [2.1–3.1]	7.1 [6.1–8.2]	4.2 [3.9–4.6]
Other HNPCC cancer	2.1 [1.7–2.5]	1.4 [1.1–1.8]	1.8 [1.6–2.0]
Family history			
CRC in first/second degree[a]	2.3 [2.1–2.5]	3.0 [2.8–3.3]	2.6 [2.5–2.7]
CRC 2 in first degree	3.1 [2.6–3.6]	4.2 [3.6–4.8]	3.6 [3.4–3.8]
Endometrial cancer first/ second degree[a]	2.7 [2.4–3.2]	2.7 [2.3–3.1]	2.6 [2.4–2.8]
Endometrial cancer 2 in first degree	6.5 [1.8–24]	26 [6.0–113]	12 [6.3–23]
Other HNPCC cancer	1.5 [1.4–1.7]	1.4 [1.4–1.6]	1.5 [1.4–1.6]
Age at diagnosis			
CRC[b]	1.5 [1.5–1.5]	1.4 [1.4–1.4]	1.4 [1.4–1.4]
Endometrial cancer[c]	1.3 [1.2–1.4]	1.4 [1.3–1.4]	1.3 [1.3–1.4]
Model performance			
c statistic	0.79 [0.76–0.83][d]	0.80 [0.76–0.84][e]	0.80 [0.77–0.83][d]
Mean observed versus predicted	14% versus 14%	15% versus 13%[e]	15% versus 15%
Calibration slope	0.85[d]	1.26 [1.03–1.49][e]	0.94[d]

[a]Family history coded as first-degree + 0.5 second-degree relatives, with first-degree relatives coded as 0 or 1 and second-degree relatives coded as 0, 1, 2+
[b]Age effect for colorectal cancer and/or adenoma in probands, and colorectal cancer in first- and second-degree relatives
[c]Age effect for endometrial cancer in probands, in first-degree and in second-degree relatives
[d]Internal validation by bootstrapping for *c* statistic and calibration slope
[e]External validation for *c* statistic, mean observed and predicted probabilities, and calibration slope

17.3.3   Geographic Validation

With geographic validation, we evaluate a predictive model according to site or hospital. Geographic validation can be seen as a variant of cross-validation. It could be labeled "leave-one-center-out cross-validation" [546]. Importantly, standard cross-validation makes splits in the data at random; with geographic validation the splits are not at random. Some examples are shown in Table 17.4. Geographic validation is often possible with collaborative studies, and more meaningful than a standard cross-validation procedure [473].

A drawback of such geographical validations is that validation samples may get quite small, leading to unreliable results. Setting-specific results should not be overinterpreted, for example, as showing that "the model was not valid for hospital X", or for "cohort #4" in an individual patients data meta-analysis [457]. For example, in the testicular cancer case study, we found overall adequate calibration for patients treated in each of the participating studies (Fig. 17.6) [645]. The overall intercept may have been too low for study #6 however. Note that we perform multiple, small, subgroup analyses, with multiple testing. Emphasis should be on quantifying the amount of heterogeneity beyond chance [30, 31, 457]. Differences between settings will always seem to be present with small numbers (Chap. 21). On the other hand, remarkable findings for a specific setting may indicate a need for further validation and updating before applying the model in this setting (see Chap. 20) and trigger further research.

17.3.4   Fully Independent Validation

Finally, we discuss external validation by independent investigators ("fully independent validation"). Other investigators may use slightly different definitions of predictors, outcome, and study patients that were differently selected compared to the development setting. An example of that is a prostate cancer model developed for clinically seen patients and validated in patients selected by a systematic screening program (European Study on Prostate Cancer, ERSPC) [562]. Here,

Table 17.4 Examples of studies with external validation according to site ("leave-one-center-out cross-validation")

Model	Development	Validation	Site
Testicular cancer [551]	6 × 5 groups	6 × 1 group	A group consisted of a single hospital or a previously published patient series
Chlamydia trachomatis [192]	4 × 3 regions	4 × 1 region	Municipality health centers organizing regional case finding
DRASTIC study [314]	5 × 4 hospitals	5 × 1 hospital	Large hospitals participating in an RCT+ a category "other"

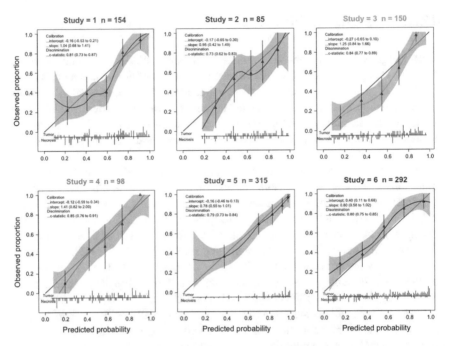

Fig. 17.6 Results of external validation by study group (internal-external validation) [473, 546] for the testicular cancer prediction model for prediction of residual tumor based on development and validation sets (*n* = 1094 total). We note *c* statistics around 0.8 for all studies, with overall minor miscalibration [645]

case-mix seemed similar, but a severe underestimation of relatively innocent ("indolent") cancer probability was found (Table 17.5). This phenomenon was addressed by a new logistic model intercept, while keeping the regression coefficients close to their original values.

Similarly, it was found that a prediction model for the selection of patients undergoing in vitro fertilization for single embryo transfer needed an adjustment when a model developed at one hospital was applied in another center. Again, a systematic difference remained even after adjustment for well-known and important predictors [262]. This difference in average outcome ("calibration-in-the-large") is an important motivation for recalibration of model predictions as a simple but important updating technique (see Chap. 20).

Some examples of fully independent validation studies with their main conclusions are listed in Table 17.6. It seems that fully external validation studies often provide more unfavorable results than weaker tests of validity, especially more unfavorable compared to internal validation results [13, 103, 513, 666].

Table 17.5 Performance of three previous nomograms for indolent prostate cancer developed by Kattan et al. [295] validated in 247 ERSPC patients [562]

Performance parameter		Nomogram		
		Base	Medium	Full
Area under the ROC curve	Kattan et al.	0.64	0.74	0.79
	ERSPC	0.61 [0.54–0.68]	0.72 [0.66–0.78]	0.76 [0.70–0.82]
Calibration in the large	Predicted	24%	22%	15%
	Observed	49% [43–55%]	49% [43–55%]	49% [43–55%]
Calibration slope	Predicted	1	1	1
	Observed	0.78 [0.32–1.24]	0.87 [0.55–1.19]	1.07 [0.74–1.40]

Base: serum PSA + clinical stage + biopsy Gleason grade 1 and 2
Medium: Base + US volume + %positive cores
Full: Base + US volume + mm cancerous tissue + mm noncancerous tissue

Table 17.6 Examples of studies with fully independent external validation

Model	Development	Validation	Conclusions
Prostate cancer	Two hospitals [295]	Screening setting (ERSPC) [562]	Intercept problem
Aneurysm mortality	One hospital + meta-analysis [555]	UK small aneurysm trial [71] and another hospital [304]	Missing predictors; poor/moderate performance
Renal artery stenosis	RCT [314]	One French hospital [366]	"reasonably valid"

17.3.5   Reasons for Poor Validation

Unfavorable results at validation may often be explained by inadequate model development. Sample size may have been relatively small, or patients were selected from a single center. This was for example noted in a review of over 25 models in traumatic brain injury [436]. Also, statistical analysis may often have been suboptimal, e.g., with stepwise selection in relatively small samples with many potential predictors, and no shrinkage of regression coefficients to compensate for overfitting [563].

Other explanations include true differences between development and validation settings, especially in coding of predictors and outcome. Measurement error may cause invalidity [355, 414]. The problem of transportability of models that incorporate laboratory tests results was already recognized in the 80s for a prediction rule for jaundice, where lab measurement units were not consistent [500]. Indeed, the validation of a model that was previously developed by others is often more difficult than anticipated. If a nomogram is presented with some nonlinear terms, it is not so easy to derive a formula to calculate outcome predictions for new patients. So, it is quite likely that errors are made at such external validation studies. Units of measurement and the intercept value require special attention. Contacting the authors may help to prevent mistakes.

Moreover, variables required for a model may not be available at validation. A constant value can be filled in (e.g., the mean or median), but obviously this limits the external performance of a model. For example, a Dutch model for abdominal aneurysm mortality was validated in the UK small aneurysm study, while 2 of the 7 predictors were not available [71]. In a validation study with patients from Rotterdam, all predictors except 1 were available and a better external performance was found [304]. A better approach may be to use submodels for validation. Such submodels do not contain all predictors, but are readily applicable in the presence of missingness [167].

Another strategy to facilitate external validation is followed in the Observational Health Data Sciences and Informatics (OHDSI) program (https://www.ohdsi.org/). Here a common data model is used to standardize data structure and language across a wide range of data bases. An R package is available for building and validating patient level predictive models using data in common data model format [452].

17.4 Concluding Remarks

We considered several approaches to internal and external validation. For internal validation, bootstrapping appears most attractive, provided that we can replay all modeling steps. This may sometimes be difficult, e.g., when decisions on coding of predictors and selection of predictors are made in the modeling process. Several variants of bootstrapping are under study, which may be more efficient than the standard procedure.

Any internal validation technique should be seen as validating the modeling *process* rather than a specific *model* [232]. For example, when a split-sample validation is followed, e.g., to convince physicians who are skeptical of modern developments, the final model should still be derived from the full sample. It would be a waste of precious information if the final model were only based on a random part of the sample [533]. Differences in regression coefficients will generally be small, since the split was at random, and the data have overlap, but the estimates of the full sample will be more stable. If a stepwise selection procedure was followed in the random part of the study, it should be repeated in the full study sample. This may result in a different model specification. Arguably, this is preferable to sticking to results from only part of the available data.

The same reasoning holds for cross-validation and bootstrap validation. Especially with bootstrap validation we may well illustrate the instability of stepwise selection procedures (see Chap. 11). The final model may only be selected in a few of the bootstrap samples [27, 563]. Such model uncertainty has to be taken into account in the optimism estimate for the final model.

If external validation has been performed, we may similarly define the final model from the combined data set (development plus validation). This was done in the Lynch syndrome case study (Table 17.3) [40]. The regression coefficients in the final model are a compromise between the estimates in the development and validation sample. This combination of data assumes that the two samples represent the same population, which is not necessarily the case (Chap. 20). If relevant differences are found, a setting-specific intercept, or setting-specific interaction terms for predictor effects, may be included (see Chaps. 20 and 21).

Questions

17.1. Stability of internal validation techniques (Table 17.1)

    (a) Split-sample validation is notoriously unstable. In contrast, apparent validation and bootstrap validation share stability in the estimation of model performance. Do you agree?

    (b) Cross-validation eventually uses 100% of the sample for validation; why might multi-fold cross-validation help?

17.2 Interpretation of external validation (Fig. 17.6)

Figure 17.6 can be interpreted in different ways. One perspective is to emphasize the similarity in performance between settings. Alternatively, we might focus on specific subset, which shows a systematic miscalibration. What would be your view on the performance of these subsets? Consider a fixed effect and random effect perspective (see also Chap. 20).

17.3 Problems with internal validation [67]

Interpret the published results on "internal validation" in Table 2 from an Ann Int Med paper (http://www.annals.org/cgi/reprint/143/4/265.pdf).

    (a) What do you think went wrong?

    (b) What do you think of the interpretation provided in the text?

    (c) What do you think about the "corrected Table 2", published as an erratum? http://www.annals.org/cgi/reprint/144/8/620.pdf.

Chapter 18
Presentation Formats

Background The presentation of a prediction model deserves careful attention. Epidemiologic regression analyses commonly concentrate on estimation of relative effects, with presentation of tables with odds ratios or hazard ratios, and their confidence intervals. Such tables are usually not sufficient to calculate absolute risks, which require a baseline risk. This is a model intercept for continuous or binary outcomes or a baseline hazard for survival outcomes. We need to separate presentations that generate predictions ("prediction models") from presentations that generate advice for a decision ("decision rules") . Various presentation formats are possible for such prediction models and for decision rules, some of which will be discussed in this chapter. We illustrate the creation of some formats at a technical level for the testicular cancer case study.

18.1   Prediction Models Versus Decision Rules

A clinical prediction model provides an estimate of absolute risk, based on the combination of several patient characteristics. For a good prediction model, the prediction for an individual patient can span a wide range, from relatively low to relatively high. The interpretation of the predictions and any actions is left to the treating physician and/or the patient. We can also present a decision rule, where a specific course of action is suggested depending on the combination of patient characteristics. Decision rules are hence not synonymous with prediction models [451]. Decision rules require more subject matter input, e.g., from clinical experts, especially on the choice of a cutoff point for predictions (see Chap. 16).

Some have argued that presentation as a decision rule leads more easily to a wide application of a model. Examples include decision rules for traumatic injuries to the ankle/foot, knee, cervical spine, and head ("Ottawa rules"). The developers of the rules suggest substantial impact, and conclude that emergency physicians should adopt these clinical decision rules to standardize care and reduce costs [437]. Decision rules may also be a natural extension of heuristic rules that humans tend to use [182].

© Springer Nature Switzerland AG 2019
E. W. Steyerberg, *Clinical Prediction Models*, Statistics for Biology and Health, https://doi.org/10.1007/978-3-030-16399-0_18

We discuss several options for presentation of prediction models and clinical decision rules (Table 18.1). Formats differ on aspects such as the medium by which they are presented (on paper or electronically), the level of detail in the predictions (rough indications of risk or exact probabilities), presence of indicators of

Table 18.1 Some examples of presentation formats for clinical prediction models and clinical decision rules

Rule	Characteristics	Pros	Cons	Example
Prediction models				
Regression formula	Simple, follows directly from analysis	Can be implemented in computerized format	Leaves work to the user; difficult to calculate confidence intervals	Predicted response dose, formula in abstract [265]
Spreadsheet	Includes exact calculations, exact 95% confidence intervals	Standard software, familiar to many	Needs user to open specific file	Survival after surgery for lung cancer [52]
Web application	Includes exact calculations, exact 95% confidence intervals	Easy to use from www	Storing previous cases may not be so easy	PREDICT (https://www.predict.nhs.uk/) to asses benefit of treatment for breast cancer [87]
Nomogram	Includes quite exact calculations, approximate 95% confidence intervals	Quite exact predictions	Difficult to understand at first sight	Prostate cancer recurrence [294]
Score chart	Includes approximate calculations, approximate 95% confidence intervals	Easy to understand	Approximate predictions	DRASTIC prediction rule for renal artery stenosis [314]
Table	Includes averaged calculations, approximate 95% confidence intervals can be added	Very easy to understand and use have to be categorized	Predictions by predictor combination; continuous predictors	Framingham risk equation to identify candidates of statin therapy [674]
Specific formats	Based on specific interest of audience	Should appeal specifically to target audience	Less easy to understand for nontarget audience	Relevance of pre- and postchemotherapy mass size in testicular cancer, for radiologists [553]

(continued)

Table 18.1 (continued)

Rule	Characteristics	Pros	Cons	Example
Decision rules				
Regression tree	Simple, large groups	Very easy to understand and use	Unstable if based on raw data	Goldman diagnostic index for acute MI [188]
Score chart rule	Score based on highly rounded coefficients	Rule simple to understand	Inaccurate predictions	CT rule for minor head injury [519]
Survival by group	Simple, large groups	Very easy to understand and use	Stable but cutoffs based on distribution of risk rather than decision-analytic considerations	IGCC classification for testicular cancer [4]
Meta-model tree	Simple, large groups	Easy to understand and use	Continuous predictors have to be categorized	Testicular cancer group with >70% benign tissue [552]

uncertainty (e.g., 95% confidence intervals around predictions), and user-friendliness (simple to complex formats).

> **Box 18.1 Regression Formula for Prediction of the Individual Follicle-Stimulating Hormone Threshold [265]**
>
> FSH response dose = 4 body mass index (in kg/m^2) + 32 clomiphene citrate resistance (yes = 1 or no = 0) + 7 initial free insulin-like growth factor-I (in ng/mL) + 6 initial serum FSH level (in IU/L) − 51.

18.2   Presenting Clinical Prediction Models

Clinical prediction models provide probabilities of diagnostic or prognostic outcomes. We discuss detailed presentations with a regression formula, a nomogram, or a score chart (Table 18.1).

18.2.1   Regression Formulas

Clinical prediction models can be presented in various formats. The simplest form is to present the final regression formula. An example is the regression formula presented in the abstract of a study in anovulatory infertile women (Box 18.1) [265].

Calculation of predictions with a regression formula incorporates two steps. The first step is to calculate the linear predictor. The linear predictor is central to regression models such as linear, logistic, polytomous, Cox, and many parametric survival models. In the linear predictor, we multiply regression coefficients with predictor values. Definitions and encoding of the predictors have to be clear to the user. For binary predictors, a 0/1 coding is convenient, which makes that patients without a characteristic have a score of zero. For categorical predictors, dummy variables are usually constructed. The reference category for these dummy variables can be based on frequency (e.g., the most common category is the reference), or on clinical considerations. For continuous variables, the units have to be clear. For example, units for concentrations are important (by weight, e.g., mg/dl, or molecular count, e.g., mmol/l). Also, continuous predictors are sometimes centered to the mean value, which should then be subtracted from the original value when using the regression formula. For interpretation of relative effects, scaling may be different from that in the prediction formula, e.g., with age per 10 years, or blood pressure per 10 mmHg. Continuous predictors are sometimes standardized by dividing by the standard deviation in the sample; this may seem attractive but hampers transportability to other settings.

The second step is to translate the linear predictor values to units on the outcome scale. For a logistic model, we use the logistic transformation to estimate probabilities of the outcome ($p(y = 1)$). For survival, we can estimate survival probabilities, e.g., at 1, 2, or 5 years, median survival, or other quantiles of survival. With a Cox model, we need the baseline hazard function to estimate these survival probabilities $S(t)$: $S(t) = h_0(t) * \exp(\text{linear predictor})$, where $h_0(t)$ indicates the baseline hazard function for time t. Some parametric survival models have one or two constants to define baseline risk similar to other regression models. Predictions from such parametric models are straightforward to calculate and are more stable at the end of follow-up (Chap. 4).

Shrinkage can be incorporated in the translation from linear predictor to predictions. One way is to standardize predictor values, such that the average of the linear predictor is zero [627]. We can then multiply the linear predictor with the shrinkage factor. The average of the predictions will then remain reasonably correct. However, a systematic error will arise when the range of predictions is wide, or the shrinkage severe, because of the nonlinearity in the translation from linear predictor to prediction. As an alternative, we can shrink regression coefficients and re-estimate the intercept for proper calibration-in-the-large.

Regression formulas can serve as the basis for computerized implementation, in mobile phones, hospital information systems or electronic patient records, web pages, or spreadsheets (see www.nomograms.org). One example is a spreadsheet to show survival after surgery for lung cancer, where a model is presented including seven predictors. The predicted survival curve was calculated according to the individual predictor values, with an approximate 95% confidence interval [52].

Web-based calculators become more and more common. From R, Shiny applications can be set up for WWW presentation. Specific websites are available for detailed calculation of predictions, some with the option to estimate the impact of treatment. For example, the PREDICT tool shows how breast cancer treatments after surgery might improve survival rates (www.predict.nhs.uk). Once details about the patient and their cancer have been entered, the tool shows how different treatments would be expected to improve survival rates up to 15 years after diagnosis. These individualized estimates of benefit of treatment rely on available data on prognostic effects and on the effectiveness of treatment. The optimal combination of prognosis and treatment effect is a vivid area of research [300, 333, 630].

18.2.2 Confidence Intervals for Predictions

Uncertainty around predictions for linear regression models can be presented with *confidence* intervals and *prediction* intervals. Confidence intervals indicate the uncertainty around the average and become very small with very large sample size. For example, a growth curve predicting length by age will have a very tight confidence interval when based on millions of adolescents. Prediction intervals for individual subjects will however remain of substantial size because of the variability in the population.

For predicted probabilities, the fact that a probability is estimated reflects the inherent uncertainty of the prediction process. Confidence intervals around predicted probabilities can become quite small with large sample size, but the prediction for an individual remains a probability. With regression analysis, predictions can approach, but never reach, 0 or 1.

Uncertainty in survival can be indicated around probabilities at time points in follow-up. We can also indicate uncertainty around survival duration, e.g., median survival surrounded by 2.5, 25, 75, and 97.5% quantiles. The latter quantiles will cover a substantial width, even with infinite sample size, similar to the prediction intervals in linear regression.

Confidence intervals are only a valid indication of the uncertainty of the prediction model if there is no systematic bias in the predictions. The total uncertainty in a prediction is the sum of systematic and random errors. Miscalibration of predictions is an example of a systematic error, which may be due to various differences between the development setting and the setting where the model is applied, e.g., coding of predictors, missed predictors with different distributions, and truly differential effects (Chaps. 17 and 19). Hence, we must be cautious in the interpretation of predictions when the confidence interval is small because of a large sample size. On the other hand, a model derived from a small data set will show large confidence intervals, which is a useful warning against overinterpretation of predictions.

Meta-analyses commonly quantify variability between studies in random effect analyses. Inclusion of the between-study heterogeneity leads to wider confidence intervals for a treatment effect than a fixed effect estimate that ignores such between-study heterogeneity [246]. Similar to treatment effects, we may include between-study heterogeneity in prediction intervals for predictions for individuals.

Furthermore, one might argue that the values of the predictions remain of primary interest for decision-making, and uncertainty is less relevant [295]. If we cannot make a better estimate than the one provided by the model, following that estimate is the best we can do, even when the estimate is uncertain.

Technically, confidence intervals are calculated with the standard error (SE) of a prediction. The standard error is calculated from the covariance matrix of the regression model. If shrinkage was applied, it may be reasonable to still use the covariance matrix of the original, unshrunken, model. With a penalized model, we can use the covariance matrix of the penalized model, which will result in slightly smaller standard errors of predictions than the original model.

Every combination of predictor values leads to a different standard error of the prediction. The same linear predictor value can have a different standard error, since different combinations of predictor values may lead to the same sum. This is handled easily in a regression formula, in a spreadsheet, or web-based calculation, but more complicated in paper-based presentation formats such as nomograms and score charts. In the latter formats, using the mean or median standard error can be considered to indicate uncertainty for a given linear predictor value [225].

If we want to communicate uncertainty, we might try to estimate the effective number of patients similar to the patient where the prediction is made. This assessment can be based on a comparison of SEs: the SE for an individualized prediction will be larger than the SE for a prediction for the full sample. This ratio is more unfavorable with more extreme covariate patterns, where uncertainty for a prediction is large.

18.2.3   Nomograms

Nomograms are graphical presentations of a prediction model. Nomograms have a long history in the pre-computer era, with a more recent role as presentation format of a clinical prediction model [353]. Again, two steps are discerned. The calculation of the linear predictor is essentially as for a regression formula: each predictor value corresponds to a regression weight. The nomogram has a reference line for reading scoring points (e.g., 0–100 or 0–10, Fig. 18.1). The user manually totals the points and the total corresponds linearly to the linear predictor. The second step is the transformation of the linear predictor to predictions, which can be read at the bottom of the nomogram. Predictions can be in the form of a probability, median survival, or other quantities. Harrell's nomogram function is a valuable tool to develop these presentations [225].

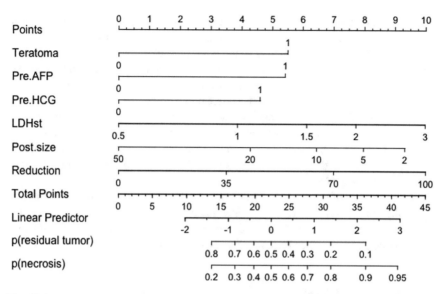

Fig. 18.1 Nomogram for prediction of the nature of residual histology based on six predictors in a penalized logistic regression model. Teratoma: absence of teratoma elements in the primary tumor; Pre.AFP: prechemotherapy AFP normal; Pre.HCG: prechemotherapy HCG normal; LDHst: standardized prechemotherapy LDH (LDH divided by upper limit of normal values; one means values equal to upper normal); Post.size: postchemotherapy mass size in mm. Reduction: % Reduction in size during chemotherapy, e.g., 50–10 mm = 80%

Box 18.2 Instruction to physicians using the model in their care:

Determine the patient's value for each predictor, and draw a straight line upward to the points axis to determine how many points toward benign histology the patient receives. Sum the points received for each predictor and locate this sum on the total points axis. Draw a straight line down to find the patient's predicted probability of residual tumor or necrosis (benign histology).

Box 18.3 Instruction to patient:

"Mr. X, if we had 100 men exactly like you, we would expect that the chemotherapy was fully successful in approximately <predicted probability from nomogram * 100>, as reflected in fully benign disease at surgical resection of your abdominal lymph nodes." (Text based on Kattan et al. [295]; note that the number 100 may be debated, since the effective sample size for some covariate patterns may be far less.)

Nomograms have especially been promoted for urological tumors, such as prostate cancer [97, 467]. Advantages are several. The relative importance of the predictors can be judged by the length of the lines with nomogram scores, provided that the predictor values on the lines are based on the distribution of the predictor in the data under study. Hence, the reader obtains a visual impression of the relevance of a predictor in the model, relative to the other predictors. Furthermore, interaction terms can be handled. Separate lines are constructed usually, such that only one axis has to be read to obtain a score corresponding to a predictor value. Complex models, e.g., survival models with time-dependent covariates can also be presented as nomograms [296]. The translation of the total points to the probability or survival scale is relatively easy. Scales can be extended with approximate confidence intervals (e.g., with the median standard error per tenth of predicted risk), or additional scales for the outcome, e.g., 25 and 75 survival percentiles [225]. Color versions are also possible [596].

Disadvantages of nomogram presentations include the relative complexity at first sight, the inaccuracy of readings when many predictors are included, and the inaccuracy of translation to the final outcome. It is not clear yet whether clinicians prefer nomograms to other formats such as score charts.

18.2.4   Score Chart

Score charts are another simple presentation format for clinical prediction models. The first step is to round regression coefficients to scores. A simple approach is to multiply coefficients by 10 and round them. However, we can often find lower numbers for multiplication that still allow for a sufficiently refined prediction. Some analysts define scores by dividing through the smallest coefficient of a binary predictor, which then has by definition a score of 1. The other predictors get rounded scores. This procedure is suboptimal, since it capitalizes on the estimate of one coefficient. This leads to unnecessary extra uncertainty in the rounded coefficients. It is preferable to search for a common denominator across all coefficients. A score chart for the testicular cancer model is shown in Table 18.2, with corresponding probabilities in Fig. 18.2.

18.2.5   Tables with Predictions

Predictions can sometimes be presented in table format, but this may require some simplifications of the model. Especially, we need to categorize continuous predictors, which implies a loss of information (see for an example from the Framingham Heart Study [674]. Also, the adult treatment panel III (ATP III) presents a number of tools for detailed calculations on the web (http://www.cvriskcalculator.com/). An interactive risk assessment tool is presented to estimate 10-year risk for "hard" coronary heart disease outcomes (myocardial infarction and coronary death), and calculators are downloadable for local use.

Table 18.2 Score chart for estimation of the probability of benign tissue after chemotherapy for metastatic testicular cancer with continuous predictors

Characteristic	Scores						Sum score
Primary tumor							
No teratoma elements	1						
Prechemotherapy tumor markers							
AFP normal	1						
HCG normal	1						
LDH times normal							
Values	0.6	1	1.6	2.5	4	6	
Scores[a]	−0.5	0	0.5	1	1.5	2	
Postchemotherapy size (mm)							
Values	<5	10	20	40	70		
Scores[a]	+0.5	0	−0.5	−1	−1.5		
Reduction in size							
Values	Increase	0%	50%	100%			
Scores[a]	−1	0	1	2			
Total score (add all)							...
Probability of benign tissue and 95% CI from Fig. 18.2							... % [...% - ...%]

[a]Intermediate scores can be estimated with linear interpolation

Fig. 18.2 Probability of necrosis (benign tissue) in relation to the sum score from Table 18.2. Number of patients with each score are indicated at the bottom, and reflected in the size of the dots. 95% confidence intervals are shown around the predicted probabilities

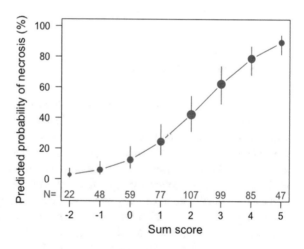

A simple table has been successful in providing indications for statin treatment. This table defines absolute 10-year risks of cardiovascular events by smoking status, hypertension, diabetes, cholesterol to HDL-cholesterol ratio, and sex. Moreover, colors were added corresponding to treatment advice: treat with a statin, do not treat with a statin, or treat in the presence of a family history of cardiovascular disease [195].

Table 18.3 Probability of benign tissue in relation to the sum of five favorable characteristics and mass size for the testicular cancer case study. P(Nec): Probability of necrosis

	Sum of favorable characteristics*					
Residual mass size	0	1	2	3	4	5
0 – 9 mm			p>60%	p>70%	p>80%	Follow-up
10 – 19 mm	Resection					P(Nec) > 90%
20 – 29 mm				p>60%		
30 – 49 mm					p>70%	p>80%
>= 50 mm, or increased mass	P(Nec) <= 60%					

[a]Sum of five characteristics: Primary tumor teratoma negative; prechemotherapy AFP normal; prechemotherapy HCG normal; prechemotherapy LDH elevated; and reduction in mass size $\geq 70\%$

A tabular presentation was considered as a simple way to present the testicular cancer model [550]. The advantage is that decisions can easily be coupled to the predictions. In this case, a clear treatment advice was linked to predictions over 90% (follow-up) and prediction below 60% (resection, Table 18.3). In between is a gray area, where treatment decision-making is not straightforward and may depend on various factors, such as feasibility of close follow-up, experience of surgeon, and the technical difficulty of the surgery. All patients with a large (≥ 50 mm) or increased mass should undergo resection, as well as all with less than two favorable characteristics. This tabular format however implies a severe loss of overall discriminative ability (c decreases from 0.839 to 0.773).

18.2.6   Specific Formats

Specific formats may appeal to certain audiences. For example, radiologists are important in the monitoring of treatment of cancer. They usually compare images obtained during or after treatment with images made before treatment. Hence, a presentation of prediction model might focus on the information in such images. This was attempted for the relevance of pre- and postchemotherapy mass size in the testicular cancer prediction example (Fig. 18.3) [553]. We created iso-probability curves for combinations of pre- and postchemotherapy mass size, based on the underlying logistic regression function. The graph shows that the postchemotherapy size was more relevant than the prechemotherapy size; probabilities increase sharply with smaller postchemotherapy size. This is caused by a direct effect of postchemotherapy size, in combination with a strong effect of reduction in size (larger reductions with smaller postchemotherapy sizes).

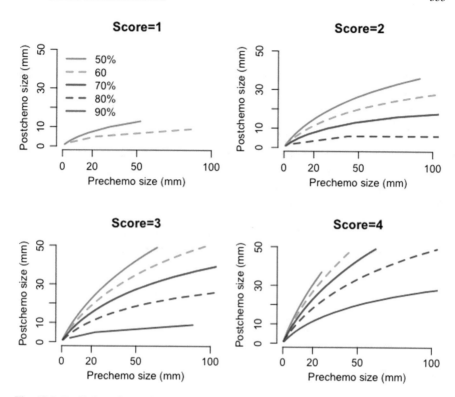

Fig. 18.3 Predictions for benign histology based on prechemotherapy and postchemotherapy mass size, and by score of four prognostic characteristics (no teratoma elements in primary tumor, normal AFP, normal HCG, or elevated LDH). Lines indicate probabilities of 50–90 of benign tissue. Patients with a score of zero always had predicted probabilities below 50%. For example, a postchemotherapy size of 20 mm after a prechemotherapy size of 100 mm results in a probability around 90% when the score is 4, but a probability around 65% when the score is 2

18.2.7   Black-Box Presentations

Machine learning (ML) models will increasingly be used to develop prediction models. Some methods, such as the LASSO or elastic net, are extensions of traditional regression methods. Models developed with these methods can transparently be presented. Availability of a formula is important to allow for validation and updation of models by other researchers.

Model availability is also important for models developed with artificial intelligence (AI) methods, such as neural nets and black-box algorithms such as deep learning. These may not be presented explicitly in a formula. In the field of ML and AI, the need to transparency typically focuses on interpretability of the algorithm [444]. The more important issue to allow for external validation studies by independent researchers. Apart from potential overfitting due to small sample size or very flexible modeling, predictive performance, and especially calibration, is expected to vary across time and place [504]. In addition, performance tends to vary depending on characteristics of measurement tools, such as biomarker assay kits or imaging machines [181]. Also, electronic health record (EHR) data handling depends on location. As a result, there is no guarantee that any predictive algorithm will work as advertised, even when the development study included an external validation or when the algorithm received regulatory approval [444, 504].

For validation, we need to have access to the algorithm to generate predictions. Proprietary issues may make this difficult. For updating, an option is to do reverse engineering, with model predictions generated by an algorithm for a wide combination of predictor values. A regression model can then be fitted on these predictions as a meta-model, with fine-tuning to a specific setting (Chaps. 20 and 21). Alternative approaches are possible, also for methods such as support vector machines (SVM) [597]. These approaches include the interval coded scoring (ICS) system, which imposes that the effect of each variable on the estimated risk is constant within consecutive intervals [598]. Such an approach makes that complex models can still be used in clinical encounters.

18.3   Case Study: Clinical Prediction Model for Testicular Cancer Model

18.3.1   Regression Formula from Logistic Model

In the testicular cancer case study, we concentrate on prediction of a benign histology ("necrosis") after chemotherapy for metastatic disease; the complement of prediction of residual tumor. A logistic regression model with five or six predictors was fitted. Bootstrapping suggests a uniform shrinkage factor of s of approximately 0.95. Further, a penalty factor of four was used in a penalized maximum likelihood procedure (Table 18.4).

The formula with shrunk coefficients is

$$lp_{shrunk} = -0.95 + 0.83 * Teratoma + 0.82 * Pre.AFP + 0.71 * Pre.HCG + 0.89 * \ln(LDHst)$$
$$-0.26 * sqrt(Post.size) + 0.014 * Reduction,$$

where Teratoma = 1 if teratoma elements were present in the primary tumor, 0 otherwise; Pre.AFP = 1 if prechemotherapy AFP was elevated, 0 if normal; Pre. HCG = 1 if prechemotherapy HCG was elevated, 0 if normal; ln(LDHst) refers to the natural logarithm of the prechemotherapy LDH value, standardized to the upper limit of local normal limits; sqrt(Post.size) refers to the square root of the postchemotherapy size in mm; Reduction refers to the reduction is size during chemotherapy in %.

Table 18.4 Regression coefficients in logistic regression models for postchemotherapy histology in testicular cancer, with uniform shrinkage ($s = 0.95$), penalized ML estimation (penalty factor $l = 4$), and the scores for a score chart (multiplication by 10 or 10/8 to achieve simpler scores)

Predictor	$Coef_{orig}$	$Coef_{shrunk}$	$Coef_{pen}$	$10* Coef_{pen}$	$10/8* coef$
Teratoma	0.909	0.825	0.873	9	1
Pre.AFP	0.903	0.819	0.860	9	1
Pre.HCG	0.783	0.710	0.729	7	1
Log(LDHst)	0.985	0.894	0.884	9	1
Sqrt(Post.size)	−0.292	−0.264	−0.261	−3	0
Reduction (%)	0.016	0.014	0.016	0	0

The formula with penalized coefficients is

$$lp_{penalized} = -1.09 + 0.87 * Teratoma + 0.86 * Pre.AFP + 0.73 * Pre.HCG + 0.88 * \ln(LDHst)$$
$$-0.26 * sqrt(Post.size) + 0.016 * Reduction.$$

The formula to calculate predicted probabilities is simply:

$$P = 1/\left(1 + e^{(-lp)}\right).$$

If we want to calculate confidence intervals, we need the covariance matrix, which looks like

```
            Intercept Teratoma  Pre.AFP   Pre.HCG    LDHst Post.size Reduction
Intercept      0.3700 -3.1e-02 -3.0e-02 -1.4e-02  0.04200  -0.04300  -2.7e-03
Teratoma      -0.0310  4.6e-02  5.7e-03 -2.4e-03 -0.00150   0.00100   5.6e-05
Pre.AFP       -0.0300  5.7e-03  5.4e-02 -9.2e-03  0.00320   0.00130   8.6e-05
Pre.HCG       -0.0140 -2.4e-03 -9.2e-03  5.3e-02  0.01100  -0.00160   8.0e-06
LDHst          0.0420 -1.5e-03  3.2e-03  1.1e-02  0.04400  -0.00970  -4.1e-04
Post.size     -0.0430  1.0e-03  1.3e-03 -1.6e-03 -0.00970   0.00660   3.1e-04
Reduction     -0.0027  5.6e-05  8.6e-05  8.0e-06 -0.00041   0.00031   2.7e-05
```

The square root of the diagonal indicates the variance of the regression coefficients. The off-diagonal numbers are used for calculation of the variance of specific combinations of predictor values: $SE_{prediction}$ = transpose(X) * covariance matrix * X. A detailed example is provided for the EuroSCORE, which predicts cardiac operative risks [375]. The predictions for the testicular cancer histology are presented with 95% confidence in an Excel spreadsheet, which is available at www.clinicalpredictionmodels.org.

18.3.2 Nomogram

A nomogram can easily be constructed with Harrell's rms library:

```
# Make a penalized model
full <- lrm(Necrosis ~
      Teratoma+Pre.AFP+Pre.HCG+log(LDHst)+sqrt(Post.size)+Reduction,
      data=n544,...) # 5-predictor model
p       <- pentrace(full, c(0,1,2,3,4,5,6,7,8,10,12,14,20))
full.pen <- update(full, penalty=p$penalty) # Optimal penalty factor 4
# Make nomogram from penalized model
nom <- nomogram(full.pen,  fun=c(function(x)(1-plogis(x)), plogis),
      lp=T,lp.at=c(-2,0,2,4),
      LDHst=c(.5,1,1.5,2,3,4), Post.size=c(50,20,10,5,2),
      Reduction=c(0,35,70,100),
      fun.at=c(seq(.1,.9,by=.1),0.95),
      funlabel=c("p(residual tumor)", "p(necrosis)"),  vnames="lab",
      maxscale=10)
plot(nom)
```

We used a maximum of 10 points in Fig. 18.1, accepting some loss in accuracy in summing the points corresponding to each predictor value. The total points correspond linearly to the linear predictor, which correspond to p(residual tumor) and to p(necrosis) (or benign histology) through the logistic transformation (plogis).

18.3.3   *Score Chart

A score chart for the testicular cancer prediction model was shown in Table 18.2. We considered the following steps with some technical details:

(1) Multiply and round regression coefficients of binary predictors and dummy variables of categorical predictors.
(2) Search for score for continuous predictors, continuous or categorized.
(3) Estimate the multiplication factor for the scores.
(4) Estimate the intercept corresponding to the scores; check the deterioration in discriminative performance; present as score chart.

These steps are explained with R code at www.clinicalpredictionmodels.org.

For point (4), we note that the discriminative ability would deteriorate substantially if we would categorize the continuous predictors. A drop in c statistic from 0.839 to 0.808 (Table 18.5). The tabular presentation in Table 18.3 leads to an even larger drop (to 0.77). Hence, categorization made for a simplified presentation at the cost of performance, while rounding had limited effect.

Table 18.5 Discriminatory ability of different formats of presentation the testicular cancer prediction model

Format	Table/Figure	C statistic
Logistic formula/nomogram/graphical	Table 18.4/Fig. 18.1/Fig. 18.3	0.839
Rounded scores	Table 18.2/Fig. 18.2	0.838
Categorized scores	Tables at website	0.808
Tabular	Table 18.3	0.773

18.3.4   Summary Points

- Many presentation formats are possible, as illustrated for the testicular cancer model that predicts the presence of tumor versus benign tissue after chemotherapy.
- User-friendliness may vary, and empirical evidence on what formats clinicians prefer is limited.
- The discriminative ability may suffer from overly simple presentations.
- Web-based presentations and apps become increasingly popular.
- Predictive algorithms in medicine should be free and easily available to allow independent validation and updating for different settings, irrespective of their development by traditional regression, machine learning, or artificial intelligence methods.

18.4   Presenting Clinical Decision Rules

18.4.1   Regression Tree

Some modeling techniques, such as regression and classification trees, more naturally lead to decision rules. A regression tree classifies patients according to a (usually limited) number of characteristics (Chap. 4). It is therefore often possible for clinical experts to link treatment recommendations to the various groups defined by the tree. Once these treatments have been defined, the tree can often be reformatted for easier application. This was done for the Goldman diagnostic index for acute MI. Based on a tree analysis of 482 patients suspected of acute MI, a decision protocol was constructed in the format of a simple flowchart considering nine clinical factors [188]. Tree presentations are generally considered to be easy to understand. However, as discussed before, deriving a stable, reliable tree requires large amounts of data: trees are very data-hungry and may often have suboptimal performance; their use for prediction modeling should be discouraged [20, 23, 612, 613].

18.4.2   Score Chart Rule

Scores can be based on severely rounded coefficients, e.g., counting each predictor as one point. This may be reasonable when the actual regression coefficients are similar in magnitude. When coefficients vary in magnitude, an alternative is to define minor and major risk factors [519]. Such major rounding of coefficients leads to less accurate predictions than the original rule. Especially, calibration may suffer [376]. The advantage of severe rounding is that it is possible to remember such decision rules by heart, in contrast to more refined prediction models [36].

A simple rule can be defined as that exceeding a certain score is an indication for a certain action. An example is the difficult issue of which patients should have a CT scan after minor head injury (defined as having sustained blunt injury to the head, with normal or minimally altered level of consciousness upon presentation, i.e., a Glasgow Coma Scale score of 13–15). In one recent study, a detailed prediction model was developed, from which a simple decision rule was derived. Major and minor risk factors were defined based on rounding of the regression coefficients from a logistic model, and categorization of continuous predictors (such as age: <40: zero score; 40–59: minor; ≥ 60: major). The decision rule was CT scan in case of presence of at least one major or two minor risk factors (out of a list of ten major and eight minor risk factors) [519]. With this rule, the sensitivity was 100% for neurosurgical interventions (at apparent validation). This high sensitivity was important, since patients requiring neurosurgical interventions should not be missed. Internal validation by bootstrapping showed however that we should not expect 100% sensitivity in new patients. The average sensitivity from a bootstrap validation procedure was 96%, with 100% sensitivity in 56% of the bootstrap samples. On the other hand, many CT scans would still be made in those without an important outcome (specificity only 25%, or a false-positive CT scan rate of 75%). Implementation of the decision rule was expected to reduce the number of CTs by approximately 25%. Hence, most patients with minor head injury should have a CT scan if we want to exclude serious injury.

18.4.3   Survival Groups

Results from survival analyses are often presented by grouped predictions, e.g., quarters. Such grouping can be linked to treatment recommendations. Survival can also be shown in relation to specific combinations of risk factors, similar to a regression tree. This approach was followed for the IGCC classification [4]. Five predictors were considered: two were coded as dichotomous predictors (poor versus good), and three tumor markers were coded as low, intermediate, and high according to their level. A good prognosis group contained patients without intermediate or poor risk characteristics. An intermediate group contained patients with intermediate levels of tumor markers, but no poor risk characteristics. A poor prognosis group contained patients with at least one high tumor marker or a poor risk factor. The numbers of patients were approximately 50%, 35%, and 15%, with 5-year survival of 92%, 80%, and 50%, respectively. The choice of risk group definitions was motivated by the idea to study more aggressive new therapy in the poor risk group (e.g., stem cell therapy), and less aggressive therapy in the good prognosis group (e.g., three instead of four cycles of chemotherapy) [125].

Such risk classifications present predictions for groups of patients, which is expected to lead to stable predictions at a group level. Note that the definition of the risk groups is often motivated by the distribution of risk rather than by decision-analytic considerations [615].

18.4.4 Meta-Model

Another option is to develop a meta-model, which describes an underlying, more complex model with a certain level of accuracy. A meta-model is a model that predicts the predictions from an underlying model. It aims to capture the general patterns and inherits any shrinkage of coefficients from the underlying more complex model [227]. For a decision rule, we may categorize the predictions from the underlying model at a relevant cutoff, e.g., as needing treatment versus no treatment. Subsequently, we can predict membership of either category. The meta-model can be presented in various forms, for example, as a tree. A tree may be an attractive format for this step because of its intuitive communication, although we risk some refinement in risk predictions (see, e.g., Fig. 18.4 [552]).

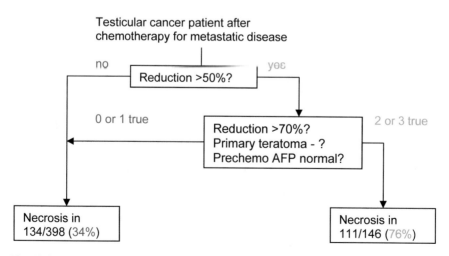

Fig. 18.4 Decision rule for patients with testicular cancer [552]. Resection is advised if necrosis (benign histology) is unlikely (34% vs. 76%)

18.5   Concluding Remarks

The presentation format is an important issue in prediction modeling. The overview in this chapter intends to give inspiration for presentation of prediction models and decision rules. The format should match with the intended audience; some clinical areas have a more quantitative orientation than others. Also, some formats have become more or less standard in certain areas, for example, nomograms for prostate cancer, and survival curves by quarter in oncology in general [97]. Graphical presentations may sometimes be considered, e.g., to show predictions in relation to a single continuous predictor and one or two categorical predictors. There is no convincing evidence on the preference of certain presentation formats over others for optimal communication of individualized predictions [580].

We can imagine that the ongoing automatization, e.g., with electronic patient records, will enable the direct and easy availability of predictions from detailed and rather complex prediction models. Hence, computerized presentations have the future, both for prediction models and decision rules. Especially attractive is the combination of prognostic evidence as summarized in a prediction model with evidence on the relative effect of a treatment as found in a randomized controlled trial or summarized in a meta-analysis [300, 630]. A positive example is the PREDICT model [87]. A serious point of attention is the transparency of machine learning and AI models, where proprietary interests may conflict with openness, and hence obstruct assessment of generalizability (part III).

Questions

18.1. Testicular cancer presentation formats

Calculate predicted probabilities for a man with a postchemotherapy mass of 12 mm, which was 24 mm before chemotherapy, who had no teratoma elements in his primary tumor, elevated AFP, normal HCG, and three times normal LDH levels, using

(a) the nomogram (Fig. 18.1),
(b) the score chart (Table 18.2 with Fig. 18.2),
(c) the simplified table (Table 18.3),
(d) the graphs for radiologists (Fig. 18.3),
(e) the penalized regression formula (Sect. 18.3.1), and
(f) the classification tree (Fig. 18.4).

18.2. Continuous predictors in a score chart (Sect. 18.3.3)

(a) What specific challenges are posed by continuous predictors in a score chart?
(b) What is the disadvantage of categorizing scores for a score chart (see Table 18.5)?

18.3. Odds ratios or regression coefficients for scores [388]

Several investigators have used odds ratios to derive scores for logistic regression models, which are added in a sum score.

(a) Why is this incorrect?
(b) What kind of deviations will occur if some odds ratios are small and some very large?

18.4. Prediction models and decision rules

(a) What is the difference between a prediction model and a decision rule?
(b) How can we derive a decision rule from a prediction model?

Part III
Generalizability of Prediction Models

Generalizability refers to the external validity of predictions from a model. The quality of predictions can be quantified by various performance measures, e.g., related to calibration, discrimination, and clinical usefulness. These measures reflect the validity of regression coefficients and the specific case-mix of the external setting.

For generalizability, internal validity is a minimum prerequisite. To achieve internal validity, we need to follow the seven steps outlined in Part II. In Part III, we first consider differences between populations that may affect generalizability (Chap. 19). Next, we consider approaches to updating of a prediction model for a specific setting (Chap. 20). Finally, we consider the situation that a prediction model is applied in multiple settings. Detection of differences between settings may then actually be the purpose of the analysis, for example, the comparison of quality of care providers, such as hospitals, in a league table ("provider profiling", Chap. 21).

Chapter 19
Patterns of External Validity

Background Generalizability depends on the quality of the prediction model as developed for the development setting (internal validity), and on characteristics of the population where the model is applied (validity of regression coefficients, and distribution of predictor values). The general framework of the validity of predictions was discussed in Chap. 17 (see in particular Fig. 17.1). Here, we first consider a number of typical situations that we may encounter when a prediction model is applied externally. Theoretical relations are illustrated with a large sample simulation and findings in some case studies. Approximate power calculations are given for tests of invalidity of a prediction model.

19.1 Determinants of External Validity

We concentrate on the external validity of predictions for a binary outcome y. We consider a number of differences between populations that determine this external validity, related to case-mix and regression coefficients β (Table 19.1).

19.1.1 Case-Mix

With case-mix, we refer to the distribution of predictors X that are included in the regression model $y \sim X$, as well as the distribution of predictors that are not included in the model, either observable or unobservable. Predictors not included in the model are referred to as "missed predictors" ("Z"), despite the fact that some may, in fact, be observable. Since the linear predictor (lp) is a linear function of the

© Springer Nature Switzerland AG 2019
E. W. Steyerberg, *Clinical Prediction Models*, Statistics for Biology and Health, https://doi.org/10.1007/978-3-030-16399-0_19

Table 19.1 Potential differences between populations that determine external validity

Scenario	Characteristic	Differences	Example
Case-mix	Distribution of observed predictors X	Different selection, e.g., more severe patients are selected; or inclusion criteria smaller/wider	Validation in the referral center; validation in/outside RCT
	Distribution of missed predictors Z	Different selection based on predictors not considered in the model	Validation in different settings
	Distribution of outcome y	Retrospective sampling of cases and controls	Case–control design
Coefficients	Coefficients β smaller than expected	Overfitted model is validated	Validation of model from small development sample
	Coefficients β different	Truly different population	Validation in different settings

predictors X, we will for simplicity consider one predictor x in the model $y \sim x$. Here, x represents a linear combination of X. Similarly, the missed predictors Z are represented as one variable z in the regression model $Y \sim x + z$.

19.1.2 Differences in Case-Mix

A different case-mix may be encountered because the setting differs compared to the development situation; e.g., model development in secondary care, and validation in a primary or tertiary care setting. Or a model was developed in patients participating in a randomized controlled trial (RCT) and is applied in a less selected population. Such situations make that the distribution of observed predictors X is different between development and validation setting. The distribution of missed predictors Z may also differ when we apply a model in a different setting; per definition, such differences cannot be excluded a priori. Missed predictors Z may be fully independent of X, or be correlated. Finally, the design of a study may cause differences in the incidence of the outcome y, and may hence influence the case-mix. For example, a case–control design can be followed, where the ratio of cases to controls is different than in the underlying population.

19.1.3 Differences in Regression Coefficients

Regression coefficients β can be different between settings because of true differences between populations. Various reasons can be thought of, including definitions of predictors, the definition of the outcome, and a different selection of patients.

In practice, the coefficients β are not known for the development setting, but only estimated from a finite sample size. The same holds for a validation sample from a validation setting. This makes that it is virtually impossible that exactly the same regression coefficients are found when a regression model is re-estimated in a validation sample. Even if the underlying coefficients are identical, some of the re-estimated coefficients will be larger and some smaller than in the development sample due to sampling error.

Another problem is that regression coefficients may on average have been overestimated because of overfitting in the development data set. Such overfitting is most likely for models developed in small data sets with a relatively large number of (candidate) predictors (see, e.g., Chaps. 5, 11 and 13). Specifically, if models have been developed with stepwise selection methods, or variants, we must fear that the regression coefficients were estimated too extremely [94, 267, 541, 563]. Shrinkage or penalization of coefficients at model development may limit the risk of overestimation of coefficients for predictive purposes (Chap. 13). Shrinkage or penalization methods, however, have not been applied for many currently available prediction models.

19.2 Impact on Calibration, Discrimination, and Clinical Usefulness

In the following, we will consider various scenarios for differences between populations (Table 19.1). We will study the impact of these differences on calibration, discrimination, and clinical usefulness of prediction models for binary outcomes. We simulate an outcome y which depends on x and a missed predictor z (both with standard Normal distribution). In the development population, we estimate a logistic regression model with an intercept β_0 and coefficient β_1 for x, while in fact the outcome y is determined by x and z. The missed predictor z and x are uncorrelated, weakly correlated, or moderately correlated (Pearson correlation coefficients r 0, 0.33, 0.5, Table 19.2 and Fig. 19.1).

19.2.1 Simulation Setup

We create a validation population to apply a previously developed model. Various differences are simulated for the validation population compared to the development population. We first consider populations ($n = 500,000$) and later samples of smaller size to illustrate sampling variability and statistical power. We consider a scenario inspired by the testicular cancer case study, with an average prevalence of residual tumor tissue close to 50%, and a decision threshold for the probability of residual tumor of 30% (Chaps. 15 and 16). We consider a good discriminating model, with c statistic of 0.81. This c statistic is achieved with a logistic regression

Table 19.2 Design of simulations with predictor x and missed predictor z, for a logistic regression model $y \sim x + z$ ("adjusted analysis") and $y \sim x$ ("unadjusted analysis")

Correlation $x - z$	Adjusted coefficients	Unadjusted coefficient
Pearson $r = 0$, $R^2 = 0\%$	$2.1 * x + 1.5 * z$	$1.5 * x$
Pearson $r = 0.33$, $R^2 = 11\%$	$1.5 * x + 1.5 * z$	$1.5 * x$
Pearson $r = 0.5$, $R^2 = 25\%$	$1.2 * x + 1.5 * z$	$1.5 * x$

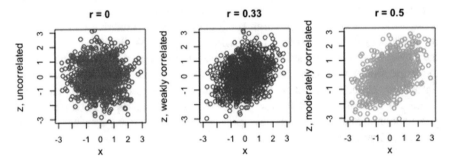

Fig. 19.1 Correlation between x (represented in the linear predictor) and z (a missed predictor), with no to moderate correlation. Illustration above with $n = 1000$; $n = 500,000$ in further simulations

model with a single predictor x, with x normally distributed and regression coefficient β 1.5. We can hence define the linear predictor as $lp = 1.5 * x$.

We generate the outcome y with the inclusion of the missed predictor z (uncorrelated or correlated). In the underlying model, the lp is a function of x and z. With uncorrelated $x - z$, we define the lp as $lp = 2.1 * x + 1.5 * z$. The adjusted regression coefficient for x is 2.1 rather than 1.5. This may be surprising. It is related to the "stratification" or "conditioning" effect in nonlinear models such as logistic regression and Cox regression models, or "non-collapsibility of odds ratios" [210]. In nonlinear models, adjusted effects are more extreme than unadjusted effects when a covariate is considered that is related to the outcome, but uncorrelated to other covariates. This is well known in the analysis of randomized clinical trials (see Chaps. 2 and 22) [174, 233, 463, 537]. In unadjusted analysis, the coefficient for x is 1.5 (Table 19.2).

For moderately correlated $x - z$ data ($r = 0.5$, Fig. 19.1), we define the lp as $lp = 1.2 * x + 1.5 * z$. Now the adjusted regression coefficient β is 1.2 rather than 1.5, which is caused by the positive correlation between x and z. This is classical confounding: the confounding effect of this correlation was stronger than the stratification effect. The adjusted coefficient is smaller than the unadjusted coefficient (1.2 vs. 1.5, Table 19.2). An intermediate situation was identified by trial and error, where the correlation between x and z was 0.33, such that the negative effect of confounding and positive effect of stratification on z are exactly balanced in the adjusted analysis. The true model was $lp = 1.5 * x + 1.5 * z$.

In both development and validation settings, we study predictions only in relation to x, since z is a missed predictor. The observed relation is $lp = 1.5 * x$ at development, with a c statistic of 0.81. At validation, we hope to see $y = 0 + 1 * lp$ in a logistic regression model (see Chap. 15 and 21 for more background on this "recalibration model") [114]. The relation between y and lp may be influenced by changes in the distribution of the x, z, or y, or differences in the regression coefficients that determine the lp (see Table 19.1).

19.2.2 Performance Measures

We concentrate on a limited number of indicators of calibration, discrimination, and clinical usefulness, although many more performance measures can be considered for validation of predictions for binary outcomes (see Chaps. 15 and 16). For calibration we consider calibration-in-the-large (intercept given that slope b is set to 1, $a|b = 1$) and the calibration slope (b). Both are determined in logistic regression models: $y \sim lp$. The linear predictor lp is entered as an offset variable ($a|b = 1$), or as the only predictor (slope b) in a logistic regression model estimated in the validation data. The c statistic is used to indicate discriminative ability (Chap. 15). For clinical usefulness, we calculate the net benefit (NB), with the formula $NB = (TP - w\,FP)/n$, where TP is the number of true positive classifications, FP the number of false positive classifications, and w is a weight equal to the odds of the threshold (cutoff/(1 − cutoff)), or the ratio of harm to benefit (see Chap. 16). We compare the NB of the model with a cutoff at 30% with the strategy with the next best NB ("treat all", or "treat none"). With an incidence of the outcome at 50% and a threshold of 30%, "treat all" has the next best NB: for every 100 patients, 50 true positive classifications are made, and 50 false positive classifications (which are weighted as 3/7). The NB of "treat all" hence is $50 - 3/7 * 50 = 28.6/100$ patients. A clinically useful model should have a NB higher than this reference value.

Together, these performance measures may be referred to as "ABCD". The letters relate to performance measures as: (A) for the intercept given that slope b is set to 1, $a|b = 1$; (B) for the calibration slope b; (C) for the c statistic; (D) for decision-analytic, the Net Benefit [565].

When the considered model is applied in the development population, the calibration is perfect ($a|b = 1 = 0$; slope $b = 1$) and discrimination good ($c = 0.81$, Fig. 19.2). The increase in NB by 0.055 means that 5.5 more true positive classifications are obtained per 100 patients, at the same number of false positive classifications (see Chap. 16). The model performance is identical whether uncorrelated or correlated missed predictors are present, since the model is always $y = 1.5 * x$ (Table 19.2).

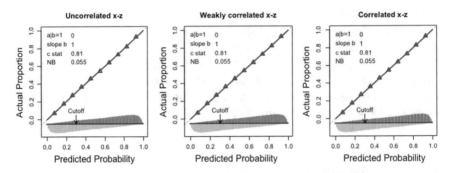

Fig. 19.2 Calibration, discrimination, and clinical usefulness when the prediction model is applied in a population with an identical distribution of predictor *x* and missed predictor *z* (from left to right: r = 0, r = 0.33, r = 0.5; n = 500,000). *a|b* = 1: intercept given slope *b* is 1; slope *b*: calibration slope in a calibration model *y* ~ *lp*; *c* stat: *c* statistic indicating discriminative ability; NB: Net Benefit compared to "treat all". The value of 0.055 means that 5.5 more true positive classifications are made per 100 patients, at the same number of false positive classifications (see Chap. 16). Triangles represent tenths of patients grouped by similar predicted probability. The distribution of patients is indicated with spikes at the bottom of the graph, separately for those with and without the outcome

19.3 Distribution of Predictors

We consider various selection mechanisms based on observed predictors *X* and missed predictors *Z*. Such selection is an example of missing not at random (MNAR, Chap. 7). We know that the regression coefficient of a single predictor *x* remains unbiased with a *MNAR* mechanism (Chap. 7). Hence, calibration will be unaffected. Of interest is any influence on discrimination and clinical usefulness.

19.3.1 More or Less Severe Case-Mix According to X

Subjects may be more likely to be included in the validation setting because they have higher *x* values ("more suspect cases"). For example, we may assume that only the higher *x* values are represented (correlation with missingness status *r* = 0.62, R^2 39%). This leads to a more severe case-mix at validation.

```
n      <- 500000
x      <- rnorm(n)                            # standard normal x
xM     <- ifelse(rnorm(n=n,sd=.8) < x, x, NA) # 50% missing, r=0.62
```

In our particular simulation, the more severe case-mix is associated with somewhat less spread in predictions, and hence a lower *c* statistic (0.77 instead of 0.81, Fig. 19.3). Moreover, only a few patients have predictions below the

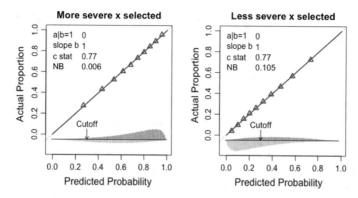

Fig. 19.3 Influence of selection of more or less severe cases according to predictor *x*. 50% of the subjects were selected, with higher or lower likelihood of selection with higher *x* values. Validation with a less severe case-mix makes the prediction model clinically more useful by having more predictions below the cutoff (right panel)

threshold of 30%, reducing the NB to 0.006 instead of 0.055. The prediction model would be judged of very limited utility in this validation setting. If the missingness was even more selective ($r > 0.75$), the NB would become zero, meaning that "treat all" would be as good a policy as using the prediction model. In contrast, a less severe case-mix led to a higher NB (NB 0.104, Fig. 19.3, right panel) . This is explained by the fact that the risk threshold now falls approximately in the middle of the risk distribution, which compensates for the lower c statistic. The patterns in Fig. 19.3 were identical with uncorrelated or correlated z.

19.3.2   *Interpretation of Testicular Cancer Validation*

These findings are important for the interpretation of the external validity of the testicular cancer example presented in Chaps. 15 and 16. When applied in more severe patients treated at a tertiary referral center (Indiana University Medical Center [644], we noted a decrease in clinical usefulness of the prediction model. But we have to realize that not all testicular cancer patients undergo surgical resection; there is "verification bias" [45]. Typically a selection is made toward those with a suspicion of residual tumor (e.g., larger residual masses). If all testicular cancer patients were considered, the model would also indicate resection in some of the patients who were not candidates for resection under current policies. Clinical usefulness would hence be judged higher.

19.3.3   More or Less Heterogeneous Case-Mix According to X

Another situation is that a more heterogeneous setting is considered, which is fully represented by the X values. For example, inclusion criteria may be wider in surveys of patients with traumatic brain injury (TBI) compared to randomized controlled trials (RCTs) [465]. RCTs typically have a list of inclusion and exclusion criteria. If these criteria apply to predictors that are all considered in the prediction model, the distribution of X values will be more heterogeneous in surveys. Note that the selection on X values may lead to extrapolation of model predictions in the validation data beyond observed X values in the development data.

The heterogeneity in case-mix translates into a higher discriminative ability; we can distinguish more patients with very low or very high prediction (c statistic 0.90 instead of 0.81, Fig. 19.4 left panel). More patients have predictions below the postulated threshold of 30%, doubling the NB (0.104 instead of 0.055). The prediction model would be judged quite useful in this more heterogeneous validation setting. The reverse is found for validation in a setting with less heterogeneity (lower c statistic, 0.75; lower NB, 0.03, Fig. 19.4, right panel). These patterns were identical with uncorrelated or correlated z.

19.3.4   More or Less Severe Case-Mix According to Z

Similar to distributions of observed predictors, distributions of missed predictors Z may also differ between development and validation settings. We will see that the correlation between observed predictors X and missed predictors Z is especially relevant for calibration.

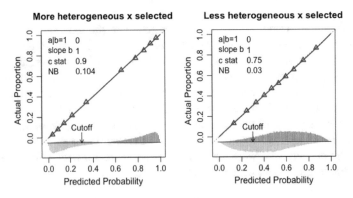

Fig. 19.4 Influence of selection of more or less heterogeneous cases according to observed predictor values. Approximately 35% of the subjects were selected, with a higher or lower likelihood of selection with more extreme x values. Validation with a more heterogeneous case-mix makes the prediction model more discriminatory and clinically more useful (left panel)

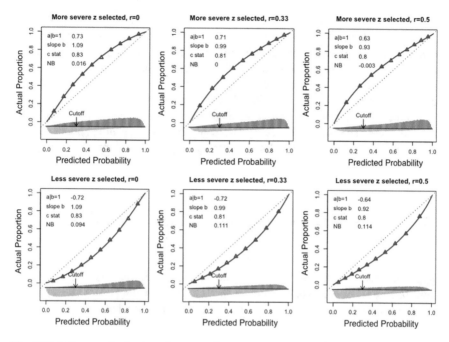

Fig. 19.5 Influence of selection of more or less severe cases according to a missed predictor ($x - z$ correlation 0, 0.33 or 0.5). 50% of the subjects were selected, with higher or lower likelihood of selection with higher z values

The first situation is that a prediction model is applied in a setting of more or less severe cases, according to predictors which are not (or not fully) captured in the prediction model. A more severe case-mix mainly causes a systematic miscalibration of predictions (Fig. 19.5, top row). The calibration-in-the-large ($a|b = 1$) values are around 0.7, which reflects that approximately twice as many cases are found than predicted (odds ratio $\exp(0.7) = 2.0$). The calibration slope is around 1. Without correlation between x and z ($r - 0$, Fig. 19.5, upper left panel), the slope is 1.1, which is explained by the reduced stratification effect of z in the regression model. In the development setting, the stratification effect was such that the adjusted coefficient was 2.1 for an unadjusted coefficient of 1.5 for x; with less stratification, the unadjusted coefficient is $1.1 * 1.5 = 1.65$. With moderate correlation ($r = 0.5$, Fig. 19.5, upper right panel), the confounding effect was weaker, leading to an unadjusted coefficient of $0.93 * 1.5 = 1.4$ for x.

The discrimination follows the same pattern as the calibration slope, with values around the original estimate of $c = 0.81$. The poor calibration causes the model to have at most small clinical usefulness. The NB of the model may even become negative (-0.003 in Fig. 19.5, upper right panel). This means that worse decisions are made with the model than the reference strategy of "treat all". This can be understood by realizing that the model assigns patients with a prediction under 30% to "no treatment", while predictions are systematically too low. Many among those with a prediction under 30% have actual probabilities over 30% and should have been classified for "treat". On balance, the loss of inappropriately withholding treatment from those with actual probabilities over 30% was larger than the gain of reducing false positive classifications (100% with a "treat all" strategy).

The reverse pattern is noted when selection is on less severe patients according to some missed predictor (Fig. 19.5, lower row). Calibration-in-the-large is the main problem. Interestingly, the clinical usefulness is now increased, despite this miscalibration. The various impacts of miscalibration on clinical usefulness can be examined in Daan Nieboer's online ShinyApp: https://dcacalibration.shinyapps.io/dcacalibration/.

19.3.5 More or Less Heterogeneous Case-Mix According to Z

Similar to observed predictors, we can imagine that missed predictors Z may have a more or less heterogeneous distribution in a validation setting. Such distributional changes affect the calibration slope, but not calibration-in-the-large (Fig. 19.6). The

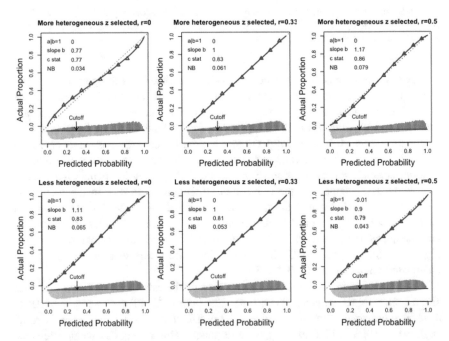

Fig. 19.6 Influence of selection of more or less heterogeneous cases according to a missed predictor z ($x - z$ correlation 0, 0.33 or 0.5). Approximately 35% of the subjects were selected, with higher or lower likelihood of selection with more extreme z values

specific patterns in calibration again reflect the balance of stratification and confounding effects. Discrimination and clinical usefulness were better with higher calibration slopes.

19.4 Distribution of Observed Outcome *y*

A case–control design allows for separate sampling of cases ($y = 1$) and controls ($y = 0$). Cases and controls should come from the same underlying populations, as would be considered in a cohort study (Chap. 3). In the examples thus far, the ratio of cases and controls was 1:1 (50% incidence of the outcome *y*). The effect of manipulating the outcome incidence is reflected in calibration-in-the-large. With a ratio of 2 cases to 1 control, the odds ratio of the intercept is 2. Indeed, the coefficient is 0.69, or log(2) (Fig. 19.7, left panel). Conversely, a ratio of 1 case to 2 controls leads to an intercept of −0.69. With a proper case–control design, the effects of predictors remain identical (calibration slope = 1), as well as the *c* statistic (0.81). Calculation of clinical usefulness is only sensible after correction of the intercept, which can be seen as translating a case–control design back to clinical practice [302].

In a traditional case–control design, the number of controls in the population is unknown. This makes it impossible to correctly adjust the intercept. In a *nested* case–control design, we sample the cases and controls from a defined underlying cohort. The number of controls is known in such a design, which makes it straightforward to adjust the intercept, for example by weighting the controls by the inverse of their sampling ratio.

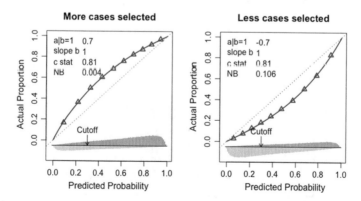

Fig. 19.7 Influence of a case–control design on the model intercept; calibration slope and discrimination remain unaffected. The ratio of cases to controls was set to 2:1 (left,) and 1:2 (right panel), corresponding to the miscalibration of +log(2) and log(0.5)

19.5   Coefficients β

19.5.1   Coefficient of Linear Predictor < 1

Overfitting is a major problem of predictive modeling (Chaps. 4–18). At external validation, we may often find a less predictive effect of the linear predictor lp. This reduced effect might have been detected already at internal validation. It should have led to the incorporation of a shrinkage or a penalty factor to compensate for overfitting. True differences in predictive effects may also play a role, for example, caused by definition and selection issues.

A typical shrinkage factor found at internal validation is 0.8; more severe overfitting might lead to a shrinkage factor of 0.6. At external validation, we find that such patterns of overfitting lead to a reduction in discriminative ability (c 0.77 or 0.72 instead of 0.81) and a reduction in clinical usefulness (Net Benefit 0.037 or 0.014 instead of 0.055, Fig. 19.8).

19.5.2   Coefficients β Different

In addition to being overestimated on average, regression coefficients may truly differ between development and validation settings. Various causes can be imagined, all related to the validation population not being "plausibly related" anymore to the development population [285]. Terrin et al. considered various scenarios of different effects of predictors in a validation setting. In simulation studies, they simulated weaker effects of predictors, motivated by clinical scenarios, and found reductions in c statistic from 0.75 to 0.72 [578].

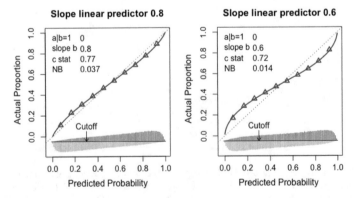

Fig. 19.8 Influence of overfitting in model development. The slope of the linear predictor is 0.8 or 0.6, with lower discriminative ability (c = 0.77 or 0.72), and lower clinical usefulness (net benefit 0.037 or 0.014)

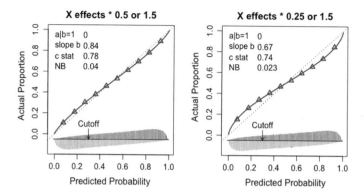

Fig. 19.9 Influence of differences in regression coefficients between development and validation setting. Regression coefficients were 0.5 smaller or 1.5 times as large in the left panel (overall effect: slope 0.84), and 0.25 or 1.5 times as large in the right panel (overall effect: slope 0.68). In the right panel, discriminative ability and clinical usefulness were affected substantially (*c* statistic 0.74, net benefit only 0.023)

In Chap. 5, we used an arbitrary example of differences in predictor effects, with predictors having 0.5 or 1.5 times the effect of the development setting: $x = 0.5 * x1 + 1.5 * x2 + \cdots + 0.5 * x9 + 1.5 * x10$. We use this example here for illustration, and a more extreme situation, with very small effects at validation (5 x variables with effect 0.25). These misfits led to calibration slopes of 0.84 and 0.67, and lower discriminative ability and clinical usefulness (Fig. 19.9). Hence, differences between effects in the development setting versus the validation setting may seriously deteriorate model performance.

19.6 Summary of Patterns of Invalidity

We summarize the patterns of invalidity in Table 19.3.

- Calibration

In the development setting, the calibration was perfect, the *c* statistic 0.81 and the Net Benefit of applying the model 0.055. Calibration remained perfect when the validation setting consisted of more or less severe patients according to predictor values, or more or less heterogeneous patients according to observed or missed predictor values. Calibration can be systematically disturbed by a more or less severe distribution of missed predictor values (*z*, e.g., intercept +0.7 or −0.7). A similar disturbance can be caused by a case–control design; however, the case–control ratio is under the influence of the researcher, while the distribution of a missed predictor usually is not. Miscalibration can also be caused by overfitting at model development (e.g., slope 0.8 or 0.6), or truly differential predictive effects

Table 19.3 Patterns of invalidity for a prediction model for binary outcomes in relation to differences between development and validation populations

Scenario	Characteristics	Differences	$a\|b = 1$	b	c stat	NB
Development setting	$y = 1.5 * x$ ($x \sim N$ (0,1))	–	0	1	0.81	0.055
Case-mix in validation setting	Distribution of observed predictors X	More severe patients	0	1	0.77	0.006
		Less severe patients	0	1	0.77	0.104
		More heterogeneous	0	1	0.90	0.104
		Less heterogeneous	0	1	0.75	0.030
	Distribution of missed predictors Z	More severe patients[a]	log(2)	1	0.81	0.001
		Less severe patients[a]	−log(2)	1	0.81	0.109
		More heterogeneous[a]	0	1	0.83	0.062
		Less heterogeneous[a]	0	1	0.81	0.053
	Distribution of outcomes y	2 times more cases	log(2)	1	0.81	NA
		2 times less cases	−log(2)	1	0.81	NA
Coefficients in validation setting	Coefficients β smaller than expected	Slope 0.8	0	0.8	0.77	0.037
		Slope 0.6	0	0.6	0.72	0.014
	Coefficients β different	X effects * 0.5 or 1.5	0	0.84	0.78	0.040
		X effects * 0.25 or 1.5	0	0.68	0.74	0.023

[a]For correlation $x - z$ of 0.33; detailed results in Figs. 19.5 and 19.6
$a\|b = 1$: intercept given that calibration slope b is 1, indicating "calibration-in-the-large"; b: calibration slope; c stat: concordance statistic to indicate discriminative ability; NB net benefit; *NA* not applicable

(coefficients of individual predictors 0.25/0.5/1.5 times as large, details at www. clinicalpredictionmodels.org).

- Discrimination

Discriminative ability is mathematically related to the calibration slope, with a lower c statistic associated with a lower calibration slope at validation [629]. Another reason for a lower c statistic is a less heterogeneous case-mix (e.g., slope = 1, but $c = 0.75$ instead of 0.81, Fig. 19.4, right panel). Indeed, a high c statistic such as 0.90 was found for a more heterogeneous setting (Fig. 19.4, left panel). More heterogeneity in missed predictors had only small effects (Fig. 19.6). These examples illustrate that discrimination is determined by the combination of validity of estimated regression coefficients β and case-mix. Poor discrimination can hence result from both aspects (i.e., poor calibration, and/or relatively homogeneous case-mix).

- Clinical usefulness

Tables 19.3 and 19.4 highlight the importance of calibration for clinical usefulness. A systematic miscalibration, e.g., caused by a more severe case-mix according to a missed predictor z, may lead to a model without clinical usefulness. With incorrect calibration, we can make systematically wrong decisions. This is not the case if predictions are moderately calibrated [606]. Discrimination and calibration slope are linked, and a lower calibration slope or lower discrimination are hence both associated with a lower clinical usefulness.

Perfect calibration and good discrimination protect us against negative clinical usefulness [602]. Discrimination is important; better discrimination may lead to better decision-making. If a model has no discriminative ability, it cannot improve upon a default strategy of treating all/none. Discrimination is hence a necessary but not sufficient condition for clinical usefulness.

When applying the model in more or less severe patients, the c statistic was 0.77 for both settings, but clinical usefulness was only 0.006 for a more severe setting and 0.104 for a less severe setting. These findings are in line with the lack of clinical usefulness of the testicular cancer case study in Chap. 16, where we noted that few patients had a prediction below the threshold of 30% for the probability of tumor tissue at external validation.

Case-mix is also very relevant, especially for variables that are not in the model (Z). The case-mix in observed predictors (X) affects clinical usefulness through the

Table 19.4 Combinations of differences between development and validation populations and their impact on the validity of a prediction model for binary outcomes

Scenario	x	z	Coefficients	a|b = 1	b	c stat	NB
Change of setting	–	More severe	X effects * 0.5 or 1.5	0.67	0.87	0.78	−0.008
				−0.67	0.87	0.78	0.098
	–	Less severe					
RCT versus survey	More heterogeneous	More severe	X effects * 0.5 or 1.5	0.64	1.04	0.88	0.027
				0.69	0.59	0.65	−0.036
	Less heterogeneous	More severe		−0.68	1.03	0.88	0.167
				−0.68	0.59	0.65	0.037
	More heterogeneous	Less severe					
	Less heterogeneous	Less severe					

distribution of predictions around the decision threshold, while leaving calibration largely intact. The case-mix in missed predictors (Z) may predominantly affect clinical usefulness through poor calibration-in-the-large

19.6.1   Other Scenarios of Invalidity

Thus far, we considered one element at a time for differences between development and validation populations. All simulation results depend on the specific parameters chosen; with more extreme parameter settings, differences will be larger. We can consider other scenarios that are also plausible at validation of a prediction model, where we combine differences in the distribution of x, z, and regression coefficients β (Table 19.4). Detailed results are provided at www.clinicalpredictionmodels.org.

19.7   Reference Values for Performance

Two types of reference values are useful to interpret the validity of a prediction model [629]:

1. The performance if the model would be fully valid, given the case-mix in the validation sample: a model-based performance estimate.
2. The performance with coefficients optimized for the validation data: a refitted model.

Such reference values are useful to obtain insight into what is happening at validation: are there merely differences in case-mix or differences in regression coefficients compared to the development setting?

19.7.1   Model-Based Performance: Performance
         if the Model Is Valid

The distribution of predictors X should be taken into account to indicate a model's performance under the condition that the model predictions are valid in the validation sample. For a regression model, this means that the regression coefficients for predictors X and the model intercept are fully correct for the validation setting.

For calibration, obvious reference values are 0 for calibration-in-the-large, and 1 for the calibration slope. For discrimination, a practical approach is to simulate the outcome y for the observed case-mix in X, given that the prediction model is correct. This is simply obtained by first calculating the predictions for each subject in the validation data, and subsequently randomly assigning an outcome y based on this prediction. With at least 100 repetitions for each patient, a stable estimate of the reference values is obtained. We illustrate the calculation below for 1000 repetitions per patient in a logistic regression model.

Analytic alternatives are available. The Gonen and Heller c statistic was originally proposed for Cox regression models, estimating performance if the model is valid [190]. This approach was extended by Van Klaveren to logistic regression and other types of models. The expected c statistic for the situation that the model is correct is labeled the model-based concordance ("*mbc*") [629].

19.7.2   Performance with Refitting

Another type of reference value is the performance obtained by refitting the model in the validation data. The regression coefficients are then optimized for the validation data, and hence provide an upper bound for the performance, which would be obtained if the coefficients from the development setting were exactly equal to those in the validation setting. This upper bound does not only depend on case-mix, but also on the effects of predictors in the validation setting. It is hence not simple to compare performance between development and validation settings: differences may be attributable to both case-mix and/or coefficients.

19.7.3   *Examples: Testicular Cancer and TBI

We apply the calculation of reference values to the testicular cancer and traumatic brain injury (TBI) case studies (Table 19.5). Prediction models were developed with $n = 544$ testicular cancer patients ($n = 245$, 45%, with benign histology), and $n = 2036$ TBI patients ($n = 798$, 39%, with an unfavorable 6-month outcome). The 544 testicular cancer patients are mostly from secondary care centers [551], while external validation was in 273 patients from a tertiary care center [644]. A benign outcome was less frequent among these patients (n = 76/273, 28%). The 2036 TBI

Table 19.5 Examples of reference values for performance of two prediction models, developed in one setting and applied in another setting

Example	Measure	Apparent	Internally validated	Externally validated	Model-based	Refitted
Testicular cancer: secondary care → tertiary referral	c stat R^2	0.818 38.9%	0.812 37.4%	0.785 26.7%	0.824 37.0%	0.819 34.2%
Traumatic brain injury: RCT → surveys	c stat R^2	0.767 27.9%	0.765 27.3%	0.816 37.1%	0.804 35.3%	0.819 38.0%

patients were from the Tirilazad randomized controlled trials [259], with validation in three largely unselected series (UK 4 center study, European Brain Injury Consortium survey, Traumatic Coma Databank, $n = 2090$) [357]. These patients more often had an unfavorable outcome at 6 months ($n = 1249/2090$, 60%) compared to the development sample.

In the testicular cancer case study, the apparent c statistic was 0.818, with 0.006 optimism according to a bootstrap procedure. At external validation, the c statistic was 0.785, while 0.824 was expected based on the case-mix of the predictor variables (the mbc, "model-based", Table 19.5). When the model was refitted, the performance was slightly lower than this reference value (c statistic 0.819 vs. 0.824). A similar pattern was noted for the R^2 statistic. We might test the statistical significance of these differences in performance but concentrate here on the point estimates.

In the TBI case study, the apparent c statistic was 0.767, with negligible optimism. Surprisingly, the c statistic was higher at external validation (0.816), while 0.804 was expected based on the case-mix of the predictor variables. When the model was refitted, the performance was higher again (refitted c 0.819 vs. mbc 0.804). A similar pattern was noted for the R^2 statistic.

The interpretation of Table 19.5 is a follows:

1. Internal validation corrects for the statistical problem of overfitting in the development setting; case-mix is unchanged.
2. External validation tests the model in a sample from a new setting, where both case-mix and coefficients may be different than in the development sample.
3. The reference performance corrects for the new case-mix according to predictor values in the validation sample, while keeping the coefficients at the values from the development setting.
4. The refitted performance corrects for the new case-mix and estimates optimal regression coefficients in the validation sample.

The poorer external performance of the testicular cancer model is not explained by case-mix, at least not in the distribution of observed predictor values, since the reference performance was very similar to that in the development sample. The poorer external validity should hence be attributed to differences in regression coefficients between the settings. The refitted performance was similar to the reference performance, indicating that the predictors had similar predictiveness in both settings when refitted.

The better external performance of the TBI model is partly explained by case-mix, since the reference performance was higher than in the development sample. The surprisingly good external validity should further be attributed to differences in regression coefficients between the settings; predictive effects were overall stronger in the validation setting (calibration slope 1.08), in line with the even better refitted performance ("refitted" c 0.819, Table 19.5).

19.7.4   *R Code for reference values

```
# fit in development data
fit          <- lrm(y ~ x1+x2+ ..., data=dev.data, linear.predictors=T)
# refit in validation data: refitted reference performance
fit.val      <- update(fit, data=val.data)

# linear predictor for validation data
lp           <- predict(fit,newdata=val.data)
# External validation
val.prob.ci.2(logit=lp,y=val.data$y, ... ) # with confidence intervals

# Reference value if model valid: simulation of outcomes
n            <- nrow(validation.data)
nsamples     <- 1000      # for stable results
perf.m       <- matrix(nrow=nsamples*n, ncol=2)
perf.m[,1]   <- rep(lp, nsamples) # repeat linear predictor nsamples times
# Generate y for validation data
perf.m[,2]   <- ifelse(runif(length(perf.m[,1]))<=plogis(perf.m[,1]), 1, 0)
# Determine reference values
perf.ref     <- val.prob(logit=perf.m[,1],y=perf.m[,2], ... )

# Alternative: use analytical solution for the model-based c statistic
https://github.com/David-van-Klaveren/mbc
```

19.8   Validation Sample Size

Thus far, we examined theoretical patterns of invalidity with very large simulated samples. The testicular cancer and TBI case studies (Sect. 19.7.3) considered more limited sample sizes for model development and validation; differences in model performance might at least partly be attributed to chance. Performance parameters for calibration (model intercept, $a|b = 1$; calibration slope, b), and discrimination (c statistic), and decision-analytic measures of clinical usefulness (Net Benefit, NB) are subject to sampling error in real life.

19.8.1   Uncertainty in Validation of Performance

We first illustrate some of the empirical behavior of measures for calibration and discrimination of logistic regression models. The prediction model is the same as before, with a linear predictor in the logistic regression model defined by 10 normally distributed X variables, each with a regression coefficient of 0.76 (see Sect. 19.5.2). The model has a c statistic of 0.812. We consider small to large sample sizes for model development ($N_{dev} = 100$ to $N_{dev} = 10,000$) and for model validation ($N_{val} = 100$ to $N_{val} = 10,000$), with outcome incidence 50% or 10%. Simulations are first performed under the Null hypothesis, i.e., that both samples originate from the same underlying population (Table 19.6). Case-mix and

Table 19.6 Estimation of calibration and discrimination of logistic regression models in small to large sample sizes for model development and for model validation

Scenario	Events/N_{dev}	Events/N_{val}	Estimated performance at validation (mean ± SE)		
			$a\|b = 1$	Slope b	c statistic
Incidence 50% Large sizes	5000/10,000	5000/10,000	0 ± 0.03	1.00 ± 0.03	0.81 ± 0.004
Small development samples	50/100	5000/10,000	0 ± 0.28	0.64 ± 0.15	0.77 ± 0.017
	100/200		0 ± 0.17	0.82 ± 0.13	0.79 ± 0.010
	250/500		0 ± 0.12	0.92 ± 0.09	0.80 ± 0.006
	500/1000		0 ± 0.08	0.95 ± 0.07	0.81 ± 0.005
	1000/2000		0 ± 0.06	0.97 ± 0.05	0.81 ± 0.004
Small validation samples	5000/10,000	50/100	0 ± 0.24	1.06 ± 0.24	0.82 ± 0.043
		100/200	0 ± 0.16	1.03 ± 0.17	0.81 ± 0.030
		250/500	0 ± 0.11	1.01 ± 0.10	0.80 ± 0.018
		500/1000	0 ± 0.08	1.00 ± 0.07	0.81 ± 0.014
		1000/2000	0 ± 0.06	1.00 ± 0.05	0.81 ± 0.009
Small development samples, **half size** validation	50/100	25/50	0 ± 0.52	0.71 ± 0.31	0.77 ± 0.070
	100/200	50/100	0 ± 0.34	0.83 ± 0.25	0.79 ± 0.048
	250/500	100/200	0 ± 0.20	0.95 ± 0.18	0.80 ± 0.030
	500/1000	250/500	0 ± 0.13	0.98 ± 0.11	0.81 ± 0.018
	1000/2000	500/1000	0 ± 0.10	0.99 ± 0.09	0.81 ± 0.014
Small development samples, **equal size** validation samples	50/100	50/100	0 ± 0.44	0.66 ± 0.23	0.77 ± 0.051
	75/150	75/150	0 ± 0.32	0.77 ± 0.22	0.78 ± 0.039
	100/200	100/200	0 ± 0.27	0.82 ± 0.19	0.79 ± 0.033
	175/350	175/350	0 ± 0.19	0.89 ± 0.15	0.80 ± 0.023
	250/500	250/500	0 ± 0.15	0.93 ± 0.13	0.80 ± 0.019
	500/1000	500/1000	0 ± 0.11	0.97 ± 0.09	0.81 ± 0.014
	1000/2000	1000/2000	0 ± 0.08	0.99 ± 0.07	0.81 ± 0.010
Incidence 10% Large sizes	1000/9000	1000/9000	0 ± 0.05	1.00 ± 0.05	0.83 ± 0.007
Selected combinations of development and validation sample sizes	50/450	50/450	0 ± 0.25	0.85 ± 0.18	0.81 ± 0.033
		100/900	0 ± 0.23	0.85 ± 0.15	0.81 ± 0.021
		200/1800	0 ± 0.19	0.86 ± 0.14	0.81 ± 0.018
		1000/9000	0 ± 0.18	0.86 ± 0.14	0.81 ± 0.010
	100/900	50/450	0 ± 0.22	0.93 ± 0.17	0.82 ± 0.032
		100/900	0 ± 0.18	0.93 ± 0.13	0.82 ± 0.021
		200/1800	0 ± 0.15	0.93 ± 0.11	0.82 ± 0.015
		1000/9000	0 ± 0.13	0.93 ± 0.11	0.82 ± 0.008
	200/1800	50/450	0 ± 0.19	0.95 ± 0.15	0.82 ± 0.031
		100/900	0 ± 0.18	0.96 ± 0.13	0.82 ± 0.022
		200/1800	0 ± 0.11	0.97 ± 0.10	0.83 ± 0.017
		1000/9000	0 ± 0.09	0.96 ± 0.07	0.82 ± 0.007
	1000/9000	50/450	0 ± 0.17	1.01 ± 0.15	0.83 ± 0.030
		100/900	0 ± 0.13	0.99 ± 0.10	0.83 ± 0.021
		200/1800	0 ± 0.09	1.00 ± 0.07	0.83 ± 0.015

Numbers are mean ± standard error (SE) in validation samples, as observed in simulations (100–1000 repetitions for sufficiently stable results)

regression coefficients were hence identical in both settings, and estimates may vary only because of finite sample sizes at the development and/or validation. Finite sample size implies a risk of overfitting at model development, and limited precision both at development and validation.

With 50% incidence of the outcome in very large development and validation sizes (N_{dev} = 10,000 and N_{val} = 10,000), the standard errors (SE) are small: the SE around the calibration-in-the-large and calibration slope b is 0.03, the SE around the c statistic is 0.004. With 10% incidence, N_{dev} = 10,000 and N_{val} = 10,000, the SEs are larger, corresponding to the lower number of events (1000 instead of 5000).

(a) We find that the average calibration-in-the-large is approximately 0 in all scenarios; the standard error (SE) depends on the size of the development sample and the size of the validation sample. With only 100 subjects for model development, the SE is 0.28 if validation is in 10,000 subjects; if validation is in 50 or 100 subjects, the SE is much larger (±0.52 and ±0.44, respectively). A quite low SE (±0.06) is found with at least n = 2000 for model development and 10,000 for model validation, or with a reversal of this design (development n = 10,000, validation n = 2000).

(b) The calibration slope b is below 1 when small samples are used for model development (e.g., average b = 0.65 with N_{dev} = 100 and N_{val} = 10,000, reflecting a clear need for shrinkage of coefficients, or use of penalization, see Chap. 13). In contrast, small validation samples lead to an upward bias for the slope (e.g., average b = 1.08 with N_{dev} = 10,000 and N_{val} = 100). The SE is somewhat larger with small validation samples than with small development samples (e.g., N_{dev} = 100: SE ± 0.15; N_{val} = 100: SE ± 0.25).

(c) The discriminative ability (c statistic) was 0.81 in the population, but smaller with small development samples (e.g., c = 0.77 with N_{dev} = 100, N_{val} = 10,000). Again, small validation samples led to an upward bias (e.g., c = 0.82 with N_{dev} = 10,000 and N_{val} = 100). The SE was markedly higher with small validation samples (e.g., N_{dev} = 100: SE ± 0.017; N_{val} = 100: SE ± 0.043). Apparently, small development samples lead to poor discriminating models, which can reliably be quantified with large validation samples. Small validation samples lead anyway to uncertain estimates of discrimination.

19.8.2   *Estimating Standard Errors in Validation Studies

In Table 19.6, we calculated standard errors (SEs) empirically by studying the distribution of coefficients over samples. In Table 19.7, we use the asymptotic SE for the performance measures. The SE of calibration-in-the-large and calibration slope are obtained from the variance estimates in the logistic regression models which have the linear predictor as the only independent variable. We may assume that the parameters a and b are Normally distributed, such that the SE can directly

Table 19.7 Required differences between development and validation settings (effect sizes) for 80% power when validating a logistic regression model in a setting with 50 or 10% incidence of the outcome

Scenario	Events/N val	$a\|b = 1 \Leftrightarrow 1$[a]	slope $b < 1$[b]	$c < c_{reference}^b$
Incidence 50%	50/100	±0.67, OR = 1.96	<0.40	<−0.107
	100/200	±0.45, OR = 1.57	<0.58	<−0.077
	250/500	±0.31, OR = 1.36	<0.75	<−0.045
	500/1000	±0.22, OR = 1.25	<0.83	<−0.035
	1000/2000	±0.17, OR = 1.18	<0.88	<−0.022
Incidence 10%	50/450	±0.45, OR = 1.61	<0.63	<−0.075
	100/900	±0.34, OR = 1.44	<0.75	<−0.052
	200/1800	±0.25, OR = 1.29	<0.83	<−0.037

OR odds ratio

[a]2-sided statistical test in a logistic regression model with the linear predictor based on the development sample as an offset variable

[b]1-sided test in a logistic regression model with the linear predictor as the only predictor

be used for a 95% confidence interval. If calibration-in-the-large is expressed as an observed over expected ratio, it needs a log transformation, which makes it a univariate logistic regression coefficient [521].

The SE of the c statistic is calculated with standard formulas for rank order statistics [223]. We found that the asymptotic SEs agreed rather well with the empirical estimates, although one might consider the logit transformation when calculating 95% confidence intervals for the c statistic [521].

19.8.3 Summary Points

- Variability is substantial with small development samples, and especially with small validation samples.
- The effective sample size is largely determined by the number of events rather than the total sample size.
- We can base 95% confidence intervals directly on SE estimates for calibration-in-the-large and calibration slope, while the c statistic may benefit from a logit transformation.

19.9 Design of External Validation Studies

The variability in performance has implications for the design and power of validation studies [438, 520]. We have seen in Chap. 17 that the bootstrap is generally useful for internal validation purposes. Despite its inefficiency, some researchers may like a split-sample approach to convince their readership. This design has severe limitations: in small samples, we should aim to estimate internal validity, which is better done by bootstrapping or cross-validation, e.g., 10 × 10-fold (Chap. 17). In large samples, we should aim to estimate external validity and assess heterogeneity in performance, which is well possible with a leave-one-out cross-validation by site, study, or another meaningful nonrandom split [30, 31, 473, 546].

If a split is considered, a common ratio is 2/3 of the sample for model development and 1/3 for validation. According to Table 19.6, a lower variability of performance is obtained with a 50:50 split-sample design; but this design has more optimism in calibration slope and discrimination. A 2:1 ratio may be a reasonable balance between optimizing bias and variability.

For external validation we may sometimes choose a temporal validation design [285]. We then face the same question on how to choose the size of the development data set versus the size of the more recent validation set. With spatial validation, e.g., "leave-one-center-out" cross-validation, the validation sets may be much smaller than the development set. The results in Table 19.6 show that this makes the performance quite uncertain in each validation part per se. The heterogeneity in performance over splits may, however, be of particular interest, and can be estimated by using multiple splits.

Another situation is that a model was published, and we simply wish to externally validate this model for our setting. Then, we do not have access to the development data. We set up a fully independent external validation study, and wonder about a reasonable sample size, accepting the developed model as reasonable to test. This design requires some estimates of statistical power to detect relevant differences in performance.

19.9.1 Power of External Validation Studies

Traditional power calculations depend on various quantities: statistical Type I and Type II error; the variability in the quantity we want to test, and the "clinically relevant" difference we do not want to miss. Type I error is conventionally set at 5%, and type II error at 20% (power 80%). The variability of performance measures is shown in Table 19.6. Note that these are empirically derived standard errors for 1 specific logistic regression model (with 10 normally distributed predictors). In practice, we may only know the asymptotic (i.e. estimated) standard error of some measures such as the model intercept, which depends on the event rate and numbers of events [460]. Clinically relevant differences may be context-dependent. For logistic regression models we might consider a systematic over or underestimation by 1.5 times the odds of the outcome (intercept + or − ln(1.5)), a calibration slope less than 0.8 (difference 0.2 with ideal slope of 1), and a decrease in c statistic by more than 0.05 (given the same case-mix). These numbers are arbitrary, and some may consider a decrease in c statistic by 0.02 already relevant.

Some specific issues come up in power calculations for validation studies. The first is whether we should perform one-sample or two-sample tests. If we consider the prediction model as a fixed system generating predictions, a one-sample test is reasonable to test whether the validation performance deviates from hypothesized values. For calibration, these values are obvious: 0 for calibration-in-the-large, and 1 for calibration slope. For the c statistic, we may consider the reference value assuming identical case-mix in the validation setting (model-based performance estimate, see Sect. 19.7).

Alternatively, we might consider a two-sample test, including uncertainty in the estimate from the development setting. This is natural for the c statistic, and in fact also for calibration statistics such as intercept (reference: 0) and calibration slope (reference: 1), since the reference values of 0 and 1 are estimates in the development setting rather than fixed quantities.

A further issue is whether we should perform 1-sided or 2-sided tests. Calibration-in-the-large asks for a 2-sided test, since the incidence in the validation setting may be higher or lower than predicted. But for calibration slope, we could test for slope $b < 1$, rather than slope $<> 1$, assuming we are primarily interested in overfitting. Similarly, only a decrease in discrimination is an interesting alternative hypothesis. Finally, one might argue that we should consider the assessment of validity as an assessment of equivalence in model performance: is the observed performance in the validation in line with our expectations? This implies that we change the Null hypothesis to stating that the model is invalid, and test whether the model performance is within reasonable limits from the expected value. The reasonable limits may be context-dependent, similar to defining "clinically relevant" differences in traditional sample size calculations.

19.9.2 *Calculating Sample Sizes for Validation Studies

We first approximate the statistical power given the standard error under the null hypothesis, i.e., the model was actually valid in the development and validation setting. We consider standard errors for model development with a large development sample size, such that the predominant source of variability is the validation sample size in Table 19.7. We might then use 1-sample tests for all performance measures. In situations with relatively small development size, a 2-sample test might be more appropriate.

One and two-sided tests may be used as follows:

- For calibration-in-the-large, it may reasonable to use a 2-sided test for: $a|$ $b = 1 <> 1$.
- For calibration slope, a 1-sided test may be used to test slope $b < 1$.
- For the c statistic, a 1-sided test may be used for deterioration in performance $(c < c_{reference})$.

Table 19.8 Power for testing slope < 1 (true value 0.84) and a *c* statistic decrease of −0.043 (true decrease 0.821–0.778)

Scenario	Events/N_{val}	Slope *b* 0.84 SE, power	*c* statistic −0.043 SE, power
Incidence 50%	50/100	0.20; 15%	0.046; 11%
	100/200	0.14; 25%	0.032; 24%
	250/500	0.088; 50%	0.021; 57%
	500/1000	0.062; **78%**	0.014; **87%**
	1000/2000	0.044; 97%	0.010; 99%

Bold: example discussed in the text

The critical values[1] for power calculations are determined by Type I and Type II error, which we set at 5% (1-sided or 2-sided) and 20% (1-sided). The critical value is 1.96 + 0.84 = 2.80 for 2-sided tests, and 1.64 + 0.84 = 2.49 for 1-sided tests. We multiply these critical values with the SE to obtain the minimum differences that can be detected with 80% power (Table 19.7).

As expected, small validation sizes only reach 80% power to detect quite a substantial invalidity. For example, if we validate a model in a sample with 50 events and 50 nonevents, we have 80% power to detect a calibration-in-the-large problem with approximately twice too high, or twice too low predictions (Odds Ratio 1.96); a dramatically poor calibration slope (less than 0.4), and a decrease in *c* statistic over 0.1 (Table 19.7). To detect a more modest calibration-in-the-large problem, such as 1.25 times too low or too high predictions, we would need at least 500 events and 500 nonevents (total *n* > 1000). This sample size would also have 80% power for a slope less than 0.83, and a decrease in *c* by 0.035. With more nonevents (incidence of outcome 10%), the picture is slightly better in terms of the number of events required, but the total sample size should be at least 2000 (200 events) for reasonable power.

In further analysis, we simulate power in the case that the developed prediction model is invalid for the validation setting. We create a model with coefficients 0.76 for 10 normally distributed predictors *x*1 to *x*10, and validate this model in a setting where the coefficients are 0.5 or 1.5 times as large. In the validation setting, calibration-in-the-large is fine (average 0), but the slope is 0.84 instead of 1, and the *c* statistic is 0.778 instead of 0.821 in the development setting (change −0.043).

If we validate this model with 500 events among 1000, Table 19.7 suggests that we may expect 80% power if the slope would be <0.83 in the validation setting; this is confirmed in Table 19.8 (78% power to detect a deterioration in slope, if slope *b* < 0.84). For a decrease in *c* statistic by −0.043, we expect that more than 250 events and 250 nonevents are required (Table 19.7). Indeed, the statistical power is 87% with 500 events (Table 19.8).

---

[1]Critical value: the value that a test statistic must exceed for the null hypothesis to be rejected.

19.9.3 Rules for Sample Size of Validation Studies

Various studies have suggested rules of thumb for sample sizes of validation studies. These often relate to the number of events required, which is the limiting factor for the effective sample size with low event rates. As noted in Chap. 3, the total number of patients n is also relevant; combined the numbers of events and total n determine the event rate. So, 100 events among 1000 imply more statistical power than 100 among 200 patients. The number of events is the key factor for validation studies in low incidence settings.

Most studies support the claim that at least 100–200 events are required for reasonable statistical power [104, 423, 533, 643]. Another study suggested a formula that allows the user to specify the sample size, with a focus on an expected calibration index (ECI) [416]. This index is based on the squared difference between the observed risk (obtained by smooth calibration curves) and the risk predicted by the model. If a model is well calibrated, it will have a low ECI value. If we require the calibration index to be under some value, such as ECI < 1.25, the required sample size was 69 events among 640. With 100 events (among 938), calibration performance could more reliably be determined. A recent simulation study started from a reported split-sample validation with only 3 events among 10 patients [533]. Such as low number is obviously too low for any meaningful interpretation. Expanding validation sizes to 100 events or 500 events showed a much narrower variance of the c statistic for models with true c statistics of 0.7, 0.8, or 0.9 (Fig. 19.10).

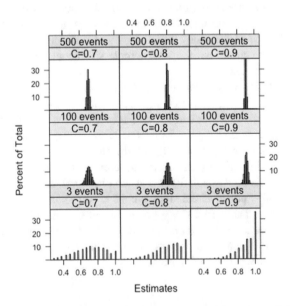

Fig. 19.10 Estimates of c statistics in 100,000 simulations of validation of a prediction model with a true c-statistic (indicating discriminative ability) of either 0.7, 0.8, or 0.9, in a situation with 500 events (1167 nonevents), 100 events (233 nonevents), or 3 events (7 nonevents). We note an extremely wide distribution of estimates with 3 events, with a spike at 1.0 (perfect separation) [533]

19.9.4 Summary Points

- The variability of external validation assessments depends on the size of the development sample and the size of the validation sample.
- For statistical testing, we may accept the prediction model as given, and hence perform 1-sample tests, with one-sided testing for a calibration slope < 1 and a decrease in c statistic.
- For such tests to have reasonable power, we need at least 100 events and at least 100 nonevents in external validation studies, but preferably more (>250 events). With lower numbers the uncertainty in performance measures is large.

19.10 Concluding Remarks

The performance of a prediction model in a new setting ("generalizability", or "transportability") essentially depends on two aspects: (1) the validity of the regression coefficients, and (2) the case-mix in the validation setting.

(1) The validity of regression coefficients can be assessed by comparing regression coefficients between settings. Indeed, we note that some validation studies report on the coefficients in their validation sample and compare these to the previous estimates from a development sample. With relatively small development and validation samples, it would be highly coincidental if coefficients agreed perfectly. Even if the two samples came from exactly the same underlying population, chance processes will cause the coefficients in both samples to differ from each other to some extent, with some coefficients larger and some smaller than expected from the development sample. Moreover, correlations between predictors may make that differences in estimated coefficients have ultimately limited impact on estimated probabilities. True differences in coefficients between settings may be due to differences in selection of patients, the definition of predictors and outcome, and other reasons.

(2) Differences in case-mix between development and validation setting are usually considered informally, by comparing patient characteristic in a kind of "Table 19.1". One usually makes only informal comparisons to the case-mix in the development sample. Some rather simple statistical measures have previously been proposed for an assessment of comparability, such as the "M statistic" to compare trauma populations [70]. With this approach, predicted probabilities of patients are grouped, for example as 0–25%, 26–50%, 51–75%, 76–90%, 91–95%, and 96–100%. The fraction of patients in these groups at validation is compared to the fraction at model development. The smaller of the

two fractions is summed over all groups. This creates a number ranging from 0 to 1. M-values close to 1 indicate a perfect match with the development case-mix, while 0 indicates a total discrepancy between the two samples. An arbitrary cutoff point of 0.88 has been suggested, and studies with M-values below 0.88 should be "interpreted cautiously" [70].

A more interesting approach is to develop a membership model, if we have access to both the development and validation data. We can then predict membership of the validation sample in contrast to the development sample [130]. If such prediction is well possible, as reflected in a high membership c statistic, the validation sample differs substantially from the development data. If the validation and development sample arose at random from the same underlying population, the expected membership c statistic is 0.5.

We followed a simple and systematic approach to study the influence of differences in case-mix and regression coefficients on validated model performance. Differences in predictor distributions ("X") do not affect calibration, and only discrimination aspects, as long as the model is correctly specified for the range of X values examined. If nonlinearities and/or interactions had been missed at model development, we can imagine that shifting to another predictor distribution may impact on calibration as well. Furthermore, we may assume that a very different distribution in X implies that differences in missed predictors ("Z") are also likely. Differences in missed predictors between settings may severely invalidate a prediction model, both with respect to calibration (especially calibration-in-the-large) and discrimination. When predictions are systematically miscalibrated, we can make systematically wrong decisions based on the model [606]. This may lead to a negative Net Benefit of using the model, compared to a default policy without using the model. It is therefore important to perform external validation studies [56, 451].

We also noted that the distribution of predictors can formally be taken into account in the calculation of reference values for model performance, given that the model is valid in the validation sample. This may be very useful to obtain insight into what is happening at validation: differences in case-mix and/or differences in regression coefficients?

Finally, we studied design issues of validation studies for prediction models for binary outcomes. If a temporal split is made, a 2:1 ratio may be reasonable. This limits overfitting at development, and still gives reasonable power at validation. As a rule of thumb, the validation data set should contain at least 100 events and 100 nonevents for reasonable power [104, 643]. For the detection of smaller but still quite relevant invalidity, higher sample sizes are advisable, e.g., 250 events and 250 nonevents, or 100 events and 900 nonevents. More theoretical approaches are discussed elsewhere for specific contexts [614, 683].

Can we anticipate poor validity? The PROBAST (Prediction model Risk Of Bias ASsessment Tool) group recently proposed a set of 20 signaling questions across 4 domains (participants, predictors, outcome, and analysis) to assess the risk of bias and applicability concerns [389]. The intent is to support systematic reviews of prediction modeling studies, where it is important to examine the risk of bias and applicability to the intended population and setting. The 20 questions were based on expert opinion, and no support is available as yet that poor scores relate to poor validity (see Chap. 24). This is in contrast to therapeutic [679] and diagnostic [337, 480] studies, where specific design characteristics have been found to relate to bias.

Questions

19.1 Differences between populations (Table 19.1)
Consider a model that is developed with logistic regression analysis in a sample of 100 patients in a clinical setting. The model is validated in a screening setting.

(a) What would you expect for the event rate (prevalence of outcomes)?
One characteristic is measured more precisely in the screening setting, with a lower detection threshold for being labeled a "positive" predictor value. What differences would you expect with respect to:
(b) Case-mix, i.e., the distributions of predictor values
(c) Regression coefficients

19.2 Validity of a model
What would happen to the calibration and discrimination of a prediction model if

(a) units of measurement were wrong, e.g., mg/dl versus mmol/L?
(b) a simpler measurement device was used, with random deviations compared to the measurements in the development setting;
(c) a more heterogeneous case-mix was present in the validation setting;
(d) a treatment was used which was very effective for all patients;
(e) a treatment was used which was very effective for one subgroup;

19.3 Influence of case-mix on clinical usefulness
A less severe case-mix led to a higher Net Benefit than a more severe case-mix (NB 0.104 vs. 0.006, Fig. 19.3). How do you explain this finding?

19.4 Disturbance of calibration
We found that calibration was not disturbed when the validation setting consisted of (1) more or less severe patients according to predictor values, or (2) more or less heterogeneous patients according to observed or missed predictor values.

(a) What does disturb calibration-in-the-large?
(b) What does disturb the calibration slope?

19.5 Discrimination and clinical usefulness

(a) Why is discrimination a *necessary but not sufficient* condition for clinical usefulness?

19.6 Reference values for performance (Sect. 19.7)
Reference values indicate a model's performance under the condition that the model predictions are valid in the validation sample.

(a) How is it possible that the reference value for performance can be better than the performance estimate in the development setting?

19.7 Power of validation studies (Table 19.7)

Suppose we wish to detect a possible deterioration in calibration-in-the-large with an odds ratio of 1.5, and a calibration slope < 0.8.

(a) What sample size is required with 50% event rate for each of these performance measures?

(b) What sample size would you recommend?

Chapter 20
Updating for a New Setting

Background A prediction model ideally provides valid predictions of outcome for individual patients at another setting than where the model was developed, e.g., differing in time and place. The validity of predictions can be assessed by comparing observed outcomes and predictions when empirical data from this external setting are available. Various patterns of invalidity may, however, be observed as we have seen in Chap. 19. Detection of calibration-in-the-large problems should have top priority since miscalibration can cause systematically wrong decision-making with the model (negative net benefit). Obviously, we may subsequently aim to update the model to improve predictions for future patients from the new setting. We discuss several approaches for updating a previously developed model. The risk is that simply re-estimating all regression coefficients in a model might replace reliable but slightly biased estimates by unbiased but very unreliable ones, particularly if the validation data set is relatively small.

We start with considering updating methods that focus on recalibration (reestimation of the intercept, and/or updating of the slope of the linear predictor). Next, we turn to more structural model revisions (re-estimation of some or all regression coefficients, model extension with more predictors). For illustration, we consider case studies with updating of a previously developed logistic regression model, a regression tree, and a previously developed Cox regression model. We conclude that parsimonious updating methods may often be preferable to more extensive model revisions, which should only be attempted with relatively large validation samples, in combination with shrinkage or penalization of differences between the updated model and the previously developed model.

© Springer Nature Switzerland AG 2019
E. W. Steyerberg, *Clinical Prediction Models*, Statistics for Biology and Health, https://doi.org/10.1007/978-3-030-16399-0_20

20.1   Updating Only the Baseline Risk

The external validity (or generalizability) of model predictions is important when a previously developed model is applied in another setting, such as another medical center, and/or in a more recent time period. When empirical data are available, we can assess the external validity according to measures such as calibration and discrimination. Also, we may consider updating a previously developed model, such that the prediction model is adjusted to local and/or contemporary circumstances.

The first issue to consider is calibration-in-the-large. The mean observed outcome should be equal to the mean of the predicted outcomes; for a survival outcome, the number of observed deaths should agree with the predicted number. Calibration-in-the-large is controlled by the model intercept for continuous and dichotomous outcomes and by the baseline hazard function in a survival model. Several approaches can be followed to adjust the intercept for a new setting.

20.1.1   Simple Updating Methods

A simple approach is to consider the mean observed outcome in the new setting, and compare this to the mean of the development setting. The difference is used to update the baseline risk. This is a naïve Bayesian approach, based on a univariate comparison of outcomes incidences in the development and validation setting. This approach has been shown to work reasonably well in a number of case studies, suggesting that differences in mean outcome are often largely attributable to factors outside the model [92, 392].

Similarly, it is possible to present a prediction model with the explicit option to use a setting-specific intercept. An example is the score chart for operative mortality for elective aortic aneurysm surgery (Chap. 14) [555]. Another example is a model to guide the indication for a CT scan in patients with minor head injury [519]. The model was developed in a setting with 243 of 3181 (7.6%) presenting with intracranial traumatic lesions. The model was presented with a range from 2.5 to 15% for the "prior probability" of an intracranial traumatic lesion. Such a simple adjustment is directly applicable if the case-mix between development and validation samples is fully comparable with respect to the predictors in the model. A variant is to use the mean outcome and the mean of predictor values in the calculation of the required update of the intercept [348]. The intercept adjustment reflects differences between settings in other aspects than captured by the predictors; these were referred to as Z variables in the previous chapter, in contrast to the predictors X in the model.

A special case is infectious disease prediction, where seasonal patterns are important and epidemics occur. These background incidences have an impact on the intercept of prediction rules for infectious diseases [162, 455].

20.2 Approaches to More Extensive Updating

In addition to calibration-in-the-large, further aspects of calibration need to be considered. These may conveniently be studied in the context of a general recalibration model, where the linear predictor based on the previously developed model is the only covariate, as discussed in previous chapters [114]. This model has only two free parameters: intercept α and calibration slope $\beta_{overall}$. A simple updating method might focus on recalibration, i.e. that the updated model has a new intercept α and new regression coefficients based on the multiplication of the original coefficients with $\beta_{overall}$. This recalibration approach has been followed for updating of a previously developed model in the context of risk-adjustment [131, 272] and prediction [176, 380, 514, 623]. We may also consider more extensive updating methods ("model revision"), such as reestimation of regression coefficients of some or all predictor variables, [515, 584] and considering more covariables for the inclusion of the model ("model extension", following terminology proposed by Van Houwelingen) [623]. These approaches are illustrated in the following section with a case study in the GUSTO-I data.

20.2.1 Eight Updating Methods for Predicting Binary Outcomes

We consider 8 updating methods for predictions of binary outcomes (Table 20.1). For illustration, we assume that a previously developed logistic regression model is available with 8 predictors, but that 8 more are of interest as potential predictors for the validation setting. The described methods generalize to updating of any previously developed prediction model. The methods are ordered according to the number of parameters that are estimated for updating of the original model [536].

- **No updating**

  The first method is not to allow for any updating, that is to keep all regression coefficients fixed at their original value, including the intercept. The linear predictor lp for method 1 (lp_1) is calculated as

$$lp_1 = \alpha_{orig} + \beta_{orig} * X_{1..8},$$

where α_{orig} indicates the intercept from the original study; β_{orig} the regression coefficients from the original study; and $X_{1...8}$ the 8 predictors in the new (validation) sample. This method provides a reference upon which improvement should be obtained with any updating method.

Table 20.1 Updating methods considered for a previously developed TIMI-II logistic regression model with 8 predictors in GUSTO-I where 8 more predictors were available [536]

Nr	Label	Notation	Predictors considered	Parameters tested	Parameters estimated
	No updating				
1	Apply original prediction model	–	8	0	0
	Recalibration				
2	Update intercept	α	8	0	1
3	Recalibration of intercept and slope	α + calibration slope $\beta_{overall}$	8	0	2
	Model revision				
4	Recalibration + selective reestimation	$\alpha + \beta_{overall} + \gamma_{1..8\mid}$ $_{p \leq 0.05}$	8	8	2–9
5	Reestimation	$\alpha + \beta_{1..8}$	8	0	9
	Model extension				
6	Recalibration + selective reestimation + selective extension	$\alpha + \beta_{overall} + \gamma_{1..8\mid}$ $_{p \leq 0.05}$ $+$ $\beta_{9..16\mid}$ $_{p \leq 0.05}$	16	16	2–17
7	Reestimation + selective extension	$\alpha + \beta_{1..8} + \beta_{9..16\mid}$ $_{p \leq 0.05}$	16	8	9–17
8	Reestimation + extension	$\alpha + \beta_{1..16}$	16	0	17

- **Recalibration**

   The second and third methods are simple recalibration methods. Updating of the intercept α intends to correct "calibration-in-the-large", i.e. to make the average predicted probability equal to the observed overall event rate:

$$lp_2 = \alpha_{new} + lp_1.$$

   Hereto we may fit a logistic regression model in the validation sample with the intercept α as the only free parameter and the linear predictor lp_1 as an offset variable (i.e., the slope is fixed at unity).

   In method 3, we update both the intercept α and the overall calibration slope $\beta_{overall}$ by fitting a logistic regression model in the validation sample with lp_1 as the only covariable:

$$lp_3 = \alpha_{new} + \beta_{overall} lp_1.$$

   This method has also been labeled "logistic calibration" [227].

- **Model revision**

   Methods 4 and 5 reestimate more parameters in the model, referred to as "model revision". With method 4, we first perform method 3, and then test whether predictors have an effect that is clearly different in the validation sample. We hereto perform likelihood ratio tests of model extensions in a forward stepwise manner, considering the predictor with the strongest difference first. We may extend the revised model until all differences in predictive effects have $p > 0.05$ for each predictor (or another p-value, or use AIC). As a maximum, 7 predictors could be selected, since $\beta_{overall}$ was always included in the model. The number of estimated parameters could hence vary between 2 and 9. The linear predictor becomes

$$lp_4 = \alpha_{new} + \beta_{overall}lp_1 + \gamma_{1..8|p \leq 0.05} * X_{1..8|p \leq 0.05},$$

where a maximum of 7 out of the 8 predictors is selected, and γ_i indicates the deviation from the recalibrated coefficient: $\gamma_i = \beta_i - \beta_{overall}\, lp_1$. We estimate γ_i with a logistic regression model in the validation sample with the recalibrated linear predictor lp_3 as an offset variable (i.e. the slope is fixed at unity).

With method 5 we fit the 8-predictor model in the validation data:

$$lp_5 = \alpha_{new} + \beta_{new} * X_{1..8},$$

where α_{new} and β_{new} indicate the intercept and 8 regression coefficients for the validation sample. Note that method 4 falls in between method 3 and 5: if selection of γ_i is extremely stringent (p-value of 0), method 4 is equal to method 3 (no individual coefficients reestimated), and if selection is extremely liberal (p-value of 1), method 4 is equal to method 5 (all individual coefficients reestimated). We label method 4 recalibration + selective reestimation.

• **Model extension**

Methods 6–8 consider additional predictors: "model extension" methods. Method 6 is a variant of method 4: we recalibrate the original model with an intercept α and the overall calibration slope $\beta_{overall}$, and test 16 predictors for statistically significant effects. The linear predictor becomes

$$lp_6 = \alpha_{new} + \beta_{overall}lp_1 + \gamma_{1..8|p \leq 0.05} * X_{1..8|p \leq 0.05} + \gamma_{9..16|p \leq 0.05} * X_{9..16|p \leq 0.05},$$

where at most 15 out of the 16 predictors are selected.

Method 7 is a variant of method 5, where we reestimate the original model and selectively extend the model with more predictors $X_{9..16}$ that have statistically significant predictive effects in the validation sample:

$$lp_7 = \alpha_{new} + \beta_{new} * X_{1..8} + \gamma_{9..16|p \leq 0.05} * X_{9..16|p \leq 0.05}.$$

With method 8 we fit a model with 16 predictors, i.e., 8 from the original model and 8 additional predictors:

$$lp_8 = \alpha_{new} + \beta_{new} * X_{1..16}$$

20.3   Validation and Updating in GUSTO-I

For an illustration of updating methods, we consider a prediction model for patients with acute MI that was developed with logistic regression analysis in the TIMI-II trial [395]. This trial included 3339 patients treated in 50 US centers between 1986 and 1988 [583]. The model was developed with backward stepwise selection methods and some continuous predictors were dichotomized. Although these approaches may be considered quite suboptimal for model development [563], we might consider the "TIMI-II model" relevant for generating predictions in GUSTO-I.

The TIMI-II model included eight dichotomous predictors: shock, age > 65 years, high risk (anterior infarct location or previous MI), diabetes, hypotension (systolic blood pressure < 100 mmHg), tachycardia (pulse > 80 beats per minute), relief of chest pain > 1 h, female gender. The outcome was 42-day mortality, in contrast to 30-day mortality in GUSTO-I [1, 329]. We first validated this model in patients from the GUSTO-I trial (n = 40,830, Fig. 20.1).

20.3.1   Validity of TIMI-II Model for GUSTO-I

We note that the observed mortality in GUSTO-I is systematically lower than predicted (Fig. 20.1). This may be attributed to the slight difference in outcome definition (30-day mortality in GUSTO-I versus 42-day mortality in TIMI-II) and improvements in care for acute MI patients.

The validity is further assessed by comparing the regression coefficients between TIMI-II and GUSTO-I (Table 20.2). We note that the coefficients are reasonably

Fig. 20.1 Calibration plot of the TIMI-II model (developed in n = 3339) [395] to predict 30-day mortality after acute myocardial infarction in GUSTO-I (*n* = 40,830) [329]. Triangles are based on tenths of patients with similar predicted probabilities. The distribution of predicted probabilities is shown at the x-axis (vertical lines, stratified by 30-day status). We note that the predicted risks are systematically too high; e.g., the highest tenth has a mean predicted probability of 35% while the observed frequency is 27% [536]

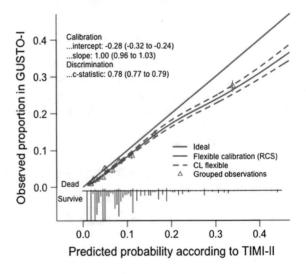

Table 20.2 Logistic regression coefficients ± standard error in the TIMI-II data and in parts of the GUSTO-I data [536]

Predictors	TIMI-II n = 3339	GUSTO-I Total n = 40,830	GUSTO-I US patients n = 23,034	GUSTO-I W region n = 2188	GUSTO-I Sample 5 n = 429
Shock	1.79 ± 0.29	1.60 ± 0.08	1.56 ± 0.11	2.39 ± 0.41	2.96 ± 0.92
Age > 65	0.99 ± 0.18	1.43 ± 0.05	1.34 ± 0.06	1.64 ± 0.22	1.37 ± 0.49
High risk	0.92 ± 0.26	0.71 ± 0.04	0.70 ± 0.06	0.85 ± 0.21	0.76 ± 0.50
Diabetes	0.74 ± 0.19	0.28 ± 0.05	0.31 ± 0.07	0.07 ± 0.25	−0.11± 0.64
Hypotension	0.69 ± 0.27	1.19 ± 0.06	1.19 ± 0.07	1.22 ± 0.25	1.39 ± 0.57
Tachycardia	0.59 ± 0.16	0.62 ± 0.04	0.61 ± 0.06	0.65 ± 0.20	0.88 ± 0.49
Time to relief	0.53 ± 0.20	0.50 ± 0.05	0.51 ± 0.06	0.26 ± 0.21	0.68 ± 0.54
Sex	0.47 ± 0.19	0.43 ± 0.04	0.47 ± 0.06	0.62 ± 0.20	−0.04 ± 0.51
Intercept	−4.47 ± 0.35	−4.82 ± 0.06	−4.84 ± 0.09	−5.09 ± 0.30	−5.19 ± 0.72

similar, although the coefficients of Age > 65 and Hypotension are somewhat larger in GUSTO-I, and those of Shock, High risk, and Diabetes smaller.

We further study the estimated coefficients in smaller parts of the GUSTO-I data set (Table 20.2). A total of 23,034 patients are included from the US. Within the US, 2188 patients are from the West region, including 429 patients in "sample 5". The logistic regression coefficient of diabetes is close to zero in the West region and negative in sample 5. The effect of sex has vanished in the smallest sample.

20.3.2 Updating the TIMI-II Model for GUSTO-I

We illustrate the application of the updating methods 2, 3, and 4 in Table 20.3. Corresponding to the observed miscalibration in Fig. 20.1, the intercepts are negative (around −0.3) when method 2 is applied, with somewhat more extreme estimates in the smaller validation sets. The corresponding odds ratios are between 0.63 in sample 5 (OR = e $^{0.47}$, $p = 0.03$) and 0.76 in the total GUSTO-I data set (OR = e $^{-0.28}$, $p < 0.001$), indicating that the predicted probabilities are approximately 1.3–1.6 times too high. The calibration slopes are close to 1 (method 3).

Method 4 updates the original model as in method 3 plus an estimation of coefficients that are clearly different from overall recalibrated values. We find that the differences in effects of Age > 65, High risk, Diabetes, Hypotension, and Tachycardia are statistically significant in the total GUSTO-I data set. No statistically significant deviations are observed in the smallest sample, obviating a clear need for reestimation of individual coefficients (Table 20.3).

The results of method 5, reestimating all model coefficients, were already shown in Table 20.2. For updating methods 6–8, 8 additional predictors are considered. These are height, weight, hypertension, smoking, hypercholesterolemia, previous angina, family history, and ST elevation in > 4 leads. These 8 additional predictors are to some extent correlated to the 8 TIMI-II predictors. In a 16-predictor model,

Table 20.3 Illustration of updating of the TIMI-II model in parts of the GUSTO-I data according to calibration methods (method 2 and 3) and model revision with statistically significant different coefficients (method 4)

	GUSTO-I Total n = 40,830	GUSTO-I US patients n = 23,034	GUSTO-I Region 1 n = 2188	GUSTO-I Sample 5 n = 429
Recalibration: Method 2				
α: intercept	-0.28 ± 0.02	-0.34 ± 0.03	-0.36 ± 0.09	-0.47 ± 0.22
Method 3				
α: intercept	-0.28 ± 0.03	-0.39 ± 0.05	-0.10 ± 0.16	-0.26 ± 0.47
$\beta_{overall}$: calibration slope	0.99 ± 0.02	0.98 ± 0.03	1.13 ± 0.09	1.11 ± 0.22
Model revision: Method 4[a]				
α: intercept	-0.76 ± 0.15	-0.62 ± 0.17	-0.25 ± 0.36	-0.26 ± 0.47
$\beta_{overall}$: calibration slope	0.91 ± 0.04	0.94 ± 0.04	1.14 ± 0.12	1.11 ± 0.22
γ_1: shock	+0	+0	+0	+0
γ_2: age > 65	$+0.53 \pm 0.06$	$+0.42 \pm 0.07$	$+0.49 \pm 0.24$	+0
γ_3: high risk	-0.12 ± 0.06	-0.17 ± 0.07	+0	+0
γ_4: diabetes	-0.39 ± 0.06	-0.38 ± 0.08	-0.79 ± 0.27	+0
γ_5: hypotension	$+0.56 \pm 0.07$	$+0.52 \pm 0.08$	+0	+0
γ_6: tachycardia	$+0.09 \pm 0.05$	+0	+0	+0
γ_7: time to relief	+0	+0	+0	+0
γ_8: sex	+0	+0	+0	+0

[a]The updated regression coefficients β_i can be calculated as $\beta_{overall} * \beta_{i,\ TIMI} + \gamma_i$

the 8 additional predictors are each statistically significant ($p < 0.01$) in the full GUSTO-I data set ($n = 40,830$) and the US part ($n = 23,034$), but their predictive effects are smaller than those of the 8 predictors from the TIMI-II model. In the West region, only weight and ST elevation have statistically significant incremental effects, while HTN and ST elevation had statistically significant effects in the smallest sample.

20.3.3   Performance of Updated Models

We hope that updating improves the performance of the prediction model. The calibration problem as noted in Fig. 20.1 is solved when the intercept is updated (all methods except method 1). The c index of the TIMI-II model was around 0.78 with methods 1–3 (Table 20.4). Updating of some (method 4) or all (method 5) of the coefficients led to a somewhat higher apparent discriminative ability (c around 0.80 in the larger samples). The extension of the TIMI-II model with more predictors increased the apparent discriminative ability further, although the increase was small in the total data set (from 0.79 to 0.80).

Table 20.4 Number of parameters estimated and apparent performance of updated versions of the TIMI-II model in parts of the GUSTO-I data. Results are shown for methods 1–8 as defined in Table 20.1

	Method	GUSTO-I Total n = 40,830	GUSTO-I US patients N = 23,034	GUSTO-I W region n = 2188	GUSTO-I Sample 5 n = 429
Parameters estimated	1	0	0	0	0
	2	1	1	1	1
	3	2	2	2	2
	4	7	6	4	2
	5	9	9	9	9
	6	17	13	5	3
	7	17	17	11	11
	8	17	17	17	17
Discrimination (c statistic)	1	0.782	0.780	0.795	0.776
	2	0.782	0.780	0.795	0.776
	3	0.782	0.780	0.795	0.776
	4	0.793	0.791	0.810	0.776
	5	0.793	0.790	0.819	0.793
	6	0.802	0.800	0.819	0.790
	7	0.802	0.800	0.828	0.828
	8	0.802	0.800	0.830	0.852

Since the apparent performance may be a severely optimistic estimate of performance in new patients, we studied the internal validity of the updated prediction models as identified with method 3, 5, and 8 for the smallest sample ($n = 429$). Models were developed in 500 bootstrap samples (drawn with replacement from the validation sample) and tested in the validation sample to estimate the optimism in apparent performance measures. The optimism was smallest for the 2-parameter model (method 3), and largest with the 17 parameter model (method 8), where discrimination was expected to decrease from 0.85 to 0.77. The highest internal validity was found for method 3, with optimism-corrected c 0.77. This suggests that a model with updating of fewer parameters may perform better in independent data than a more extensively updated model. This issue is systematically studied in Sect. 20.4.

20.3.4   *R Code for Updating Methods

We start with defining 2 models in the GUSTO-I sample (sample 5, n = 429):

```
full8s <- lrm(DAY30~SHO+A65+HIG+DIA+HYP+HRT+TTR+SEX,data=gustos,x=T,y=T)
fulls  <- update(full8s, .~.+HEI+WEI+HTN+SMK+LIP+PAN+FAM+ST4)
```

The 8 coefficients in TIMI-II model were

```
timi8.par <- c(-4.465, 1.79, 0.99, 0.92, 0.74, 0.69, 0.59, 0.53, 0.47)
```

For method 1, we calculate the linear predictor:

```
lp1 <- full8s$x %*% timi8.par[-1] + timi8.par[1]
```

For methods 2 and 3, we update the intercept or recalibrate the model:

```
lp2 <- lrm.fit(y=full8s$y, offset=lp1)$linear.predictor
lp3 <- lrm.fit(y=full8s$y, x=lp1)$linear.predictor
```

For method 4, we test for deviations of effects, while always updating the intercept and slope:

```
for (i in 1:8) # 8 predictors, examine each for different effect gamma
     {fit4 <- lrm.fit(y=full8s$y, x=cbind(full8s$x[,i], lp1))
     ... } # some printing of results of fit4
```

For methods 5 and 8, we simply refit the model

```
lp5 <- full8s$linear.predictor
lp8 <- fulls$linear.predictor
```

For methods 6 and 7 we again examine contributions of predictors beyond the effect of lp1. For example, method 7 works like

```
for (i in 9:16) # 8 more predictors, examine effects
     {fit7 <- lrm.fit(y=fulls$y, x=cbind(fulls$x[,i], full8s$x))
     ... } # some printing of results of fit7
```

20.4   Shrinkage and Updating

Traditionally, regression coefficients are shrunken towards zero (see Chap. 13). For model updating, we may consider shrinkage of regression coefficients of revised models towards their recalibrated values [536, 623]. This implies that some regression coefficients are pulled to higher values rather than towards zero.

In traditional model development, a simple heuristic shrinkage factor can be defined as (model $\chi^2 - df$)/model χ^2 (see Chap. 13) [109]. Here model χ^2 refers to the difference in -2 log-likelihood between a model with and without predictors, and df refers to the degrees of freedom used by the predictors. We can use the same formula in the context of model revision (method 4 and 5) and model extension (methods 6–8, Table 20.1). The model χ^2 then refers to the difference in -2 log-likelihood between a model with reestimated predictors and the recalibrated model, and df corresponds to the difference in degrees of freedom of these models. Regression coefficients can be pulled towards their recalibrated values as obtained with method 3. A motivation for this shrinkage approach was developed by Van Houwelingen and is presented at www.clinicalpredictionmodels.org.

20.4.1   Shrinkage Towards Recalibrated Values in GUSTO-I

We apply shrinkage towards recalibrated values as obtained with method 3 for the TIMI-II model, when applied in GUSTO-I. Re-estimated coefficients for the first 8 predictors are pulled towards $\beta_{overall} * \beta_{i,TIMI}$ with methods 4 and 5. The coefficients of the additional 8 predictors considered in methods 6–8 are shrunken towards zero, since these predictors were not included in the TIMI-II model. The intercept of the shrunken model was re-estimated to ensure that the sum of predicted probabilities equaled the sum of observed outcomes (in our case: deaths). When stepwise regression is applied to select predictors for the model, the degrees of freedom of the candidate predictors should be considered in the formula [227, 627].

As an alternative, we may shrink coefficients towards the original TIMI coefficients. This is also straightforward with penalized maximum likelihood for model re-estimation. Hereto we use the original model predictions as an offset variable in the re-estimated logistic regression model.

For illustration, we consider updating of the TIMI-II model for the West region in GUSTO-I ($n = 2188$, Table 20.5). Here, re-estimated coefficients were somewhat different from the recalibrated coefficients, with larger effects for Shock, Age, and Hypotension, and smaller effects for Diabetes and Time to relief. The recalibrated model χ^2 was 170, which increased by 24 to 194 for the re-estimated model. The traditional shrinkage factor is (model $\chi^2 - df$)/χ^2 = (194–8)/194 = 0.96. This factor is used to shrink coefficients towards zero. The recalibration shrinkage factor is (24–7)/24 = 0.71. This factor is used to shrink coefficients towards the recalibrated values:

$$\text{model5s} = \alpha_{new} + \beta_{overall} * \beta_{TIMI, 1..8} + s * \left(\beta_{West, 1..8} - \beta_{overall} * \beta_{TIMI, 1..8} \right);$$

Here, α_{new} is the new model intercept, $\beta_{overall}$ is the recalibration slope, $\beta_{TIMI, 1..8}$ are the 8 coefficients from the TIMI model, s is the shrinkage factor, and $\beta_{West, 1..8}$ are the coefficients optimized for the West region.

Table 20.5 Logistic regression coefficients in updated models for the West region of GUSTO-I ($n = 2188$)

Predictor	Reestimated	Recalibrated	TIMI	Shrunken towards			Penalized towards	
				zero	recal	TIMI	zero	TIMI
Shock	2.40	2.02	1.79	2.30	2.29	2.21	2.37	2.38
Age > 65	1.64	1.12	0.99	1.57	1.49	1.44	1.53	1.60
High risk	0.85	1.04	0.92	0.81	0.90	0.87	0.80	0.85
Diabetes	0.07	0.84	0.74	0.07	0.29	0.27	0.07	0.10
Hypotension	1.22	0.78	0.69	1.17	1.09	1.06	1.16	1.19
Tachycardia	0.65	0.67	0.59	0.62	0.65	0.63	0.61	0.64
Time to relief	0.26	0.60	0.53	0.25	0.36	0.34	0.25	0.28
Female sex	0.62	0.53	0.47	0.60	0.60	0.58	0.61	0.62

Shrinkage and penalization were applied towards zero or towards (recalibrated) values of coefficients from the TIMI-II model

Equivalently, we can write the shrunk model as a weighted sum of recalibrated and TIMI coefficients:

$$\text{model5s} = \alpha_{new} + s * \beta_{West,\,1..8} + (1-s) * \beta_{overall} * \beta_{TIMI,\,1..8}.$$

With $s = 0.71$, it is clear that the new model coefficients $\beta_{West,\,1..8}$ as estimated in the West region are more relevant than the coefficients $\beta_{TIMI,\,1..8}$ from TIMI (weight $1 - 0.71 = 0.29$).

We can also examine the improvement of re-estimated coefficients over using the original TIMI coefficients; this appears to be associated with an increase in model χ^2 by 27. With $df = 8$, the shrinkage factor towards the original TIMI coefficients becomes (model $\chi^2 - df)/\chi^2 = (27–8)/27 = 0.70$.

The final coefficients are surprisingly similar when shrunken to zero or pulled to recalibrated values. The largest discrepancy is for Diabetes, where the re-estimated coefficient was close to zero (0.07), while the recalibrated value was much higher (0.84, Table 20.5). Shrinkage towards zero leaves the coefficient at 0.07, but pulling towards the recalibrated value of 0.84 leads to a value of 0.29. Pulling towards TIMI-II coefficients leads to slightly smaller coefficients. Shrinkage towards zero is in the spirit of Bayesian analysis with an uninformative prior (coefficients are assumed to be zero); Pulling toward (recalibrated) coefficients assumes that the TIMI-II model is relevant for the new setting (coefficients are assumed to be close to the TIMI-II values).

For comparison, we examine results from penalized maximum likelihood procedures (Table 20.5). In the re-estimated 8-predictor model, the optimal penalty factor is 6. The same value is found when the TIMI coefficients are used as an offset variable in the logistic regression model. The resulting penalized coefficients in the standard formulation of the penalized model are quite similar to the "shrunken to zero" coefficients. When penalized towards TIMI-II values, all coefficients are slightly larger, and closer to the re-estimated coefficient values.

20.4.2 *R Code for Shrinkage and Penalization in Updating

We start with reestimating the 8-predictor model in the West region

```
full8        <- lrm(DAY30~SHO+A65+HIG+DIA+HYP+HRT+TTR+SEX,data=West,x=T,y=T)
```

The original TIMI coefficients are in linear predictor 1, lp1

```
timi8.par    <- c(-4.465, 1.79, 0.99, 0.92, 0.74, 0.69, 0.59, 0.53, 0.47)
lp1          <- full8$x %*% timi8.par[-1] + timi8.par[1]
```

Coefficients with traditional heuristic shrinkage are calculated as $(\chi^2 - df)/\chi^2$

```
s.orig        <- (full8$stats[3]-full8$stats[4]) / full8$stats[3]
full8.coef.s.orig <- s.orig * full8$coef[-1]
```

Shrinkage towards recalibrated values is calculated as

```
full3        <- lrm.fit(y=full8$y, x=lp1)  # recalibration model
model.chi2   <- deviance(full3)[2] - deviance(full8)[2] # delta χ2
df3          <- full8$stats[4]-full3$stats[4] # delta df (8-1=7)
s.recal      <- (model.chi2 - df3)/model.chi2 # shrinkage towards recal TIMI
coef.s       <- s.recal*full8$coef[-1] +       # wsum of full8 and recal TIMI
                (1-s.recal)*full3$coef[2]*timi8.par[-1]
```

Shrinkage towards TIMI-II values is calculated as

```
full8.off    <- update(full8, offset=lp1)  # offset model
s.off        <- (full8.off$stats[3]-full8.off$stats[4]) / full8.off$stats[3]
coef.s.off   <- s.off * full8.off$coef[-1] + timi8.par[-1]
```

Standard penalized maximum likelihood estimation is as

```
p            <- pentrace(full8, c(0,2,3,4,5,6,7,8,10,14,20), maxit=50)
full.p       <- update(full8, penalty=p$penalty)
```

Penalization towards TIMI-II values is calculated as

```
p.o          <- pentrace(full8.off, c(0,2,3,4,5,6,7,8,10,14,20), maxit=50)
full.o.p     <- update(full8.off, penalty=p.o$penalty) # optimum lambda 6
coef.o.p     <- full.o.p$coef + timi8.par
```

20.4.3   Bayesian Updating

Another approach, similar to shrinkage (see Chap. 13), is to use Bayesian estimation methods for model updating. We assume that the development and validation samples come from an underlying superpopulation with some heterogeneity between settings. We may attempt to use the estimated heterogeneity to obtain Bayesian estimates of updated coefficients. An updated intercept $\alpha_{updated}$ can be obtained with a simple formula [393]:

$$\alpha_{updated} = \alpha_{overall} + \tau^2 / \left(\tau^2 + \sigma^2_{estimated}\right) * \left(\alpha_{estimated} - \alpha_{overall}\right),$$

where $\alpha_{overall}$ is the overall mean estimate for the intercept; τ^2 is the variance between development and validation settings ("heterogeneity"); and $\alpha_{estimated}$ and $\sigma^2_{estimated}$ are the estimated intercept and its variance in the validation sample. A relatively large sampling uncertainty (large $\sigma^2_{estimated}$) implies substantial shrinkage for $\alpha_{estimated}$ towards the overall mean α. In contrast, large heterogeneity (large τ^2) implies that $\alpha_{estimated}$ is not much shrunken towards the overall mean α. The extreme is that τ^2 is infinity, i.e., each $\alpha_{estimated}$ is used as estimate for $\alpha_{updated}$. Every setting is considered as unique and should have its own intercept. The latter is implausible and argues for some form of Bayesian analysis. The challenge of such a Bayesian analysis is especially that we need to specify a value for τ^2.

A full Bayesian approach is to elicit τ^2 from experts; they may, for example, state that it is unlikely that the incidence of the outcome (adjusted for the prediction model) is more than 4 times lower or higher than the original incidence [202, 203]. Interpreting these limits as 95% credibility intervals means that $\tau \approx \log(4)/2 = 0.69$, and $\tau^2 = 0.48$. Stating that the limits are 2 times lower to 2 times higher incidence implies $\tau \approx \log(2)/2 = 0.35$, and $\tau^2 = 0.12$, leading to more shrinkage. The Empirical Bayes approach is to estimate τ^2 from the distribution of intercepts in different validation samples. This approach will be followed in Chap. 21.

In addition to the baseline risk, we can in principle consider all model parameters in a Bayesian framework, for example, the calibration slope or individual regression coefficients [128]. A previously developed model serves as a prior which is combined with new patient data using the likelihood function and Bayes rule to obtain posterior estimates of the regression coefficients in the prediction model [573]. If new data are observed, Bayes theorem can be used to update the prior distribution to a posterior distribution $\pi(\beta | \text{new data})$ using the likelihood of the observed data $l(\text{new data} | \beta)$

$$\pi(\beta | \text{new data}) = \frac{l(\text{new data} | \beta)\pi(\beta)}{\int l(\text{new data} | \beta)\pi(\beta)d\beta}$$

We may use independent normal distributions as prior distributions for the regression coefficients β of our prediction model with means from the previously developed model and a standard deviation of $\log(4)/2$. This means that we are 95%

sure that the regression coefficients in the new situation lie between ¼ and 4 times the original values on the odds scale [203]. The choice of prior variance determines the amount of shrinkage of the regression coefficients towards the mean of the prior distribution. We might also use the variance–covariance matrix of log odds ratios from the development sample, and multiply by the sample size of the development sample for an appropriate prior [573]. When applying the Bayesian approach the variance should align with the expected degree of heterogeneity between the development and update population.

20.5   Sample Size and Updating Strategy

The choice of updating method depends on various factors. The first requirement is that it is reasonable to apply the previously developed model in the new setting from a clinical point of view. The model should not evidently be overfitted, include predictors with plausible effects, and have been developed with adequate statistical methods given the sample size. Some other signaling questions are proposed in the PROBAST checklist [389]. The relevance of the model should be supported by reasonable validity in the sample from the new setting, i.e., some correlation should be present between predictions and outcomes. If this not the case, we should not consider updating methods, but may essentially consider the situation as developing a new model [626]. Also, the size of the development sample may have been too small to consider updating seriously. Possibly we can then start our updated model with the selection as considered in the previous model, but directly re-estimate coefficients (method 5, Table 20.1).

In the situation of a large development sample, we may have good confidence in the previously estimated regression coefficients. If we only have a small validation sample size, we should be modest in updating the model and recalibration may be sufficient (methods 2 and 3, Table 20.1). In contrast, if we have a large validation sample, more rigorous updating is reasonable. These hypotheses were examined in a large simulation study within GUSTO-I, following the design shown in Fig. 20.2.

20.5.1   *Simulations of Sample Size, Shrinkage, and Updating Strategy

Simulation studies were performed in GUSTO-I to increase our insights in the link between sample size and updating strategy (Fig. 20.2). Validation sample sizes ranged from $n = 200$ to $n = 1000$ in Fig. 20.3, and from $n = 1000$ to $n = 10,000$ in Fig. 20.4. We find that a modest improvement in discriminative ability was achieved by model reestimation and model revision (methods 4–8), if validation sample sizes are relatively large and shrinkage is used. But with a relatively small

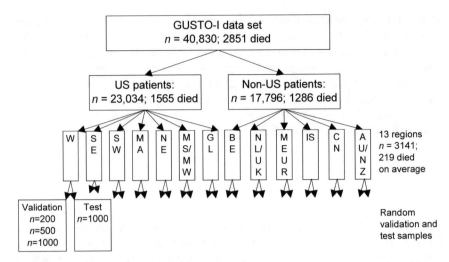

Fig. 20.2 Schematic presentation of the sampling design of a simulation study in GUSTO-I. The GUSTO-I data was split into 13 regions. The 7 US regions were West (W), South–East (SE), South–West (SW), Massachusetts (MA), New England (NE), Mid-South/Mid-West (MS/MW), and Great Lakes (GL). The 6 non-US regions were Belgium (BE), the Netherlands/United Kingdom (NL/UK), middle Europe—including France, Spain, Germany, Poland-(MEUR), Israel (IS), Canada (CN), and Australia/New Zealand (AU/NZ). Updating methods 1–8 were applied in random samples from each region with sizes of 200, 500, or 1000 patients. Updated models were tested in independent test samples with 1000 patients from the same region as where the validation sample originated from

validation sample, we should only attempt to improve calibration, i.e., with updating of the model intercept (method 2) and calibration slope (method 3). Shrinkage is essential to prevent overfitting in updated models from small validation samples (Figs. 20.3 and 20.5).

More extensive updating is beneficial if the previous model was based on a relatively small sample ($n = 500$ instead of $n = 3339$), while a relatively large validation sample was available (Fig. 20.5). See www.clinicalpredictionmodels.org for more details [536].

20.5.2   A Closed Test for the Choice of Updating Strategy

As discussed above, sample size is important to balance the amount of evidence for updating in the new patient sample and the danger of overfitting. An approximately closed test can be considered to define the extensiveness of the updating to increase progressively from a minimum (the original model) to a maximum (a completely revised model) [640]. The procedure involves multiple testing with maintaining approximately the chosen type I error rate. The closed test is similar to the testing

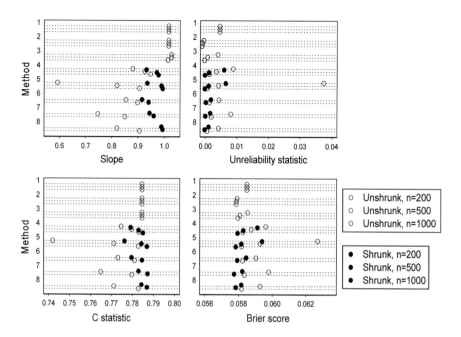

Fig. 20.3 Dotcharts showing the average results for 8 updating methods (numbers 1–8, Table 20.1) with or without application of shrinkage in the updating of regression coefficients. For methods 1–5, validation sample sizes were 200, 500, or 1000 (3 rows). For methods 6–8, validation sample sizes were 500 or 1000 (2 rows). Validation samples were drawn from 13 regions within the GUSTO-I study (Fig. 20.2). Slope: calibration slope; Unreliability statistic: chi-square test for calibration intercept and slope. Performance was determined in independent test samples with $n = 1000$

procedure in the setting of fractional polynomials [477]. The testing procedure consisted of the following steps for methods 5, 3, and 1 as discussed in Sect. 20.2.1:

1. Test the refitted model (*method 5*) against the original model (*method 1*); if the refitted model provides a significantly better fit: continue, otherwise keep the original model.
2. Test the refitted model (*method 5*) against the model with an updated intercept (*method 2*); if the refitted model provides a significantly better fit: continue, otherwise use the model with an updated intercept.
3. Test the refitted model (*method 5*) against the recalibrated model (*method 3*); if the refitted model provides a significantly better fit: use the refitted model, otherwise use the recalibrated model.

Standard statistical tests can be used for each step, such as the difference in the -2 log-likelihood between the models that are compared.

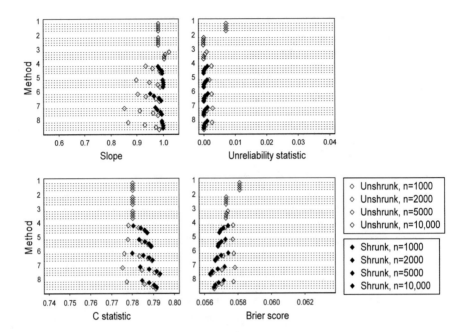

Fig. 20.4 Dotcharts showing the results of simulation studies in the US patients from the GUSTO-I study. Average results are shown for 8 updating methods (numbers 1–8), with or without application of shrinkage in the updating of regression coefficients. Validation sample sizes were 1000–10,000 (4 rows for each method), with test sample sizes of $n = 10,000$

20.6   Validation and Updating of Tree Models

Prediction models developed with CART methods, or recursive partitioning, are attractively presented as trees (see Chap. 4). Usually, predicted outcomes are presented for each branch. Validation can then be performed in different ways.

A radical validation approach is to redevelop a new tree in a validation sample, and compare the structure. For example, we redeveloped a tree for the survival of 456 testicular cancer patients with a poor prognosis according to the International Germ Cell Cancer Collaborative Group (IGCCCG) [616]. The statistically optimal tree was very different from the tree as developed in a sample of 332 German patients [310]. This approach to validation is similar to redeveloping a model with stepwise methods in a validation sample, if stepwise methods were applied in a development sample. It is highly unlikely that such a model building strategy results in the same selection of predictors (Chap. 11). Model redevelopment gives insight into the instability of the modeling procedure, but does not directly answer the question to what extent the outcomes in the validation data are adequately predicted by the old model.

A better validation strategy could be to accept the tree structure, but to re-estimate the predictions of the outcome. For a binary outcome, these estimates

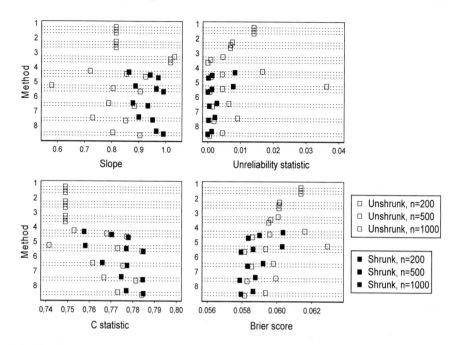

Fig. 20.5 Dotcharts showing the results of simulation studies with smaller development samples ($n = 500$ instead of $n = 3339$ for the original TIMI-II model). Average results are shown for 8 updating methods (numbers 1–8), with or without application of shrinkage in the updating of regression coefficients. For methods 1–5, validation samples contained 200, 500, or 1000 patients (3 rows). For methods 6–8, sample sizes were 500 or 1000 (2 rows)

are simply the observed frequencies of the outcome in the branches. This is analogous to updating *method 5* (model reestimation while accepting the model structure, see Sect. 20.2.1). An illustration is in Fig. 20.6. Survival was generally better at development than in the validation sample. A total of 125 patients was expected to have died by 2 years, while the observed number was 199 (i.e., 1.6 times more deaths). Some revision of the tree structure might be inspired by the validation findings. For example, no difference is noted between those with or without Abdominal metastases in Fig. 20.6 (53% vs. 56% 2-year survival). This split might be omitted for future predictions.

A more parsimonious strategy is to use a recalibration model, similar to method 3 (Table 20.1). For a binary outcome we model the outcome y as a function of a new intercept α and calibration slope $\beta_{overall}$:

$$y \sim \alpha + \beta_{overall} * \hat{y},$$

where y is the outcome, α the updated intercept, $\beta_{overall}$ the calibration slope, and $\hat{y}$ the predicted outcome by the original tree. If the outcome is binary, we may transform $\hat{y}$ to log(odds($\hat{y}$)); for survival outcomes we could use the log(cumulative hazard) of the Kaplan–Meier estimates at certain time points during follow-up: log

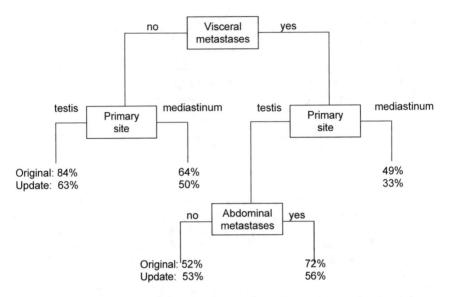

Fig. 20.6 Regression tree as developed for poor prognosis patients with non-seminomatous germ cell cancer. The 2-year survival is shown for the development sample ("Original", *n* = 332) and for the validation sample ("Update", *n* = 456) [616]

$(-\log(S(t|branch)))$, with $S(t|branch)$ indicating survival at time *t* in a branch of the tree. This approach preserves the relative effects, but updates the predictions to obtain calibration-in-the-large, and compensates for overfitting.

In the testicular cancer example, we assessed the calibration slope in the model:

$$\log(-\log(S_{IGCCCG}(t|branch))) = \alpha + \beta_{overall} * \log(-\log(S_{development}(t|branch))),$$

where $S(t|branch)$ refers to the observed Kaplan–Meier survival probabilities for tree branch, and $\beta_{overall}$ is the calibration slope. We found $\alpha = -0.19$, and $\beta_{overall} = 0.46$. The predictive effects in the IGCCCG data were hence much less than at model development ($\beta_{overall} < 1$), consistent with the hypothesis that the original tree was overfitted. This same pattern was noticed from a comparison of the discriminative ability. The *c* statistic was 0.63 at model development, and only 0.56 at validation.

20.7   Validation and Updating of Survival Models

Predictions of survival models involve a time dimension, e.g. for the fraction of patients surviving 1, 2, or 5 years after the start of follow-up. The most common prognostic model in medical research is the Cox proportional hazards model, which can combine multiple prognostic factors to predict survival at different time points:

$$S(t|X) = S_0(t)^{\exp(\beta X)},$$

where $S(t|X)$ denotes the probability of being alive at time t for a patient with predictors X; $S_0(t)$ denotes the baseline survival function for time t (usually for the average of predictor values), and βX indicates the linear predictor (multiplication of regression coefficients β with predictor values X). We can also write the survival function based on the baseline cumulative hazard $H_0(t)$ as $S(t|X) = \exp(-H_0(t) * \beta X)$. The baseline cumulative hazard $H_0(t) = -\log(S_0(t))$.

Hence, making predictions with the Cox model for individual patients requires that we know the baseline survival (or baseline cumulative hazard) function as well as the regression coefficients β [471].

- The full baseline survival function is usually not specified in publications, but sometimes survival at clinically relevant time points is provided (e.g. 1, 2, and 5-year survival). Also Kaplan–Meier curves can provide the baseline survival function graphically.
- The regression coefficients β are often provided in a table as hazard ratios (exp (β)). This makes it possible to calculate a linear predictor for new patients. Sometimes a simplified version of the model is presented as a "prognostic index", e.g., based on a sum score, or a count of the number of adverse prognostic factors.

In the following, we discuss a case study on updating of a survival model, where limited results were reported from the developed model, i.e., only 2- and 5-year survival estimates for four prognostic groups.

20.7.1 *Validation of a Simple Index for Cancer Survival

A Cox regression model for overall survival for aggressive non-Hodgkin's lymphoma was developed by an international group of investigators [2]. Five pretreatment clinical characteristics were considered: age, Karnovsky score, Ann Arbor stage, extranodal sites and LDH scores. The five predictors are dichotomized for use in the "international prognostic index" (IPI). The IPI score counts the number of unfavorable predictors. The more extreme categories 0 and 1, and 4 and 5 are combined, resulting in groups with IPI 1–4. The 2-year survival probabilities was reported to range from 34 to 84%, and the 5-year probabilities from 26 to 73% (Table 20.6).

The validity of the IPI was studied in a Dutch cohort from a population-based registry of non-Hodgkin's lymphoma patients [623]. Kaplan–Meier curves for each of the 4 IPI groups showed a clear separation, while the observed survival probabilities were lower than expected (Table 20.6). This discrepancy was attributed to the selection of patients: clinical trials at model development versus a population-based registry at model validation. The validation cohort was less selected, e.g., with respect to age.

Table 20.6 Validity of the original and updated IPI for a Dutch cohort of 426 non-Hodgkin's lymphoma patients

IPI	2-year survival			5-year survival		
	Original (%)	K–M (%)	Recalibrated (%)	Original (%)	K–M (%)	Recalibrated (%)
1 ($n = 148$)	84	78	78	73	61	58
2 ($n = 110$)	66	54	55	51	35	31
3 ($n = 85$)	54	39	41	43	15	23
4 ($n = 83$)	34	24	21	26	10	9

Updating was with Kaplan–Meier curves (Sect. 20.7.2) for the 4 IPI groups and a recalibration procedure (Sect. 20.7.3, for groups by time points) [623]

The Kaplan–Meier curves answer the qualitative question of whether the discriminative ability of the original model was retained in an external setting. More quantitative questions relate to calibration: is there as a systematic difference between predicted and observed survival for all IPI groups, and what is the predictive strength of the IPI in the validation setting? These questions were studied in the recalibration framework [623].

20.7.2   Updating the Prognostic Index

The observed Kaplan–Meier probabilities can be considered as updated estimates of survival for future Dutch non-Hodgkin's lymphoma patients (Table 20.6). However, this update only considers the grouping of the IPI. The Kaplan–Meier curves are nonparametric, and allow for nonproportional hazards of the IPI risk groups. Identical results can be obtained from a Cox regression model in the validation sample with the 4 IPI groups as strata.

Recalibration of the IPI probabilities is an alternative approach, which may be especially valuable in relatively small validation samples. The Dutch cohort of 426 patients may be considered too small for the Kaplan–Meier approach, since the standard error around the survival estimates in Table 20.6 is around 5%, with 95% confidence intervals of ±10% around the Kaplan–Meier survival probabilities in Table 20.6.

20.7.3   Recalibration for Groups by Time Points

Simple recalibration is possible for the 2 time points (2 and 5 years), comparing the predicted survival with the observed survival for groups of patients in a calibration model on the log hazard scale:

Table 20.7 Updating approaches for the IPI classification in non-Hodgkin's lymphoma

Method	Approach	Proportionality assumption and baseline hazard	β_{IPI}
–	Kaplan–Meier	Nonproportional, free	Free
2	Kaplan–Meier recalibration	Nonproportional, free	Original
3a	Cox, recalibrate IPI	Proportional, free	Recalibrated
3b	Weibull, recalibrate IPI	Proportional, recalibrated	Recalibrated

$$\log(-\log(S(t|g))) = \alpha + \beta * \log(-\log(S_{model}(t|g))),$$

where $S(t|g)$ refers to the observed Kaplan–Meier survival probabilities for the groups g, and $S_{model}(t|g)$ to the predicted survival probabilities for these groups. Setting β to 1 means that we accept the hazard ratios for the 4 IPI groups as estimated in the development data set. This is analogous to method 2 for logistic regression models (Tables 20.1 and 20.7).

With $\beta = 1$, Van Houwelingen reports that $\alpha = 0.37$ at 2 years, and $\alpha = 0.56$ at 5 years [623]. Hence, we make somewhat different corrections on the log hazard scale for the 2 time points. The recalibrated survival probabilities are shown in Table 20.6, calculated with the formula

$$S_{cal}(t|g) = \exp(-\exp(\alpha + \log(-\log(S_{model}(t|g))).$$

20.7.4 Recalibration with a Regression Model

A further validity assessment is to study the calibration slope $\beta_{overall}$ in a Cox regression model:

$$S_{cal}(t|\beta X) = S_{0,new}(t)^{\exp(\beta_{overall} * \beta X)},$$

where $S_{cal}(t|\beta X)$ refers to the recalibrated survival, $S_{0, new}(t)$ to the recalibrated baseline survival function, and $\beta_{overall}$ to the calibration slope for the linear predictor βX. A Cox regression with the linear predictor βX as the single covariable assumes proportional effects of the IPI during follow-up. The baseline hazard function is updated, and a calibration slope is identified to calibrate the linear predictor to the new setting. This approach is more or less analogous to method 3 for logistic regression models (Tables 20.1 and 20.7).

Such recalibration requires that we know the linear predictor for the 4 IPI classes. The original regression coefficients for the 4 IPI classes were not published, but we can approximate the coefficients from the published 2-year and 5-year survival probabilities [623]. Hereto we rewrite the Cox survival formula $S(t|X) = S_0(t)^{\exp(\beta X)}$ as $\log(-\log(S(t|X))) = \log(-\log(S_0(t))) + \beta X$.

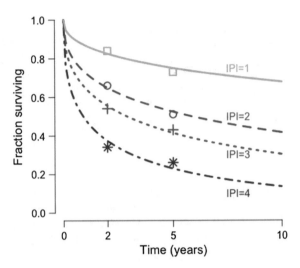

Fig. 20.7 Survival according to the International Prognostic Index (IPI) for non-Hodgkin's lymphoma patients. The reported 2- and 5-year survival probabilities are shown, with the Weibull approximation of survival with lines from 0 to 10 years of follow-up ("IPI-Weibull model") [623]

The Weibull model can be used for the baseline survival function $S_0(t)$, which specifies that $\log(-\log(S_0(t))) = \beta_0 + \beta_1 * \log(t)$. The Weibull model is attractive since it specifies the baseline survival with only 2 parameters. Other parametric models can also be used. The Weibull model reads like $\beta_0 + \beta_1 * \log(t_j) + \beta_i X_i$ with $j = 2, 5$ and $i = 1, 2, 3, 4$ for the 4 IPI groups. Since we do not have access to the original IPI data, we use a simple linear regression model to fit the parameters. The IPI-Weibull model becomes

$$\log(-\log(S_0(t))) = -0.319 + 0.439 * \log(t) + PI,$$

with PI = $-1.638; -0.824; -0.514;$ and 0 for IPI = 1–4, respectively. A reasonable fit is found for the observed 2- and 5-year estimates (Fig. 20.7). When this PI is used in a Cox regression model, the coefficient is 1.03 (SE 0.10). This indicates a very similar predictive effect of the IPI in the validation sample compared to the development sample [623]. More extensive approaches are discussed at www.clinicalpredictionmodels.org.

20.7.5   Summary Points

- The International Prognostic Index (IPI) could be updated in at least 4 ways with different freedom for the baseline hazard, with or without a proportionality assumption on the effect of the IPI, and with different assumptions on the validity of the previously estimated regression coefficients (Table 20.7).
- Kaplan–Meier estimates can be generated for the 4 IPI groups separately, which implies re-estimation of the baseline hazard, and new, separate effects for the relative effects implied by IPI.

- Kaplan–Meier estimates can also be used in a recalibration procedure per time point, preserving the original IPI effects.
- A Cox regression model can be used to re-estimate the baseline hazard, while recalibrating the IPI effects.
- A Weibull model can be used for a more parametric recalibration of the baseline hazard and the relative effects implied by IPI.

20.8   Continuous Updating

So far, we assumed that a validation sample with a fixed size was available for model updating. The updating strategy then depends, among other considerations, on the size of this validation sample, and on the size of the development sample. We can also imagine a more dynamic situation, where a previously developed model is applied in a new setting, with a continuous accumulation of patient numbers over time [514, 515, 573]. The prediction model might gradually adapt to the new setting as a self-learning system [119, 120]. It is reasonable to start with parsimonious updating methods, such as recalibration, and gradually move to model revision and model extension following the framework set out in Table 20.1.

The extensiveness of updating approaches can be guided by testing of specific model parameters, or by the closed test, as described in Sect. 20.5.2. A note of caution is that repeated testing as data accumulate implies multiple testing with a higher likelihood of rejecting the validity of the previously developed prediction model.

20.8.1   *Precision and Updating Strategy

The question is when to move on to more extensive updating in the dynamic situation with gradually increasing numbers of patients. We should not use more extensive updating methods too early, since updated predictions may then be unbiased but quite imprecise, and lead to poorer model performance instead of better performance for the new setting [536]. Statistically, we can try to set a minimum number of patients before thinking about updating the intercept. In Table 19.6, we reported standard errors (SEs) for the intercept for different sample sizes in the situation that the prediction model was fully valid for the validation setting. With 50 events among 100 or 500 subjects, the SEs were 0.24 and 0.17; with 100 events 0.16 and 0.13, respectively. So, if we would start early with updating the intercept, considerable variability would be introduced. A compromise is to consider statistical testing of the difference in the intercept. Testing is technically already possible after a few events have occurred. An important issue is the p-value to consider for updating; we may use $p < 0.05$ as a default selection rule, but we should feel free to use higher p-values, such as implied by Akaike's Information Criterion (AIC, equal to $p < 0.157$ with 1 df). This holds for a specific test for intercept updating and for the closed test (Sect. 20.5.2).

A similar discussion holds for the calibration slope. In Table 19.6 we found that the SE was between 0.10–0.15 for 50–100 events. Again, we may test for a deviation from the ideal value of 1, and requiring $p < 0.05$ before updating the slope. If the model was developed in a small sample, a slope below 1 is likely in the validation data, arguing for a higher p-value and/or a one-sided test for the alternative hypothesis "slope < 1".

20.8.2   *Continuous Updating in GUSTO-I

For illustration we consider continuous updating of the TIMI-II model in the West region of GUSTO-I. Tests for model improvement can be considered for increasingly complex models (Table 20.8). We consider the dynamic situation of increasing sample size for a self-learning system. Sample size refers in this context to the number of patients with predictors and the outcome known. In the GUSTO-I example, the outcome is 30-day mortality, which is hence known to the analyst without much delay. If a more long-term outcome is specified, e.g., 1-year survival, the delay is obviously longer before updating analyses can start. We arbitrary start testing for a difference in intercept from a sample size after including 100 patients in the validation sample, which implies at least approximately 7 events with an incidence of 30-day mortality of 7% in GUSTO-I. Inclusion is supposed to increase with calendar time. We note that the p-value for a different intercept is still high at $n = 100$ ($p = 0.64$ in this example, Fig. 20.8). The p-value decreases rapidly, to $p < 0.05$ at $n = 170$ in this example. The calibration slope is not statistically different from 1 in the full sample of $n = 2188$; in the dynamic situation, the p-value was over 0.50 for $n < 500$. From $n = 500$, we also start testing for model revision and model extension. The "model extension" method approaches statistical significance around $n = 650$, while model revision does so only at $n > 1500$ (Fig. 20.8). Around $n = 650$, we might only recalibrate the effects of the first 8 predictors, and extend the model with shrunken effects for 8 more predictors. Model extension is not statistically significant between $n = 700$ and $n = 2000$; with shrinkage of regression coefficients, the difference would anyway be small between

Table 20.8 Possible tests for model improvement in a dynamic updating strategy for the TIMI-II model in GUSTO-I

Method	Label	Parameter	df_{model}	$df_{model\ improvement}$
2	Update intercept	Intercept	1	1 (vs. TIMI-II model)
3	Recalibration	Intercept and slope	2	1 (vs. updated intercept)
5	Model revision	Reestimate coefficients	9	7 (vs. recalibrated model)
Closed	Closed test procedure	Reestimation/slope/ intercept	–	–
8	Model extension	Reestimation + extension	17	8 (vs. reestimated model)

Fig. 20.8 Continuous updating with accumulating numbers of patients in the West region from GUSTO-I. The *p*-value for the validity of the intercept is significant from *n* > 170; the *p*-value for the calibration slope does not reach significance even at *n* = 2188 (the total West region); model revision and model extension are statistically significant from *n* > 1500 and *n* > 2000

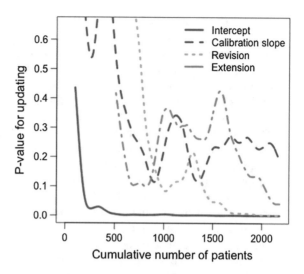

predictions with or without the 8 additional predictors. From *n* > 1500 we would re-estimate the effects of the first 8 predictors.

This example illustrates how continuous updating can be applied. Somewhat higher *p*-values might also be used for testing of updating parameters. We may furthermore rely on shrinkage methods to prevent "over-updating", just as shrinkage prevents overfitting in standard model development.

20.8.3 *Other Dynamic Modeling Approaches

Various alternative approaches are possible for dynamic model updating, including dynamic model averaging [447]. For example, an extended Kalman filter was applied in a case study to adjust the regression coefficients of a model describing the factors associated with the type of operation children with appendicitis received [370]. This approach is similar to Bayesian logistic regression, but also introduces a "forgetting" factor allowing older data to have less heavy weight compared to newer data when updating the model. In the empirical example, the dynamic model showed similar model fit to the best static models measured using the Brier score.

A challenge in methodological comparisons of updating approaches is that a fair assessment of validity should be performed for the updated model [575]. This is easy for the situation that we have two data sets: development and validation, where validation is repeatedly split in a part for updating and for testing (using cross-validation or bootstrapping). For a dynamic situation with a continuous accumulation of patient data, such validation is less straightforward. Overall, any more refined updating method, such as closed testing, Bayesian updating, and Kalman filtering, is expected to perform better than naïve refitting of a prediction model to be self-learning in the more recent data [575]. Some examples are discussed below.

- Three case studies were examined, which all confirmed that the closed testing procedure performed well [640]. The examples were on patients with prostate cancer, traumatic brain injury and children at risk of a serious infection presenting with fever. The need for updating the prostate cancer model was completely driven by a different model intercept in the update sample. Separate testing of model revision against the original model showed statistically significant results, but led to overfitting (calibration slope at validation = 0.86). The closed testing procedure selected recalibration in the large as update method, without overfitting. The advantage of the closed testing procedure was confirmed by the other two examples.
- Updating approaches have also been applied in prediction models for mortality after cardiac surgery [245, 514, 575]. Previously developed prediction models severely overestimated the mortality rates in more recent patients. All studied updating approaches showed similar performance at validation. Extensive updating methods should not be applied in smaller subgroups of type of surgery since these methods showed poor performance at validation, while recalibration and Bayesian approaches performed adequately.

- Another study considered yearly data from five international prostate biopsy cohorts (3 in the US, 1 in Austria, 1 in England) [573]. Six methods for annual risk updating were compared:

1. Static use of the online US-developed Prostate Cancer Prevention Trial Risk Calculator (PCPTRC; equivalent to *method 1* before);
2. recalibration of the PCPTRC (*method 3*);
3. revision of the PCPTRC; building a new model each year using logistic regression (*method 5*);
4. Bayesian updating;
5. Random forests (a variant of *method 5*).

All methods performed similarly with respect to discrimination, except for random forests, which performed worse. All methods except for random forests greatly improved calibration over the static PCPTRC. This case study confirmed that a simple annual recalibration of a general online risk tool for prostate cancer could improve its accuracy with respect to the local patient practice at hand.

- Machine-learning and more traditional regression-based models all benefited from dynamic updating in case studies on hospital-acquired acute kidney injury [120] and 30-day hospital mortality [119].

20.9 Concluding Remarks

Recalibration methods are attractive because of their stability, which is related to the fact that few parameters are estimated [114, 623]. The disadvantage of simple recalibration methods is a potential for bias in the individual regression coefficients.

In contrast, the model revision may lead to a lower bias but higher variance in the updated model, since more parameters are estimated [536]. Re-estimation of coefficients and model extension with new predictors should not be considered too early, since our simulations indicated that the predictive performance of an updated model can be worse than the original model (e.g. a lower discriminative ability) [536].

Some shrinkage or penalization is hence required. Bayesian and dynamic modeling approaches also effectively combine evidence from new data with an existing prediction model. Shrinkage methods in model updating may not only improve calibration, but also discrimination. This is in contrast to traditional model development, where shrinkage does merely improve calibration and has no substantial impact on discrimination. Note that the shrinkage factor is zero unless the chi-square is larger than the df used in model estimation ($s = $ (model $\chi^2 - df$)/ model χ^2). This sets an effective limit to the p-values for testing; e.g. with 8 df, the chi-square has to be larger than 8, which is equivalent to $p < 0.43$.

We can also envision a combination of selection and shrinkage of updated effects through the application of the LASSO. This would limit overfitting and accept the coefficients from the original model until sufficient evidence is gathered in support of differential effects.

From a clinical perspective, the key question is whether a previously developed model is reasonable to apply in a new setting. Some further examples are in Table 20.9. The question of applicability requires subject knowledge. From a statistical perspective, the sample sizes of both the validation data set and the development data set are crucial in the choice of an updating method. Our simulations in Figs. 20.3, 20.4 and 20.5 and other studies support the idea that substantial sample sizes are required before an improvement in discriminative ability is achieved by updating of regression coefficients.

A specific situation of model updating is that we consider a new predictor, which was not part of a previously developed model. For example, a new biomarker may be promising, with the prognostic value shown in a meta-analysis. If we know the correlation of this biomarker with traditional predictors, we may update the regression coefficients in a multivariable model with both the traditional predictors and the biomarker. An illustration is available for coronary heart disease [258]. If individual patient data are available, updating of a previously developed model with a biomarker may be achieved by imputation of the missing biomarker in those patients with missing values [405].

20.9.1 Further Illustrations of Updating

Approaches to validation and updating of prediction models have been applied in various medical studies. Extensive practical examples include

- A research line on increasingly improving the prediction of Lynch syndrome based on personal and family cancer history. An initial model ("PREMM1,2")

Table 20.9 Examples of updating of previously developed prediction models

Patients	Outcome	Development	Validation	Updating
Patients with suspect personal or family burden of cancer [40]	Lynch syndrome	First series of tested patients ($n = 898$)	Second series of tested patients ($n = 1016$)	Combined model with intercept from second series
Children with growth hormone deficiency [124]	Growth	Kabi Pharmacia International Growth Study database ($n = 593$)	Dutch Growth Foundation database ($n = 136$)	$\hat{Y}_c = \hat{Y}_o + (2.15 - 0.19 * \hat{Y}_o)$, where $\hat{Y}_c$ and $\hat{Y}_o$ are the calibrated and original predictions
Men undergoing prostatectomy for prostate cancer [562]	Indolent cancer	Clinical series ($n = 409$) [295]	European randomized study on screening for prostate cancer ($n = 247$)	Recalibration of intercept and rounding of coefficients for score chart
Patients with stable chest pain [176]	Coronary artery disease	Literature review	14 hospitals ($n = 2260$) and 18 hospitals ($n = 5677$)	Model revision was necessary to correct overestimation especially in women
Patients undergoing cardiac surgery [514]	In-hospital death	EuroSCORE database ($n = 13,302$) [404]	16 Dutch hospitals ($n = 95,240$)	Improved calibration-in-the large

was developed using logistic regression in a cohort of 898 individuals and subsequently prospectively validated in 1016 patients, with updating of the intercept [40]. This model was extended subsequently to PREMM1,2,6 [291] and PREMM5 [292], with some further updating attempts [193]. A large scale, international external validation was also performed [290], and assessment of impact in clinical practice [632].

- A model to predict growth in children with growth hormone deficiency was updated with Dutch data [124].
- Various studies focused on the validity and updating options for prediction models in the field of prostate cancer [405, 562, 573].
- Diagnosing coronary artery disease among patients with stable chest pain [176, 177] with some large scale validation studies [145, 178] and model extensions [144].
- Validation and updating of the EUROSCORE for prediction of in-hospital death after cardiac surgery [245, 514, 575].

Questions

20.1 Simple updating of model intercept
Suppose a model predicts an average operative mortality for elective aortic aneurysm surgery of 8%, but we observe 10 deaths out of 200 (5%) in another series from another hospital.

  (a) What would be the most naïve update of the model intercept?
  (b) What problems should be considered in such a naïve update?

20.2 Model updating framework (Table 20.1)
Which updating methods can be seen as nested models, i.e., that a next updating method is an extension of a previous, simpler, method?

20.3 Updating strategies (Table 20.1)
What updating strategy makes sense when major improvements in care have taken place

  (a) for all patients
  (b) for a subgroup of patients

20.4 Shrinkage and recalibration (Table 20.5)
We note that the shrunken coefficients for female sex are very similar, whatever method is applied (0.60, 0.60, and 0.58 for shrinkage towards zero, recalibrated coefficients, or TIMI coefficients, respectively). How is this possible?

20.5 Performance of updated models (Table 20.4 and Figs. 20.3, 20.4 and 20.5).
We note that the c statistic for method 8 (Reestimation + extension, 16 predictors) seems to perform best in all parts of GUSTO-I. Performance seems especially good in the smallest sample (sample5, $n = 429$, $c = 0.852$).

  (a) How do you explain this high apparent c statistic?
  (b) How is it possible that reestimation can lead to a poorer performing model at validation in independent patients (Fig. 20.3)?
  (c) Does consideration of 8 more predictors in methods 6–8 lead to better models compared to method 5 in Figs. 20.3, 20.4 and 20.5?

20.6 Continuous updating (Fig. 20.8)
In Fig. 20.8, we note that the p-value for updating of the intercept decreases quickly to small, statistically significant, values. How do you explain this pattern?

20.7 Validation and updating of a Framingham model
Consider the paper by D'Agostino on the validity of the Framingham risk function to other populations [118]. What is the essential strategy for validation and updating of predictions?

Chapter 21
Updating for Multiple Settings

Background Updating of a prediction model should be considered after validation for a single new setting as discussed in Chap. 20. We can also consider updating for a range of settings, such as multiple hospitals. We can consider such settings as parts of an underlying superpopulation. This makes the settings to some extent related, while on the other hand, patients are more similar within settings. We may first quantify the distribution of differences between settings, and subsequently update the model to setting-specific values considering this distribution. This approach is well possible with random effects models or Empirical Bayes estimation. We illustrate the approach for logistic regression models.

We may specifically be interested in differences between centers in the context of quality assessment. We illustrate some methods for estimation of differences and rank ordering between centers for patients with stroke ("provider profiling"), where adjustment for predicted risk is needed before meaningful interpretation is possible.

21.1 Differences in Outcome

21.1.1 Testing for Calibration-in-the-Large

We first concentrate on systematic differences between settings in outcome, reflected in calibration-in-the-large. We consider the situation of differences between hospitals in logistic regression models, and subsequently turn to survival models. For logistic regression models, we can simply include "hospital" as a categorical variable in a prediction model, and test for statistical significance of the differences between hospitals. Such an analysis can be performed without adjustment for predictors ("unadjusted", or "crude" comparison), or with adjustment for important predictors of outcome ("adjusted" comparison). The differences that remain after adjustment are of interest, both from the viewpoint of the applicability

© Springer Nature Switzerland AG 2019
E. W. Steyerberg, *Clinical Prediction Models*, Statistics for Biology and Health, https://doi.org/10.1007/978-3-030-16399-0_21

of a prediction model across centers, and from the viewpoint of provider profiling (the comparison of the quality across centers) [62].

A theoretical objection to this "fixed-effect" approach is that "hospital" is actually measured at a higher level than at the patient level. This argues for using a multilevel (or "mixed") model, where hospital is at the first level, and patients are considered within hospitals [131]. The hospital is defined as a random factor, and patient characteristics are considered as fixed factors (within hospitals). We then estimate the distribution of the random effects, and can test for significance of this distribution, i.e., that the distribution is wider than expected based on chance alone.

21.1.2   *Illustration of Heterogeneity in GUSTO-I

Several prediction models can be considered for application in patients suffering from an acute myocardial infarction (MI). We focus on the TIMI-II model, as defined before (Chap. 20). This model includes eight dichotomous predictors [395]. We apply the TIMI-II model in patients from the GUSTO-I trial, with special attention to the validity in geographic groups [539]. Patients were entered in GUSTO-I between 1990 and 1993 at 1 of 1082 participating hospitals in 14 countries. We distinguished 16 geographical regions within the GUSTO-I trial (Fig. 20.2): 8 in the United States, 6 in Europe (based on combinations of neighboring countries), and 2 other regions (Canada and Australia/New Zealand). These regions included on average 2552 patients and 178 deaths. Furthermore, we performed more detailed analyses based on geographically related groups of hospitals. The number of patients per hospital was too low for meaningful analyses at the hospital level (average $n = 38$, expected 2.4 deaths). Grouping resulted in 121 small and 48 large groups, consisting of on average 9 and 23 hospitals and at least 20 and 50 deaths, respectively. The distinction in 16 regions, 48 large groups, and 121 small groups were considered to study regional heterogeneity.

We first test for regional differences in logistic regression models that included dummy variables for each region or group of hospitals. All such tests were highly statistically significant, indicating that the regional differences in 30-day mortality could not reasonably be explained by chance (Table 21.1). We used the TIMI-II model in 2 ways: as an offset variable, and with refitting of the regression coefficients. With an offset, the regression coefficients were kept at the values as estimated in TIMI-II, and the intercept and center effects were the free parameters. We found slightly higher χ^2 statistics if the original TIMI-II coefficients were used (as shown in Table 21.1) rather than refitted coefficients (not shown).

Second, we test for regional differences in a random effects logistic regression model, where region or groups of hospitals are considered as a random factor, and the TIMI-II coefficients are considered in an offset variable. We may try to compare models with the random effect to models without the random effect, although some worry that the log likelihood may not be fair to compare. If a likelihood ratio test is calculated, a 2-sided p-value may be obtained by dividing by 2 [518].

Table 21.1 Testing for heterogeneity in mortality across groups in GUSTO-I, with adjustment according to the TIMI-II model. Groups refer to testing of intercept differences, slopes refer to testing of differential calibration slopes by group

	Groups	Groups as fixed effects	Slopes as fixed effects
Regions	16	$\chi^2 = 69$, 15 df, $p < 0.0001$	$\chi^2 = 18$, 15 df, $p = 0.24$
Large subsamples	48	$\chi^2 = 102$, 47 df, $p < 0.0001$	$\chi^2 = 53$, 47 df, $p = 0.25$
Small subsamples	121	$\chi^2 = 197$, 120 df, $p < 0.0001$	$\chi^2 = 117$, 120 df, $p = 0.56$

An advantage of the random effects model is that we can interpret the values of the heterogeneity between groups (variance: τ^2). The standard deviation (τ) reflects differences between groups on the original scale (here: the logistic scale), corrected for random noise. We find that τ^2 is around 0.025 (τ around 0.16). The heterogeneity was similar between small or large subsamples and between the 16 regions. The between center variance can be expressed in various ways, including the median odds ratio for logistic regression models [24], and the median hazard ratio for survival differences [32].

21.1.3   Updating for Better Calibration-in-the-Large

If differences in outcome between centers are relevant (e.g., statistically significant and with substantial magnitude), we may want to update the prediction model with center-specific estimates of the intercept [626]. In the traditional, fixed effects, approach we could simply use the intercepts per center after adjusting for patient characteristics as center-specific estimates (Table 21.2). These estimates may often be quite unstable, and show a relatively wide distribution. This will especially occur when many small settings are considered, i.e., with relatively few patients and/or events.

Alternatively, we consider the hospital effects as a distribution, commonly specified as a normal distribution with a mean and standard deviation reflecting the heterogeneity between hospitals. This leads to Empirical Bayes (EB) estimation (Table 21.2) [626]. The formula for EB adjusted center effects is [393]

$$\alpha_{EB} = \mu + \tau^2/(\tau^2 + \sigma_i^2) * (\alpha_i - \mu),$$

Table 21.2 Approaches for testing and estimation of differences between settings to correctly estimate average outcomes

Approach	Testing	Estimation
Fixed effects	Setting as categorical variable	Adjusted intercepts
Random effects	Heterogeneity across settings	Empirical Bayes (direct or two-step)

where μ is the overall mean estimate; τ^2 is the variance between settings ("heterogeneity"); and α_i and σ_i^2 are the estimated hospital-specific intercepts and their variances. The traditional fixed effect estimates α_i are shrunken towards the overall mean μ. The extent of shrinkage depends on τ^2 and σ_i^2. A relatively large sampling uncertainty (large σ_i^2) implies substantial shrinkage for α_i towards the overall mean μ. In contrast, large heterogeneity (large τ^2) implies that α_i is not much shrunken towards the overall mean μ. An infinite value for τ^2 implies that the fixed effect estimates α_i are used as estimates for α_{EB}. Every setting is then considered as unique and needs its own intercept.

21.1.4   Empirical Bayes Estimates

There are two broadly applied approaches to EB estimation: a direct, one-step, and a two-step approach [83]. The direct approach is to use a random effects model, where the distribution of random effects and the updated intercepts are estimated in one step. This model may have difficulties in the joint estimation of random effects for multiple differences between centers. For example, we may want to estimate heterogeneity in both intercept and calibration slope, but find that the model estimation does not converge.

The two-step approach starts with a traditional fixed effect analysis of between center differences. We may choose one large center as the reference category for comparison of intercepts, but preferably we compare differences to the average outcome. Technically, this can be achieved by studying each center while including an offset variable based on predictions for all centers. For each center, we obtain an estimate of the difference to the average outcome, and a standard error (SE). For the second step, we use the center-specific estimates as outcomes in a linear random effects model for continuous outcomes, with weights according to the variance of the fixed effect estimates. With this second step, we estimate the heterogeneity between centers for use in the EB formula. The uncertainty in determining the heterogeneity is ignored in this two-step procedure, while it is included in the direct approach. Several examples of the two-step approach are available for medical prediction problems [83, 518, 539, 626].

21.1.5   *Illustration of Updating in GUSTO-I

We may wonder how large the differences between centers are relative to each other, and whether a simple overall update of the intercept from the TIMI-II model would be sufficient in GUSTO-I [539]. We use the TIMI-II model as an offset variable for updating in the GUSTO-I data.

With a fixed effects approach, we estimate the difference in intercept for each group within GUSTO-I compared to the predicted log odds from TIMI-II. We also

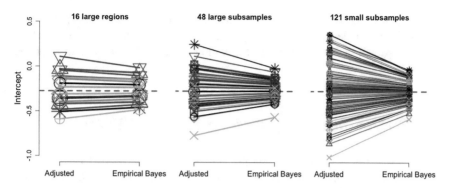

Fig. 21.1 Updating of intercepts of the TIMI-II model for subsamples in GUSTO-I. The overall intercept adjustment is –0.27 (dotted line - - -). We note a substantial variability in fixed effect adjusted intercept estimates for the smaller groups (121 small subsamples), which are shrunken towards the average with Empirical Bayes estimation in a random effects model. Also among the 16 regions, we note that smaller regions have more shrinkage of their model intercepts towards the overall intercept

obtain standard errors for these differences. The R code is shown in Sect. 21.4. With a random effects model (e.g., `glmer` function in the `lme4` package in R), we can directly obtain EB estimates of the intercepts per group.

We find that the overall intercept should be updated with the value –0.27. Regional differences as estimated with traditional fixed effect methods were substantially reduced in the Empirical Bayes estimation, whether 16 regions, 48 large subsamples, or 121 small subsamples were considered (Fig. 21.1). The EB estimates for the two extreme regions are –0.49 and –0.02, while the fixed effect estimates are – 0.59 and +0.11. Hence, we would traditionally estimate that one region had a much lower mortality than observed in TIMI-II (–0.59), and one region a slightly higher mortality (+0.11). With EB estimation, these estimates are shrunken towards the average of –0.27. Not surprisingly, these two extremes had the smallest and second smallest sample size among the regions. The same patterns are observed for groups of hospitals, with shrinkage to values between –0.56 and –0.02 for large and between – 0.58 and –0.002 for small subsamples. We can conclude that a substantial part of the variability in adjusted intercepts of the smaller groups can be attributed to chance. Adjusted estimates correct for case-mix differences according to the TIMI-II model, while EB estimates additionally adjust for chance.

21.1.6   Testing and Updating of Predictor Effects

Next to the intercept, an obvious question is whether the effects of predictors differ by setting. A simple approach is to test for interactions between predictor effects by setting. This is the traditional fixed effects approach. We can also consider the effect of one or more predictors as having distributions across settings in a random effects model.

It is more parsimonious to study interactions by setting for the linear predictor of the prediction model, since the linear predictor summarizes the effects of predictors. The assessment of heterogeneity in calibration slope is also possible in a random effects model.

21.1.7   *Heterogeneity of Predictor Effects in GUSTO-I

We study the calibration slope for the (log odds of the) TIMI-II predictions of 30-day mortality for regional groups in GUSTO-I. We hereto use the linear predictor based on the TIMI-II model as the only predictor for updating in the GUSTO-I data.

We find that the calibration slope should be updated to the value 1.00; overall, there is no need for updating of the slope. In a fixed effect analysis, we test interactions with groups and find that there is overall no such interaction within GUSTO-I (Table 21.1). This finding is confirmed in random effect models, where a very small distribution is estimated around the overall recalibration slope. The EB estimates of the slopes are very close to the overall slope of 1.00.

In addition, we tested for fixed effect interactions of effects of individual predictors by group, e.g., age * setting, and shock * setting [539]. None of these overall tests for interaction were statistically significant, suggesting that is it reasonable to assume a single effect of each predictor across the geographical areas in GUSTO-I.

We conclude that the variability in the effects of predictors is small in GUSTO-I. Hence, no updating by group is necessary beyond the simple update of the model intercept (with –0.27). This small variability may potentially be explained by the fact that predictors were registered according to uniform definitions, were relatively objective characteristics with limited measurement error (e.g., age), and that the quality of data collection was controlled well in this large-scale trial. Indeed, neither did we find heterogeneous predictor effects in a registry of 14,857 heart failure patients [31]. In contrast, comparisons across less controlled settings may show less consistency with respect to the effects of predictors, e.g., in meta-analyses of studies with quite different definitions of predictors.

21.1.8   *R Code for Random Effect Analyses in GUSTO-I

The essential R code for some of the random analyses in GUSTO-I is shown below, with a full script at the web.

```
library(lme4)     # linear and generalized linear random effect models
timi8.par <- c(-4.465, 1.79, 0.99, 0.92, 0.74, 0.69, 0.59, 0.53, 0.47)
full8 <- lrm(DAY30~SHO+A65+HIG+DIA+HYP+HRT+TTR+SEX, data=gusto, x=T)
lp1   <- full8$x %*% timi8.par[-1] + timi8.par[1] # lp1 based on TIMI-II
```

Test differences between regions (Table 21.1).

Fixed and random effects with lp1 (including TIMI-II coefficients) as offset for 16 regions:

```
full.o       <- glm(gusto$DAY30~1, offset=lp1, family=binomial) # α -.27
full8.REGL.o <- glm(gusto$DAY30~gusto$REGL,offset=lp1,family=bin) # fixed
fullr.REGL.o <- glmer(gusto$DAY30~1+(1|gusto$REGL), offset=lp1,
                    family=binomial) # random effects for region
```

Estimate calibration slopes between centers (Table 21.1).

```
full8.REGL.lp <- lrm(DAY30~as.factor(gusto$REGL)*lp1, data=gusto) # fixed
fullr.lp.REGL <- glmer(DAY30~lp1 + (1|REGL) + (0+lp1|REGL),
                    family=binomial, data=gusto) # α -.27, β 1.00
```

21.2   Provider Profiling

The applicability of prediction models across centers requires an assessment of differences between centers [30, 31]. Differences between centers are also central in comparisons of the quality of centers as part of provider profiling[408]. Provider profiling often includes outcomes such as mortality and morbidity, but may also include measures such as patient satisfaction, and organizational issues such as procedures and processes of delivering care [135]. In addition to testing and estimation of differences between centers, a specific aspect of provider profiling is that we may want to rank centers according to their performance in league tables [189]. Such ranking would enable patients and other stakeholders to choose the best provider for a specific health problem. Moreover, a relatively poor performance might be an incentive for a provider to critically review the processes of care delivery, and stimulate improvements. Such feedback should lead to a continuous quality improvement [556]. Provider profiling according to the outcome is surrounded by many methodological problems [367, 407, 505, 507, 518, 539]. Observational data are analyzed, which generally need to be interpreted with more caution than an experimental study. Some argue that we should concentrate on the direct measurement of adherence to clinical and managerial standards [338]. If we aim to compare outcome across centers, two methodological issues are essential: (1) case-mix adjustment and (2) dealing with statistical uncertainty.

1. Case-mix adjustment should appropriately capture differences between centers in patient characteristics that are outside the influence of actions in the center. Instead of predictors, we now consider these patient characteristics as confounders, since they may be both related to setting and outcome. Some centers may treat more severe patients, which hampers a fair comparison with a center with less severe patients. We want to compare centers after adjusting for confounding factors. Choosing an appropriate adjustment model is not easy, and may be limited by the type of data that is available. For example, administrative databases may not include all potential confounders, and have problems in coding. For example, postoperative complications may be miscoded as comorbidities [224]. Moreover, end points assessment is often nonstandardized [506].

2. Second, substantial differences between centers may appear in traditional, fixed effect analysis, with or without adjustment for confounders. But this picture is noisy. We have seen that EB estimation is a more conservative solution, compensating for the randomness in the fixed effect analysis. EB estimates hence allow for a better interpretation of any differences between centers that remain after adjustment for case-mix [338, 367, 407, 505, 507, 518, 539].

21.2.1 Ranking of Centers: The Expected Rank

The first attempts of provider profiling already included league tables: rankings were made for physician-specific mortality after coronary artery bypass grafting surgery in New York State [199]. There is ample experience with the ranking of schools [189]. Ranking is also very popular in the lay press [660].

Many argue that the uncertainty in differences between centers needs to be reflected in such league tables. The key problem with ranking is that one center has to be first and one has to be last. One approach was illustrated for league tables of in vitro fertilization clinics, where the uncertainty in rank was indicated with a 95% confidence interval around the rank [367]. If ranking is very noisy, the confidence intervals are very wide.

Another approach is to use expected ranks [320, 624], which is similar to the idea of using a median rank from a distribution of ranks [189]. The expected rank is determined by the probability that the performance at center i is better than at another center j: $P(\alpha_{EB, i} > \alpha_{EB, j})$. We use the EB estimates of differences α_i and α_j, since these are considered better reflections of any true differences between centers. Practically, we can calculate this probability from the standardized difference in performance estimates:

$$(\alpha_{EB,i} - \alpha_{EB,j}) / \sqrt{(var(\alpha_{EB,i}) + var(\alpha_{EB,j}))}.$$

We take the sum of these probabilities over all comparisons with centers j : $\sum P(\alpha_{EB,i} > \alpha_{EB,j})$, where j $\neq$ i. The expected rank ER is estimated as

$$ER_i = 1 + \sum P(\alpha_{EB,i} > \alpha_{EB,j})$$
$$= 1 + \sum \Phi(\alpha_{EB,i} - \alpha_{EB,j}) / \sqrt{(var(\alpha_{EB,i}) + var(\alpha_{EB,j}))},$$

where j $\neq$ i, and Φ is the normal distribution function. We assume that low values of α_{EB} are good; if the low value is quite certain, the rank should be close to 1. Indeed, we note that if the summed probability that center i has worse outcomes than any other center j is low, the rank remains close to 1. If this probability is high, the rank becomes high (poor performance). Such ranking is possible if the differences $\alpha_{EB,\ i} - \alpha_{EB,\ j}$ are large relative to the SE of this difference ($\sqrt{var(\alpha_{EB,i}) + var(\alpha_{EB,j})}$). If the standardized differences are close to zero, this corresponds to overlap between posterior probability intervals, and expected ranks are around the mid-rank.

For better interpretation, we can scale the expected ranks ER between 0 and 100%:$PCER_i = 100 * (ER_i - 0.5) / Ncenters$,

where PCER stands for "PerCentiles based on Expected Ranks". The $PCER_i$ can be interpreted as the probability that the performance in center i is better than in any randomly selected other center. If the ER is 1 for a center, this indicates a much better performance than the other centers. If the comparison is with 9 other centers (Ncenters = 10), the PCER becomes 5%; if the comparison is with 99 other centers (Ncenters = 100), the PCER becomes 0.5%. The definition, hence, accounts for the discrete nature of the number of centers.

In summary, the ER and PCER incorporate both the magnitude of the difference of a particular center compared to other centers and the uncertainty in this difference. These measures for ranking need further empirical support for their applicability. We illustrate the ranking of centers in a case study of outcome after stroke, after considering traditional and EB estimation for between center differences.

21.2.2 *Example: Provider Profiling in Stroke

We consider differences in outcome between 10 hospitals in the Netherlands [341]. The participating sites comprised 1 small (<400 beds), 4 intermediate (400–800 beds), and 5 large centers (>800 beds). Two centers were university hospitals. All but 1 hospital had a stroke unit, 8 were participating in a regional stroke service, and 9 were equipped for thrombolytic therapy. The sample consisted of 505 patients with complete data on potential confounders and outcome. The distributions of age and stroke subtype varied substantially by hospital (Table 21.3).

Table 21.3 Characteristics of 10 hospitals treating 505 patients with acute brain ischemia

Hospital	n	Age (years)	Sex (male) (%)	Stroke subtype (Brain infarction) (%)	Poor outcome (%)
1	39	77	46	97	59
2	92	73	54	95	72
3	31	69	61	97	35
4	41	65	59	80	44
5	22	74	55	91	73
6	24	65	67	63	29
7	99	68	65	94	39
8	37	70	41	92	78
9	50	71	56	88	54
10	70	72	47	81	46
Total	505	71	55	89	53

At 1 year, 268 (53%) patients had a poor outcome (dead: $n = 143$, Rankin scale score 3, 4, or 5: $n = 125$). The fraction of patients with a poor outcome varied between centers in unadjusted analysis, with apparently best results in hospital 6 (29% poor outcome) and worst in hospital 8 (78%, Table 21.3). These differences were highly significant in a traditional fixed effects analysis of differences between hospitals ($\chi^2 = 48$, 9 df, $p < 0.0001$, Table 21.4), and were partly explained by a higher age of patients in hospitals with worse outcome. For example, hospitals 2, 5, and 8 had over 70% poor outcome, but mean ages of 73, 74, and 70 years (Table 21.3). Adjusting for all 12 potential confounders led to halving of the differences seen in unadjusted analysis ($\chi^2 = 23$ instead of 48, Table 21.4). This pattern was also seen in the random effect analysis, where the estimated τ^2 (indicating heterogeneity between centers) with adjustment for 12 confounders was half that of the unadjusted τ^2 (0.17 vs. 0.34).

Table 21.4 Traditional fixed effect and Empirical Bayes (EB) estimates for differences in poor outcome between 10 hospitals, adjusted for 12 confounders. Values are logistic regression coefficients

Hospital	n	Unadjusted $\chi^2 = 48$	Adjusted $\chi^2 = 23$	EB_{adj} $\tau^2 = 0.17$
1	39	0.24	−0.29	−0.18
2	92	0.81	0.24	0.31
3	31	−0.72	0.32	−0.49
4	41	−0.37	−0.39	−0.22
5	22	0.86	0.91	0.3
6	24	−1.01	−0.47	−0.19
7	99	−0.55	−0.15	−0.11
8	37	1.17	1.16	0.53
9	50	0.04	0	0
10	70	−0.29	−0.09	−0.07

21.2.3   *Estimating Differences Between Centers

We can estimate the differences between centers in logistic regression models, where we compare each center to the average. The traditional fixed effects change considerably between an unadjusted and an adjusted analysis with 12 confounders. Hospital 1 seems to perform relatively poorly in unadjusted analysis (positive coefficient), while an adjusted analysis indicates that this hospital performs relative good (negative coefficient, Fig. 21.2). Changes for other hospitals were only noted quantitatively, without changing sign, with adjusted differences generally closer to zero. Further changes were seen with Empirical Bayes estimation of differences. All differences were reduced, especially for smaller centers (e.g., hospital 5: deviation +0.91 to +0.33).

The uncertainty around the estimated differences between centers is indicated in Fig. 21.2 for the adjusted and Empirical Bayes (EB) analyses. We note that EB estimation does not affect the point estimate nor the confidence interval for the larger centers, such as hospitals 2 and 7. For smaller centers, such as hospitals 5, 6, and 8, the point estimates for the deviation from the average are shrunken, and the confidence intervals smaller. None of the centers has a deviation that is significantly away from zero in the EB estimation, while the overall heterogeneity is statistically significant (Table 21.4).

Differences between centers can be summarized in a median odds ratio (MOR) [322]. The MOR is defined as the median of the odds ratios for two patients with the same covariates from different hospitals, comparing the patient at higher risk of the outcome and the patient at the lower risk of the outcome. The MOR hence reflects the typical difference between providers. Differences in risk may be quantified by the cluster-specific random effects, assuming a normal distribution:

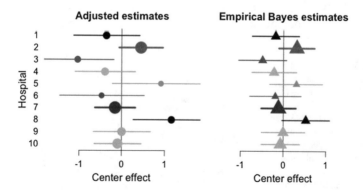

Fig. 21.2 Differences in poor outcome between 10 centers with traditionally adjusted, fixed effect, estimates, and Empirical Bayes estimates. We note that estimates of relatively small centers (e.g., 5, 6, and 8) are shrunk substantially towards to average with EB estimation

$$MOR = \exp\left(\sqrt{(2\tau^2)} \times \Phi^{-1}(0.75)\right),$$

where $\Phi - 1(0.75) = 0.6745$; the 75th percentile of a standard normal distribution [24]. For the stroke patients, τ^2 was estimated as 0.17, and hence, the MOR was exp $(\sqrt{(2 * 0.17)} * 0.67) = \exp(0.39) = 1.48$. Hence, in half such comparisons, the odds of poor outcome would be less than 1.5 for a patient at the hospital at higher risk compared to a similar patient (with the same predictor values) at the hospital at lower risk.

We can also consider ranges for the effect distribution (τ^2), e.g., the 95% range $[-1.96 * \tau$ to $+1.96 * \tau]$. We then find that the best centers at the 2.5% percentile would have 0.45 times the average risk, and the worst centers at the 97.5% percentile 2.2 times the average risk, so a 95% range of 0.45–2.2 for the odds ratio of poor outcome after acute brain ischemia (a fivefold difference).

21.2.4   *Ranking of Centers*

We can rank hospitals in unadjusted, adjusted and EB analyses (Fig. 21.3). The EB analyses are preferable for estimation of the magnitude of differences between hospitals. Ranking of hospital based on EB estimates does, however, not circumvent the problem that one hospital has to be at the top and one at the bottom of a league table. We should also incorporate the uncertainty in the ranking, since there can still be substantial variability in the EB estimates of differences between hospitals. We, therefore, may consider the Expected Rank (ER) and Percentile Expected Rank (PCER) of each hospital (formulas in Sect. 21.2.2) [320, 624].

The Expected Rank (ER) can be calculated with consideration of the probability that a hospital is worse than any other hospital. Figure 21.3 shows that this approach leads to shrinkage of the ranks towards the median rank of 5.5 for the 10 hospitals [344]. Hospital 8 has rank 10 (poorest performance) in unadjusted, adjusted and EB analyses, but the ER or EPC is 9.1 or 9.2, respectively, meaning that approximately 1 out of 10 centers is expected to be worse than this center

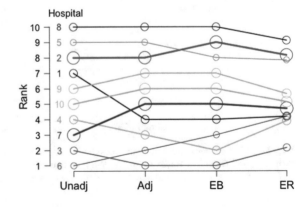

Fig. 21.3 Ranks of the 10 hospitals in unadjusted, adjusted, Empirical Bayes (EB) analyses, and the Expected Rank (ER). Dot size is based on the square root of the sample size per hospital. According to all analyses, hospital 8 ranks as the poorest. Hospital 6 seemed to do best in unadjusted analysis (rank 1), shifted to rank 2 in adjusted analysis, to rank 3 in EB analysis, and has an ER around 4

(Fig. 21.3). Hospital 6 seemed to do best in unadjusted analysis (rank 1), shifted to rank 2 in adjusted analysis, to rank 3 in EB analysis, and has an ER around 4.

We can also express these shrunk ranks on a 0–100% scale in the PCER. Hospital 8 has a PCER of 86%, which means that there is a 86% probability that the performance in hospital 8 is worse than any randomly selected other center. Hospital 6 has PCER 36%. Hospital 3 ranks highest, with PCER 17%, meaning that there is only 17% probability that any randomly selected other center is better than this center. Note that all these estimates are under the implausible assumptions that the statistical model is fully correct, the data are reliable, and that no residual confounding is present.

21.2.5   *R Code for Provider Profiling

Some of the R code for the analyses in the stroke example is shown below; a full script is available at www.clinicalpredictionmodels.org. We use the lme4 library in R; many other implementations are available, which may give different results with small sample sizes [335].

Estimate differences between centers (Table 21.4) and rank centers (Fig. 21.3).

```
# Fit a full model 12 predictors (only patient characteristics)
full <- lrm(RANKI1J2~AGE+ ... 11 char,data=cva)
# Use offset for effect estimation; approximate; not fully correct
full.ZH.o <- glm(cva$RANKI1J2~cva$ZHCLUCO, offset=full$linear.predictors,
                 family=binomial) # chi2 22.7, p=0.007
# with random effect: tau 0.396; lme4 package
fullr.ZH.Laplace.o <- glmer(RANKI1J2~(1|ZHCLUCO),
offset=full$linear.predictors, family=binomial, data=cva)

# posterior center effects
coef(fullr.ZH.Laplace.o)[[1]][,1] # coef
# the SE of the posterior center effects can be extracted
attr(ranef(fullr.ZH.Laplace.o,condVar=TRUE)$ZHCLUCO,"postVar") # SE


ER  <- rep(NA,10) # Expected Rank (ER)
for (i in 1:10) { # coef and SE are in Rtable
ER[i] <- 1+ (sum(pnorm((Rtable[i,1] - Rtable[,1][-i]) /
                       sqrt(Rtable[i,4]^2+Rtable[-i,4]^2)))) }
ER # 10 ranks: [1] 4.13 8.50 1.96 ...
PCER   <- 100*(ER-0.5)/10 # Percentile Expected Rank

# Results for Fig 21.3
      unadj adjusted EB   ER   EPC
      unadj adjusted EB   ER   EPC
[1,]    7           4   4 4.18 4.03
[2,]    8           8   9 8.15 8.05
[3,]    2           1   1 2.16 2.10
...
```

21.2.6   Guidelines for Provider Profiling

Some guidelines have been suggested for statistical methods for public reporting of health outcomes. A list with seven preferred attributes of the statistical modeling was suggested [315]:

(1) clear and explicit definition of patient sample,
(2) clinical coherence of model variables,
(3) sufficiently high-quality and timely data,
(4) designation of a reference time before which covariates are derived and after which outcomes are measured,
(5) use of an appropriate outcome and a standardized period of outcome assessment,
(6) application of an analytical approach that takes into account the multilevel organization of data,
(7) disclosure of the methods used to compare outcomes, including disclosure of performance of risk-adjustment methodology in derivation and validation samples.

Attributes 1–5 are more general in nature than attributes 6 and 7 [505]. We have focused in this chapter on the latter 2 attributes, especially attribute 6 ("multilevel organization of data", implying random effects analysis and EB estimation) [24, 32, 407, 408].

21.2.7   Concluding Remarks

We started this chapter with some considerations on the local applicability of prediction models. Specifically, we studied the influence of place of treatment ("center") on calibration of predictions. Calibration-in-the-large can be improved by adjusting the intercept in a regression model. The intercept is equivalent to the baseline hazard function in a survival model. The two main approaches to updating of the baseline risk are a fixed effect and a random effects approach.

If we consider only one specific setting, a fixed effect approach is most natural, although we might also perform some type of Bayesian updating of the intercept (see Chap. 20). If we consider multiple settings, such as multiple hospitals, Empirical Bayes updating has advantages, as illustrated with the GUSTO-I and stroke examples. Many more applications have been published over recent years. EB estimation is attractive whether we update the intercept, calibration slope, or effects of individual predictor effects per center.

There may be some confusion about naming and notation in traditional and random effect models. We refer to adjusted estimates in line with standard epidemiological nomenclature, where crude estimates are synonymous to unadjusted, fixed effect estimates. Furthermore, random effects models are also known as mixed effect models, hierarchical, or multilevel models. A random effects model for between center differences may also be labeled a "random intercept model with common slopes" for the predictor effects.

The methodological issues around multicenter applicability of prediction models are very similar to issues in provider profiling. For provider profiling, we assume that the predictor effects are identical across settings, similar to traditional confounder correction in epidemiology. This is similar to assuming a "global model" in meta-analysis of prediction models: predictor effects are assumed to be common across settings while the baseline risk may vary [83]. If predictor effects differ by setting, the comparison between settings becomes conditional on the specific values of the predictor, similar to the interpretation of predictive effects in the presence of statistical interaction. The randomness of estimates per setting can also be included in the ranking, as was illustrated with the "Expected Rank" and related measures.

Finally, we note that many of the assessments of heterogeneity between hospitals, regions, or other types of clusters are similar to assessments of heterogeneity between studies in the context of a meta-analysis. In meta-analysis, the minimum conditioning is for study, equivalent to allowing the baseline risk to vary across prediction models. More flexibility can be considered in meta-analyses of prediction models, by allowing the calibration slope to vary by study, and even the predictor effects. The focus in meta-analyses may be on summary estimates of predictor effects, while we focused here primarily on the validity of the predictions from the model across multiple settings.

21.2.8   *Further Literature*

Accurate registration and case-mix adjustment have received substantial attention in debates around provider profiling. The issues of estimation of differences and ranking under uncertainty have only more recently received more attention. Indeed, the uncertainty in estimates per center has a large impact on the interpretation of provider profiling attempts. A summary measure may be to estimate "rankability": $\tau^2/(\tau^2 + \text{median}(\sigma)^2)$ [618]. This measure is an example of a variance partition coefficient (VPC), where various variants have been described of the form $VPC = \tau^2/(\tau^2 + \sigma^2)$ [24]. Such VPC measures may assist in interpreting between center differences, in addition to measures such as the median odds ratio (MOR) [322]. Austin and others caution against naïve interpretation of the change in between center heterogeneity with and without predictors: the nonlinear nature of logistic and Cox regression models makes that τ^2 can increase if predictors are added to a model that are associated with risk in poorer performing centers [24].

Individual centers are often too small to reliably determine whether they are an outlier (either good or bad) [24, 33, 166, 339, 408, 409]. The uncertainty in per center estimates can be examined in various ways, including bootstrapping [189]. Various graphical possibilities have emerged to indicate performance while taking into account uncertainty. One key presentation is the funnel plot [526]. Funnel plots avoid spurious ranking of centers into league tables by plotting control limits around the estimated performance based on the precision of the estimates [498]. Furthermore, the performance of a center over time can be monitored in a CUSUM graph [211].

Questions

21.1   Heterogeneity across GUSTO-I (Table 21.1)

   (a) The estimate of regional variability, τ^2, is larger when we consider
        the smaller subsamples (0.033 versus 0.025 for regions). What
        might be an explanation for this larger τ^2?
   (b) How do you explain the much larger spread between adjusted,
        fixed effect, intercepts between the 121 small subsamples com-
        pared to the 16 regions? Why are these shrunk more?
   (c) Consider a subsample where we estimate a logistic regression
        coefficient of 0.4 for the difference to the (adjusted) average
        outcome (SE of estimate: 0.5, traditional fixed effect analysis).
        What is the EB estimate if the heterogeneity τ^2 across centers is
        0.2, 0.5, or 2? Use the formula from section 21.1.3 for α_{EB}.

21.2   Provider profiling (Sect. 21.2)

   (a) Mention at least two key problems of ranking providers, such as
        hospitals.
   (b) Why is ranking especially difficult for relatively small hospitals?

21.3   Case-mix adjustment (Table 21.3)
       Verify (1) that centers with a many good outcomes of stroke had mostly
       lower aged patients in Table 21.3, and (2) that case-mix adjustment halves
       the apparent heterogeneity between centers in Table 21.4.

21.4   Rankability of stroke outcomes

   (a) The heterogeneity in the stroke outcomes is substantial and sta-
        tistically significant (Table 21.4). Nevertheless, the Expected
        Ranks of quite some centers are close to the median rank of 5.5 in
        Fig. 21.3. How do you explain this modest rankability?
   (b) Calculate the rankability according to the formula $\rho = \tau^2 / \tau^2 +$
        median(s^2), with s^2 indicating the between center variance. Use
        the τ^2 estimate from Table 21.3. Use Fig. 21.2 to determine the
        median(s) (and median(s^2)).

Part IV
Applications

In this final part, we apply the framework to model development and validation as set out in parts II and III to two case studies. In Chap. 22, we discuss prediction modeling for patients with an acute myocardial infarction as enrolled in the GUSTO-I trial. In Chap. 23, we present a case study on prediction in survival data, with the extra complication of model selection in multiply imputed data sets. Finally, we give some practical advice on the main issues in prediction modeling, discuss reporting guidelines (specifically: TRIPOD), and describe the medical problems used throughout the text with the available data sets (Chap. 24).

Chapter 22
Case Study on a Prediction of 30-Day Mortality

Background Binary outcomes are encountered in many medical prediction problems, including diagnostic problems (presence of disease) and prognostic outcomes (occurrence of complications, short-term mortality). In this book, one key example of a binary outcome is 30-day mortality in patients suffering from an acute myocardial infarction. A prediction model was developed in over 40,000 patients from the GUSTO-I trial. We review the development of this model according to the seven steps of the checklist for developing valid prediction models presented in Part II. Moreover, we discuss the design and results of a number of methodological studies that were performed in the GUSTO-I data set.

22.1 GUSTO-I Study

22.1.1 Acute Myocardial Infarction

Acute myocardial infarction ("heart attack") is caused by the formation of a clot in one of the coronary arteries that supply blood to the heart muscle. Acute MI is a major public health problem. Mortality is substantial in the period immediately after the event, and also during the years after surviving the initial infarction. Some patients die before reaching the hospital. Patients seen in hospitals are reported to have an average mortality within 30 days around 6–15%, with improvement over time [316].

The risk of 30-day mortality strongly depends on various prognostic factors (Table 22.1). In younger patients, risks are much lower than in older patients. Other patient demographics are also important (gender, length, weight), as well as the presence of risk factors (hypertension, diabetes, smoking, family history) and the history of previous cardiovascular events (previous MI, angina, stroke, bypass surgery). Relevant presenting characteristics include the location of the infarction and the extent of ECG abnormalities. Very important is the acute state of the patient

© Springer Nature Switzerland AG 2019
E. W. Steyerberg, *Clinical Prediction Models*, Statistics for Biology and Health, https://doi.org/10.1007/978-3-030-16399-0_22

Table 22.1 Categories of predictors for 30-day mortality in acute MI [329]

Categories	Examples
Demographics	Age, sex, weight, height, geographical site
Risk factors	Diabetes, hypertension, smoking status, hypercholesterolemia, family history of MI
Other history	Previous MI, angina, cerebrovascular disease (e.g., stroke), bypass surgery, angioplasty
Cardiac state	Location of infarction, electrocardiogram abnormalities
Presenting characteristics	Systolic and diastolic blood pressure, heart rate, left ventricular function (e.g., presence of shock, Killip class)

as reflected by blood pressure, heart rate, and left ventricular function (e.g., presence of shock).

22.1.2 *Treatment Results from GUSTO-I

Various drugs and treatments are nowadays available for acute MI, including drugs that attack the clot ("thrombolytics") and acute revascularization, such as percutaneous interventions ("PTCA") [297]. GUSTO-I is one of the major randomized controlled trials that compared alternative treatments for acute MI. Specifically, the comparison was on efficacy of four intravenous thrombolytic regimens [1]. Earlier studies had shown that a new and more expensive thrombolytic drug, tissue plasminogen activator ("tPA"), restored blood flow through the coronary arteries more quickly and more often than alternative drug regimens. The hypothesis in GUSTO-I was that tPA would show a 1% absolute reduction in 30-day mortality [1]. Treatments in the three other arms included streptokinase (SK), an older and less expensive thrombolytic drug, which was given with two different regimens of heparin (a drug that helps keep the coronary artery open after the initial breakup of the clot by a thrombolytic drug), and a combination of tPA and streptokinase. The trial enrolled 41,021 patients admitted to 1081 hospitals in 15 countries. The trial convincingly showed a benefit of tPA treatment ($p < 0.001$).

The GUSTO-I trial provides a rich and unique source of information. Various substudies have been reported, often in major general and cardiovascular journals. The large number of patients from all over the world make for a good base to draw reliable conclusions. GUSTO-I has, hence, contributed to major progress in our knowledge of acute MI.

22.1.3 Prognostic Modeling in GUSTO-I

In the GUSTO-I trial, a comprehensive set of prognostic factors was collected, which was first used for prognostic modeling by Dr Kerry Lee at Duke University,

representing a team of GUSTO-I investigators [329]. The Lee et al. paper in
Circulation is quite extensive compared to other prognostic studies published in
medical journals. It provides many statistical details on several predictive modeling
issues for logistic regression [329]. The paper is freely available from the
Circulation website [328]; the Abstract is in Box 22.1. We review the paper with
the model development checklist (Table 22.2).

Table 22.2 Checklist for developing valid prediction models applied to the GUSTO-I analysis by
Lee et al. in Circulation [328, 329]

Step	Specific issues	GUSTO-I model
General considerations		
Research question	Aim: predictors/prediction?	Both
Intended application	Clinical practice/research?	Clinical practice
Outcome	Clinically relevant?	30-day mortality
Predictors	Reliable measurement? comprehensiveness	Standard clinical workup; extensive set of candidate predictors
Study design	Retrospective/prospective? cohort; case control	RCT data: prospective cohort
Statistical model	Appropriate for research question and type of outcome?	Logistic regression
Sample size	Sufficient for aim?	>40,000 patients; 2851 events: excellent
Seven modeling steps		
1. Preliminary	Inspection of data Missing values	Table 1 (here: Table 22.3) Single imputation
2. Coding of predictors	Continuous predictors Combining categorical predictors Combining predictors with similar effects	Extensive checks of transformations for continuous predictors Categories kept separate
3. Model specification	Appropriate selection of main effects? Assessment of assumptions (distributional, linearity and additivity)?	Stepwise selection Additivity checked with interaction terms, one included
4. Model estimation	Shrinkage included? External information used?	Not necessary No
5. Model performance	Appropriate measures used?	Calibration and discrimination
6. Model validation	Internal validation including model specification and estimation? External validation?	Bootstrap and 10-fold cross-validation No external validation
7. Model presentation	Format appropriate for audience	No; formula in appendix; later paper focused on clinical application
Validity		
Internal: overfitting	Sufficient attempts to limit and correct for overfitting?	Large sample size, predictors from literature
External: generalizability	Predictions valid for plausibly related populations?	Large set of predictors, representing important domains; not assessed in this study

Box 22.1 Predictors of 30-Day Mortality in the Era of Reperfusion for Acute Myocardial Infarction: Results From an International Trial of 41,021 Patients. Lee et al., Circulation 1995; 91:1659–1668 [328, 329]

Background Despite remarkable advances in the treatment of acute myocardial infarction, substantial early patient mortality remains. Appropriate choices among alternative therapies depend on an estimate of the patient's risk. Individual patients reflect a combination of clinical features that influence prognosis, and these factors must be appropriately weighted to produce an accurate assessment of risk. Prior studies to define prognosis either were performed before the widespread use of thrombolysis or were limited in sample size or spectrum of data. Using the large population of the GUSTO-I trial, we performed a comprehensive analysis of relations between baseline clinical data and 30-day mortality and developed a multivariable statistical model for risk assessment in candidates for thrombolytic therapy.

Methods and Results For the 41,021 patients enrolled in GUSTO-I, a randomized trial of four thrombolytic strategies, relations between clinical descriptors routinely collected at initial presentation, and death within 30 days (which occurred in 7% of the population) were examined with both univariable and multivariable analyses. Variables studied included demographics, history and risk factors, presenting characteristics, and treatment assignment. Risk modeling was performed with logistic multiple regression and validated with bootstrapping techniques. Multivariable analysis identified age as the most significant factor influencing 30-day mortality, with rates of 1.1% in the youngest decile (<45 years) and 20.5% in patients >75 (adjusted $\chi^2 = 717$, $P < 0.0001$). Other factors most significantly associated with increased mortality were lower systolic blood pressure ($\chi^2 = 550$, $P < 0.0001$), higher Killip class ($\chi^2 = 350$, $P < 0.0001$), elevated heart rate ($\chi^2 = 275$, $P < 0.0001$), and anterior infarction ($\chi^2 = 143$, $P < 0.0001$). Together, these five characteristics contained 90% of the prognostic information in the baseline clinical data. Other significant though less important factors included previous myocardial infarction, height, time to treatment, diabetes, weight, smoking status, type of thrombolytic, previous bypass surgery, hypertension, and prior cerebrovascular disease. Combining prognostic variables through logistic regression, we produced a validated model that stratified patient risk and accurately estimated the likelihood of death.

Conclusions The clinical determinants of mortality in patients treated with thrombolytic therapy within 6 h of symptom onset are multifactorial and the relations complex. Although a few variables contain most of the prognostic information, many others contribute additional independent prognostic information. Through consideration of multiple characteristics, including age, medical history, physiological significance of the infarction, and medical treatment, the prognosis of an individual patient can be accurately estimated.

22.2 General Considerations of Model Development

22.2.1 Research Question and Intended Application

The title of the paper mentions "Predictors of 30-day mortality ...", and indeed insight in prognostic effects is an aspect that receives much attention in this paper. But the text also states that the goal of the study was to develop a multivariable statistical model "with patient data routinely collected at initial presentation that would be clinically useful in managing patients who are candidates for thrombolytic therapy" [329]. So, research questions relate both to insight in the relevance of predictors and to obtaining predictions, as is common in prediction research [508]. "Managing patients with acute MI" likely refers to making appropriate decisions among alternative therapies, including the more expensive thrombolytic drug (tPA) and the cheaper drug (streptokinase). The authors argue rightly that these choices should depend on an estimate of the patient's risk. This issue is further expanded on in a subsequent paper by Califf et al. [86]. The key role of baseline risk for decision-making is illustrated on acute MI treatment by thrombolytics in at least two other publications [184, 298].

The authors provide statements on the requirements for such a prognostic model: "To be broadly useful, a risk-assessment algorithm should include all clinically relevant prognostic indicators and should be derived from a population that represents the types of patients seen in clinical practice so that stable estimates of true risk relations can be assessed. A useful model should appropriately weight clinically relevant predictors and be validated in a population with a broad spectrum of patients and hospital settings". According to the authors, the GUSTO-I trial data set fulfills these requirements.

22.2.2 Outcome and Predictors

The outcome was 30-day mortality. This is a "hard" end point, and it was the primary end point in the analysis of treatment efficacy in this trial [329]. For decision-making on therapy, mortality, and quality of life in the longer term may be more relevant. The gain by using a more expensive thrombolytic drug (tPA) is then reflected in a better (quality adjusted) life expectancy [60].

The study considers many potential predictors. A comprehensive set of approximately 25 characteristics was considered, based on subject matter knowledge (input from expert clinicians, literature). An overview of the main characteristics is provided in Table 22.3, with their relations to 30-day mortality in univariate logistic regression analyses.

Table 22.3 Illustration of the effects of some key prognostic factors in predicting 30-day mortality in acute MI. The χ^2 statistics are based on the difference in -2 log likelihood between a logistic regression model with one predictor and a model without the predictor

Predictor	Overall n = 40,830		Deaths n = 2,851		Unadjusted χ^2
	Median [25–75p]		Median [25–75p]		
Age (years)	62 [52–70]		72 [64–78]		2099 (1 df)
Systolic BP (mmHg)	130 [112–144]		120 [100–140]		733 (1 df)[a]
	n	col%	n	row%	
Killip					1388 (3 df)
I	34,825	85%	1,773	5.1%	
II	5,141	13%	716	14%	
III	551	1.3%	181	33%	
IV	313	0.6%	181	58%	
Location of infarction					354 (2 df)
Anterior	15,900	39%	1,582	9.9%	
Inferior	23,704	58%	1,181	5.0%	
Other	1,226	3%	88	7.2%	
Previous MI	6,726	16%	807	12%	271 (1 df)
Diabetes[b]	6,005	15%	653	11%	146 (1 df)
Smoking[b]					483 (2 df)
Current	17,543	43%	736	4.2%	
Ex-smoker	11,210	27%	805	7.2%	
Never smoked	12,077	30%	1,310	11%	
Thrombolytic therapy[b]					15 (3 df)
SK + iv hep	10,377	25%	770	7.4%	
SK + subcut hep	9,796	24%	705	7.2%	
tPA + SK	10,504	26%	723	7.0%	
tPA + iv hep	10,344	25%	653	6.3%	
Total n	40,830	100%	2,851	7.0%	–

MI myocardial infarction; *SK* Streptokinase; *tPA* tissue plasminogen activator; *hep* heparin
[a]Systolic BP with winsorizing above 120 mmHg
[b]Data corrected compared to the original publication [329]

22.2.3   Study Design and Analysis

The data come from a RCT. Data collection was prospective, with rigorous quality control on predictor information and outcome assessment. The inclusion criteria for GUSTO-I were relatively liberal, making the findings probably well generalizable to other acute MI patients.

The choice of the statistical model does not receive much attention in the paper; logistic regression is assumed to be suitable for this situation with a dichotomous outcome (dead/alive). The model can approach nonlinear models by including interactions and nonlinear terms, which were examined.

A total of 2,851 patients had died by 30 days. Thirty-nine percent of the deaths (1125) occurred within 24 h; more than half (55%) occurred within 48 h of randomization. This number of events provides an exceptional and excellent basis for prognostic modeling.

22.3   Seven Modeling Steps in GUSTO-I

22.3.1   Preliminary

An overview of the data is provided in Table 22.3 [329]. The outcome (30-day mortality) was complete for 40,830 of the 41,021 patients (99.5%). Distributions of some candidate predictors were quite skewed, e.g., for Killip class (a measure of left ventricular function). Categories III or IV were present in only 2% of the patients; these categories represent patients in shock.

Missing values occurred for various candidate predictors, but usually only in a small fraction. Missing values were imputed for further statistical analysis ("single imputation", see Chaps. 7 and 8). Imputation was based on the correlation among predictors, which were exploited with flexible functions (transcan function in S + software, the pre-R era). Details on the missing values were not provided, nor were analyses repeated with complete cases only.

22.3.2   Coding of Predictors

Much attention was given to the transformations of continuous predictors. Linear and restricted cubic spline functions were used to describe the relations between predictor and mortality (see Chap. 10). For further analysis, some simplifying transformations were chosen, including winsorizing of values (for example for systolic blood pressure).

For categorical variables, detailed categorizations were kept as such for statistical analysis, which was reasonable given the large sample size. For example, many studies consider the location of infarction as anterior versus other. In GUSTO-I, the coding was as anterior (39%), inferior (58%), or other (3%), where "other" included posterior, lateral and apical locations. Also, Killip class was considered as a categorical variable, despite that class III and class IV each contained only 1% of the patients. The ordinal nature of this predictor was ignored in the analyses.

22.3.3   Model Specification

The authors state that they aimed to identify which variables were most strongly related to short-term mortality. This answers a research question related to hypothesis testing, rather than prediction per se [508]. The specific technique used for selection is not explicitly stated, but likely only statistically significant variables were considered as predictors ($p < 0.05$).

The authors tested interactions among the predictors, i.e., they examined whether the prognostic relation of a predictor differed by levels of other predictors ("additivity assumption", Chap. 12). In the Results, the authors state:

> Only one interaction among these factors was significant to the degree that it was appropriate to include in the model—the interaction between age and Killip class.

Linearity of predictors was assessed in detail; transformations chosen at univariate analysis were also used in multivariable analysis.

22.3.4   Model Estimation

Regression coefficients were estimated with standard logistic regression analysis, which maximizes the log likelihood of the fit of the model to the data. More advanced methods are available (Chap. 13), but these modern estimation methods are less relevant in very large data sets such as GUSTO-I.

22.3.5   Model Performance

Discrimination and calibration were studied to indicate model performance. The area under the receiver operating characteristic curve (AUC, equivalent to the c statistic) was used to study discrimination. The authors explain that the AUC measures the concordance of predictions with actual outcomes (how well the predictions rank order patients with respect to their outcomes) and that AUC is a simple transformation of Somer's D rank correlation between the model predictions and actual outcomes.

Calibration of the model predictions was assessed graphically and by comparison of the average model prediction to the observed mortality rate across tenths of risk. The latter grouping procedure is often used in the Hosmer–Lemeshow goodness of fit test, which we discourage to use (Chap. 15). Further, the authors compared predictions and observed mortality within specific subgroups of patients with different risk levels. This method is not often performed to study calibration of prediction models [602]. First, it is only reasonable with large numbers of patients in the subgroups, as in GUSTO-I. More importantly, it is only a check on marginals of predictions according to predictor values. The comparison with observed outcomes will only show violations of nonlinearity for continuous variables. It is insensitive to having missed interactions in the model. We discussed various other measures for calibration in Chap. 15. Clinical usefulness was not evaluated explicitly.

22.3.6 Model Validation

GUSTO-I is a very large data set. This makes that the performance of the model can be assessed reliably in a simple and direct way, i.e., on the same patients that were used to develop the model. Optimism in performance would be a problem in relatively small data sets, i.e., either that many predictors were considered, or that relatively few events were available for the logistic regression analysis. Both are not the case in GUSTO-I. Nevertheless, the authors embarked on attempts to validate the predictive performance of the model, especially the AUC. The authors explain their approach clearly:

> First, 10-fold cross validation was performed: the model was fitted on a randomly selected subset of 90% of the study patients, and the resulting fit was tested on the remaining 10%. This process was repeated 10 times to estimate the extent to which the predictive accuracy of the model (based on the entire sample) was overoptimistic. Second, for each of 100 bootstrap samples (samples of the same size as the original population but with patients drawn randomly, with replacement, from the full study population), the model was refitted and then tested on the original sample, again to estimate the degree to which the predictive accuracy of the model would be expected to deteriorate when applied to an independent sample of patients [329].

A more extensive description of these validation techniques was provided in Chap. 17. Model optimism was negligible, both in the 10-fold cross-validation procedure and with bootstrapping. This was as expected, since the sample size was very large with a relatively small number of predictors.

22.3.7 Presentation

Results of the modeling process were presented in various ways. The relevance of each predictor was shown by an ANOVA table, where the contribution of each predictor was indicated by the drop in an adjusted χ^2 statistic. A simple table is obtained in R (rms library) for the five prognostic factors that were considered most important [86]:

```
> anova(fit1)
                    Wald Statistics           Response: DAY30

    Factor                                      Chi-Square d.f. P
    AGE   (Factor+Higher Order Factors)            1392     4  <.0001
     All Interactions                                31     3  <.0001
    KILLIP  (Factor+Higher Order Factors)           434     6  <.0001
     All Interactions                                31     3  <.0001
    SYSBP120                                        567     1  <.0001
    PULSE                                           317     1  <.0001
    MILOC                                           144     2  <.0001
    PMI                                              92     1  <.0001
    AGE * KILLIP   (Factor+Higher Order Factors)     31     3  <.0001
    TOTAL                                          3154    12  <.0001
```

A graphical illustration is more attractive (Fig. 22.1, plot(anova(fit))). It appears that age with interactions with Killip is associated with a contribution to the χ^2 statistic of 1392; if analyzed as a main effect the contribution was 1380. Killip contributes 434 (389 in a model without interaction). Systolic blood pressure (with winsorizing at 120 mmHg) and a high pulse also contribute substantially. The interaction between age and Killip class is of relatively minor importance ($\chi^2 = 31$).

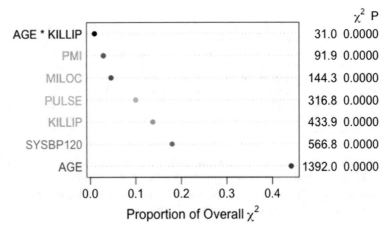

Fig. 22.1 Prognostic importance of five key predictors for 30-mortality in GUSTO-I [86]. Age stands out as the dominant prognostic factor (χ^2 1392, plus interaction effect χ^2 31)

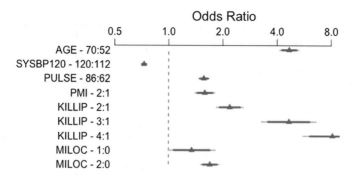

Fig. 22.2 Odds ratios for five key predictors for 30-mortality in GUSTO-I [86]. 95 and 99% confidence intervals are shown. Age and Killip class have very strong relative effects, and all confidence intervals are small

Interestingly, the choice of thrombolytic therapy had an adjusted χ^2 of only 15 in the prediction model [86], which is small compared to the importance of the other predictors. This phenomenon is observed in many prognostic evaluations of RCTs: treatment has a statistically significant impact on outcome, but its relevance is small compared to other prognostic factors.

Odds ratios (ORs) for the effect of predictors were shown graphically [329]. Odds ratios are calculated from the logistic regression coefficients as OR = exp (coef). An OR larger than 1 indicates that the risk of mortality is increased, while an OR smaller than 1 indicates that the risk of mortality is decreased (e.g., lower risk with higher systolic blood pressure, Fig. 22.2). For continuous variables, the ORs were presented as the odds of death for patients at the 75th percentile of the distribution of the predictor versus patients at the 25th percentile. We show ORs on the log scale for easier interpretation of the relative magnitude of effects. At a log scale, an OR of 4 is twice as far away from 1 as an odds ratio of 2, consistent with a doubling in prognostic effect.

22.3.8   Predictions

The Appendix of the Circulation paper lists a formula which can be used to calculate the probability of 30-day mortality for an individual patient [329]. This formula is difficult to follow because it includes cubic spline transformations. A far easier presentation was done for the model with five key predictors (Table 22.4) [86].

Table 22.4 Score chart to estimate 30-day mortality after acute MI [86]. Note that the interaction between age and Killip is represented in a table for easy application

Predictor	Values	Points			
Age (years)		Killip class			
		I	II	III	IV
	40	28	42	54	59
	50	38	49	59	65
	60	47	56	64	70
	70	57	63	70	76
	80	66	70	75	82
	90	75	77	81	88
	100	85	84	86	94
Systolic BP (mmHg)	40	34			
	80	17			
	120+	0			
Heart rate (beats/ min)	10	9			
	30	5			
	50	0			
	90	9			
	130	17			
Infarct location	Anterior	6			
	Inferior	0			
	Other	3			
Previous MI	Yes	5			
Total	Add points	…			

Box 22.2 Formula from the Appendix of the Lee et al. paper [328, 329] Risk Model for 30-Day Mortality

Probability of death within 30 days $= 1/[1 + \exp (-L)]$, where $L = 3.81 + 0.0762$ age $-0.0398 \min(SBP, 120) + 2.08$ [Killip class II] $+ 3.62$ [Killip class III] $+ 4.04$ [Killip class IV] $- 0.0211$ heart rate $+ 0.0394$ (heart rate $- 50)_+ - 0.0397$ height $+ 0.000184$ (height $- 154.9)^3_+ - 0.000898$ (height $- 165.1)^3_+ + 0.00159$ (height $- 172.0)^3_+ - 0.00107$ (height $- 177.3)^3_+ + 0.000194$ (height $- 185.4)^3_+ + \dots$.

Explanatory notes:

1. Brackets are interpreted as $[c] = 1$ if the patient falls into category c, $[c] = 0$ otherwise.
2. $(x)_+ = x$ if $x > 0$, $(x)_+ = 0$ otherwise.
3. For systolic blood pressure (SBP), values >120 mmHg are winsorized.

22.4 Validity

22.4.1 Internal Validity: Overfitting

Overfitting was of limited relevance, because of the very large sample size. Quite extensive checks of assumptions were performed for a substantial number of candidate predictors, but this "data hungry" approach was reasonable in such a huge data set. Overfitting was assessed by cross-validation and bootstrapping, and found to be irrelevant.

22.4.2 External Validity: Generalizability

Will predictions be valid for plausibly related populations? External validity was not assessed in the paper. We note however that a large set of predictors was considered and included in the model, representing important domains of predictors.

Various other models have been developed to predict short-term mortality after acute MI, some before and some after the development of the GUSTO-I model. Usually, large sample sizes were available, such that model development could start de novo. Examples of models developed earlier were the TIMI-II model [395], the GISSI-II model [361], and a model from a Belgium center [142].

Interestingly, we found that these different models for acute MI may have a similar performance, e.g., an AUC around 0.8, but provide very different predictions for individual patients [540]. These differences were attributable to choice of predictors rather than to differences in regression coefficients, highlighting the importance of model selection issues (Chap. 11).

22.4.3 Summary Points

- The Lee et al. paper is an excellent illustration of many of the essential steps in developing a valid prediction model
- Nowadays, we can readily deal with missing values in a slightly more sophisticated way than single imputation, although single imputation is much better than a complete case analysis (Chap. 7)
- A limitation of the model is the translation into clinical practice of the full model; an easily applicable format was used for a reduced model with 5 key predictors [86]

- Moreover, generalizability to current clinical practice is doubtful since the treatments have changed substantially since the years that patients were enrolled in GUSTO-I (early 1990s). We expect a need for model updating, at least of the model intercept.

22.5   Translation into Clinical Practice

The model presented in Circulation is not easily applicable in the presented form. Many predictors were included, while it was found that 90% of the prognostic information was contained in five variables:

> A perspective on the overall contribution of various components of the baseline clinical data to the prediction of mortality can be obtained by use of the global chi-square statistic from the logistic model as an index of prognostic information. This index from the full model can be compared with reduced models containing a smaller number of variables. The likelihood ratio chi-square statistic for the full model containing all of the prognostic factors was 4379. In contrast, this statistic for a model containing age alone was 2099, meaning that age provides nearly half the prognostic information. Adding other variables provides an increased proportion of information; combining age, systolic blood pressure, Killip class, heart rate, infarct location, and age-by-Killip-class interaction provides approximately 90% of the total prognostic information contained in this array of baseline clinical characteristics [329].

Further, the presentation in the Appendix as a formula is probably frightening to most clinicians. A simpler format was required. Both issues were addressed in a later publication, which focused on decision-making on thrombolytic therapy [86].

22.5.1   Score Chart for Choosing Thrombolytic Therapy

Five predictors were considered and presented in a table to derive a summary score for a patient (see Chap. 18). Age and Killip class were included as main effects and with interaction terms. The interaction effect is nicely illustrated in Table 22.4 and Fig. 22.3. At younger ages, Killip class makes a substantial difference. Equivalently, age matters among those with Killip class I, but less among those with higher Killip classes. At the end of the age range (age 100 years), some strange patterns arise, with Killip class I patients having a higher score than those with Killip class II or III. This is a biologically implausible pattern. It illustrates that even in a huge data set such as GUSTO-I, artifacts can show up. These artifacts may be due to the specification of the logistic model with a linear interaction term, or to the specific sample. The implausible pattern could have been prevented by placing some restrictions on the interactions, as was done for a prediction model for renal

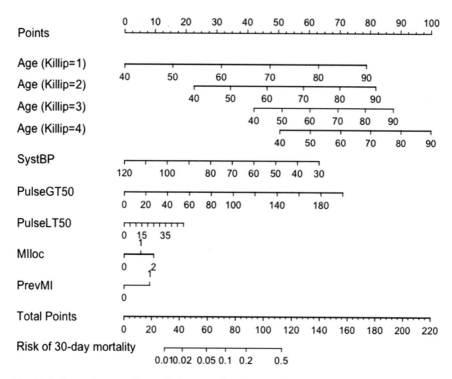

Fig. 22.3 Score chart to estimate 30-day mortality after acute MI, presenting the same model as in Table 22.4. Note that the interaction between age and Killip is represented as age effects per Killip category for easy application in practice

artery stenosis [314] and illustrated in Chap. 12 for age effects in the Lynch syndrome model.

22.5.2   From Predictions to Decisions

The score from Table 22.4 corresponds to a probability of 30-day mortality with or without tPA treatment (Table 22.5). We can, hence, determine the benefit of administering tPA instead of streptokinase from this table. A substantial benefit should be estimated before treating with tPA since this drug is expensive and has a substantial risk of side effects (especially bleeding) [184, 298]. Note that the tPA reduction shows an increase with the score on an absolute scale (Fig. 22.4). The relative reduction was, however, more or less constant at 15% on the odds scale (odds ratio 0.81 in a model with five key predictors). So, the same relative benefit

Table 22.5 Translation of score from Table 22.4 into estimated mortality with streptokinase (SK) or tPA treatment [86]

Score	SK mortality (%)	tPA mortality (%)	tPA reduction (%)
30	0.4	0.4	–
40	0.8	0.8	0.01
50	1.7	1.4	0.3
60	3.5	2.8	0.8
70	10	8.3	1.7
80	20	17	3
90	40	35	5

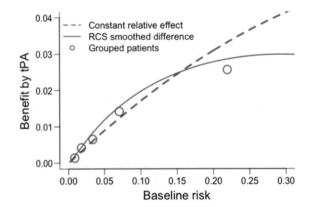

Fig. 22.4 Absolute benefit in 30-day mortality by accelerated tPA treatment compared to streptokinase (SK) in relation to baseline mortality risk. We note that the absolute benefit increases with increasing baseline risk, while we assume a constant relative risk effect (Odds Ratio for tPA 0.81 in a logistic model with 5 key predictors, 95% CI 0.73 − 0.90). Dots reflect difference in proportions of patients who died in groups defined by quantiles of predicted risk, comparing tPA versus SK. Solid line represents the differences between two rcs fits with 5 knots (4 df) for those randomized to tPA and those randomized to SK [86]

leads to substantially different absolute benefits [300]. This observation has been made for many other diseases as well (see Chap. 2).

As an example, we consider the score for a hypothetical 65-year-old male. The score would be 60 points for the combination of age 65 and Killip class II, 8 points for a systolic blood pressure of 100 mmHg, 5 points for heart rate 75 bpm, 6 points for anterior infarct location, and no points for previous MI. The total is 79 points. When treated with tPA, his 30-day mortality risk is estimated as approximately 16%, while SK would be predicted to lead to a mortality of approximately 19%. So, tPA would be expected to reduce mortality by approximately 3%.

22.5.3 Covariate Adjustment in GUSTO-I

The effects of adjustment for predictors have been described for the GUSTO-I data in at least two methodological studies [332, 537]. Both studies considered the effect of tPA versus streptokinase. The first study considered adjustment for age or a comprehensive set of 17 predictors (age plus 16 other baseline characteristics) [537]. The second study used another approach and adjusted for the 5 most important predictors [86, 332].

In the first analysis, it was found that patients were 0.17 years older in the tPA group (61.03 years, $n = 10,348$) than in the two SK groups (60.86 years, $n = 20,162$) [537]. This difference should be fully attributed to chance, and a formal test to compare the ages makes no sense if a proper randomization procedure was followed [501]. However, we know that age is a very strong predictor. The univariate regression coefficient for age was 0.082 per year. We estimated the difference in treatment effect that was attributable to age imbalance by multiplying the difference in mean age with the regression coefficient: $0.17 * 0.082 = 0.014$. The 0.17 years older age of the tPA group made that the treatment effect was underestimated by 0.014 on the logistic scale. The adjusted treatment effect corrects for this imbalance. But it also provides a stratified estimate, which has an expectation further from zero [174, 463]. This stratification effect was calculated as the remaining part of the difference between unadjusted and adjusted treatment effect [537].

The unadjusted treatment effect was an OR of 0.853 (coefficient −0.1586), and the adjusted estimate was an OR 0.829 (coefficient −0.1878, 18% more extreme). Age imbalance explained −0.014 or 9% of the difference, leaving another 9% attributable to stratification. Some argue that unadjusted treatment effects are biased if we are interested in more personalized treatment effect estimates [174, 233].

The key treatment comparison in tPA versus streptokinase we made in 30,510 patients [86]. It was estimated that an adjusted analysis with 26,900 patients would have the same power as the original unadjusted analysis of 30,510 patients. Such a 12% reduction in sample size is a major argument in favor of adjusted analyses to test for treatment effect [537]. Either sample sizes could be reduced, or the sample size could be kept at the number based on a traditional, unadjusted, analysis, while the actual analysis would give more statistical power.

Much more can be said on the modeling of treatment effects in randomized clinical trials, which is mostly beyond the scope of this book. Adjusted analyses were the primary analysis in about half of recently reported RCTs across various fields [18]. Advantages are that adjusted analyses have more power, and that adjusted treatment effects may be more relevant for clinical practice. Note that adjusted p-values of a particular trial do not necessarily have to be more extreme than those from an unadjusted analysis [332]. However, since we are more interested in the adjusted than the unadjusted effect, the adjusted p-value is arguably preferable. The actual gain in power depends on the strength of the prognostic relations of predictors to outcome. Some argue that adjusted analyses make sense once a specific type of correlation exceeds 0.2 [441]. Finally, any adjustment procedure should be prespecified in the trial protocol, to prevent a search for the adjustment model that gives the most impressive estimate or most extreme p-value for the treatment effect.

22.6   Concluding Remarks

The GUSTO-I case study illustrates many of the steps that need to be considered in the development of a valid prediction model [329]. It is fortunate that the paper is freely accessible [328], and that we can make parts of this rich data set available for practical experience in prediction modeling (Chap. 24, data courtesy: Duke Clinical Research Institute, Durham, NC). The decision-making implications were well addressed in another study [86], which used a slightly simplified prediction model.

Questions

22.1 Estimate 30-day mortality (Table 22.4, and spreadsheet)
Consider a male patient with Killip class I, a systolic blood pressure of 100 mmHg, heart rate 80 bpm, anterior infarct location, and with a previous MI. Use the simple table (Table 22.4) to estimate 30-day mortality and compare this estimate to the more exact calculation with the full regression formula (spreadsheet at www.clinicalpredictionmodel.org).

(a) What is the risk of mortality from acute MI if this patient is 55 years old?
(b) What if he were 75 years old?

Now consider decision-making on tPA treatment.

(c) What is the impact of age on prioritizing tPA treatment based on the reduction in 30-day mortality?
(d) What might be the priority if we consider gain in life expectancy instead of 30-day mortality?
(e) What is the threshold for the ratio between life expectancies of a 75 versus a 55-year-old patient in this example?

22.2 Stratification and treatment effects
We study the effect of a hypothetical treatment, with and without stratification for gender. The Table with results is presented below. We compare 30-day mortality ("Dead") between treatments A and B.

Table: hypothetical treatment effect in a randomized controlled trial, with stratification by gender.

Treatment	Men		Women	
	Dead	Survived	Dead	Survived
A	10	80	72	18
B	18	72	80	10

(a) What is the odds ratio for the treatment effect (A vs. B) among men?
(b) And among women?
(c) What is the OR for treatment if we do not stratify by gender?
(d) Is treatment balanced by gender?
(e) How do you explain these findings?
(f) What is the OR of gender, ignoring treatment?
(g) What is the OR of gender, conditional on treatment?
(h) What would happen if gender had no prognostic effect, i.e., the OR for gender was 1?
(i) How do these results explain the impact of covariate adjustment in GUSTO-I? Specifically, the unadjusted OR was 0.853 and the adjusted OR 0.829, while imbalance only accounted for a difference of −0.014 on the log odds scale?

Chapter 23
Case Study on Survival Analysis: Prediction of Cardiovascular Events

Background Survival is an important long-term outcome in prognostic research, including medical areas such as cardiovascular disease and oncology. We consider a model for the occurrence of vascular events in patients with symptomatic cardiovascular disease. Patient data were from the Second Manifestations of ARTerial disease (SMART) study. We go through the seven steps of the checklist for developing valid prediction models, as presented in Part II. Specific focus is on the combination of models specification and estimation with the LASSO in combination with multiple imputation of missing values. The data set and R code are made available at the book's website (www.clinicalpredictionmodels.org).

23.1 Prognosis in the SMART Study

The SMART study is an ongoing prospective cohort study coordinated by University Medical Center Utrecht, the Netherlands, and initiated by Prof. Van der Graaf and colleagues [137, 512]. Many prediction models in the field of cardiovascular disease are developed with data from subjects without clinically manifest atherosclerosis [666]. These include the Framingham risk score, PROCAM, and SCORE [17, 590, 674]. These models may be able to rank patients with clinically manifest disease according to risk, but would be expected to underestimate absolute risk in patients with clinically manifest cardiovascular disease [151].

Assessment of absolute risk is important for secondary prevention. According to the current guidelines, all patients who experienced a symptomatic cardiovascular event should be considered as at high risk (more than 20% absolute risk on a future event in the next 10 years). No further categorization is available.

© Springer Nature Switzerland AG 2019
E. W. Steyerberg, *Clinical Prediction Models*, Statistics for Biology and Health, https://doi.org/10.1007/978-3-030-16399-0_23

Relevant outcomes in patients with cardiovascular disease (coronary artery disease, cerebral artery disease, peripheral arterial disease, and abdominal aortic aneurysm) include stroke, myocardial infarction or cardiovascular death. Hard outcomes are generally preferred because they lead to better comparability between studies and hence a better generalizability. The aim in the current study was to develop a prediction model for patients with cardiovascular disease. We estimate the 1-, 3-, and 5-year risks on the occurrence of vascular events (stroke, myocardial infarction, or cardiovascular death).

23.1.1   Patients in SMART

We consider 3873 patients who were enrolled in the study in the period of September 1996 and March 2006; the cohort has since been expanded [609]. Patients had a clinical manifestation of atherosclerosis (transient ischemic attack, ischemic stroke, peripheral arterial disease, abdominal aortic aneurysm, or coronary heart disease). After written informed consent, they underwent a standardized vascular screening including a health questionnaire for clinical information, laboratory assessment and anthropometric measurements at enrolment. During follow-up, patients were biannually asked to fill in a questionnaire on hospitalizations and outpatient clinic visits. The end points of interest for the present study were (acute) vascular death, (non-)fatal ischemic stroke or (non-)fatal myocardial infarction, and the composite end point of any of these vascular events (Table 23.1). If a patient had multiple events, the first recorded event was used for analysis. Data were available on 14,530 person-years collected during a mean follow-up of 3.8 years (range 0–9 years). A total of 460 events occurred, corresponding to a 5-year cumulative incidence of 14.2% (1–0.858 free of events). The 9-year incidence was 1–0.725 = 27.5%, so already above the clinically defined threshold of 20% 10-year risk (Fig. 23.1).

23.2   General Considerations in SMART

23.2.1   Research Question and Intended Application

The aim was to develop a prediction model for long-term outcome. Given the available follow-up, 1-, 3-, and 5-year risks could be assessed reliably. Achieving adequate predictions was more prominent than insight in the predictor effects per se (Table 23.1). The intended application was inpatient counseling; a high absolute risk might motivate patients to change inappropriate lifestyles and to comply with their medication regimens.

Table 23.1 Checklist for developing a valid prediction model in the SMART study

Step	Specific issues	SMART model
General considerations		
Research question	Aim: predictors/prediction?	Emphasis on prediction
Intended application	Clinical practice/research?	Clinical practice
Outcome	Clinically relevant?	Hard cardiovascular events
Predictors	Reliable measurement? Comprehensiveness	Detailed workup; comprehensive set of candidate predictors
Study design	Retrospective/prospective? Cohort; case control	Prospective cohort
Statistical model	Appropriate for research question and type of outcome?	Cox regression
Sample size	Sufficient for aim?	3873 patients, 460 events: very good
7 modeling steps		
1. Preliminary	Inspection of data Missing values	Table 23.3 Multiple imputation
2. Coding of predictors	Continuous predictors Combining categorical predictors Combining predictors with similar effects	Winsorizing and splines for continuous predictors Sum score for cardiovascular history
3. Model specification	Appropriate selection of main effects? Assessment of assumptions (distributional, linearity and additivity)?	Stepwise selection with high p-value and LASSO Additivity checked with interaction terms Proportional hazards checked
4. Model estimation	Shrinkage included? External information used?	Penalized estimation with LASSO No
5. Model performance	Appropriate measures used?	Focus on discrimination
6. Model validation	Internal validation including model specification and estimation? External validation?	Bootstrap within imputed set including all modeling stepsm such as cv for LASSO optimal penalty No external validation
7. Model presentation	Format appropriate for audience	Nomogram
Validity		
Internal: overfitting	Sufficient attempts to limit and correct for overfitting?	Large sample size, predictors from literature, LASSO for selection and shrinkage
External: generalizability	Predictions valid for plausibly related populations?	Large set of predictors, representing important domains; not assessed in this study

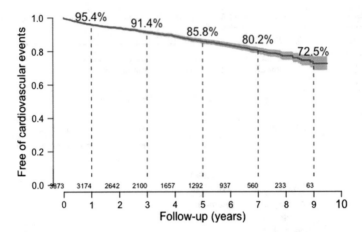

Fig. 23.1 Overall fraction of patients free of events during 9 years of follow-up. In total, 460 patients had a cardiovascular event, for a 5-year risk of cardiovascular events of 14.2% (1 − 0.858)

23.2.2   Outcome and Predictors

The primary outcome was any cardiovascular event, comprising cardiovascular death, nonfatal stroke, and nonfatal myocardial infarction. Combining different events is a common approach in vascular research to increase statistical power. A cardiovascular event occurred in 460 patients during follow-up.

The selection of predictors was motivated by characteristics included in Framingham and SCORE models. The relation with future events has also been established for several traditional risk factors, including hyperhomocysteinemia, intima–media thickness, and creatinine. Other candidate predictors were demographics (sex and age), and risk factors for vascular events in the general population (smoking, alcohol use, body mass index (BMI), diastolic and systolic blood pressure, lipids, and diabetes).

It is well conceivable that indicators of the extent of atherosclerosis are very relevant to predict events in patients with symptomatic atherosclerosis. Such indicators are the location of symptomatic vascular disease (cerebral, coronary, peripheral arterial disease, or AAA), and markers of the extent of atherosclerosis (homocysteine, creatinine, albumin, intima–media thickness (IMT), and presence of a carotid artery stenosis, Table 23.2).

Table 23.2 Potential predictors in the SMART study data set ($n = 3{,}873$). Relatively many missing values were present for different ways to measure blood pressure

Characteristics	
Demographics	
Female sex ("SEX", n, 0 missing)	975 (25%)
Age ("AGE", in years, 0 missing)	60 [52–68]
Classical risk factors	
Smoking ("SMOKING", n (%), 25 missing)	
Never	693 (18%)
Former	2711 (70%)
Current	444 (12%)
Packyears ("PACKYRS", in years, 21 missing)	20 [6–34]
Alcohol ("ALCOHOL", n (%), 25 missing)	
Never	751 (20%)
Former	408 (11%)
Current	2689 (69%)
Body mass index ("BMI", in kg/m^2, 3 missing)	26.7 (24–29)
Diabetes ("DIABETES", n (%), 40 missing)	846 (22%)
Blood pressure	
Systolic, by hand ("SYSTH", in mmHg, 1498 missing)	140 (126–155)
Systolic, automatic ("SYSTBP", in mmHg, 1223 missing)	139 (127–154)
Diastolic, by hand ("DIASTH", in mmHg, 1499 missing)	82 (75–90)
Diastolic, automatic ("DIASTBP", in mmHg, 1221 missing)	79 (73–86)
Lipid levels	
Total cholesterol ("CHOL", in mmol/L, 18 missing)	5.1 [4.4–5.9]
High-density lipoprotein cholesterol ("HDL", mmol/L, 30 missing)	1.17 [0.96–1.42]
Low-density lipoprotein cholesterol ("LDL", mmol/L, 216 missing)	3.06 [2.39–3.83]
Triglycerides ("TRIG", mmol/L, 28 missing)	1.54 [1.12–2.23]
Previous symptomatic atherosclerosis	
Cerebral ("CEREBRAL", n (%), 0 missing)	1147 (30%)
Coronary ("CARDIAC", n (%), 0 missing)	2160 (56%)
Peripheral ("PERIPH", n (%), 0 missing)	940 (24%)
Abdominal aortic aneurysm ("AAA", n (%), 0 missing)	416 (11%)
Markers of atherosclerosis	
Homocysteine ("HOMOC", µmol/L, 463 missing)	12.8 [10.3–15.7]
Glutamine ("GLUT", µmol/L, 19 missing)	5.7 [5.3–6.5]
Creatinine clearance ("CREAT", mL/min, 17 missing)	89 [78–101]
Albumin ("ALBUMIN", n (%), 207 missing)	
No	2897 (79%)
Micro	655 (18%)
Macro	114 (3%)
Intima–media thickness ("IMT", mm, 98 missing)	0.88 [0.75–1.07]
Carotid artery stenosis >50% ("STENOSIS", n (%), 93 missing)	722 (19%)

23.2.3   Study Design and Analysis

The SMART study is designed as an ongoing, prospective dynamic cohort study. Patients are enrolled when presenting at the hospital, with follow-up starting from study inclusion. We used the Cox regression model, which is the default statistical model for survival outcomes. This model is appropriate for prediction of an outcome at relatively short term such as 5-year cumulative incidence of cardiovascular events. For long-term predictions (e.g., 10-year incidences), a parametric model might be preferable such as a Weibull model. A Weibull model provides more stable estimates at the end of the follow-up [89].

With respect to sample size, the balance of 460 events and approximately 25 candidate predictors is quite reasonable (Table 23.2). This implies 18 events per variable (EPV).

23.3   Preliminary Modeling Steps in the SMART Cohort

Missing values were an important issue in the development of the prediction model. We first discuss patterns of missing values, followed by strategies for imputation.

23.3.1   Patterns of Missing Values

Many missing values were noted among four variables that relate to blood pressure measurements (two for diastolic and two for systolic pressure, >30% missing, Fig. 23.2). In the first years of the study, blood pressure was measured combined with measurement of the distensibility of the carotid artery wall ("SYSTBP" and "DIASTBP" variables). Four years after the start of the study, it was decided to measure blood pressure with the conventional sphygmomanometry as well ("by hand"). This measurement is considered in most current guidelines. Hence, conventional diastolic and systolic measurements ("SYSTH" and "DIASTH" variables) are obvious candidate predictors for our model rather than the automated measurements. Nearly, all patients had at least one type of blood pressure measurement, with Pearson correlation coefficients 0.69 and 0.59 for systolic and diastolic blood pressure measurements in 1155 and 1156 patients with conventional as well as automatic measurements available, respectively. This correlation enabled a reasonably accurate imputation of the "SYSTH" and "DIASTH" variables.

The variable homocysteine ("HOMOC") had 463 missings (12%, Table 23.3, Fig. 23.2, upper left panel). In the early years of the study, both homocysteine ("HOMOC") and conventional sphygmomanometry blood pressure measurements ("SYSTH" and "DIASTH" variables) were not performed, leading to some correlation of missingness between these variables (Fig. 23.3).

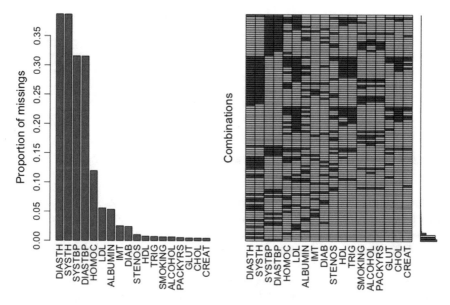

Fig. 23.2 Patterns of missing data in the SMART study ($n = 3873$, VIM library)

Table 23.3 Impact of various transformations of predictors in a univariate Cox regression models for the SMART study; complete case analysis

Predictor	Coding	Wald χ^2	df
Age	Linear	97	1
	Squared	125	2
	$(Age-55)_+$: linear effect after age 55	119	1
	$(Age-50)_+^2$: squared effect after age 50	130	2
	Restricted cubic spline, 3 df	125	3
	<50, 50–59.9, 60–69.9, ≥ 70	93	3
	<60, ≥ 60	72	1
Creatinine	Linear	93	1
	Restricted cubic spline, 3 df	116	3
	Restricted cubic spline, 2 df	99	2
	Log	131	1
Blood pressure (conventional reading)	Linear systolic	15	1
	Restricted cubic spline systolic, 2 df	15	2
	Linear diastolic	0.7	1
	Restricted cubic spline diastolic, 2 df	2	2
Previous symptomatic atherosclerosis	Sumscore 0–4	96	1
	Sumscore 0–5 (AAA = 2)	119	1
	Separate terms	123	4
	Cerebral	36	1
	Coronary	19	1
	Peripheral	23	1
	Abdominal Aneurysm Aorta	97	1

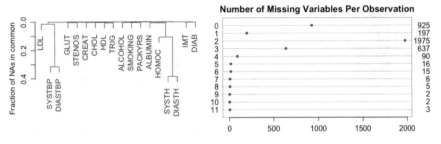

Fig. 23.3 Patterns in the combinations of missing values in the SMART study

For the other variables, we assume also that missingness was more related to logistic reasons, because all patients underwent the same screening protocol. The decision to measure variables was not obviously dependent on other observations (no MAR mechanism), the values of the characteristic itself, or characteristics not available in our dataset (no MNAR mechanisms).

Only 925 patients had no missing values among the 18 potential predictors (Fig. 23.2, right panel and Fig. 23.3, right panel). A total of 975 had 2 missings values (mostly: 1 type of blood pressure measurement not performed). A few patients had many missings (18 with 7 or more missings, Fig. 23.3, right panel).

23.3.2   Imputation of Missing Values

Missing data per predictor would lead to a substantial loss of information if only complete cases were used in the multivariable model. We, therefore, used multiple imputation techniques. We compared two main strategies:

1. Single imputation: The set of first imputations from the `mice` object was used for analyses (single imputation, SI). We also compared imputations generated by `aregImpute`. As a check for stability, we repeated the SI procedure for another set of imputations.
2. Multiple imputation: We used the `fit.mult.impute` function to combine model estimates over the m imputed data sets. We used $m = 10$ for the number of imputations. Next, we created a stacked data set of weighted observations: We put each imputed set below each other, with weight $1/m$ for each patient. So, in our case, the stacked data set had $n = 38730$ records, each with weight 0.1. The stacked data set allowed for model selection more easily than working with the results over each separate, completed data set. This was important for stepwise selection and for the LASSO.

The imputation with `mice` led to quite reasonable replacements for the missing values (Fig. 23.4). Especially, the distributions were very similar for the four blood pressure measurements. Similar results were noted with `aregImpute`.

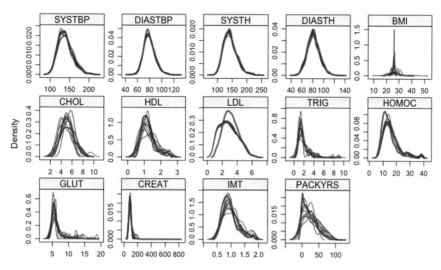

Fig. 23.4 Distribution of imputed and original values with mice in the SMART study

23.3.3 R Code for Missing Values and Imputation

Overall survival is easy to plot:

```
survplot(npsurv(S1 ~ 1), n.risk=T, conf="band", ...) # Fig 23.1
```

Important insights in missing values are obtained with the aggr function in the VIM package:

```
aggr(SMART, sortVars=T, col=c("green", "red")) # End Fig 23.2
```

The patterns of missings can also be studied with the na.patterns function from rms:

```
na.patterns <- naclus(SMART) # for 18 selected variables
plot(na.patterns, ylab="Fraction of NAs in common", ...) # Fig 23.3 left
naplot(na.patterns, which=c('na per obs'), ...)           # Fig 23.3 right
```

Imputation with aregImpute:

```
SMARTM  <-
    aregImpute(~I(TEVENT)+EVENT+SEX+I(AGE)+SYSTBP+DIASTBP+SYSTH+DIASTH+
        DIABETES+CEREBRAL+CARDIAC+AAA+PERIPH+STENOSIS+I(LENGTH)+I(WEIGHT)+
        I(BMI)+I(HISTCARD)+ I(CHOL)+I(HDL)+I(LDL)+I(TRIG)+I(HOMOC)+
        I(GLUT)+I(CREAT)+I(IMT)+ALBUMIN+SMOKING+I(PACKYRS)+ALCOHOL),
        n.impute=5, data=SMART)
SMARTc <- SMART
imputed <-impute.transcan(SMARTM, imputation=1, data=SMART, ...)
SMARTc[names(imputed)] <- imputed # Imputed set with aregImpute
```

Imputation with `mice`:

```
gm <- mice(SMART, m=10, seed=1 ) # transformations are chosen based on type
densityplot(gm) # Fig 23.4
```

Create SI set:

```
SMART1 <- complete(gm, 1)
```

Create stacked set:

```
SMART10 <- complete(gm, 1)
for (i in 2:m) { # add sets 2:10
  SMART10 <- rbind(SMART10, complete(gm, i)) } # n=38730
SMART1$w <- 1/m  # weight 0.1
```

23.4   Coding of Predictors

23.4.1   Extreme Values

Before any modeling started, the distributions of all potential predictors were carefully examined for extreme values. Biologically implausible values were set to missing values, and remaining extreme values were winsorized by shifting the values approximately below the 1st centile and above the 99th centile to "truncation points" (Chap. 9).

As an example, we consider intima–media thickness (IMT, Fig. 23.5). The mean IMT was 0.94 mm, but some patients had measurements as high as 4 mm. These high values are the result of plaque formation in the carotid artery, and may have an unduly large influence on estimates of cardiovascular event risk. A total of 51 values higher than 1.83 were shifted to 1.83 (the upper truncation point), and 13 values below 0.47 were shifted to 0.47 (the lower truncation point). We note a substantial effect of this winsorizing procedure on the relation between IMT and outcome (Fig. 23.5, right panel). A restricted cubic spline based on the original IMT values flattens off with high IMT (>1.5 mm), while a restricted cubic spline based on the winsorized IMT values is very close to a straight line. This finding illustrates that winsorizing may obviate the need for a nonlinear transformation. Before winsorizing, the Cox regression coefficient for a linear IMT variable was 0.91, while it was 1.36 after. The univariate model χ^2 improved from 61 before to 75 (1 df). Similarly, we winsorized body mass index, lipids (Cholesterol, HDL, LDL, Triglycerides), homocysteine and creatinine levels by shifting values below the 1st and above the 99th centile to the truncation points.

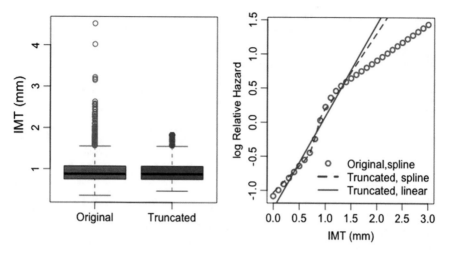

Fig. 23.5 Distribution of intima–media thickness (IMT, in mm, left panel) before and after truncation, and a plot of the effect of IMT on cardiovascular events in a univariate Cox regression model (right panel). The original IMT values are sometimes extremely high, leading to a spline with flattens off with high IMT values. The winsorized IMT values have a smaller range and lead to a quite linear relation (solid line, linear term; dotted line, spline)

23.4.2 Transforming Continuous Predictors

Age is an important predictor in cardiovascular disease. We considered several age transformations (Fig. 23.6, Table 23.3). In our cohort, the Wald χ^2 of the linear fit was 97. Adding age^2 increased the χ^2 to125, but there was a biologically implausible increased risk below age 40 years. Based on visual inspection, it may be judged reasonable to assume no age effect till age 55, and a linear effect for age >55 years ("(Age–55)$_+$" variable, χ^2 119). A transformation such as (Age–50)$_+^2$ led to an even better model (χ^2 130, Fig. 23.6). A restricted cubic spline with 3 df (4 knots) did not describe the relation of age to outcome better (χ^2 125). Categorizing by quartiles has a clearly lower performance (χ^2 93). Such categorization should not be used because jumps in predictions are unnatural. Dichotomizing at age 60 years (close to the median of 61 years) led to an even more substantial decrease performance (χ^2 72, Table 23.3), illustrating that dichotomization is "a bad idea" [472].

Other continuous predictor variables were examined in a similar way; some examples are shown in Table 23.3. For creatinine, a log transformation gave the best fit. A linear coding of systolic blood pressure was reasonable, and diastolic blood pressure had no effect when we analyzed the conventional blood pressure measurements together ("SYSTH" and "DIASTH" variables).

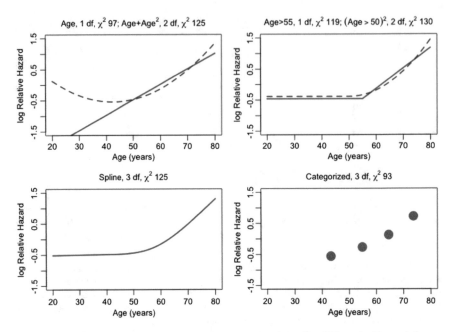

Fig. 23.6 Transformations of age in univariate analysis of the SMART study. Upper left: age linear and age plus age squared; Upper right: age linear after 55 years ("Age–55)$_+$)" and age squared above 50 years ("Age–50)$_+^2$)"; Lower left: restricted cubic spline, 4 knots, 3 *df*; Lower right: age categorized in 4 groups (3 *df*)

23.4.3   Combining Predictors with Similar Effects

Combining predictors with similar effects can be an effective way to limit the degrees of freedom of predictors in a model (Chap. 10). In atherosclerotic patients, several variables reflect the extent of atherosclerosis. The affected organs reflect the load of atherosclerosis in one particular patient. The location of symptomatic events (cerebral, coronary, abdominal aortic aneurysm (AAA), peripheral artery disease) can be entered separately in the model. For each parameter we would spend 1 *df*, resulting in a model χ^2 of 123 (4 *df*, Table 23.3). If we combine the presence of previous vascular events in 1 variable, simply by assuming equal weights for each condition, the model χ^2 is 96 (1 *df*). The difference of the two models is a χ^2 of 27, which is highly significant at 3 *df*. Separate terms hence lead to a much better fit. When we test for the separate contributions of each localization it appears that the contribution of AAA is considerably higher than the contribution of the other localizations. Once we attribute 2 points for the presence of an AAA, the sumscore performs remarkable better (range 0–5, model χ^2 119, close to 123 for separate terms, Table 23.3).

23.4.4   R Code for coding

IMT with and without winsorizing

```
IMTOfit <- cph(Surv(TEVENT,EVENT) ~ rcs(IMTO,5), data=SMARTo) #original
plot(x=seq(0,3,.1),y=predict(IMTOfit,newdata=seq(0,3,.1)),
     ylab="log Relative Hazard", xlab="IMT (mm)", ...) # plot
IMTfit <- cph(Surv(TEVENT,EVENT) ~ rcs(IMT,5), data=SMART) # winsorized
lines(x=seq(0,3,.1), y=predict(IMTfit,newdata=seq(0,3,.1)), ...)
IMTfitlin <- cph(Surv(TEVENT,EVENT) ~ IMT, data=SMART) # linear fit
lines(x=seq(0,3,.1), y=predict(IMTfitlin,newdata=seq(0,3,.1)), ...) # Fig 23.5
```

Age effects

```
S <- Surv(SMART$TEVENT, SMART$EVENT) # Short-cut; no missings in predictors
AGEfit <- S ~ AGE, data=SMART) # linear
pred <- seq(20,80,1) # range for predictions
plot(x=pred, y=predict(AGEfit, pred), ...)
anova(AGEfit) # chi-square statistic
AGEfit2 <- cph(S~pol(AGE,2), data=SMART) # age + age^2
AGEfit3 <- cph(S~ifelse(AGE>55, (AGE-55),0), ...) # age>55+
AGEfit4 <- cph(S~ifelse(AGE>50, (AGE-50)^2,0), ...) # age>50+^2)
AGEfit5 <- cph(S~rcs(AGE,4), data=SMART) # rcs, 3 df
```

Previous symptomatic atherosclerosis

```
# Score with individual terms, 4 df
fitsum  <- cph(S~CEREBRAL+CARDIAC+AAA+PERIPH, data=SMART)
anova (fitsum) # total chi-square 123, Table 23.4
 Wald Statistics          Response: Surv(TEVENT, EVENT)
 Factor      Chi-Square d.f. P
 CEREBRAL     35.73       1   <.0001
 CARDIAC      19.11       1   <.0001
 AAA          96.62       1   <.0001
 PERIPH       23.13       1   <.0001
 TOTAL       122.61       4   <.0001
```

```
# Score with each affected organ seperately in a score, assuming equal
weight
SMART$HISTCARD  <- SMART$CEREBRAL+SMART$CARDIAC+SMART$AAA+SMART$PERIPH
fitsum2  <- cph(S ~ HISTCARD, data=SMART)
anova(fitsum2) # total chi-square 96, Table 23.4
# Score with each affected organ separately in a score, AAA doubled
SMART$HISTCAR2  <- SMART$CEREBRAL+SMART$CARDIAC+2*SMART$AAA+SMART$PERIPH
fitsum3  <- cph(S~HISTCAR2, data=SMART)
anova(fitsum3)) # total chi-square 119, Table 23.4
# Deviations from linear score HISTCAR2, start with AAA
> anova(update(fitsum3, .~.+AAA)) # no change in chi-square, weight 2
perfect
```

```
 Factor      Chi-Square d.f. P
 HISTCAR2     44.05       1   <.0001
 AAA           0.00       1   0.9966
 TOTAL       119.40       2   <.0001
```

23.5   Model Specification

23.5.1   A Full Model

A full, main effects model was defined which included the common demographics age and sex, important classical risk factors (smoking status, alcohol use, body mass index, blood pressure, lipid levels, and diabetes), the sum score for previous symptoms of atherosclerosis, and finally markers of the extent of the atherosclerotic process (including hyperhomocysteinemia, creatinin, intima–media thickness of the carotid artery, carotid artery stenosis, and albuminuria). We focused on systolic blood pressure since recent publications stress the more important role of systolic rather than diastolic blood pressure in predicting cardiovascular events [571]. Indeed, the effect of systolic blood pressure was stronger than that of diastolic blood pressure in univariate analysis (Table 23.3).

The full model consisted of 14 predictors. We show the results across the 10 imputed sets in Table 23.4. Several predictors had rather limited contributions to model χ^2. Predictors with a large prognostic strength were age and the sumscore for symptoms of atherosclerosis (each χ^2 33). The marker of renal damage creatinine had a χ^2 of 13. Other characteristics had smaller prognostic relevance, with some impact of the general marker of atherosclerosis intima–media thickness (χ^2 7), and a minor contribution of homocysteine. The classical risk factors had at most a χ^2 of 5.6 (for HDL) and hence hardly contributed to the model predictions (Table 23.5).

We tested interactions between the predictors and sex by including cross-product terms with predictors in the full model (overall χ^2 17.5, 16 df, $p = 0.35$). The strongest interaction was between sex and the sumscore for previous symptomatic atherosclerosis (χ^2 6.7, 1 df, $p = 0.01$). In all, the interactions were not considered relevant enough to include an interaction term with sex in the model. We also tested proportionality of hazards over follow-up time. The overall test was not statistically significant (overall χ^2 26, 17 df, $p = 0.07$, cox.zph function), with some non-proportionality suggested for age and smoking.

23.5.2   Impact of Imputation

Fitting the full model was repeated in the complete cases ($n = 2053$), and with variants of imputation. We compare the fits obtained with the complete cases; single imputations (aregImpute or mice, two sets of SI analyses); and multiple imputations (weighted analysis in stacked data, or Rubin's rules with fit.mult. impute). The regression coefficients were estimated mostly quite consistently between approaches (Fig. 23.7). The two strongest predictors were age and the sumscore (HISTCAR2), which had no missings, and hence had very similar estimates of the regression coefficients. Estimates differed most for predictors with many missings and weak prognostic effects, such as systolic blood pressure

Table 23.4 Hazard ratios (HR) and contribution to Cox regression model (χ^2 and *df*) of the predictors in a full model for 3873 patients in the SMART study. Results are from 10 imputed data sets

Predictor	HR [95% CI]*	χ^2	*df*
$(\text{Age}{-}50)^2_+$ (68 vs. 52 years)	1.5 [1.3–1.7]	33	1
Gender (male)	0.9 [0.7–1.2]	0.2	1
Classical risk factors			
Smoking		1.6	2
Never	0.8 [0.6–1.1]		
Former	1		
Current	1.1 [0.7 –1.6]		
Alcohol		1.2	2
Never	1.1 [0.9–1.4]		
Former	1		
Current	1.0 [0.7–1.3]		
Body mass index (kg/m^2, 29 vs. 24)	0.9 [0.8–1.0]	2.7	1
Systolic blood pressure (mmHg, 156 vs. 127)	1.0 [0.9–1.2]	0.7	1
HDL (1.42 vs. 0.96)	0.8 [0.7–1.0]	5.6	1
Diabetes	1.2 [1.0–1.5]	2.7	1
Previous symptomatic atherosclerosis			
Sumscore (AAA 2 points, per 1 point)	1.4 [1.3–1.6]	33	1
Markers of atherosclerosis			
Homocysteine (mmol/l, 16 vs. 10.5)	1.0 [0.9–1.1]	0.4	1
Creatinine (mmol/l, 101 vs. 78)	1.2 [1.1–1.2]	13	1
Albumin		9	2
No	1.0		
Micro	1.3 [1.0–1.6]		
Macro	1.8 [1.2–2.7]		
Intima–media thickness (mm, 1.07 vs. 0.75)	1.2 [1.0–1.3]	7.4	1
Carotid artery stenosis >50%	1.2 [1.0–1.5]	2.6	1

* Hazard ratio [95% confidence interval] refers to interquartile range for continuous predictors

(SYSTH) and homocysteine (HOMOC). The effect of SEX was very small. Estimates were close to zero in CC and imputation analyses, albeit contrary in sign.

We also studied the standard errors of the coefficients (Fig. 23.8). As expected, the standard errors were largest in the CC analysis. The variants of SI gave similar results. Analysis of stacked data provided a kind of average over SI sets; it provided a lower variance estimate than Rubin's rules. So, the stacked data approach worked fine for estimation of coefficients, but underestimated the variance over imputations.

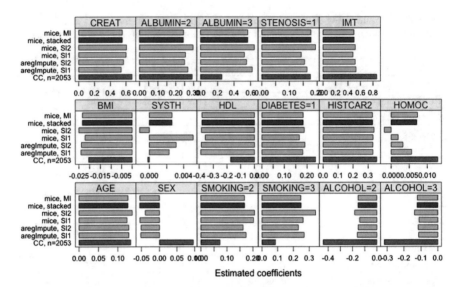

Fig. 23.7 Estimated coefficients in Cox regression models with complete case (CC) analysis ($n = 2053$), or analyses with some form of imputation. SI1 and SI2: 2 sets of single imputations, with `aregImpute` or `mice` algorithms. A weighted regression was performed in stacked data ("mice, stacked") and the mean over 10 imputed sets was taken ("mice, MI"; using `fit.mult.impute`)

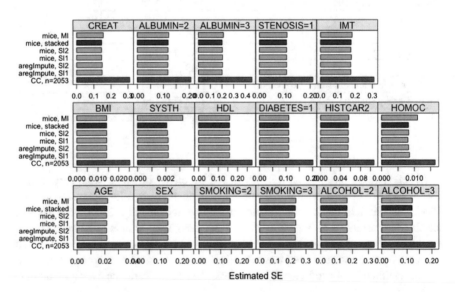

Fig. 23.8 Estimated standard error in Cox regression models with complete case (CC) analysis ($n = 2053$), or analyses with some form of imputation, as in Fig. 23.7. mice, MI applied Rubin's rules for appropriate estimation of the variance (with `fit.mult.impute`)

23.5.3   R Code for Full Model with Imputation

The full model in complete data, without imputation:

```
Frequencies of Missing Values Due to Each Variable
AGE   SEX SMOKING ALCOHOL BMI SYSTH HDL DIABETES HISTCAR2
0     0    25      25    3   1498  30   40         0
HOMOC   CREAT ALBUMIN STENOSIS IMT
463     17    207     93       98

Cox Proportional Hazards Model
 cph(formula = Surv(TEVENT, EVENT) ~
    ifelse(AGE>50, (AGE/10-5)^2, 0) +SEX +SMOKING +ALCOHOL +BMI +SYSTH +HDL +
     DIABETES +HISTCAR2 +HOMOC +log(CREAT) +ALBUMIN +STENOSIS+IMT, data = SMART,
 ...)

                        Model Tests       Discrimination Indexes
    Obs       2053    LR chi2    104.34    R2       0.080
    Events    142     d.f.           14    Dxy      0.401
    Center 3.6122     Pr(> chi2) 0.0000
```

The full model in 10 imputed data sets:

```
cph(.~..., data=SMART10, ..., weights=w) # stacked data
cox01.m <- fit.mult.impute(.~..., fitter=cph, xtrans=gm, ...) # Rubin's
rules
```

Compare various estimates of coefficients:

```
mcoef <- rbind(coef(cox0), ... , coef(cox01.m)) # coefficients in matrix
barchart(mcoef,group=rownames(matcoef),scales=list(x="free"), ...) # Fig
23.6
```

23.6   Model Selection and Estimation

23.6.1   Stepwise Selection

We judged our sample size as large enough to allow for some model reduction for easier practical application (460 events, full model with 17 *df*, ignoring that the coding of predictors also consumed some effective degrees of freedom). One approach was to apply a backward selection procedure with a higher than standard p-value. We used Akaike's Information Criterium (AIC), which implies $p < 0.157$ for selection of predictors with 1 *df* [14]. A promising alternative is to apply the LASSO method, which achieves selection of predictors by shrinking some coefficients to zero by setting a constraint on the sum of the absolute standardized coefficients [582].

Both the stepwise selection and LASSO methods were applied in the stacked data set [678]. The application of the backward stepwise procedure was relatively straightforward. We rely on estimates of the coefficients in the weighted regression,

Table 23.5 Cox regression coefficients in the full model, in a stepwise selected model (using Akaike's Information Criterion), and in the LASSO model

Predictor	Full (mice, MI)	Stepwise (AIC)	LASSO
$(Age-50)_+^2$ (years above 50)	0.13	0.13	0.12
Gender (male)	−0.05	not selected	not selected
Smoking			
Never	0	not selected	not selected
Former	0.17		
Current	0.25		
Alcohol		not selected	not selected
Never	0		
Former	−0.15		
Current	−0.12		
Body mass index (kg/m^2)	−0.023	−0.025	−0.01
Blood pressure (/10 mmHg)	0.026	not selected	0.019
HDL	−0.38	−0.40	−0.27
Diabetes	0.18	0.18	0.11
Previous vascular disease	0.33	0.35	0.33
Homocysteine (/10 mmol/l)	0.073	not selected	0.070
Log(creatinine) (mmol/l)	0.55	0.71	0.55
Albumin			
No	0	0	0
Micro	0.24	0.29	0.21
Macro	0.57	0.60	0.51
Intima–media thickness (mm)	0.50	0.55	0.49
Carotid artery stenosis >50%	0.18	0.21	0.16

and realize that we may slightly underestimate the variance of predictors with many imputed values. The alternative was to use the `fit.mult.impute` procedure multiple times to drop candidate predictors sequentially. In both cases, we selected a model with 9 predictors out of the original 14. The regression coefficients from the selected model were very similar when estimated in the stacked data or with Rubin's rules (Table 23.5).

23.6.2   LASSO for Selection with Imputed Data

The LASSO model requires a search for the optimal penalty factor (λ). This may be performed by a cross-validation procedure for a single imputed data set (Fig. 23.9). This cross-validation did not work properly with weighted regression in the stacked

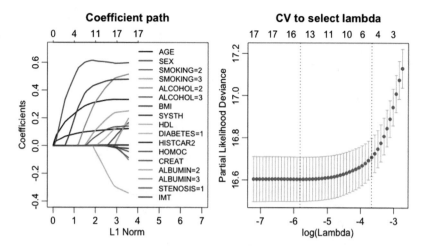

Fig. 23.9 LASSO in the first data set where missing values were completed by `mice`. The coefficient path shows that more coefficients remain in the model with less penalty (a higher L1 Norm, the sum of the absolute standardized coefficients). The optimal penalty according to cross-validation was 0.003; log(Lambda) = log(0.003) = −5.8 (right graph)

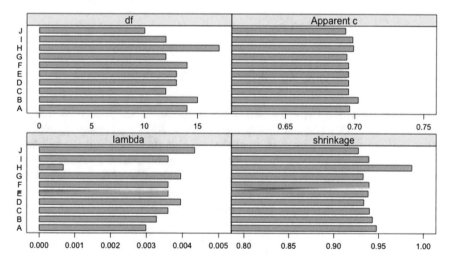

Fig. 23.10 Results of the LASSO procedure per imputed data set. Row A indicates the first imputed set, with lambda = 0.003 as shown in Fig. 23.9

data set. As a pragmatic alternative, the optimal penalty (lambda) was determined within each imputed set. The lambda values were found to vary considerably (Fig. 23.10). The mean effective shrinkage factor was 0.94; the typical degrees of freedom 13 (range 10–17), and the mean apparent discriminative ability 0.697 (range 0.6930–0.703) across the 10 imputed sets.

The mean penalty was 0.0034 and used in the stacked data set to fit a LASSO model. This model included one component of the smoking and one of the alcohol variables. To drop these, we may slightly increase the penalty to 0.004 rather than 0.0034; alternatively, the grouped LASSO might be used. The final LASSO model then resembled the stepwise model, with 11 predictors left, and slightly shrunk coefficients (Table 23.5).

23.7   Model Performance and Internal Validation

Discrimination of the full model was indicated by the c statistic, which was 0.697. The apparent performance of the stepwise model and the LASSO model were very similar: 0.694 and 0.695 respectively. More relevant is the optimism-corrected performance. We hereto performed a bootstrap procedure within each imputed data set. This is a pragmatic approach to the combination of model selection in imputed data, which may provide quite reasonable estimates op optimism-corrected performance [401]. The optimism was determined as usual within each imputed data set, and results averaged to provide the overall optimism-corrected performance estimates. All model selection and estimation steps were repeated within each bootstrap sample.

23.7.1   Estimation of Optimism in Performance

More specifically, the following steps were followed, in line with what was discussed in Sect. 5.3.4 (*Calculation of optimism-corrected performance*). We also show the key R commands. We label the imputed data set *I* and the bootstrap sample within an imputed set *Bi*. The samples *Bi* are created by an index *j*, drawn with replacement from *I*. We focus on the internal validation of the LASSO model, since the internal validation of the full model and the stepwise model can be done per imputed set *I* with the `validate` function in `rms`:

```
data1 <- as.data.frame(complete(gm,i)) # this is set I
S1    <- Surv(time=data1$TEVENT, event=data1$EVENT) # for later use
```

0. Consider an imputed data set *I* with imputation *i* out of 1:*m* imputed sets, as above.

rms:

```
for (i in 1:m) { # m imputed sets
data1    <- as.data.frame(complete(gm,i)) # this is set I
S1       <- Surv(time=data1$TEVENT, event=data1$EVENT)
cox01.1 <-cph(S1 ~ ..., data=data1, x=T, y=T) # full model in I
validate(cox01.1, B=200) # 200 bootstraps per imputed sets
validate(cox01.1, B=200, bw=T, rule='aic') } # end over m imputed sets
```

1. Construct a LASSO model in the imputed sample *I*

```
cv.glmmod <- cv.glmnet(x=cox01.1$x, y=S1, alpha = 1, family="cox")
model.L1 <- glmnet(x=cox01.1$x, y=S1, alpha = 1,
lambda=cv.glmmod$lambda.min, family="cox") # use optimum penalty
lp1      <- cox01.1$x %*% coef(model.L1)   # for apparent performance
```

2. Draw a bootstrap sample *Bi* with replacement from the imputed sample

```
j     <- sample(nrow(data1), replace=T) # for sample Bi
S1j   <- Surv(data1[j,"TEVENT"],data1[j,"EVENT"]) # for cph fit
```

3. Construct a model in sample *Bi* replaying every step that was done in the imputed sample *I*, especially model specification steps such as selection of predictors. Determine the bootstrap performance as the apparent performance in sample *Bi*.

```
cv.j <- cv.glmnet(x=cox01.1$x[j,], y=S1j, alpha = 1, family="cox")
model.L1j <- glmnet(x=cox01.1$x[j,], y=S1j, alpha=1,
lambda=cv.j$lambda.min, family="cox") # use optimum penalty from Bi
lp1j <-   cox01.1$x[j,] %*% coef(model.L1j) # apparent performance in Bi
App <- rcorr.cens(-as.numeric(lp1j),S1j)[2] # apparent Dxy for Bi
```

4. Apply model from *Bi* to the original sample *I* without any modification to determine the test performance

```
lp1   <- cox01.1$x %*% coef(model.L1j)       # validated performance in I
Test <- rcorr.cens(-as.numeric(lp1),S1)[2] # test Dxy in I; c=D/2+.5
```

5. Calculate the optimism as the difference between bootstrap performance and test performance

```
Opt   <- (App-Test) / 2 # optimism in c statistic
```

6. Repeat steps 1–4 many times, at least 200, to obtain a stable mean estimate of the optimism.

```
B <- 200
```

7. Subtract the mean optimism estimate (step 6) from the apparent performance in each imputed set *I* to obtain the optimism-corrected performance estimate

The validated performance across the imputations follows the pattern for the

```
AppI <- rcorr.cens(-as.numeric(lp1),S1)[2]/2 + .5  # # apparent c for I
Opt.mean.Bi <- mean(Opt) # optimism over 200 bootstrap samples B
CoptI <- AppI - Opt.mean.Bi # optimism-corrected for set I
Opt.mean.i  <- mean(CoptI) # optimism over 10 imputed sets m
```

apparent performance, where the concordance statistics for the full, stepwise and LASSO models were 0.697, 0.694, and 0.695, respectively (Fig. 23.11). Validated concordance statistics (c) confirm that the full model has the best performance according to bootstrapping within each imputed set. The mean of the optimism-corrected c statistics was 0.687. The mean optimism was 0.014; when we apply this to the apparent fit over the stacked data the optimism-corrected estimate is 0.683. The LASSO performance is second best in most imputed sets (mean c 0.682), and backward stepwise selection based on AIC is not much worse (mean c 0.677, Fig. 23.11). Overall, we may expect a c statistic around 0.68 in similar patients as used for development of the SMART prediction model.

We also evaluated the calibration slope that may be expected after the LASSO procedure. The LASSO led to effective shrinkage by a factor of 0.94. According to

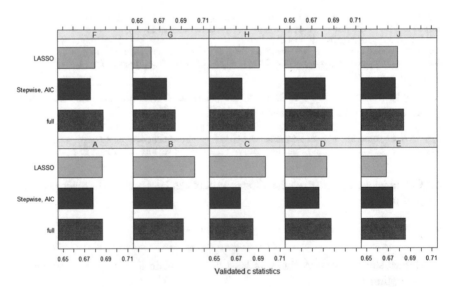

Fig. 23.11 Validated concordance statistics for different modeling approaches in each of the 10 imputed data sets. The full model has the best performance according to bootstrapping within each imputed set; and the LASSO is second best in most imputed sets, and backward stepwise selection based on AIC is not much worse

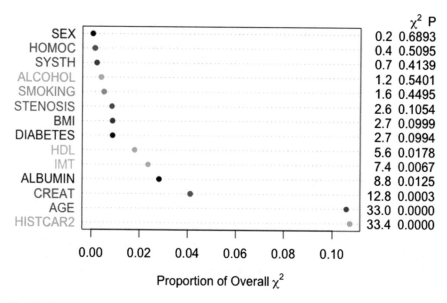

Fig. 23.12 Relative contribution of each predictor to the full prediction model, using the chi-square statistics information as presented in Table 23.4

bootstrap validation, the expected calibration was 0.99, so very close to the perfect value of unity.

23.7.2   *Model Presentation*

The results of the modeling process can be presented in various ways. From Table 23.4, we learn about the relative contributions of each predictor to the model; a graphical depiction is shown in Fig. 23.12. For a survival model such as the SMART prediction model, we may summarize the discriminative ability by a grouped Kaplan–Meier plot (Fig. 23.13). Finally, we may present the LASSO model as a nomogram (Fig. 23.14). In the nomogram, we can judge the relative importance of each predictor by the number of points attributed over the range of the predictor, and we can calculate 3-year and 5-year survival estimates. Survival relates here to the probability of being free of a cardiovascular event.

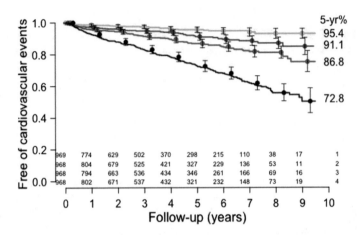

Fig. 23.13 Fractions of patients free of events in 4 groups according to prognostic risk profile from the LASSO model. In group 1, only 33 of 969 had a cardiovascular event, for a 5-year risk of cardiovascular events of 4.6% (1–0.954). In group 4, 247 of 968 had a cardiovascular event, for a 5-year risk of 27% (1–0.73)

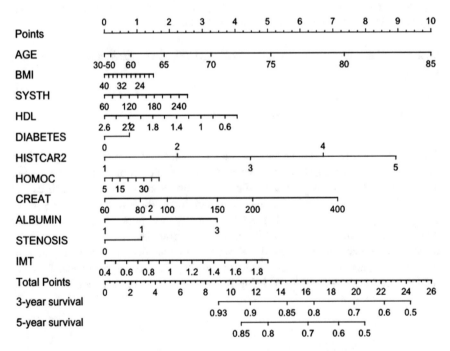

Fig. 23.14 Nomogram for the LASSO model developed with multiple imputation in the SMART study (*n* = 3873) to predicted 3-year and 5-year survival (probability of being free of a cardiovascular event). For example, a 75-year-old patient, with a BMI of 28, HDL 1, no diabetes, previous aortic aneurysm but no other symptoms of atherosclerosis (HISTCAR2 = 2), a creatinine value of 100, low albumin, no carotid stenosis, IMT of 1 mm, has a total points score of 5 + 1 + 3 + 0 + 2 + 2 + 0 + 0 + 2 = 15. This corresponds to predicted 3- and 5-year survival of approximately 85% and 75% respectively

23.7.3 R Code for Presentation of a Survival Model

Relative contributions of each predictor in full model

```
plot(anova(cox01.multfit), what='proportion chisq', ...) # Fig 23.11
```

Nomogram for the LASSO model; copy coefficients to a cph object

```
LASSOsel <- update(cox01.multfit, .~. -SEX - ALCOHOL - SMOKING, surv=T)
coefL     <- as.numeric(coef(model.L1) # extract coefs from LASSO fit
LASSOsel$coefficients <- coefL[abs(coefL)>0] # select non-NULL
surv  <- Survival(LASSOsel) # Predicted survival from model
surv3 <- function(x) surv(3*365.25,lp=x)
surv5 <- function(x) surv(5*365.25,lp=x)
plot(nomogram(LASSOsel, fun=list(surv3, surv5), AGE=c(30,seq(50,85,5)),
CREAT=c(60,80,100,150,200,400), funlabel=c('3-year survival', '5-year
survival'), maxscale=10, ...)) # Fig 23.13
```

Four prognostic groups in Kaplan–Meier curve, which are as follows:

```
S1 <- Surv(SMART$TEVENT/365.25, SMART$EVENT) # survival time in years
g4 <- cut2(LASSOsel$linear.predictors, g=4)  # 4 groups
levels(g4) <- 1:4
survplot(npsurv(S1 ~ g4), n.risk=T, conf="bars", ...)   # Fig 23.12
```

23.8 Concluding Remarks

This case study illustrates how a prediction model can be developed and internally validated for a survival analysis problem, with an advanced modeling procedure (LASSO) in multiply imputed data. Some further methodological work is needed to improve on the somewhat pragmatic choices on combining LASSO with imputation. Most modeling steps could be considered in the bootstrap procedure for internal validation.

This case study also confirms the distinction between risk factors in the general population (without cardiovascular disease) and prognostic factors in patients with symptomatic disease. Classical risk factors such as smoking, alcohol use, BMI, blood pressure, HDL, and diabetes, had very limited prognostic value in the clinical setting. These characteristics are hence not useful to predict future events once the cardiovascular disease has developed. Indicators of previous symptomatic cardio-vascular disease and the extent of atherosclerosis were more useful. This finding is similar to findings in the GUSTO-I study (Chap. 22), where e.g., smoking was associated with a better outcome after acute MI: risk factors may not be prognostic once the disease has developed.

Questions

23.1 Composite outcomes (Sect. 23.2.2 and Table 23.1)
Outcomes were combined in the presented analyses.

   (a) What assumptions does this imply about the effects of the predictors for
       each outcome?
   (b) How could this be tested? See Glynn and Rosner [186]

23.2 Missing values (Figs. 23.2 and 23.3)

   (a) Some might argue to exclude patients with many missing values. What
       would be a reasonable number as maximum of missing values per
       patient in the current analysis?
   (b) Others might argue to exclude candidate predictors with many missing
       values. What would be a reasonable number as maximum of missing
       values per predictor in the current analysis?
   (c) We note that missing values occur together for some predictors. We could
       also choose to exclude patients with missing values ("NA") in specific
       combinations predictors. Which would you choose?

23.3 Effects of LASSO versus stepwise selection (Table 23.5)
We select largely the same predictors with a LASSO procedure as with
stepwise selection using AIC.

   (a) How is it possible to obtain the same selection with these different
       methods?
   (b) The effect of age is similar to both methods, while the effect of BMI is
       very weak according to the LASSO. How is this possible?

23.4 Variability between imputations and bootstrap samples

   (a) How large is the variability between imputations for the penalty factor
       lambda in Fig. 23.10?
   (b) Is this variation relevant?
   (c) The current internal validation settings were: 200 bootstraps within 10
       sets of imputations, with 10-fold cross-validation within each
       bootstrap. So, B = 200; m = 10; cv = 10, for a total of 20,000 model
       fits. How might we better balance these numbers?

23.5 Combining LASSO and imputation
In the case study, we estimated the mean lambda over imputed data sets, and
used the mean lambda in stacked data to fit single LASSO model. An
alternative is to fit LASSO models in every imputed set, and take the mean
coefficients across imputations [401].

   (a) What are the advantages of the latter approach (mean(coefficients))?
   (b) What are the advantages of the case study approach (coefficients | mean
       (λ))?

Chapter 24
Overall Lessons and Data Sets

Background In this final chapter, we summarize some lessons learnt on development, validation, and updating of prediction models, based on the empirical experience from case studies as described in this book, and modeling experience in other medical prediction problems. We consider the essential elements to successful modeling: appropriate methods; sufficient sample size; emphasis on validation; using, not ignoring, subject matter knowledge. We also reflect further on modern machine learning techniques. Reporting guidelines and risk of bias tools are discussed. We end this chapter with a description of the case studies used throughout this book, where data sets are available through the book's website.

24.1 Sample Size

Developing a valid prediction model from a relatively small data set has proven to be hard. Many empirical examples are availability of poor performance at external validation [13, 513]. Overfitting is a severe problem; it is common to ask too much from a small sample [563]. Asking many questions is natural: data collection in empirical studies is costly, and we are curious about what patterns emerge from our precious data. Small data sets, hence, might merely serve to explore rather than to derive firm relations. Yet, we need such firm relations for accurate predictions. Also, we need strong predictors [431]; hence, when we have only a few relatively weak predictors it is tempting to search further for additional predictors [266]. An honest internal validation procedure should reveal the optimism that is associated with the full modeling procedure, including any searches for interesting patterns [94, 535, 563, 685]. Harrell and others have observed that model uncertainty usually is more important for optimism in model performance than parameter uncertainty [225]. Hence, this step should never be forgotten, and careful reporting is needed [303]. See Chatfield [94] and others for a more theoretical but well-readable discussion on model uncertainty [34, 138, 222]. Below, we further

© Springer Nature Switzerland AG 2019
E. W. Steyerberg, *Clinical Prediction Models*, Statistics for Biology
and Health, https://doi.org/10.1007/978-3-030-16399-0_24

illustrate the impact of model uncertainty, specifically, the problematic role of stepwise selection to develop prediction models, and the harm that can be done by studying more predictors beyond a core set of predictors.

24.1.1   Model Selection, Estimation, and Sample Size

Simulations in GUSTO-I and other studies clarified the relation between model selection (use of stepwise methods vs. a full model), estimation (maximum likelihood, ML; shrinkage based on bootstrapping; penalization), and sample size [542, 543]. We first study an 8-predictor model in small and large subsamples with on average 24 and 59 events, respectively. We first focus on discriminative ability (c statistic, or area under the ROC curve, Fig. 24.1), and then on calibration (slope of the linear predictor, Fig. 24.2).

- Model selection strategies were addressed in Chaps. 10 and 11. Some pros and many cons of stepwise methods were discussed. The GUSTO-I simulations confirm that stepwise methods are rather harmful in small samples, with a median c statistic (or area under the ROC statistic) of 0.72 at validation if we use the traditional criterion of $p < 0.05$ for selection of predictors (Fig. 24.1, left panel). A full model reaches a c statistic around 0.76.
- Model estimation strategies were discussed in Chaps. 13 and 14. Penalized (or "regularized") regression can be performed with a $L2$ penalty ("ridge regression") or a $L1$ penalty (LASSO). The c statistic was not affected much by penalized estimation, although the best-validated performance was achieved by the full model with penalized regression ($c = 0.766$).

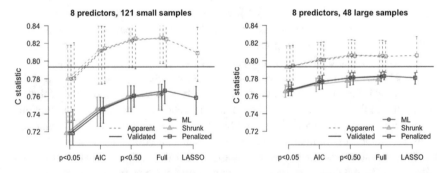

Fig. 24.1 Discriminative ability in relation to model selection, estimation, and sample size for an 8-predictor model developed in subsamples from the GUSTO-I trial (see Chap. 22). Small and large subsamples included on average 24 and 59 events, respectively (30-day mortality). Models were created with stepwise selection ($p < 0.05$, AIC ($p < 0.157$), $p < 0.50$) and with fitting a full model, with estimation by standard maximum likelihood (ML), shrinkage of regression coefficients (based on bootstrap validation), and penalized maximum likelihood. Moreover, we applied the LASSO for model selection by shrinking some parameters towards zero. Model performance was assessed in the development samples and the part of GUSTO-I that was not used for model development. Substantially better performance was noted for models derived from the larger subsamples

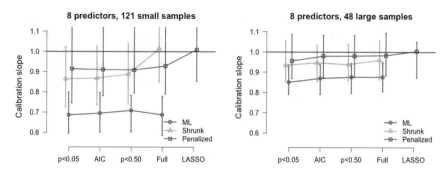

Fig. 24.2 Calibration slope in relation to model selection, estimation, and sample size for an 8-predictor model developed in subsamples from the GUSTO-I trial (see legend Fig. 24.1). Substantially better performance was noted for models with shrinkage or penalization compared to standard maximum likelihood (ML) estimation

- The key relevance of an adequate sample size for model development and validation was stressed throughout this book, and specifically in Chaps. 5, 17, 20 and 21.

   - We note a substantially better validated performance if models were constructed in larger samples (Fig. 24.1, right panel). The best performance was found for the full model with penalized regression ($c = 0.783$). The LASSO performance was close ($c = 0.781$), and stepwise with $p < 0.05$ remained suboptimal ($c = 0.767$). The performance in the full GUSTO-I data with a full model was slightly higher ($n = 40,830$, 2,851 events, $c = 0.793$).
   - We also note less variability in performance with larger sample sizes (smaller interquartile range, Fig. 24.1). The variability in apparent performance was larger than at validation, in line with the discussion in Chap. 19.
   - Sample size also affected the optimism in apparent performance estimates (dotted lines in Fig. 24.1). The optimism was around +0.06 for the small samples, and +0.02 for the larger samples.

In sum, stepwise selection led to poor discriminative ability at validation, particularly with small development samples; shrinkage or penalized estimation had limited impact; and a larger sample size alleviated the problems. The event per variable (EPV) ratio was 24/8 = 3 for the small samples and still below 10 for the larger samples (59/8 = 7.4).

24.1.2   Calibration Improvement by Penalization

All models provided on average correct predictions (calibration-in-the-large). We further focused on the calibration slope, which reflects whether predictions were too extreme (see Chap. 17). Model selection had limited impact on calibration; the slope was around 0.7 when models were developed in small samples with maximum likelihood estimation (Fig. 24.2). Shrinkage or penalization was important, bringing slopes closer to the ideal value of 1. Particularly, good calibration was noted for the LASSO. A larger sample size led to improved calibration with any of the methods, although standard ML estimation still led to too extreme predictions (slope around 0.87, Fig. 24.2, right panel).

24.1.3   Poorer Performance with More Predictors

When we study more predictors, we would expect that we could obtain better performing models. Remarkably, this was not the case in simulations in GUSTO-I [542]. A full model with 17 predictors had at most similar performance to a full 8-predictor model, when we applied penalized maximum likelihood estimation ($c = 0.783$ with 8 or 17 predictors, Fig. 24.3). Backward stepwise selection with $p < 0.05$ led to similarly poor models when 17 predictors were considered instead of 8 ($c = 0.763$ with 17 vs. $c = 0.767$ with 8 predictors). Hence, when we start with too many predictors, stepwise selection methods may not be able to save us, even if all predictors are of prognostic relevance (all $p < 0.01$ in the full GUSTO data set; $c = 0.805$ for 17 vs. $c = 0.793$ for 8 predictors). The balance between the number of predictors and number of events should be for candidate predictors, not the number of selected predictors (Chap. 4).

As expected, the calibration slope was poorer with 17 rather than 8 predictors with standard maximum likelihood (ML) estimation. This reflected more overfitting. Shrinkage or penalization resolved the calibration problem (Fig. 24.4).

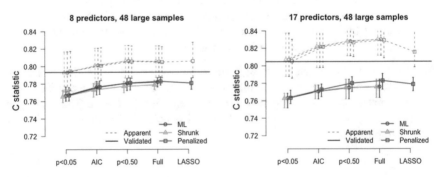

Fig. 24.3 Discriminative ability in relation to the number of predictors (see legend of Fig. 24.1). We note that models estimated with 17 rather than 8 predictors had more optimism and were not performing better at validation

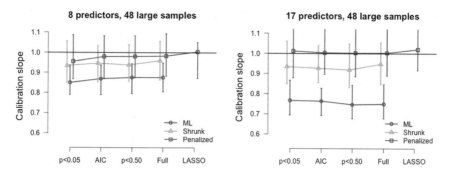

Fig. 24.4 Calibration slope in relation to the number of predictors (see legend of Fig. 24.1). We note that models estimated with 17 rather than 8 predictors suffered more from overfitting with standard maximum likelihood (ML) estimation. Shrinkage or penalization resolved the calibration problem

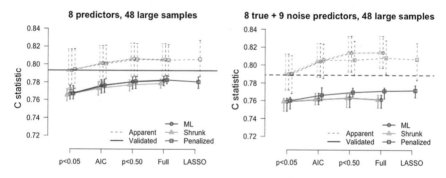

Fig. 24.5 Discriminative ability and the impact of noise predictors (see legend of Fig. 24.1). Any models estimated with 17 predictors performed worse than a model starting with 8 true predictors

24.1.4 Model Selection with Noise Predictors

Results were thus far for modeling in a context with strong to weak predictors with sets of 8 or 17 predictors. We might hope that stepwise selection would be of benefit in a situation of some true and some noise predictors. We hereto randomly permute the 9 extra predictors in the 17-predictor model compared to the 8-predictor model. The discriminative performance of this model is obviously lower than the model with true predictors ($c = 0.789$ for 8 + 9 noise vs. $c = 0.805$ for 17 true predictors). Figure 24.5 illustrates that a full model with penalized estimation is still the best choice, either with *L2* penalty (ridge) or *L1* penalty (LASSO). An even better model would arise if we did not consider any of the 9 extra predictors; whether these are true (Fig. 24.3) or noise predictors (Fig. 24.5).

Table 24.1 Problem areas with prognostic modeling, and potential solutions with their benefits

Problem	Characterization	Potential solutions	Benefits
Sample size	Asking too much from the data relative to its size	Balance research question and modeling approach with available information	Less overfitting
	Particularistic, single center samples used	Collaborative efforts	Statistical and epidemiological advantages (standard errors decrease with larger sample size; generalizability increases; cross-validation possible for external validation)
Validation	Internal validity is a minimum requirement	Bootstrap validation	Honest impression of model performance for similar patients
	External validity important as a second aim	Multicenter/ international studies for external validation	Impression of model performance in plausibly related settings
Subject matter knowledge	Use rather than ignore	Literature review; expert opinion	Model stability; less overfitting

24.1.5 Potential Solutions

A potential solution for small sample size is to perform collaborative studies (Table 24.1). For example, instead of analyzing a single-center retrospective cohort study, we may collect data from multiple centers, leading to a multicenter cohort study. Apart from simply increasing sample size other advantages occur. The multiple centers may be slightly different from each other, in local protocols for diagnostic workup, treatment choices, definition of predictors, etc. Such heterogeneity needs to be quantified to understand the generalizability of the resulting model [457]. If it were derived from a single center, the results might be typical for that setting, rather than represent "current practice". Also, cross-validation becomes possible, where we leave out one center to test a model that was developed on other centers (Chaps. 17 and 19) [546].

24.1.6 R Code for Model Selection and Penalization

The full 8-predictor is simply:

```
gusto8 <- lrm(day30~a65+sex+dia+hyp+hrt+hig+sho+ttr, data=gusto,
x=T,y=T,maxit=50)
gustoi <- gusto[gusto$grps==i,] # select a small subsample
gusto8i <- update(gusto8, data=gustoi)
```

Stepwise selection:

```
bwsel  <- fastbw(gusto8i, rule="p", type="individual", sls=.05)
fitbw <- lrm.fit(y=gusto8i$y, x=as.matrix(gusto8i$x[, bwsel$factors.kept]))
```

Shrink coefficients by bootstrapping:

```
gusto8i$coef[2:9]*validate(gusto8i, B=200)[4,5] # multiply by s factor
fitbw$coef[-1]*validate(gusto8i, bw=T, rule="p", type="individual",
sls=.05, B=200)[4,5] # multiply by s factor, included the selection per B
```

Penalized regression, *L2* penalty for ridge regression:

```
p <- pentrace(gusto8i, penalty=c(1,2,3,4,5,6,8,10,12,16,24,30),maxit=99)
update(gusto8i, penalty=p$penalty)$coef[-1]
update(fitbw,   penalty=p$penalty)$coef[-1] # same penalty after selection
```

Penalized regression, *L1* penalty for LASSO regression:

```
glmmod <- glmnet(x=gusto8i$x, y=gusto8i$y, alpha=1, family="binomial")
lambda <- rep(0.001,10)
  for (j in 1:10) { cv.glmmod <- cv.glmnet(x=fitf$x, y=fitf$y, alpha = 1,
                     family=c("binomial"))
                  lambda[j] = cv.glmmod$lambda.min }
model8.L1 <- glmnet(x=gusto8i$x, y=gusto8i$y, alpha = 1, family="binomial",
          lambda = mean(lambda)) # model fitted with lambda from 10x10 cv
```

Random permutation was by the `sample` command:

```
gustop <- gusto # use this data set as basis
gustop[,Cs(PMI,HEI,WEI, ...)] <-
      rbind(sample(gusto$PMI), sample(gusto$HEI), sample(gusto$WEI), ... )
```

24.2 Validation

Internal and external validations deserve our full attention in prediction modeling. Patterns in a data set have no meaning if these patterns are invalid outside the specific data set. First, we need to check internal validity [546]. The bootstrap is a very useful tool for this purpose, but we should be careful to apply it honestly, i.e., not secretly forget some model specification steps [535]. Second, we are concerned about external validity; if a model is only applicable in strict settings, we are astray from serious science [285].

Sample size is important both for development and validation samples. If sample size is insufficient at model development, overfitting will occur. If sample size is insufficient at model validation, we may falsely conclude that a model performs satisfactorily, while substantial invalidity may in fact exist.

24.2.1 Examples of Internal and External Validation

Some models may generalize well if developed according to the principles outlined in Part II, but other models require at least an adjustment for the average, case mix adjusted incidence of the outcome. In GUSTO-I, we noted that the variability by subsample or region was largely attributable to chance, but this was in the context of a randomized trial, with a specific protocol (Chap. 22). A previously developed model (TIMI-II) required updating of the intercept [536, 540]. In the testicular cancer example, we noted some differences between centers, but the sample sizes were not large enough to draw a firm conclusion on similarity of the intercept across settings (Chap. 19) [645]. In the stroke example, substantial differences between centers were noted that were beyond chance (Chap. 21) [341]. Systematic differences can sometimes be attributed to specific circumstances; for example, a systematically poorer than predicted outcome was noted in patients from developing and middle-income countries [435].

The internal, temporal and geographic validity was also studied for outcome prediction models in stroke [311]. Internal validation was not enough, and some form of external validation was necessary for a good impression of model performance in new patients. This was partly caused by problems to fully capture all modeling steps in the internal validation procedure, which hence resulted in still too optimistic estimates of model performance. A study in children with fever also emphasized that external validation was necessary beyond internal validation [56].

24.3   Subject Matter Knowledge Versus Machine Learning

24.3.1   Exploiting Subject Matter Knowledge

Throughout this book, using subject matter knowledge has been emphasized. Examples of valid models that were built from scratch are rare. Most successful models combine well-known predictors and limit the use of the data set to some fine-tuning of the model specification. For example, we may eliminate some main effects that do not contribute to outcome prediction. On the other hand, we may include some non-linear terms that are important to capture the relation of a continuous predictor with the outcome. We may also include some interactions, if these are very strong. The main role of the data set then is to quantify the predictor–outcome relations, and provide an impression of the performance of the model. As discussed in Chap. 1, we aim to avoid the situation that we develop a model without some knowledge on which predictors to include, in what functional form, and unknown effects (see Table 1.1).

Model updating is a formal approach to use prior knowledge (Chaps. 20 and 21). We start with assuming that a prior model is valid for a new setting. We modify coefficients and add other predictors if indicated by the data under study. Such model updating is only possible if a reasonable prior multivariable model exists. We are back at standard model development if only univariate associations are known, or qualitative statements on the strength of a predictive effects.

Several disadvantages can be mentioned for modeling with subject knowledge. First, we may miss important new predictors. We should be prepared to take this risk, since searching for new predictors has many risks of its own, including testimation bias, instability of the search, and false positive discoveries [268]. Second, we may object that we do not discover new knowledge. We only combine what is known already. This is, however, precisely the role of prediction models in medicine: they quantify what is already known. Knowledge discovery is a phase before we can start serious prediction modeling. Prediction models may have a role beyond systematic review of prognostic factors, as is starting to be promoted by the Cochrane collaboration [459]. Systematic reviews may provide summaries of relative risks; prediction models provide absolute risks.

We may be interested in a prediction model that includes new predictors, such as a genetic marker, or other types of biomarker or imaging characteristic. We first would need robust evidence on the univariate effect of the marker, and preferably also on its effect adjusted for other important predictors [373]. If this evidence is sufficient, we could study the performance of the marker when integrated into a prediction model. Of interest is the incremental value of the marker [293]. Several performance criteria can be used, such as increase in discriminative ability, reclassification, and decision curve analysis (see Chap. 16) [429, 561, 564].

Maarten van Smeden, LUMC, Leiden, published an attractive flowchart to guide model developers (Fig. 24.6) [633]. The key issues to consider include:

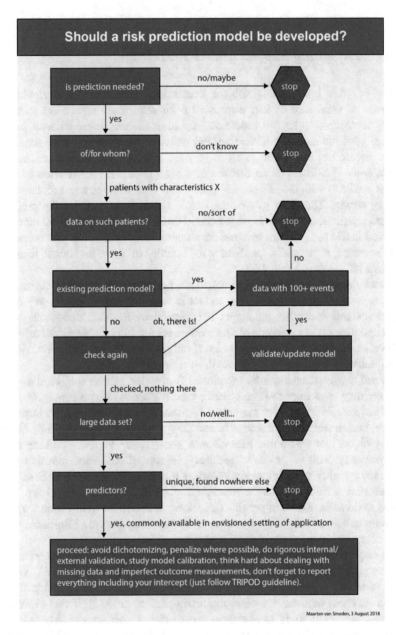

Fig. 24.6 Maarten van Smeden's flowchart for the question: should a new prediction model be developed? [633]

- Is a prediction model of interest?
- What is the audience?
- Are high-quality data from the relevant subjects available?
- Is there no existing prediction model to validate and update from?
- Is sample size adequate?
- Are predictors known and likely available in the envisioned setting?

If questions are answered with "No", prediction model development should not be pursued. Importantly if a model is developed or validated, it should be reported in a transparent way, specifically, following the TRIPOD guideline [105, 390].

24.3.2 Machine Learning and Big Data

Machine learning approaches generally follow a different philosophy (see also Chap. 4). The idea is to extract patterns from data more agnostically, with less human involvement in the modeling [283]. Very large sample sizes are then needed, which may become more and more within reach in the Big Data era [43]. One example is the OHDSI Observational Health Data Sciences and Informatics (OHDSI) program https://www.ohdsi.org/. Very large data sets are made accessible through adoption of a Common Data Model. For prediction modeling, the LASSO is used as a default [452]. The LASSO takes a nice position, since it can be regarded as an extension of traditional regression analysis, and as a prime example of machine learning.

Various other machine learning and artificial intelligence techniques are gaining popularity [181, 444]. Specifically, deep learning techniques (including convolutional neural networks) have been applied successfully for learning from radiological images [346]. Deep learning algorithms may increasingly beat humans in discovering patterns in such images and assist computerized diagnosis.

24.4 Reporting of Prediction Models and Risk of Bias

24.4.1 Reporting Guidelines

Reporting of prediction models is often unclear, with a lack of detail on methods and results. Various reporting guidelines have been proposed, following the CONSORT initiative for randomized clinical trials, STARD for diagnostic studies and REMARK for prognostic factor studies. All are readily available and maintained at http://www.equator-network.org/. In 2015, a specific reporting guideline was proposed for the development or validation of prediction models: Transparent Reporting of a multivariable prediction model for Individual Prognosis Or Diagnosis (TRIPOD) [105]. The TRIPOD initiative developed a set of recommendations for the reporting of studies developing, validating, or updating a prediction model, whether for diagnostic or prognostic purposes. The central claim is: "Only with full and clear reporting of information on all aspects of a prediction model can risk of bias and potential usefulness of prediction models be adequately assessed."

An extensive list of potential items was reduced and revised by discussion among methodologists, health care professionals, and journal editors. The resulting TRIPOD Statement is a checklist of 22 items. The TRIPOD Statement aims to improve the transparency of the reporting of a prediction model study regardless of the study methods used. Importantly, an explanation and elaboration document provides detail on many aspects of model development or validation [383].

The checklist has 22 items (Table 24.2, also available at www.tripod-statement. org). The items relate to title and abstract to enable retrieval by readers and for systematic reviews; the introduction to clarify the context and purpose of the model; the methods used and results, with items as discussed in this book; the discussion, where attention is needed on both limitations for internal and external validity since these impact on the potential clinical use of the model. Some other information is also required such as the availability of supplementary material (which should be encouraged, specifically the statistical code that was used for analysis) and the source of funding. Related checklists include:

- REporting recommendations for tumor MARKer prognostic studies (REMARK) [373]
- RiGoR: reporting guidelines to address common sources of bias in risk model development [303]
- Strengthening the reporting of Genetic RIsk Prediction Studies: GRIPS [280].

The need for transparency is recognized by many in the scientific world, including editors of journals. The practical adherence is unfortunately still limited. An underlying difficulty is whether all 22 items are really critical for the assessment of risk of bias and potential usefulness of prediction models.

24.4.2   Risk of Bias Assessment

Various tools have been proposed to assess the risk of bias in prediction models. One such tool is PROBAST ("Prediction model Risk Of Bias ASsessment Tool") [389]. This tool intends to assess the risk of bias and applicability of diagnostic and prognostic prediction model studies. Similar to TRIPOD, the tool was only informed by expert judgment. This is in contrast to therapeutic [679] and diagnostic [337, 480] studies, where various design characteristics have been found to relate to bias in estimated treatment effects or test characteristics. PROBAST is organized into 4 domains: participants, predictors, outcome, and analysis, with 20 signaling questions. Risk of bias was defined to occur when shortcomings in study design, conduct, or analysis are expected to lead to systematically distorted estimates of

Table 24.2 The TRIPOD checklist for prediction model development and validation [105]

Section/Topic	Item		Checklist item
Title and abstract			
Title	1	D;V	Identify the study as developing and/or validating a multivariable prediction model, the target population, and the outcome to be predicted
Abstract	2	D;V	Provide a summary of objectives, study design, setting, participants, sample size, predictors, outcome, statistical analysis, results, and conclusions
Introduction			
Background and objectives	3a	D;V	Explain the medical context (including whether diagnostic or prognostic) and rationale for developing or validating the multivariable prediction model, including references to existing models
	3b	D;V	Specify the objectives, including whether the study describes the development or validation of the model or both
Methods			
Source of data	4a	D;V	Describe the study design or source of data (e.g., randomized trial, cohort, or registry data), separately for the development and validation data sets, if applicable
	4b	D;V	Specify the key study dates, including start of accrual; end of accrual; and, if applicable, end of follow-up.
Participants	5a	D;V	Specify key elements of the study setting (e.g., primary care, secondary care, general population) including number and location of centers
	5b	D;V	Describe eligibility criteria for participants
	5c	D;V	Give details of treatments received, if relevant
Outcome	6a	D;V	Clearly define the outcome that is predicted by the prediction model, including how and when assessed
	6b	D;V	Report any actions to blind assessment of the outcome to be predicted
Predictors	7a	D;V	Clearly define all predictors used in developing or validating the multivariable prediction model, including how and when they were measured
	7b	D;V	Report any actions to blind assessment of predictors for the outcome and other predictors
Sample size	8	D;V	Explain how the study size was arrived at
Missing data	9	D;V	Describe how missing data were handled (e.g., complete-case analysis, single imputation, multiple imputation) with details of any imputation method
Statistical analysis methods	10a	D	Describe how predictors were handled in the analyses
	10b	D	Specify type of model, all model-building procedures (including any predictor selection), and method for internal validation
	10c	V	For validation, describe how the predictions were calculated
	10d	D;V	Specify all measures used to assess model performance and, if relevant, to compare multiple models
	10e	V	Describe any model updating (e.g., recalibration) arising from the validation, if done

(continued)

Table 24.2 (continued)

Section/Topic	Item		Checklist item
Risk groups	11	D;V	Provide details on how risk groups were created, if done
Development versus validation	12	V	For validation, identify any differences from the development data in setting, eligibility criteria, outcome, and predictors
Results			
Participants	13a	D;V	Describe the flow of participants through the study, including the number of participants with and without the outcome and, if applicable, a summary of the follow-up time. A diagram may be helpful
	13b	D;V	Describe the characteristics of the participants (basic demographics, clinical features, available predictors), including the number of participants with missing data for predictors and outcome
	13c	V	For validation, show a comparison with the development data of the distribution of important variables (demographics, predictors and outcome)
Model development	14a	D	Specify the number of participants and outcome events in each analysis
	14b	D	If done, report the unadjusted association between each candidate predictor and outcome
Model specification	15a	D	Present the full prediction model to allow predictions for individuals (i.e., all regression coefficients, and model intercept or baseline survival at a given time point)
	15b	D	Explain how to the use the prediction model
Model performance	16	D;V	Report performance measures (with CIs) for the prediction model
Model-updating	17	V	If done, report the results from any model updating (i.e., model specification, model performance)
Discussion			
Limitations	18	D;V	Discuss any limitations of the study (such as nonrepresentative sample, few events per predictor, missing data)
Interpretation	19a	V	For validation, discuss the results with reference to performance in the development data, and any other validation data
	19b	D;V	Give an overall interpretation of the results, considering objectives, limitations, results from similar studies, and other relevant evidence
Implications	20	D;V	Discuss the potential clinical use of the model and implications for future research
Other information			
Supplementary information	21	D;V	Provide information about the availability of supplementary resources, such as study protocol, Web calculator, and data sets
Funding	22	D;V	Give the source of funding and the role of the funders for the present study

*Items relevant only to the development of a prediction model are denoted by D, items relating solely to a validation of a prediction model are denoted by V, and items relating to both are denoted D;V. See also the TRIPOD Explanation and Elaboration document [383]

model predictive performance. Only limited empirical evidence is available on this relation for the suggested 20 questions. We might summarize the key risks of bias in prediction models as:

(1) application of sensible methods;
(2) adequate sample size.

Of course, application of sensible methods is not so straightforward for prediction modeling; although some red flags are easily identified, e.g. in Fig. 24.6. Neither is the definition of an adequate sample size easy.

PROBAST may prove relevant for the broader perspective of applicability of prediction models, which relates to external validity. PROBAST was designed for systematic reviews, where an earlier checklist is also available: CHecklist for critical Appraisal and data extraction for systematic Reviews of prediction Modeling Studies (CHARMS) [384]. The CHARMS checklist aims to support the design of systematic reviews of prediction model studies, and to determine what to extract and appraise in primary studies. Seven key items are listed related to the framing of the review question, and 11 domains are considered to extract and critically appraise the primary studies.

24.5 Data Sets

We considered many examples throughout the text. For some case studies, empirical data are available through www.clinicalpredictionmodels.org (Table 24.3). These case studies are discussed below in a simple format. First, we list the abstract of the key publication of the study, if relevant. We then list the contents of the data sets. The data sets are made available for didactic purposes only. If publication by any means is pursued, investigators are required to contact the authors of the original publication and the author of this book.

Table 24.3 Summary of case studies with data sets available at www.clinicalpredictionmodels. org

Case study	Characterization	N patients (events); predictors
GUSTO-I	Prediction of 30-day mortality in acute myocardial infarction	Original: n = 40,830 (2851). West region n = 2,188 (135); Sample4, n = 785 (52); Sample5, n = 429 (24); 17 predictors
SMART	Prediction of secondary cardiovascular events	n = 3873 (460); 26 predictors
Testicular cancer	Diagnosis of residual mass histology (benign vs. other, or in 3 categories)	Development, n = 544 (245 benign); validation, n = 273 (76 benign); 6 predictors
Abdominal aortic aneurysm	Prediction of perioperative mortality after elective surgery	n = 238 (18); 7 predictors
Traumatic brain injury	Prediction of 6-month outcome	n = 2159; 503 deaths, 851 unfavorable outcome; 14 predictors

Table 24.4 Data description of various subsamples from the GUSTO-I trial as considered in this book. The full GUSTO-I trial contained 40,830 patients of whom 2,851 died

Name	Description (no/yes is coded as 0/1)	GUSTO-I 2851/40830	US 1565/23034	West region 135/2188	Sample4 52/785	Sample5 24/429
AGE	Age in years (range: 19–110)	61	61	60	62	60
A65	Age >65 years (0/1)	40%	39%	38%	42%	37%
SEX	Gender (male = 0, female = 1)	25%	27%	25%	26%	27%
KILLIP	Measure for left ventricular function (1–4)	85/13/1/1%	87/11/1/1%	89/10/1/1%	78/19/3/0%	86/13/1/1%
SHO	Shock: Killip class 3/4 versus 1/2 (0/1)	2%	2%	1%	3%	2%
DIA	Diabetes (0/1)	15%	17%	14%	11%	13%
HYP	Hypotension: systolic BP < 100 (0/1)	8%	10%	10%	5%	11%
HRT	Heart rate: pulse >80 ("tachycardia", 0/1)	33%	34%	33%	27%	35%
ANT	Anterior infarct location (0/1)	39%	37%	37%	36%	36%
PMI	Previous myocardial infarction (0/1)	16%	17%	17%	18%	15%
HIG	High risk: ANT or PMI (0/1)	49%	48%	49%	46%	47%
HEI	Height in cm (range: 140–212)	171	172	172	169	172
WEI	Weight in kg (range: 36–213)	79	82	83	75	83
SMK	Smoking (1 = never; 2 = ex; 3 = current)	43/27/30%	43/28/29%	41/31/28%	33/39/28%	43/30/28%
HTN	Hypertension history (0/1)	38%	43%	40%	38%	39%
LIP	Lipids: hypercholesterolaemia (0/1)	34%	38%	40%	39%	35%
PAN	Previous angina pectoris (0/1)	37%	35%	34%	38%	31%
FAM	Family history of MI (0/1)	42%	49%	48%	41%	48%
STE	ST elevation on ECG: number of leads (range: 0–11)	4.1	4.0	4.0	4.3	4.0
ST4	ST elevation on ECG: >4 leads (0/1)	38%	37%	36%	41%	36%
TTR	Time to relief of chest pain > 1 h (0/1)	65%	66%	61%	50%	61%

24.5.1   GUSTO-I Prediction Models

The key publication of prediction in GUSTO-I is by Kerry Lee (Circulation, 1995, see Box 22.1) [329]. Many other publications are available that use the GUSTO-I data, including a practical prediction tool by Rob Califf [86]. Small parts of the GUSTO-I data set are made available: sample5 contains 429 patients, sample4 785 patients, and the West region sample 2188. The patients partly overlap, which can be identified by matching on the 17 predictors and the outcome in the data set (Table 24.4).

Several methodological studies have been performed with the GUSTO-I database. Ennis et al. compared a variety of modern learning methods, including logistic regression, Tree, GAM, and MARS methods (see Chap. 6) [153]. The GUSTO-I data set has also been instrumental to compare various aspects of predictive modeling strategies [536, 539, 540]. The large size of GUSTO-I makes that subsamples can be created where models can be developed, which can subsequently be tested on an independent part of the data set. This approach has been followed to empirically test many aspects of logistic regression modeling, such as the selection of predictors in a prognostic model and estimation of regression coefficients (Figs. 24.1, 24.2, 24.3, 24.4 and 24.5) [541−543, 547].

24.5.2   SMART Case Study

The SMART (Second Manifestations of ARTerial disease) study was discussed in detail in Chap. 23 [512]. The 7 modeling steps from part II were followed, and R code is available to perform the described analyses. A description of the data is shown in Table 24.5.

Table 24.5 SMART study data set ($n = 3,873$). The primary outcome was a cardiovascular event, which occurred in 460 patients during follow-up (5-year cumulative incidence: 14%)

Name	Description (coding: no/yes is coded as 0/1)	Development 460/3,873
Tevent	Time to cardiovascular event (days)	1370
Event	Cardiovascular event (clinical, 0/1)	460
Sex	1 = Male, 2 = Female sex	25%
Age	Age (years)	60
Diabetes	Ever diabetes (0/1)	22%
Cerebral	Ever cerebrovascular disease (0/1)	30%
Cardiac	Ever cardiovascular disease (0/1)	56%
AAA	Ever abdominal aortic aneurysm (0/1)	11%
Periph	Ever periferal vascular disease (0/1)	24%

(continued)

Table 24.5 (continued)

Name	Description (coding: no/yes is coded as 0/1)	Development 460/3,873
Stenosis	Carotic stenosis $\geq$ 50% by duplex (0/1)	19%
Systbp	Systolic blood pressure (automatic, in mmHg)	141
Diastbp	Diastolic blood pressure (automatic, in mmHg)	80
Systh	Systolic blood pressure (by hand, in mmHg)	142
Diasth	Diastolic blood pressure (by hand, in mmHg)	82
Length	Length (m)	1.74
Weight	Weight (kg)	81
BMI	Body mass index (kg/m^2)	26.7
Chol	Cholesterol level (mmol/L)	5.2
HDL	High-density lipoprotein cholesterol (mmol/L)	1.2
LDL	Low-density lipoprotein cholesterol (mmol/L)	3.1
Trig	Triglycerides level (mmol/L)	1.9
Homoc	Homocysteine level (μmol/L)	13.8
Glut	Glutamine (μmol/L)	6.3
Creat	Creatinine clearance (mL/min)	98
IMT	Intima media thickness (mm)	0.93
Albumin	Albumin in urine: 1 = No; 2 = Low; 3 = High	79%/18%/3%
Smoking	Smoking status: 1 = No; 2 = Former; 3 = Current	18%/70%/12%
Packyrs	Packyears smoked	23
Alcohol	Alcohol consumption: 1 = No; 2 = Former; 3 = Current	20%/11%/70%

24.5.3 Testicular Cancer Case Study

The key publication for clinicians is a paper in JCO in 1995 [551], with a validation study in the same journal in 1998 [545]. Some methodological aspects are discussed in a paper in *Statistics in Medicine* in 2001 (Box 24.1, Table 24.6) [566].

Box 24.1 Abstract of the methodological paper on prediction of residual mass histology in testicular cancer patients [566]. Residual mass histology in testicular cancer: development and validation of a clinical prediction rule

Ewout W. Steyerberg; Yvonne Vergouwe; H. Jan Keizer and J. Dik F. Habbema for the ReHiT study group

After chemotherapy for metastatic non-seminomatous testicular cancer, surgical resection is a generally accepted treatment to remove remnants of the initial metastases, since residual tumor may still be present (mature teratoma or viable cancer cells). In this paper, we review the development and external validation of a logistic regression model to predict the absence of residual tumor.

Three sources of information were used. A quantitative review identified 6 relevant predictors from 19 published studies (996 resections) [554]. Second, a development data set included individual data of 544 patients from 6 centers [551]. This data set was used to assess the predictive relations of 5 continuous predictors, which resulted in dichotomization for two, and a log, square root, and linear transformation for 3 other predictors. The multiple logistic regression coefficients were reduced with a shrinkage factor (0.95) to improve calibration, based on a bootstrapping procedure. Third, a validation data set included 172 more recently treated patients [545]. The model showed adequate calibration and good discrimination in the development and in the validation sample (areas under the ROC curve 0.83 and 0.82).

This study illustrates that a careful modeling strategy may result in an adequate predictive model. Further study of model validity may stimulate application in clinical practice.

Table 24.6 Description of testicular cancer development ($n = 544$) and validation set ($n = 273$). The primary outcome was a benign histology at postchemotherapy resection, which occurred in 45 and 28%, respectively

Name	Description (coding: no/yes is coded as 0/1)	Development 245/544 (45%)	Validation 76/273 (28%)
patkey	Patient ID	–	–
hosp	Institution ID	–	–
orchyr	Year of orchiedectomy (surgical removal of primary tumor)	1985	1993
histr3	Histology at resection: 1 = necrosis; 2 = teratoma; 3 – viable cancer	45%/42%/13%	28%/58%/13%
ter	primary tumor teratoma-negative? (0–1)	46%	38%
preafp	Prechemotherapy AFP normal? (0–1)	34%	25%
prehcg	Prechemotherapy HCG normal? (0–1)	38%	27%
lnldhst	Ln of standardized prechemotherapy LDH (LDH/upper limit of local normal value)	0.46 (LDHst 2.0)	NA
sqpost	Square root of postchemotherapy mass size (original mass size in mm)	5.1 (33 mm)	7.8 (70 mm)
reduc10	Reduction in mass size per 10%: (pre-pos)/ pre*10	4.5 (=45%)	1.4 (=14%)
nec	Necrosis at resection (0–1)	45%	28%
matter	Mature teratoma versus cancer, if not necrosis (0–1)	77%	82%
dev	Part of data set: 1 = Development ($n = 544$); 0 = Validation ($n = 273$)	1	0

24.5.4   *Abdominal Aortic Aneurysm Case Study*

The Leiden cohort contained 246 patients undergoing elective surgery for an abdominal aortic aneurysm; 238 were included in the analyses. Results are described in detail in a Ph.D. thesis by Dr. Alexander de Mol van Otterloo (currently working as a surgeon in The Hague). The prediction model based on the combination of the Leiden data and literature data was published in 1995 (Box 24.2, Table 24.7) [555], with methods addressed later in more detail [544].

Box 24.2 Abstract of the paper on prediction of perioperative mortality in AAA [555]. Perioperative mortality of elective abdominal aortic aneurysm surgery. A clinical prediction rule based on literature and individual patient data

Steyerberg EW, Kievit J, de Mol Van Otterloo JC, van Bockel JH, Eijkemans MJ, Habbema JD.

BACKGROUND: Abdominal aortic aneurysm surgery is a major vascular procedure with a considerable risk of (mainly cardiac) mortality.

OBJECTIVE: To estimate elective perioperative mortality, we developed a clinical prediction rule based on several well-established risk factors: age, gender, a history of myocardial infarction, congestive heart failure, ischemia on the electrocardiogram, pulmonary impairment, and renal impairment.

METHODS: Two sources of data were used: (1) individual patient data from 246 patients operated on at the University Hospital Leiden (the Netherlands) and (2) studies published in the literature between 1980 and 1994. The Leiden data were analyzed with univariate and multivariable logistic regression. Literature data were pooled with meta-analysis techniques. The clinical prediction rule was based on the pooled odds ratios from the literature, which were adapted by the regression results of the Leiden data.

RESULTS: The strongest adverse risk factors in the literature were congestive heart failure and cardiac ischemia on the electrocardiogram, followed by renal impairment, history of myocardial infarction, pulmonary impairment, and female gender. The literature data further showed that a 10-year increase in age more than doubled the surgical risk. In the Leiden data, most multivariate effects were smaller than the univariate effects, which is explained by the positive correlation between the risk factors. In the clinical prediction rule, cardiac, renal, and pulmonary comorbidity is the most important risk factors, while age per se has a moderate effect on mortality.

CONCLUSIONS: A readily applicable clinical prediction rule can be based on the combination of literature data and individual patient data. The risk estimates may be useful for clinical decision making in individual patients.

Table 24.7 Aortic aneurysm data set (*n* = 238). The primary outcome was surgical mortality, which occurred in only 18 patients (7.6%)

Name	Description (coding: no/yes is coded as 0/1)	Development 18/238 (8%)
Sex	Female sex (0/1)	9%
Age10	Age in decades	6.6 (66 years)
MI	Infarction on ECG (0/1)	24%
CHF	Congestive heart failure (0/1)	34%
Ischemia	Ischemia on ECG (0/1)	35%
Lung	Lung comorbidity (0/1)	19%
Renal	Renal comorbidity (0/1)	6%
Status	Perioperative mortality (0/1)	8%

24.5.5   Traumatic Brain Injury Data Set

Prognostic studies based on patients included in the Tirilazad trials are described in detail in a Ph.D. thesis by Chantal Hukkelhoven. The publication that presents a prognostic model is in a neurosurgical journal (Box 24.3, Table 24.8) [259]. More extensive data became available through an IPD meta-analysis project: IMPACT (see Chap. 8, led by Andrew Maas). This resulted in a range of methods intensive publications [129, 242, 340, 342, 343, 357, 358, 398, 559].

Box 24.3 Abstract of the paper on prediction of outcome in traumatic brain injury [259]. Predicting outcome after traumatic brain injury: development and validation of a prognostic score based on admission characteristics

Hukkelhoven CW, Steyerberg EW, Habbema JD, Farace E, Marmarou A, Murray GD, Marshall LF, Maas AI.

The early prediction of outcome after traumatic brain injury (TBI) is important for several purposes, but no prognostic models have yet been developed with proven generalizability across different settings. The objective of this study was to develop and validate prognostic models that use the information available at admission to estimate 6-month outcome after severe or moderate TBI. To this end, this study evaluated mortality and unfavorable outcome, that is, death, and vegetative or severe disability on the Glasgow Outcome Scale (GOS), at 6 months post-injury.

Prospectively collected data on 2269 patients from two multicenter clinical trials were used to develop prognostic models for each outcome with logistic regression analysis. We included seven predictive characteristics age, motor score, pupillary reactivity, hypoxia, hypotension, computed tomography classification, and traumatic subarachnoid hemorrhage. The models were validated internally with bootstrapping techniques. External validity was determined in prospectively collected data from two relatively unselected surveys in Europe ($n = 796$) and in North America ($n = 746$). We evaluated the discriminative ability, that is, the ability to distinguish patients with different outcomes, with the area under the receiver operating characteristic curve (AUC). Further, we determined calibration, that is, an agreement between predicted and observed outcome.

The models discriminated well in the development population (AUC 0.78–0.80). External validity was even better (AUC 0.83–0.89). Calibration was less satisfactory, with poor external validity in the North American survey ($p < 0.001$). Especially, observed risks were higher than predicted for poor prognosis patients. A score chart was derived from the regression models to facilitate clinical application.

Relatively simple prognostic models using baseline characteristics can accurately predict 6-month outcome in patients with severe or moderate TBI. The high discriminative ability indicates the potential of this model for classifying patients according to prognostic risk.

Table 24.8 Traumatic brain injury data set ($n = 2159$). Patients are from the International and US Tirilazad trials. The primary outcome was 6 months Glasgow Outcome Scale (range 1 for dead to 5 for good recovery)

Name	Description (coding: no/yes is coded as 0/1)	Development $n = 2159$
trial	Tirilazad international ($n = 1118$)/US ($n = 1041$)	–
d.gos	GOS at 6 months	
	1 = dead	23%
	2 = vegetative	4%
	3 = severe disability	12%
	4 = moderate disability	16%
	5 = good recovery	44%
d.mort	Mortality at 6 months (0/1)	23%
d.unfav	Unfavorable outcome at 6 months (0/1)	39%
age	Age (in years, median [interquartile range])	29 [21–42]
d.motor	Admission motor score (1–6, median)	4
d.pupil	Pupillary reactivity (1 = both reactive/2 = one reactive/3 = no reactive pupils)	70%/14%/16%
pupil.i	Single imputed pupillary reactivity (1/2/3)	70%/14%/16%
hypoxia	Hypoxia before/at admission (0/1)	22%
hypotens	Hypotension before/at admission	19%
ctclass	Marshall CT classification (1–6, median)	2
tsah	tSAH at CT (0/1)	46%
edh	EDH at CT (0/1)	13%
cisterns	Compressed cisterns at CT (0 = no/1 = slightly compressed/ 2 = fully compressed)	57%/26%/10%

(continued)

Table 24.8 (continued)

Name	Description (coding: no/yes is coded as 0/1)	Development n = 2159
shift	Midline shift > 5 mm at CT (0/1)	18%
glucose	Glucose at admission (mmol/l, median [interquartile range])	8.2 [6.7–10.4]
glucoset	Truncated glucose values (median [interquartile range])	8.2 [6.7–10.4]
ph	pH (median [interquartile range])	7.4 [7.3–7.5]
sodium	Sodium (mmol/l, median [interquartile range])	140 [137–142]
sodiumt	Truncated sodium (median [interquartile range])	140 [137–142]
hb	Hb (g/dl, median [interquartile range])	12.8 [10.9–4.3]
hbt	Truncated hb (median [interquartile range])	12.8 [10.9–4.3]

*'d.' variables denote: 'derived'

24.6 Concluding Remarks

In this final chapter, we considered some key elements to successful prediction modeling. Appropriate methods should be used, such as avoiding stepwise selection with the standard p-value of 0.05 in small data sets, and rather use penalization procedures, such as the LASSO. A sufficient sample size is important to avoid deterioration of model performance at validation. Compared to machine learning, sensible modeling in small data sets requires exploiting subject matter knowledge. Reporting guidelines and risk of bias tools were discussed and were found to be in need of empirical underpinning, since many items are currently only motivated by common sense.

Some data sets are made available to promote practical experience with the described techniques in this book. Many other medical data sets are available nowadays which can be used to train researchers in prediction modeling, and readers are encouraged to examine these. Data sharing initiatives may lead to a world of Big Data, where both traditional and more advanced statistical models may prove useful, including machine learning and artificial intelligence algorithms. The author welcomes any comments and suggestions for improvement of the text of this book, the questions at the end of each chapter, the practical exercises at the web, and usefulness of data sets.

Questions

24.1 Impact of sample size (Fig. 24.1).

In Fig. 24.1, we note that the validated discriminative ability (area under ROC curve, or c statistic) does increase by considering a larger sample size; but the apparent performance decreases.
(a) Why does a larger sample size lead to a lower apparent performance?
(b) And a higher validated performance?
(c) How can the validated performance be estimated?
(d) Why is the discriminative ability of models with ML estimation identical to models with shrinkage based on bootstrap validation?

24.2 Number of predictors and impact of sample size (Fig. 24.3).

Figure 24.3 does not show improvement by considering 17 rather than 8 predictors.
(a) How is it possible that considering more predictors does not increase the discriminative ability?
(b) What is the slope of the linear predictor (or calibration slope) with standard ML estimation, with 17 or 8 predictors?
(c) And what is the slope with shrinkage or penalized estimation, with 17 or 8 predictors?
(d) What would you do if 17 candidate predictors were available in a data set with approximately 50 events, and the aim was to make a model for predictions in individual patients?

References

1. An international randomized trial comparing four thrombolytic strategies for acute myocardial infarction. New England Journal of Medicine **329**, 673–682 (1993)
2. A predictive model for aggressive non-Hodgkin's lymphoma. New England Journal of Medicine **329**, 987–994 (1993)
3. A comparison of reteplase with alteplase for acute myocardial infarction. New England Journal of Medicine **337**, 1118–1123 (1997)
4. International germ cell consensus classification: a prognostic factor-based staging system for metastatic germ cell cancers. Journal of Clinical Oncology **15**, 594–603 (1997)
5. Age-specific relevance of usual blood pressure to vascular mortality: A meta-analysis of individual data for one million adults in 61 prospective studies. The Lancet **360**, 1903–1913 (2002)
6. Ahmed, I., Debray, T.P., Moons, K.G., Riley, R.D.: Developing and validating risk prediction models in an individual participant data meta-analysis. BMC Medical Research Methodology **14**, 3 (2014)
7. Allison, P.: What's the best R-squared for logistic regression? *Statistical Horizons* (2013)
8. Altman, D.G.: *Practical statistics for medical research*, 1st edn. Chapman and Hall, London (1991)
9. Altman, D.G.: ROC curves and confidence intervals: Getting them right. Heart **83**, 236 (2000)
10. Altman, D.G., Andersen, P.K.: Bootstrap investigation of the stability of a Cox regression model. Statistics in Medicine **8**, 771–783 (1989)
11. Altman, D.G., Bland, J.M.: Absence of evidence is not evidence of absence. BMJ **311**, 485 (1995)
12. Altman, D.G., Lausen, B., Sauerbrei, W., Schumacher, M.: Dangers of using "optimal" cutpoints in the evaluation of prognostic factors. Journal of the National Cancer Institute **86**, 829–835 (1994)
13. Altman, D.G., Royston, P.: What do we mean by validating a prognostic model? Statistics in Medicine **19**, 453–473 (2000)
14. Ambler, G., Brady, A.R., Royston, P.: Simplifying a prognostic model: A simulation study based on clinical data. Statistics in Medicine **21**, 3803–3822 (2002)
15. Ambler, G., Royston, P.: Fractional polynomial model selection procedures: Investigation of type I error rate. Journal of Statistical Computation and Simulation **69**, 89–108 (2001)
16. Ammar, K.A., Kors, J.A., Yawn, B.P., Rodeheffer, R.J.: Defining unrecognized myocardial infarction: A call for standardized electrocardiographic diagnostic criteria. American Heart Journal **148**, 277–284 (2004)

© Springer Nature Switzerland AG 2019
E. W. Steyerberg, *Clinical Prediction Models*, Statistics for Biology and Health, https://doi.org/10.1007/978-3-030-16399-0

17. Assmann, G., Schulte, H.: The Prospective Cardiovascular Munster (PROCAM) study: Prevalence of hyperlipidemia in persons with hypertension and/or diabetes mellitus and the relationship to coronary heart disease. American Heart Journal 116, 1713–1724 (1988)

18. Assmann, S.F., Pocock, S.J., Enos, L.E., Kasten, L.E.: Subgroup analysis and other (mis) uses of baseline data in clinical trials. The Lancet 355, 1064–1069 (2000)

19. Audigier, V., White, I.R., Jolani, S., et al.: Multiple imputation for multilevel data with continuous and binary variables. Statistical Science 33, 160–183 (2018)

20. Austin, P. C. : A comparison of regression trees, logistic regression, generalized additive models, and multivariate adaptive regression splines for predicting AMI mortality. Statistics in Medicine 26, 2937–57 (2007)

21. Austin, P. C.: Using the bootstrap to improve estimation and confidence intervals for regression coefficients selected using backwards variable elimination. Statistics in Medicine 27, 3286–300 (2008)

22. Austin, P.C., Fine, J.P.: Practical recommendations for reporting Fine-Gray model analyses for competing risk data. Statistics in Medicine 36, 4391–4400 (2017)

23. Austin, P.C., Lee, D.S., Steyerberg, E.W., Tu, J.V.: Regression trees for predicting mortality in patients with cardiovascular disease: What improvement is achieved by using ensemble-based methods? Biometrical Journal 54, 657–673 (2012)

24. Austin, P.C., Merlo, J.: Intermediate and advanced topics in multilevel logistic regression analysis. Statistics in Medicine 36, 3257–3277 (2017)

25. Austin, P.C., Steyerberg, E.W.: Events per variable (EPV) and the relative performance of different strategies for estimating the out-of-sample validity of logistic regression models. Statistical Methods in Medical Research 26, 796–808 (2014)

26. Austin, P.C., Steyerberg, E.W.: Graphical assessment of internal and external calibration of logistic regression models by using loess smoothers. Statistics in Medicine 33, 517–535 (2014)

27. Austin, P.C., Tu, J.V.: Automated variable selection methods for logistic regression produced unstable models for predicting acute myocardial infarction mortality. Journal of Clinical Epidemiology 57, 1138–1146 (2004)

28. Austin, P. C., Tu, J. V.: Bootstrap methods for developing predictive models in cardiovascular research. The American Statistician, 58, 131–137 (2004)

29. Austin, P.C., Tu, J.V., Ho, J.E., Levy, D., Lee, D.S.: Using methods from the data-mining and machine-learning literature for disease classification and prediction: A case study examining classification of heart failure subtypes. Journal of Clinical Epidemiology 66, 398–407 (2013)

30. Austin, P.C., van Klaveren, D., Vergouwe, Y., Nieboer, D., Lee, D.S., Steyerberg, E.W.: Geographic and temporal validity of prediction models: Different approaches were useful to examine model performance. Journal of Clinical Epidemiology 79, 76–85 (2016)

31. Austin, P.C., van Klaveren, D., Vergouwe, Y., Nieboer, D., Lee, D.S., Steyerberg, E.W.: Validation of prediction models: Examining temporal and geographic stability of baseline risk and estimated covariate effects. Diagnostic and Prognostic Research 1, 12 (2017)

32. Austin, P.C., Wagner, P., Merlo, J.: The median hazard ratio: A useful measure of variance and general contextual effects in multilevel survival analysis. Statistics in Medicine 36, 928–938 (2017)

33. Aylin, P., Alves, B., Best, N., et al.: Comparison of UK paediatric cardiac surgical performance by analysis of routinely collected data 1984-96: Was Bristol an outlier? The Lancet 358, 181–187 (2001)

34. Babyak, M.A.: What you see may not be what you get: A brief, nontechnical introduction to overfitting in regression-type models. Psychosomatic Medicine 66, 411–421 (2004)

35. Bach, P. B., Guadagnoli, E., Schrag, D., Schussler, N., Warren, J. L.: Patient demographic and socioeconomic characteristics in the SEER-Medicare database: Applications and limitations. Medical Care 40, IV-19–25 (2002)

36. Backus, B.E., Six, A.J., Doevendans, P.A., Kelder, J.C., Steyerberg, E.W., Vergouwe, Y.: Prognostic factors in chest pain patients: A quantitative analysis of the HEART score. Critical Pathways in Cardiology **15**, 50–55 (2016)

37. Baker, S.G.: Putting risk prediction in perspective: Relative utility curves. Journal of the National Cancer Institute **101**, 1538–1542 (2009)

38. Baker, S.G., Schuit, E., Steyerberg, E.W., et al.: How to interpret a small increase in AUC with an additional risk prediction marker: Decision analysis comes through. Statistics in Medicine **33**, 3946–3959 (2014)

39. Baker, S. G., Van Calster, B., Steyerberg, E. W.: Evaluating a new marker for risk prediction using the test tradeoff: An update. The International Journal of Biostatistics **8**, (2012)

40. Balmana, J., Stockwell, D.H., Steyerberg, E.W., et al.: Prediction of MLH1 and MSH2 mutations in Lynch syndrome. JAMA **296**, 1469–1478 (2006)

41. Bancroft, T.A., Han, C.P.: Inference based on conditional specication: A note and a bibliography. International Statistical Review **45**, 117–127 (1977)

42. Barnetson, R.A., Tenesa, A., Farrington, S.M., et al.: Identification and survival of carriers of mutations in DNA mismatch-repair genes in colon cancer. New England Journal of Medicine **354**, 2751–2763 (2006)

43. Beam, A.L., Kohane, I.S.: Big Data and machine learning in health care. JAMA **319**, 1317–1318 (2018)

44. Begg, C.B., Gray, R.: Calculation of polychotomous logistic regression parameters using individualized regressions. Biometrika **71**, 11–18 (1984)

45. Begg, C.B., Greenes, R.A.: Assessment of diagnostic tests when disease verification is subject to selection bias. Biometrics **39**, 207–215 (1983)

46. Begg, C.B., Satagopan, J.M., Berwick, M.: A new strategy for evaluating the impact of epidemiologic risk factors for cancer with application to melanoma. JASA **93**, 415–426 (1998)

47. Bensdorp, A.J., van der Steeg, J.W., Steures, P., et al.: A revised prediction model for natural conception. Reproductive BioMedicine Online **34**, 619–626 (2017)

48. Berkhemer, O.A., Fransen, P.S., Beumer, D., et al.: A randomized trial of intraarterial treatment for acute ischemic stroke. New England Journal of Medicine **372**, 11–20 (2015)

49. Bero, L., Rennie, D.: The cochrane collaboration: Preparing, maintaining, and disseminating systematic reviews of the effects of health care. JAMA **274**, 1935–1938 (1995)

50. Biesheuvel, C.J., Vergouwe, Y., Steyerberg, E.W., Grobbee, D.E., Moons, K.G.: Polytomous logistic regression analysis could be applied more often in diagnostic research. Journal of Clinical Epidemiology **61**, 125–134 (2008)

51. Binder, H., Sauerbrei, W., Royston, P.: Comparison between splines and fractional polynomials for multivariable model building with continuous covariates: A simulation study with continuous response. Statistics in Medicine **32**, 2262–2277 (2013)

52. Birim, O., Kappetein, A.P., Waleboer, M., et al.: Long-term survival after non-small cell lung cancer surgery: Development and validation of a prognostic model with a preoperative and postoperative mode. The Journal of Thoracic and Cardiovascular Surgery **132**, 491–498 (2006)

53. Blanche, P., Kattan, M. W., Gerds, T. A.: The c-index is not proper for the evaluation of t-year predicted risks. Biostatistics **20**, 347–357 (2019)

54. Blattenberger, G., Lad, F.: Separating the Brier score into calibration and refinement components: A graphical exposition. The American Statistician **39**, 26–32 (1985)

55. Bleeker, S., Derksen-Lubsen, G., Grobbee, D., Donders, A., Moons, K., Moll, H.: Validating and updating a prediction rule for serious bacterial infection in patients with fever without source. Acta Paediatrica **96**, 100–104 (2007)

56. Bleeker, S.E., Moll, H.A., Steyerberg, E.W., et al.: External validation is necessary in prediction research: A clinical example. Journal of Clinical Epidemiology **56**, 826–832 (2003)

57. Bleeker, S.E., Moons, K.G., Derksen-Lubsen, G., Grobbee, D.E., Moll, H.A.: Predicting serious bacterial infection in young children with fever without apparent source. Acta Paediatrica **90**, 1226–1232 (2001)

58. Blot, W.J., Omar, R.Z., Kallewaard, M., et al.: Risks of fracture of Bjork-Shiley 60 degree convexo-concave prosthetic heart valves: Long-term cohort follow up in the UK, Netherlands and USA. The Journal of Heart Valve Disease **10**, 202–209 (2001)

59. Boersma, E., Pieper, K. S., Steyerberg, E. W., et al. Predictors of outcome in patients with acute coronary syndromes without persistent ST-segment elevation. Results from an international trial of 9461 patients. The PURSUIT Investigators. Circulation **101**, 2557–2567 (2000)

60. Boersma, E., Steyerberg, E. W., van der Vlugt, M. J., Simoons, M. L.: Reperfusion therapy for acute myocardial infarction. Which strategy for which patient? Drugs **56**, 31–48 (1998)

61. Bos, J.M., Rietveld, E., Moll, H.A., et al.: The use of health economics to guide drug development decisions: Determining optimal values for an RSV-vaccine in a model-based scenario-analytic approach. Vaccine **25**, 6922–6929 (2007)

62. Boscarino, J.A., Adams, R.E.: Public perceptions of quality care and provider profiling in New York: Implications for improving quality care and public health. Journal of Public Health Management and Practice **10**, 241–250 (2004)

63. Bosco, J.L.F., Silliman, R.A., Thwin, S.S., et al.: A most stubborn bias: No adjustment method fully resolves confounding by indication in observational studies. Journal of Clinical Epidemiology **63**, 64–74 (2010)

64. Bossuyt, P.M., Reitsma, J.B., Bruns, D.E., et al.: Towards complete and accurate reporting of studies of diagnostic accuracy: The STARD initiative. Annals of Internal Medicine **138**, 40–44 (2003)

65. Bossuyt, P.M., Reitsma, J.B., Bruns, D.E., et al.: The STARD statement for reporting studies of diagnostic accuracy: Explanation and elaboration. Annals of Internal Medicine **138**, W1–W12 (2003)

66. Boulesteix, A.L., Binder, H., Abrahamowicz, M., Sauerbrei, W.: On the necessity and design of studies comparing statistical methods. Biometrical Journal **60**, 216–218 (2018)

67. Bower, M., Gazzard, B., Mandalia, S., et al.: A prognostic index for systemic AIDS-related non-Hodgkin lymphoma treated in the era of highly active antiretroviral therapy. Annals of Internal Medicine **143**, 265–273 (2005)

68. Box, G. E. P.: Robustness in the strategy of scientific model building. In Launer, R. L., Wilkinson, G. N., (Eds.), *Robustness in statistics: Proceedings of a workshop* (Vol. xvi, 296 pp.). New York: Academic Press (1979)

69. Box, G.E.P., Tidwell, P.W.: Transformation of the independent variables. Technometrics **4**, 531–550 (1962)

70. Boyd, C. R., Tolson, M. A., Copes, W. S.: Evaluating trauma care: The TRISS method. Trauma Score and the Injury Severity Score. The Journal of trauma **27**, 370–378 (1987)

71. Brady, A. R., Fowkes, F. G., Greenhalgh, R. M., Powell, J. T., Ruckley, C. V., Thompson, S. G.: Risk factors for postoperative death following elective surgical repair of abdominal aortic aneurysm: Results from the UK Small Aneurysm Trial. British Journal of Surgery **87**, 742–749 (2000)

72. Braitman, L.E., Rosenbaum, P.R.: Rare outcomes, common treatments: Analytic strategies using propensity scores. Annals of Internal Medicine **137**, 693–695 (2002)

73. Brakenhoff, T.B., Mitroiu, M., Keogh, R.H., Moons, K.G.M., Groenwold, R.H.H., van Smeden, M.: Measurement error is often neglected in medical literature: A systematic review. Journal of Clinical Epidemiology **98**, 89–97 (2018)

74. Brand, J., van Buuren, S., le Cessie, S., van den Hout, W.: Combining multiple imputation and bootstrap in the analysis of cost-effectiveness trial data. Statistics in Medicine **38**, 210–220 (2019)

75. Brehaut, J.C., Stiell, I.G., Visentin, L., Graham, I.D.: Clinical decision rules "in the real world": How a widely disseminated rule is used in everyday practice. Academic Emergency Medicine **12**, 948–956 (2005)

76. Breiman, L.: *Classification and regression trees*. Belmont: Wadsworth International Group (1984)

77. Breiman, L.: Better subset regression using the nonnegative Garrote. Technometrics **37**, 373–384 (1995)

78. Breiman, L.: Bagging predictors. Machine Learning **24**, 123–140 (1996)

79. Breiman, L.: Random forests. Machine Learning **45**, 5–32 (2001)

80. Breiman, L.: Statistical modeling: The two cultures. Statistical Science **16**, 199–231 (2001)

81. Brookes, S.T., Whitely, E., Egger, M., Smith, G.D., Mulheran, P.A., Peters, T.J.: Subgroup analyses in randomized trials: Risks of subgroup-specific analyses: Power and sample size for the interaction test. Journal of Clinical Epidemiology **57**, 229–236 (2004)

82. Brookhart, M.A., Schneeweiss, S., Rothman, K.J., Glynn, R.J., Avorn, J., Sturmer, T.: Variable selection for propensity score models. American Journal of Epidemiology **163**, 1149–1156 (2006)

83. Burke, D.L., Ensor, J., Riley, R.D.: Meta-analysis using individual participant data: One-stage and two-stage approaches, and why they may differ. Statistics in Medicine **36**, 855–875 (2017)

84. Burton, A., Altman, D.G.: Missing covariate data within cancer prognostic studies: A review of current reporting and proposed guidelines. British Journal of Cancer **91**, 4–8 (2004)

85. Butcher, I., McHugh, G.S., Lu, J., et al.: Prognostic value of cause of injury in traumatic brain injury: Results from the IMPACT study. Journal of Neurotrauma **24**, 281–286 (2007)

86. Califf, R.M., Woodlief, L.H., Harrell Jr., F.E., et al.: Selection of thrombolytic therapy for individual patients: Development of a clinical model. GUSTO-I Investigators. American Heart Journal **133**, 630–639 (1997)

87. Candido Dos Reis, F. J., Wishart, G. C., Dicks, E.M., et al.: An updated PREDICT breast cancer prognostication and treatment benefit prediction model with independent validation. Breast Cancer Research **19**, 58 (2017)

88. Cardoso, F., van't Veer, L. J., Bogaerts, J., et al.: 70-Gene signature as an aid to treatment decisions in early-stage breast cancer. New England Journal of Medicine **375**, 717–729 (2016)

89. Carroll, K.J.: On the use and utility of the Weibull model in the analysis of survival data. Controlled Clinical Trials **24**, 682–701 (2003)

90. Carter, J.L., Coletti, R.J., Harris, R.P.: Quantifying and monitoring overdiagnosis in cancer screening: A systematic review of methods. BMJ **350**, g7773 (2015)

91. Cepeda, M.S., Boston, R., Farrar, J.T., Strom, B.L.: Comparison of logistic regression versus propensity score when the number of events is low and there are multiple confounders. American Journal of Epidemiology **158**, 280–287 (2003)

92. Chan, S.F., Deeks, J.J., Macaskill, P., Irwig, L.: Three methods to construct predictive models using logistic regression and likelihood ratios to facilitate adjustment for pretest probability give similar results. Journal of Clinical Epidemiology **61**, 52–63 (2008)

93. Charlson, M.E., Pompei, P., Ales, K.L., MacKenzie, C.R.: A new method of classifying prognostic comorbidity in longitudinal studies: Development and validation. Journal of Chronic Diseases **40**, 373–383 (1987)

94. Chatfield, C.: Model uncertainty, data mining and statistical inference. Journal of the Royal Statistical Society: Series A **158**, 419–466 (1995)

95. Chen, C.H., George, S.L.: The bootstrap and identification of prognostic factors via Cox's proportional hazards regression model. Statistics in Medicine **4**, 39–46 (1985)

96. Chen, S., Wang, W., Lee, S., et al.: Prediction of germline mutations and cancer risk in the Lynch syndrome. JAMA **296**, 1479–1487 (2006)

97. Chun, F. K., Karakiewicz, P.I., Briganti, A., et al.: Prostate cancer nomograms: An update. European Urology **50**, 914–926 (2006)

98. Cintolo-Gonzalez, J.A., Braun, D., Blackford, A.L., et al.: Breast cancer risk models: A comprehensive overview of existing models, validation, and clinical applications. Breast Cancer Research and Treatment **164**, 263–284 (2017)

99. Clark, T.G., Altman, D.G.: Developing a prognostic model in the presence of missing data: An ovarian cancer case study. Journal of Clinical Epidemiology **56**, 28–37 (2003)

100. Clark, T.G., Bradburn, M.J., Love, S.B., Altman, D.G.: Survival analysis part I: Basic concepts and first analyses. British Journal of Cancer **89**, 232 (2003)

101. Claus, E.B., Risch, N., Thompson, W.D.: Autosomal dominant inheritance of early-onset breast cancer. Implications for risk prediction. Cancer **73**, 643–651 (1994)

102. Cleveland, W.S., Devlin, S.J.: Locally weighted regression: An approach to regression analysis by local fitting. JASA **83**, 596–610 (1988)

103. Collins, G.S., de Groot, J.A., Dutton, S., et al.: External validation of multivariable prediction models: A systematic review of methodological conduct and reporting. BMC Medical Research Methodology **14**, 40 (2014)

104. Collins, G.S., Ogundimu, E.O., Altman, D.G.: Sample size considerations for the external validation of a multivariable prognostic model: A resampling study. Statistics in Medicine **35**, 214–226 (2016)

105. Collins, G.S., Reitsma, J.B., Altman, D.G., Moons, K.G.: Transparent Reporting of a multivariable prediction model for Individual Prognosis or Diagnosis (TRIPOD): The TRIPOD statement. Annals of Internal Medicine **162**, 55–63 (2015)

106. Collins, L.M., Schafer, J.L., Kam, C.M.: A comparison of inclusive and restrictive strategies in modern missing data procedures. Psychological Methods **6**, 330–351 (2001)

107. Cook, N.R., Buring, J.E., Ridker, P.M.: The effect of including C-reactive protein in cardiovascular risk prediction models for women. Annals of Internal Medicine **145**, 21–29 (2006)

108. Cooper, G. S., Virnig, B., Klabunde, C. N., Schussler, N., Freeman, J., Warren, J. L.: Use of SEER-Medicare data for measuring cancer surgery. Medical Care **40**, IV43–48 (2002)

109. Copas, J.B.: Regression, prediction and shrinkage. Journal of the Royal Statistical Society: Series B **45**, 311–354 (1983)

110. Copas, J.B., Long, T.: Estimating the residual variance in orthogonal regression with variable selection. Statistician **40**, 51–59 (1991)

111. Coulter, A.: Partnerships with patients: The pros and cons of shared clinical decision-making. Journal of Health Services Research & Policy **2**, 112–121 (1997)

112. Courvoisier, D.S., Combescure, C., Agoritsas, T., Gayet-Ageron, A., Perneger, T.V.: Performance of logistic regression modeling: Beyond the number of events per variable, the role of data structure. Journal of Clinical Epidemiology **64**, 993–1000 (2011)

113. Cox, D.: Regression models and life-tables (with discussion). Journal of the Royal Statistical Society: Series B **34**, 187–220 (1972)

114. Cox, D.R.: Two further applications of a model for binary regression. Biometrika **45**, 562–565 (1958)

115. Croft, R.P., Nicholls, P.G., Steyerberg, E.W., Richardus, J.H., Cairns, W., Smith, S.: A clinical prediction rule for nerve-function impairment in leprosy patients. The Lancet **355**, 1603–1606 (2000)

116. Crowson, C.S., Atkinson, E.J., Therneau, T.M.: Assessing calibration of prognostic risk scores. Statistical Methods in Medical Research **25**, 1692–1706 (2016)

117. D'Agostino Jr., R.B.: Propensity score methods for bias reduction in the comparison of a treatment to a non-randomized control group. Statistics in Medicine **17**, 2265–2281 (1998)

118. D'Agostino Sr., R.B., Grundy, S., Sullivan, L.M., Wilson, P.: Validation of the Framingham coronary heart disease prediction scores: Results of a multiple ethnic groups investigation. JAMA **286**, 180–187 (2001)

119. Davis, S.E., Lasko, T.A., Chen, G., Matheny, M.E.: Calibration drift among regression and machine learning models for hospital mortality. AMIA Annual Symposium Proceedings **2017**, 625–634 (2017)

120. Davis, S.E., Lasko, T.A., Chen, G., Siew, E.D., Matheny, M.E.: Calibration drift in regression and machine learning models for acute kidney injury. Journal of the American Medical Informatics Association **24**, 1052–1061 (2017)

121. De Dombal, F.T.: *Diagnosis of acute abdominal pain.* Churchill Livingstone, Edinburgh (1980)

122. de Groot, J.A.H., Bossuyt, P.M.M., Reitsma, J.B., et al.: Verification problems in diagnostic accuracy studies: Consequences and solutions. BMJ **343**, d4770 (2011)

123. de Groot, J.A.H., Janssen, K.J.M., Zwinderman, A.H., Bossuyt, P.M.M., Reitsma, J.B., Moons, K.G.M.: Correcting for partial verification bias: A comparison of methods. Annals of Epidemiology **21**, 139–148 (2011)

124. De Ridder, M.A., Stijnen, T., Hokken-Koelega, A.C.: Validation and calibration of the Kabi Pharmacia International Growth Study prediction model for children with idiopathic growth hormone deficiency. The Journal of Clinical Endocrinology & Metabolism **88**, 1223–1227 (2003)

125. de Wit, R., Roberts, J.T., Wilkinson, P.M., et al.: Equivalence of three or four cycles of bleomycin, etoposide, and cisplatin chemotherapy and of a 3- or 5-day schedule in good-prognosis germ cell cancer: A randomized study. Journal of Clinical Oncology **19**, 1629–1640 (2001)

126. de Wreede, L.C., Fiocco, M., Putter, H.: The mstate package for estimation and prediction in non- and semi-parametric multi-state and competing risks models. Computer Methods and Programs in Biomedicine **99**, 261–274 (2010)

127. Debray, T. P., Damen, J. A., Riley, R. D., et al.: A framework for meta-analysis of prediction model studies with binary and time-to-event outcomes. *Statistical Methods in Medical Research*, ePub (2018)

128. Debray, T.P., Koffijberg, H., Nieboer, D., Vergouwe, Y., Steyerberg, E.W., Moons, K.G.: Meta-analysis and aggregation of multiple published prediction models. Statistics in Medicine **33**, 2341–2362 (2014)

129. Debray, T.P., Koffijberg, H., Vergouwe, Y., Moons, K.G., Steyerberg, E.W.: Aggregating published prediction models with individual participant data: A comparison of different approaches. Statistics in Medicine **31**, 2697–2712 (2012)

130. Debray, T.P., Vergouwe, Y., Koffijberg, H., Nieboer, D., Steyerberg, E.W., Moons, K.G.: A new framework to enhance the interpretation of external validation studies of clinical prediction models. Journal of Clinical Epidemiology **68**, 279–289 (2015)

131. DeLong, E.R., Peterson, E.D., DeLong, D.M., Muhlbaier, L.H., Hackett, S., Mark, D.B.: Comparing risk-adjustment methods for provider profiling. Statistics in Medicine **16**, 2645–2664 (1997)

132. Demler, O.V., Paynter, N.P., Cook, N.R.: Tests of calibration and goodness-of-fit in the survival setting. Statistics in Medicine **34**, 1659–1680 (2015)

133. Derksen, S., Keselman, H.: Backward, forward and stepwise automated subset selection algorithms: Frequency of obtaining authentic and noise variables. British Journal of Mathematical and Statistical Psychology **45**, 265–282 (1992)

134. Domingos, P.: The role of Occam's Razor in knowledge discovery. Data Mining and Knowledge Discovery **3**, 409–425 (1999)

135. Donabedian, A.: *The definition of quality and approaches to its assessment.* Ann Arbor: Health Administration Press (1980)

136. Donders, A.R., van der Heijden, G.J., Stijnen, T., Moons, K.G.: Review: A gentle introduction to imputation of missing values. Journal of Clinical Epidemiology **59**, 1087–1091 (2006)

137. Dorresteijn, J.A., Visseren, F.L., Wassink, A.M., et al.: Development and validation of a prediction rule for recurrent vascular events based on a cohort study of patients with arterial disease: The SMART risk score. Heart **99**, 866–872 (2013)

138. Draper, D.: Assessment and propagation of model uncertainty. Journal of the Royal Statistical Society: Series B **57**, 45–97 (1995)

139. Draper, N.R., Smith, H.: *Applied regression analysis*, 3rd edn. Wiley, New York (1998)

140. Dreiseitl, S., Ohno-Machado, L.: Logistic regression and artificial neural network classification models: A methodology review. Journal of Biomedical Informatics **35**, 352–359 (2002)

141. Dresser, G.K., Bailey, D.G.: A basic conceptual and practical overview of interactions with highly prescribed drugs. The Canadian Journal of Clinical Pharmacology **9**, 191–198 (2002)

142. Dubois, C., Pierard, L.A., Albert, A., et al.: Short-term risk stratification at admission based on simple clinical data in acute myocardial infarction. The American Journal of Cardiology **61**, 216–219 (1988)

143. Earle, C. C., Nattinger, A. B., Potosky, A. L., et al.: Identifying cancer relapse using SEER-Medicare data. *Medical care*, IV-75–81 (2002)

144. Edlinger, M., Dorler, J., Ulmer, H., et al.: An ordinal prediction model of the diagnosis of non-obstructive coronary artery and multi-vessel disease in the CARDIIGAN cohort. International Journal of Cardiology **267**, 8–12 (2018)

145. Edlinger, M., Wanitschek, M., Dorler, J., Ulmer, H., Alber, H.F., Steyerberg, E.W.: External validation and extension of a diagnostic model for obstructive coronary artery disease: A cross-sectional predictive evaluation in 4888 patients of the Austrian Coronary Artery disease Risk Determination In Innsbruck by diaGnostic ANgiography (CARDIIGAN) cohort. BMJ Open **7**, e014467 (2017)

146. Efron, B.: How biased is the apparent error rate of a prediction rule? JASA **81**, 461–470 (1986)

147. Efron, B., Morris, C.: Stein's paradox in statistics. Scientific American **236**, 119–127 (1977)

148. Efron, B., Tibshirani, R.: *An introduction to the bootstrap*. Chapman and Hall, New York (1993)

149. Efron, B., Tibshirani, R.: Improvements on cross-validation: The 632+ bootstrap method. JASA, **92**, 548–560 (1997)

150. Elmore, J.G., Fletcher, S.W.: The risk of cancer risk prediction: "What is my risk of getting breast cancer"? Journal of the National Cancer Institute **98**, 1673–1675 (2006)

151. Empana, J.P., Ducimetiere, P., Arveiler, D., et al.: Are the Framingham and PROCAM coronary heart disease risk functions applicable to different European populations? The PRIME Study. European Heart Journal **24**, 1903–1911 (2003)

152. Enders, C.K.: A primer on the use of modern missing-data methods in psychosomatic medicine research. Psychosomatic Medicine **68**, 427–436 (2006)

153. Ennis, M., Hinton, G., Naylor, D., Revow, M., Tibshirani, R.: A comparison of statistical learning methods on the GUSTO database. Statistics in Medicine **17**, 2501–2508 (1998)

154. Ensor, J.: pmsampsize: Calculate minimum sample size required for developing a prediction model. https://twitter.com/joie_ensor/status/1070971276980817921 (2018)

155. Ewald, B.: Post hoc choice of cut points introduced bias to diagnostic research. Journal of Clinical Epidemiology **59**, 798–801 (2006)

156. Fanning, J., Gangestad, A., Andrews, S.J.: National Cancer Data Base/Surveillance Epidemiology and End Results: Potential insensitive-measure bias. Gynecologic Oncology **77**, 450–453 (2000)

157. Faraway, J.J.: On the cost of data analysis. Journal of Computational and Graphical Statistics **1**, 213–229 (1992)

158. Farley, J.F., Harley, C.R., Devine, J.W.: A comparison of comorbidity measurements to predict healthcare expenditures. American Journal of Managed Care **12**, 110–119 (2006)

159. Felker, G.M., Leimberger, J.D., Califf, R.M., et al.: Risk stratification after hospitalization for decompensated heart failure. Journal of Cardiac Failure **10**, 460–466 (2004)

160. Ferket, B.S., Colkesen, E.B., Visser, J.J., et al.: Systematic review of guidelines on cardiovascular risk assessment: Which recommendations should clinicians follow for a cardiovascular health check? Archives of Internal Medicine **170**, 27–40 (2010)

161. Figueiras, A., Domenech-Massons, J.M., Cadarso, C.: Regression models: Calculating the confidence interval of effects in the presence of interactions. Statistics in Medicine **17**, 2099–2105 (1998)

162. Fine, A.M., Nigrovic, L.E., Reis, B.Y., Cook, E.F., Mandl, K.D.: Linking surveillance to action: Incorporation of real-time regional data into a medical decision rule. ournal of the American Medical Informatics Association **14**, 206–211 (2007)

163. Fine, J.P., Gray, R.J.: A proportional hazards model for the subdistribution of a competing risk. JASA **94**, 496–509 (1999)

164. Finlayson, E.V., Birkmeyer, J.D.: Operative mortality with elective surgery in older adults. Effective Clinical Practice **4**, 172–177 (2001)

165. Firth, D.: Bias reduction of maximum likelihood estimates. Biometrika **80**, 27–38 (1993)

166. Fischer, C., Lingsma, H.F., van Leersum, N., Tollenaar, R.A., Wouters, M.W., Steyerberg, E.W.: Comparing colon cancer outcomes: The impact of low hospital case volume and case-mix adjustment. European Journal of Surgical Oncology **41**, 1045–1053 (2015)

167. Fletcher Mercaldo, S., Blume, J. D.; Missing data and prediction: The pattern submodel. Biostatistics, Epub (2018)

168. Frank, T.S., Deffenbaugh, A.M., Reid, J.E., et al.: Clinical characteristics of individuals with germline mutations in BRCA1 and BRCA2: Analysis of 10,000 individuals. Journal of Clinical Oncology **20**, 1480–1490 (2002)

169. Friedenson, B.: Assessing and managing breast cancer risk: Clinical tools for advising patients. Med Gen Med **6**, 8 (2004)

170. Friedman, J.H.: Multivariate adaptive regression splines. The Annals of Statistics **19**, 1–141 (1991)

171. Gail, M.H., Brinton, L.A., Byar, D.P., et al.: Projecting individualized probabilities of developing breast cancer for white females who are being examined annually. Journal of the National Cancer Institute **81**, 1879–1886 (1989)

172. Gail, M.H., Pfeiffer, R.M.: On criteria for evaluating models of absolute risk. Biostatistics **6**, 227–239 (2005)

173. Gail, M.H., Pfeiffer, R.M.: Breast cancer risk model requirements for counseling, prevention, and screening. Journal of the National Cancer Institute **110**, 994–1002 (2018)

174. Gail, M.H., Wieand, S., Piantadosi, S.: Biased estimates of treatment effect in randomized experiments with non-linear regressions and omitted variables. Biometrika **71**, 431–444 (1984)

175. Gelman, A.: Sample size for interactions. https://andrewgelman.com/2018/03/15/need-16-times-sample-size-estimate-interaction-estimate-main-effect/ (2018)

176. Genders, T.S., Steyerberg, E.W., Alkadhi, H., et al.: A clinical prediction rule for the diagnosis of coronary artery disease: Validation, updating, and extension. European Heart Journal **32**, 1316–1330 (2011)

177. Genders, T.S., Steyerberg, E.W., Hunink, M.G., et al.: Prediction model to estimate presence of coronary artery disease: Retrospective pooled analysis of existing cohorts. BMJ **344**, e3485 (2012)

178. Genders, T.S.S., Coles, A., Hoffmann, U., et al.: The external validity of prediction models for the diagnosis of obstructive coronary artery disease in patients with stable chest pain: Insights from the PROMISE trial. JACC Cardiovascular Imaging **11**, 437–446 (2018)

179. Gertheiss, J., Tutz, G.: Penalized regression with ordinal predictors. International Statistical Review **77**, 345–365 (2009)

180. Geskus, R.B.: *Data Analysis with Competing Risks and Intermediate States*. Chapman and Hall/CRC, New York (2016)

181. Gianfrancesco, M.A., Tamang, S., Yazdany, J., Schmajuk, G.: Potential biases in machine learning algorithms using electronic health record data. JAMA Internal Medicine **178**, 1544–1547 (2018)

182. Gigerenzer, G., Edwards, A.: Simple tools for understanding risks: From innumeracy to insight. BMJ **327**, 741–744 (2003)

183. Glance, L.G., Dick, A., Osler, T.M., Li, Y., Mukamel, D.B.: Impact of changing the statistical methodology on hospital and surgeon ranking: The case of the New York State cardiac surgery report card. Medical Care **44**, 311–319 (2006)

184. Glasziou, P.P., Irwig, L.M.: An evidence based approach to individualising treatment. BMJ **311**, 1356–1359 (1995)

185. Gloeckler Ries, L.A., Reichman, M.E., Lewis, D.R., Hankey, B.F., Edwards, B.K.: Cancer survival and incidence from the Surveillance, Epidemiology, and End Results (SEER) program. Oncologist **8**, 541–552 (2003)

186. Glynn, R.J., Rosner, B.: Methods to evaluate risks for composite end points and their individual components. Journal of Clinical Epidemiology **57**, 113–122 (2004)

187. Goeman, J.J., le Cessie, S.: A goodness-of-fit test for multinomial logistic regression. Biometrics **62**, 980–985 (2006)

188. Goldman, L., Weinberg, M., Weisberg, M., et al.: A computer-derived protocol to aid in the diagnosis of emergency room patients with acute chest pain. New England Journal of Medicine **307**, 588–596 (1982)

189. Goldstein, H., Spiegelhalter, D.J.: League tables and their limitations: Statistical issues in comparisons of institutional performance. Journal of the Royal Statistical Society: Series A **159**, 385–443 (1996)

190. Gonen, M., Heller, G.: Concordance probability and discriminatory power in proportional hazards regression. Biometrika **92**, 965–970 (2005)

191. Gotz, H.M., van Bergen, J.E., Veldhuijzen, I.K., et al.: A prediction rule for selective screening of Chlamydia trachomatis infection. Sexually Transmitted Infections **81**, 24–30 (2005)

192. Gotz, H.M., Veldhuijzen, I.K., Habbema, J.D., Boeke, A.J., Richardus, J.H., Steyerberg, E. W.: Prediction of Chlamydia trachomatis infection: Application of a scoring rule to other populations. Sexually Transmitted Diseases **33**, 374–380 (2006)

193. Goverde, A., Spaander, M.C.W., Nieboer, D., et al.: Evaluation of current prediction models for Lynch syndrome: Updating the PREMM5 model to identify PMS2 mutation carriers. Familial Cancer **17**, 361–370 (2018)

194. Graf, E., Schmoor, C., Sauerbrei, W., Schumacher, M.: Assessment and comparison of prognostic classification schemes for survival data. Statistics in Medicine **18**, 2529–2545 (1999)

195. Graham, I.: European guidelines on cardiovascular disease prevention in clinical practice: Executive summary. Atherosclerosis **194**, 1–45 (2007)

196. Graham, I.D., Stiell, I.G., Laupacis, A., O'Connor, A.M., Wells, G.A.: Emergency physicians' attitudes toward and use of clinical decision rules for radiography. Academic Emergency Medicine **5**, 134–140 (1998)

197. Grambsch, P.M., O'Brien, P.C.: The effects of transformations and preliminary tests for non-linearity in regression. Statistics in Medicine **10**, 697–709 (1991)

198. Gray, R.J.: Flexible methods for analysing survival data using splines, with applications to breast cancer prognosis. JASA **87**, 942–951 (1992)

199. Green, J., Wintfeld, N.: Report cards on cardiac surgeons. assessing New York State's approach. New England Journal of Medicine **332**, 1229–1232 (1995)

200. Greenhalgh, T., Howick, J., Maskrey, N.: Evidence based medicine: A movement in crisis? BMJ **348**, g3725 (2014)

201. Greenland, S.: Quantitative methods in the review of epidemiologic literature. Epidemiologic Reviews **9**, 1–30 (1987)

202. Greenland, S.: Methods for epidemiologic analyses of multiple exposures: A review and comparative study of maximum-likelihood, preliminary-testing, and empirical-Bayes regression. Statistics in Medicine **12**, 717–736 (1993)

203. Greenland, S.: Putting background information about relative risks into conjugate prior distributions. Biometrics **57**, 663–670 (2001)

204. Greenland, S.: Bayesian perspectives for epidemiological research. II. Regression analysis. International Journal of Epidemiology **36**, 195–202 (2007)

205. Greenland, S.: The need for reorientation toward cost-effective prediction. Statistics in Medicine **27**, 199–206 (2008)

206. Greenland, S.: Variable selection versus shrinkage in the control of multiple confounders. American Journal of Epidemiology **167**, 523–529 (2008)

207. Greenland, S., Finkle, W.D.: A critical look at methods for handling missing covariates in epidemiologic regression analyses. American Journal of Epidemiology **142**, 1255–1264 (1995)

208. Greenland, S., Longnecker, M.P.: Methods for trend estimation from summarized dose-response data, with applications to meta-analysis. American Journal of Epidemiology **135**, 1301–1309 (1992)

209. Greenland, S., Mansournia, M.A., Altman, D.G.: Sparse data bias: A problem hiding in plain sight. BMJ **352**, i1981 (2016)

210. Greenland, S., Robins, J.M., Pearl, J.: Confounding and collapsibility in causal inference. Statistical science **14**, 29–46 (1999)

211. Grigg, O.A., Farewell, V.T., Spiegelhalter, D.J.: Use of risk-adjusted CUSUM and RSPRT charts for monitoring in medical contexts. Statistical Methods in Medical Research **12**, 147–170 (2003)

212. Grunkemeier, G. L., Anderson, R. P., Miller, D. C., Starr, A.: Time-related analysis of nonfatal heart valve complications: Cumulative incidence (actual) versus Kaplan-Meier (actuarial). Circulation **96**, II-70–74 (1997)

213. Grunkemeier, G.L., Jin, R., Eijkemans, M.J., Takkenberg, J.J.: Actual and actuarial probabilities of competing risks: Apples and lemons. The Annals of Thoracic Surgery **83**, 1586–1592 (2007)

214. Guyatt, G.H., Haynes, R.B., Jaeschke, R.Z., et al.: Evidence-based medicine: Principles for applying the Users' Guides to patient care. JAMA **284**, 1290–1296 (2000)

215. Habbema, J. D., Hilden, J.: The measurement of performance in probabilistic diagnosis. IV. Utility considerations in therapeutics and prognostics. Methods of Information in Medicine **20**, 80–96 (1981)

216. Habbema, J. D., Hilden, J., Bjerregaard, B.: The measurement of performance in probabilistic diagnosis. I. The problem, descriptive tools, and measures based on classification matrices. Methods of Information in Medicine **17**, 217–226 (1978)

217. Habbema, J. D., Hilden, J., Bjerregaard, B.: The measurement of performance in probabilistic diagnosis. V. General recommendations. Methods of Information in Medicine **20**, 97–100 (1981)

218. Hahn, G.J., Raghunathan, T.E.: Combining information from various sources: A prediction problem and other industrial applications. Technometrics **30**, 41–52 (1988)

219. Hakulinen, T., Abeywickrama, K.H.: A computer program package for relative survival analysis. Computer Programs in Biomedicine **19**, 197–207 (1985)

220. Hamburg, M.A., Collins, F.S.: The path to personalized medicine. New England Journal of Medicine **363**, 301–304 (2010)

221. Hand, D.J.: Statistical methods in diagnosis. Statistical Methods in Medical Research **1**, 49–67 (1992)

222. Hand, D.J.: Classifier technology and the illusion of progress. Statist Sci **21**, 1–14 (2006)

223. Hanley, J.A., McNeil, B.J.: The meaning and use of the area under a receiver operating characteristic (ROC) curve. Radiology **143**, 29–36 (1982)

224. Hannan, E.L., Racz, M.J., Jollis, J.G., Peterson, E.D.: Using medicare claims data to assess provider quality for CABG surgery: Does it work well enough? Health Services Research **31**, 659–678 (1997)

225. Harrell, F.E.: *Regression modeling strategies: With applications to linear models, logistic and ordinal regression, and survival analysis*, 2nd edn. Springer, New York (2015)

226. Harrell Jr., F.E., Lee, K.L., Califf, R.M., Pryor, D.B., Rosati, R.A.: Regression modelling strategies for improved prognostic prediction. Statistics in Medicine **3**, 143–152 (1984)

227. Harrell Jr., F.E., Lee, K.L., Mark, D.B.: Multivariable prognostic models: Issues in developing models, evaluating assumptions and adequacy, and measuring and reducing errors. Statistics in Medicine **15**, 361–387 (1996)

228. Harrell Jr., F.E., Lee, K.L., Pollock, B.G.: Regression models in clinical studies: Determining relationships between predictors and response. Journal of the National Cancer Institute **80**, 1198–1202 (1988)

229. Harrell, Jr., F. E., Slaughter, J. C.: *Introduction to biostatistics for biomedical research: Sample size for given precision.* Vanderbilt University School of Medicine (2018)

230. Hastie, T., Tibshirani, R.: *Generalized additive models.* Boca Raton: Chapman and Hall/CRC (1999)

231. Hastie, T., Tibshirani, R., Friedman, J.H.: *The elements of statistical learning: Data mining, inference, and prediction.* Springer, New York (2001)

232. Hastie, T., Tibshirani, R., Wainwright, M.: *Statistical learning with sparsity: The lasso and generalizations.* Boca Raton: Chapman and Hall/CRC (2015)

233. Hauck, W.W., Anderson, S., Marcus, S.M.: Should we adjust for covariates in nonlinear regression analyses of randomized trials? Controlled Clinical Trials **19**, 249–256 (1998)

234. Heagerty, P.J., Lumley, T., Pepe, M.S.: Time-dependent ROC curves for censored survival data and a diagnostic marker. Biometrics **56**, 337–344 (2000)

235. Heinze, G.: A comparative investigation of methods for logistic regression with separated or nearly separated data. Statistics in Medicine **25**, 4216–4226 (2006)

236. Heinze, G., Wallisch, C., Dunkler, D.: Variable selection - A review and recommendations for the practicing statistician. Biometrical Journal **60**, 431–449 (2018)

237. Hemingway, H. Prognosis research: Why is Dr. Lydgate still waiting? Journal of Clinical Epidemiology **59**, 1229–1238 (2006)

238. Hemingway, H., Croft, P., Perel, P., et al.: Prognosis research strategy (PROGRESS) 1: A framework for researching clinical outcomes. BMJ **346**, e5595 (2013)

239. Hermanek, P., Hutter, R.V., Sobin, L.H.: Prognostic grouping: The next step in tumor classification. Journal of Cancer Research and Clinical Oncology **116**, 513–516 (1990)

240. Hernandez, A.V., Boersma, E., Murray, G.D., Habbema, J.D., Steyerberg, E.W.: Subgroup analyses in therapeutic cardiovascular clinical trials: Are most of them misleading? American Heart Journal **151**, 257–264 (2006)

241. Hernandez, A.V., Eijkemans, M.J., Steyerberg, E.W.: Randomized controlled trials with time-to-event outcomes: How much does prespecified covariate adjustment increase power? Annals of Epidemiology **16**, 41–48 (2006)

242. Hernandez, A.V., Steyerberg, E.W., Butcher, I., et al.: Adjustment for strong predictors of outcome in traumatic brain injury trials: 25% reduction in sample size requirements in the IMPACT study. Journal of Neurotrauma **23**, 1295–1303 (2006)

243. Hernandez, A.V., Steyerberg, E.W., Habbema, J.D.: Covariate adjustment in randomized controlled trials with dichotomous outcomes increases statistical power and reduces sample size requirements. Journal of Clinical Epidemiology **57**, 454–460 (2004)

244. Heymans, M.W., van Buuren, S., Knol, D.L., van Mechelen, W., de Vet, H.C.: Variable selection under multiple imputation using the bootstrap in a prognostic study. BMC Medical Research Methodology **7**, 33 (2007)

245. Hickey, G.L., Grant, S.W., Caiado, C., et al.: Dynamic prediction modeling approaches for cardiac surgery. Circulation: Cardiovascular Quality and Outcomes **6**, 649–658 (2013)

246. Higgins, J.P.T., Thompson, S.G., Spiegelhalter, D.J.: A re-evaluation of random-effects meta-analysis. Journal of the Royal Statistical Society: Series A **172**, 137–159 (2009)

247. Hilden, J., Habbema, J. D., Bjerregaard, B.: The measurement of performance in probabilistic diagnosis. II. Trustworthiness of the exact values of the diagnostic probabilities. Methods of Information in Medicine **17**, 227–137 (1978)

248. Hilden, J., Habbema, J. D., Bjerregaard, B.: The measurement of performance in probabilistic diagnosis. III. Methods based on continuous functions of the diagnostic probabilities. Methods of Information in Medicine **17**, 238–246 (1978)

249. Hingorani, A.D., Windt, D.A., Riley, R.D., et al.: Prognosis research strategy (PROGRESS) 4: Stratified medicine research. BMJ **346**, e5793 (2013)

250. Hlatky, M.A., Greenland, P., Arnett, D.K., et al.: Criteria for evaluation of novel markers of cardiovascular risk: A scientific statement from the American Heart Association. Circulation **119**, 2408–2416 (2009)

251. Hoaglin, D. C., Mosteller, F., Tukey, J. W.: *Understanding robust and exploratory data analysis*. New York: Wiley (2000)

252. Hoeting, J., Madigan, D., Raftery, A., Volinsky, C.: Bayesian model averaging: A tutorial. Statistical Science **14**, 382–401 (1999)

253. Hoffmann, T.C., Montori, V.M., Del Mar, C.: The connection between evidence-based medicine and shared decision making. JAMA **312**, 1295–1296 (2014)

254. Hokken, R. B., Steyerberg, E. W., Verbaan, N., van Herwerden, L. A., van Domburg, R., Bos, E.: 25 years of aortic valve replacement using mechanical valves. Risk factors for early and late mortality. European Heart Journal **18**, 1157–1165 (1997)

255. Homs, M.Y., Steyerberg, E.W., Eijkenboom, W.M., et al.: Single-dose brachytherapy versus metal stent placement for the palliation of dysphagia from oesophageal cancer: Multicentre randomised trial. The Lancet **364**, 1497–1504 (2004)

256. Hosmer, D.W., Hosmer, T., Le Cessie, S., Lemeshow, S.: A comparison of goodness-of-fit tests for the logistic regression model. Statistics in Medicine **16**, 965–980 (1997)

257. Hosmer, D.W., Lemeshow, S.: *Applied logistic regression*, 2nd edn. Wiley, New York (2000)

258. Hu, G., Root, M.M.: Building prediction models for coronary heart disease by synthesizing multiple longitudinal research findings. European Journal of Cardiovascular Prevention & Rehabilitation **12**, 459–464 (2005)

259. Hukkelhoven, C.W., Steyerberg, E.W., Habbema, J.D., et al.: Predicting outcome after traumatic brain injury: Development and validation of a prognostic score based on admission characteristics. Journal of Neurotrauma **22**, 1025–1039 (2005)

260. Hukkelhoven, C.W., Steyerberg, E.W., Rampen, A.J., et al.: Patient age and outcome following severe traumatic brain injury: An analysis of 5600 patients. Journal of Neurosurgery **99**, 666–673 (2003)

261. Hunault, C.C., Habbema, J.D., Eijkemans, M.J., Collins, J.A., Evers, J.L., te Velde, E.R.: Two new prediction rules for spontaneous pregnancy leading to live birth among subfertile couples, based on the synthesis of three previous models. Human Reproduction **19**, 2019–2026 (2004)

262. Hunault, C.C., te Velde, E.R., Weima, S.M., et al.: A case study of the applicability of a prediction model for the selection of patients undergoing in vitro fertilization for single embryo transfer in another center. Fertility and Sterility **87**, 1314–1321 (2007)

263. Hunink, M. G. M., Glasziou, P. P.: *Decision making in health and medicine : Integrating evidence and values*. Cambridge: Cambridge University Press (2014)

264. Hutchinson, P.J., Kolias, A.G., Timofeev, I.S., et al.: Trial of decompressive craniectomy for traumatic intracranial hypertension. New England Journal of Medicine **375**, 1119–1130 (2016)

265. Imani, B., Eijkemans, M.J., Faessen, G.H., Bouchard, P., Giudice, L.C., Fauser, B.C.: Prediction of the individual follicle-stimulating hormone threshold for gonadotropin induction of ovulation in normogonadotropic anovulatory infertility: An approach to increase safety and efficiency. Fertility and Sterility **77**, 83–90 (2002)

266. Ioannidis, J.P.: Why most published research findings are false. PLoS Medicine **2**, e124 (2005)

267. Ioannidis, J.P.: Why most discovered true associations are inflated. Epidemiology **19**, 640–648 (2008)

268. Ioannidis, J.P.: Expectations, validity, and reality in omics. Journal of Clinical Epidemiology **63**, 945–949 (2010)

269. Ioannidis, J.P., Trikalinos, T.A., Khoury, M.J.: Implications of small effect sizes of individual genetic variants on the design and interpretation of genetic association studies of complex diseases. American Journal of Epidemiology **164**, 609–614 (2006)

270. Ioannidis, J.P.A.: Evidence-based medicine has been hijacked: A report to David Sackett. Journal of Clinical Epidemiology **73**, 82–86 (2016)

271. Ioannidis, J.P.A., Greenland, S., Hlatky, M.A., et al.: Increasing value and reducing waste in research design, conduct, and analysis. The Lancet **383**, 166–175 (2014)

272. Ivanov, J., Tu, J.V., Naylor, C.D.: Ready-made, recalibrated, or Remodeled? Issues in the use of risk indexes for assessing mortality after coronary artery bypass graft surgery. Circulation **99**, 2098–2104 (1999)

273. Jackson, D., White, I.R., Seaman, S., Evans, H., Baisley, K., Carpenter, J.: Relaxing the independent censoring assumption in the Cox proportional hazards model using multiple imputation. Statistics in Medicine **33**, 4681–4694 (2014)

274. Jamieson, G.G., Mathew, G., Ludemann, R., Wayman, J., Myers, J.C., Devitt, P.G.: Postoperative mortality following oesophagectomy and problems in reporting its rate. British Journal of Surgery **91**, 943–947 (2004)

275. Janssen, K.J., Donders, A.R., Harrell Jr., F.E., et al.: Missing covariate data in medical research: To impute is better than to ignore. Journal of Clinical Epidemiology **63**, 721–727 (2010)

276. Janssen-Heijnen, M.L., Houterman, S., Lemmens, V.E., Brenner, H., Steyerberg, E.W., Coebergh, J.W.: Prognosis for long-term survivors of cancer. Annals of Oncology **18**, 1408–1413 (2007)

277. Janssen-Heijnen, M. L. G., Maas, H. A. A. M., Houterman, S., Lemmens, V. E. P. P., Rutten, H. J. T., Coebergh, J. W. W.: Comorbidity in older surgical cancer patients: Influence on patient care and outcome. European Journal of Cancer **43**, 2179–2193 (2007)

278. Janssens, A.C., Aulchenko, Y.S., Elefante, S., Borsboom, G.J., Steyerberg, E.W., van Duijn, C.M.: Predictive testing for complex diseases using multiple genes: Fact or fiction? Genetics in Medicine **8**, 395–400 (2006)

279. Janssens, A.C., Deng, Y., Borsboom, G.J., Eijkemans, M.J., Habbema, J.D., Steyerberg, E. W.: A new logistic regression approach for the evaluation of diagnostic test results. Medical Decision Making **25**, 168–177 (2005)

280. Janssens, A.C., Ioannidis, J.P., van Duijn, C.M., Little, J., Khoury, M.J.: Strengthening the reporting of Genetic RIsk Prediction Studies: The GRIPS statement. PLoS Med **8**, e1000420 (2011)

281. Jennett, B., Snoek, J., Bond, M.R., Brooks, N.: Disability after severe head injury: Observations on the use of the Glasgow Outcome Scale. Journal of Neurology, Neurosurgery & Psychiatry **44**, 285–293 (1981)

282. Jolani, S., Debray, T.P.A., Koffijberg, H., van Buuren, S., Moons, K.G.M.: Imputation of systematically missing predictors in an individual participant data meta-analysis: A generalized approach using MICE. Statistics in Medicine **34**, 1841–1863 (2015)

283. Jordan, M.I., Mitchell, T.M.: Machine learning: Trends, perspectives, and prospects. Science **349**, 255–260 (2015)

284. Joyner, M.J., Paneth, N., Ioannidis, J.A.: What happens when underperforming big ideas in research become entrenched? JAMA **316**, 1355–1356 (2016)
285. Justice, A.C., Covinsky, K.E., Berlin, J.A.: Assessing the generalizability of prognostic information. Annals of Internal Medicine **130**, 515–524 (1999)
286. Kahan, B.C., Jairath, V., Doré, C.J., Morris, T.P.: The risks and rewards of covariate adjustment in randomized trials: An assessment of 12 outcomes from 8 studies. Trials **15**, 139 (2014)
287. Kallogjeri, D., Piccirillo, J.F., Spitznagel Jr., E.L., Steyerberg, E.W.: Comparison of scoring methods for ACE-27: Simpler is better. Journal of Geriatric Oncology **3**, 238–245 (2012)
288. Kaplan, E.L., Meier, P.: Nonparametric estimation from incomplete observations. JASA **53**, 457–481 (1958)
289. Kappen, T.H., van Loon, K., Kappen, M.A., et al.: Barriers and facilitators perceived by physicians when using prediction models in practice. Journal of Clinical Epidemiology **70**, 136–145 (2016)
290. Kastrinos, F., Ojha, R. P., Leenen, C., et al.: Comparison of prediction models for lynch syndrome among individuals with colorectal cancer. Journal of the National Cancer Institute **108**, djv308 (2016)
291. Kastrinos, F., Steyerberg, E.W., Mercado, R., et al.: The PREMM(1,2,6) model predicts risk of MLH1, MSH2, and MSH6 germline mutations based on cancer history. Gastroenterology **140**, 73–81 (2011)
292. Kastrinos, F., Uno, H., Ukaegbu, C., et al.: Development and validation of the PREMM5 model for comprehensive risk assessment of lynch syndrome. Journal of Clinical Oncology **35**, 2165–2172 (2017)
293. Kattan, M.W.: Judging new markers by their ability to improve predictive accuracy. Journal of the National Cancer Institute **95**, 634–635 (2003)
294. Kattan, M.W., Eastham, J.A., Stapleton, A.M., Wheeler, T.M., Scardino, P.T.: A preoperative nomogram for disease recurrence following radical prostatectomy for prostate cancer. Journal of the National Cancer Institute **90**, 766–771 (1998)
295. Kattan, M.W., Eastham, J.A., Wheeler, T.M., et al.: Counseling men with prostate cancer: A nomogram for predicting the presence of small, moderately differentiated, confined tumors. The Journal of Urology **170**, 1792–1797 (2003)
296. Kattan, M.W., Heller, G., Brennan, M.F.: A competing-risks nomogram for sarcoma-specific death following local recurrence. Statistics in Medicine **22**, 3515–3525 (2003)
297. Keeley, E.C., Boura, J.A., Grines, C.L.: Primary angioplasty versus intravenous thrombolytic therapy for acute myocardial infarction: A quantitative review of 23 randomised trials. The Lancet **361**, 13–20 (2003)
298. Kent, D.M., Hayward, R.A.: Limitations of applying summary results of clinical trials to individual patients: The need for risk stratification. JAMA **298**, 1209–1212 (2007)
299. Kent, D.M., Rothwell, P.M., Ioannidis, J.P., Altman, D.G., Hayward, R.A.: Assessing and reporting heterogeneity in treatment effects in clinical trials: A proposal. Trials **11**, 85 (2010)
300. Kent, D.M., Steyerberg, E.W., van Klaveren, D.: Personalized evidence based medicine: Predictive approaches to heterogeneous treatment effects. BMJ **363**, k4245 (2018)
301. Kerkhof, M., van Dekken, H., Steyerberg, E.W., et al.: Grading of dysplasia in Barrett's oesophagus: Substantial interobserver variation between general and gastrointestinal pathologists. Histopathology **50**, 920–927 (2007)
302. Kerr, K.F., Brown, M.D., Zhu, K., Janes, H.: Assessing the clinical impact of risk prediction models with decision curves: Guidance for correct interpretation and appropriate use. Journal of Clinical Oncology **34**, 2534–2540 (2016)
303. Kerr, K.F., Meisner, A., Thiessen-Philbrook, H., Coca, S.G., Parikh, C.R.: RiGoR: Reporting guidelines to address common sources of bias in risk model development. Biomarker Research **3**, 2 (2015)

304. Kertai, M.D., Steyerberg, E.W., Boersma, E., et al.: Validation of two risk models for perioperative mortality in patients undergoing elective abdominal aortic aneurysm surgery. Vascular and Endovascular Surgery **37**, 13–21 (2003)

305. Klabunde, C. N., Warren, J. L., Legler, J. M.: Assessing comorbidity using claims data: An overview. Medical care **40**, IV-26–35 (2002)

306. Kleinbaum, D. G., Kupper, L. L., Morgenstern, H.: *Epidemiologic research : Principles and quantitative methods*. Belmont: Lifetime Learning Publications (1982)

307. Knaus, W.A., Harrell, Jr., F. E., Lynn, J., et al.: The SUPPORT prognostic model. Objective estimates of survival for seriously ill hospitalized adults. Study to understand prognoses and preferences for outcomes and risks of treatments. Annals of internal medicine **122**, 191–203 (1995)

308. Knottnerus, J.A.: *Evidence base of clinical diagnosis*. Blackwell BMJ Books, Oxford (2002)

309. Koller, M.T., Raatz, H., Steyerberg, E.W., Wolbers, M.: Competing risks and the clinical community: Irrelevance or ignorance? Statistics in Medicine **31**, 1089–1097 (2012)

310. Kollmannsberger, C., Nichols, C., Meisner, C., Mayer, F., Kanz, L., Bokemeyer, C.: Identification of prognostic subgroups among patients with metastatic 'IGCCCG poor-prognosis' germ-cell cancer: An explorative analysis using cart modeling. Annals of Oncology **11**, 1115–1120 (2000)

311. Konig, I.R., Malley, J.D., Weimar, C., Diener, H.C., Ziegler, A.: Practical experiences on the necessity of external validation. Statistics in Medicine **26**, 5499–5511 (2007)

312. Krijnen, P., van Jaarsveld, B.C., Deinum, J., Steyerberg, E.W., Habbema, J.D.: Which patients with hypertension and atherosclerotic renal artery stenosis benefit from immediate intervention? Journal of Human Hypertension **18**, 91–96 (2004)

313. Krijnen, P., van Jaarsveld, B.C., Hunink, M.G., Habbema, J.D.: The effect of treatment on health-related quality of life in patients with hypertension and renal artery stenosis. Journal of Human Hypertension **19**, 467–470 (2005)

314. Krijnen, P., van Jaarsveld, B. C., Steyerberg, E.W., Man in 't Veld, A. J., Schalekamp, M. A., Habbema, J. D.: A clinical prediction rule for renal artery stenosis. Annals of Internal Medicine **129**, 705–711 (1998)

315. Krumholz, H.M., Brindis, R.G., Brush, J.E., et al.: Standards for statistical models used for public reporting of health outcomes. Circulation **113**, 456–462 (2006)

316. Krumholz, H.M., Wang, Y., Chen, J., et al.: Reduction in acute myocardial infarction mortality in the united states: Risk-standardized mortality rates from 1995–2006. JAMA **302**, 767–773 (2009)

317. Krumholz, H.M., Wang, Y., Mattera, J.A., et al.: An administrative claims model suitable for profiling hospital performance based on 30-day mortality rates among patients with an acute myocardial infarction. Circulation **113**, 1683–1692 (2006)

318. Kullback, S., Leibler, R.A.: On information and sufficiency. The Annals of Mathematical Statistics **22**, 79–86 (1951)

319. Kyrgidis, A., Kountouras, J., Zavos, C., Chatzopoulos, D.: New molecular concepts of Barrett's esophagus: Clinical implications and biomarkers. Journal of Surgical Research **125**, 189–212 (2005)

320. Laird, N.M., Louis, T.A.: Empirical Bayes ranking methods. Journal of Educational Statistics **14**, 29–46 (1989)

321. Landis, J.R., Koch, G.G.: The measurement of observer agreement for categorical data. Biometrics **33**, 159–174 (1977)

322. Larsen, K., Petersen, J.H., Budtz-Jorgensen, E., Endahl, L.: Interpreting parameters in the logistic regression model with random effects. Biometrics **56**, 909–914 (2000)

323. Laupacis, A., Wells, G., Richardson, W. S., Tugwell, P.: Users' guides to the medical literature. V. How to use an article about prognosis. JAMA **272**, 234–237 (1994)

324. le Cessie, S., van Houwelingen, H.C.: Testing the fit of a regression model via score tests in random effects models. Biometrics **51**, 600–614 (1995)

325. Le, C.T., Lindgren, B.L.: Computational implementation of the conditional logistic regression model in the analysis of epidemiologic matched studies. Computers and Biomedical Research **21**, 48–52 (1988)

326. Lecleire, S., Di Fiore, F., Antonietti, M., et al.: Undernutrition is predictive of early mortality after palliative self-expanding metal stent insertion in patients with inoperable or recurrent esophageal cancer. Gastrointestinal Endoscopy **64**, 479–484 (2006)

327. Lee, K.I., Koval, J.J.: Determinants of the best significance level in forward stepwise logistic regression. Communications in Statistics-Simulation and Computation **26**, 559–575 (1997)

328. Lee, K. L.: Predictors of 30-day mortality in the era of reperfusion for acute myocardial infarction. http://circ.ahajournals.org/cgi/content/full/91/6/1659 (2006)

329. Lee, K. L., Woodlief, L. H., Topol, E. J., et al.: Predictors of 30-day mortality in the era of reperfusion for acute myocardial infarction. Results from an international trial of 41,021 patients. GUSTO-I Investigators. Circulation **91**, 1659–1668 (1995)

330. Leening, M.J., Steyerberg, E.W., Van Calster, B., D'Agostino, R.B., Pencina, M.J.: Net reclassification improvement and integrated discrimination improvement require calibrated models: Relevance from a marker and model perspective. Statistics in Medicine **33**, 3415–3418 (2014)

331. Leening, M.J., Vedder, M.M., Witteman, J.C., Pencina, M.J., Steyerberg, E.W.: Net reclassification improvement: Computation, interpretation, and controversies: A literature review and clinician's guide. Annals of Internal Medicine **160**, 122–131 (2014)

332. Lesaffre, E., Bogaerts, K., Li, X., Bluhmki, E.: On the variability of covariate adjustment. experience with Koch's method for evaluating the absolute difference in proportions in randomized clinical trials. Controlled Clinical Trials **23**, 127–142 (2002)

333. Lesko, C.R., Henderson, N.C., Varadhan, R.: Considerations when assessing heterogeneity of treatment effect in patient-centered outcomes research. Journal of Clinical Epidemiology **100**, 22–31 (2018)

334. Lewington, S., Clarke, R., Qizilbash, N., Peto, R., Collins, R.: Age-specific relevance of usual blood pressure to vascular mortality: A meta-analysis of individual data for one million adults in 61 prospective studies. The Lancet **360**, 1903–1913 (2002)

335. Li, B., Lingsma, H.F., Steyerberg, E.W., Lesaffre, E.: Logistic random effects regression models: A comparison of statistical packages for binary and ordinal outcomes. BMC Medical Research Methodology **11**, 77 (2011)

336. Liao, J.G., Chin, K.V.: Logistic regression for disease classification using microarray data: Model selection in a large p and small n case. Bioinformatics **23**, 1945–1951 (2007)

337. Lijmer, J.G., Mol, B.W., Heisterkamp, S., et al.: Empirical evidence of design-related bias in studies of diagnostic tests. JAMA **282**, 1061–1066 (1999)

338. Lilford, R., Mohammed, M.A., Spiegelhalter, D., Thomson, R.: Use and misuse of process and outcome data in managing performance of acute medical care: Avoiding institutional stigma. The Lancet **363**, 1147–1154 (2004)

339. Lilford, R., Pronovost, P.: Using hospital mortality rates to judge hospital performance: A bad idea that just won't go away. BMJ **340**, c2016 (2010)

340. Lingsma, H., Roozenbeek, B., Steyerberg, E.W.: Covariate adjustment increases statistical power in randomized controlled trials. Journal of Clinical Epidemiology **63**, 1391 (2010)

341. Lingsma, H. F, Dippel, D. W., Hoeks, S., et al.: Variation between hospitals in patient outcome after stroke is only partly explained by differences in quality of care: Data from the Netherlands Stroke Survey. Journal of Neurology, Neurosurgery & Psychiatry **79**, 888–94 (2008)

342. Lingsma, H.F., Roozenbeek, B., Li, B., et al.: Large between-center differences in outcome after moderate and severe traumatic brain injury in the international mission on prognosis and clinical trial design in traumatic brain injury (IMPACT) study. Neurosurgery **68**, 601–607 (2011)

343. Lingsma, H.F., Roozenbeek, B., Steyerberg, E.W., Murray, G.D., Maas, A.I.: Early prognosis in traumatic brain injury: From prophecies to predictions. The Lancet Neurology **9**, 543–554 (2010)

344. Lingsma, H. F, Steyerberg, E. W, Eijkemans, M. J, Dippel, D. W., Scholte Op Reimer, W. J., Van Houwelingen, H. C.: Comparing and ranking hospitals based on outcome: Results from The Netherlands Stroke Survey. QJM **103**, 99–108 (2010)

345. Lipton, L.R., Johnson, V., Cummings, C., et al.: Refining the Amsterdam Criteria and Bethesda Guidelines: Testing algorithms for the prediction of mismatch repair mutation status in the familial cancer clinic. Journal of Clinical Oncology **22**, 4934–4943 (2004)

346. Litjens, G., Kooi, T., Bejnordi, B.E., et al.: A survey on deep learning in medical image analysis. Medical Image Analysis **42**, 60–88 (2017)

347. Little, R.J.A., Rubin, D.B.: Statistical analysis with missing data, 2nd edn. Wiley, Hoboken (2002)

348. Liu, J., Hong, Y., D'Agostino Sr., R.B., et al.: Predictive value for the Chinese population of the Framingham CHD risk assessment tool compared with the Chinese Multi-Provincial Cohort Study. JAMA **291**, 2591–2599 (2004)

349. Loeb, S., Bruinsma, S.M., Nicholson, J., et al.: Active surveillance for prostate cancer: A systematic review of clinicopathologic variables and biomarkers for risk stratification. European Urology **67**, 619–626 (2015)

350. Lord, S.J., Irwig, L., Simes, R.J.: When is measuring sensitivity and specificity sufficient to evaluate a diagnostic test, and when do we need randomized trials? Annals of Internal Medicine **144**, 850–855 (2006)

351. Lorenz, M.O.: Methods of measuring the concentration of wealth. JASA **9**, 209–219 (1905)

352. Lubien, E., DeMaria, A., Krishnaswamy, P., et al.: Utility of B-natriuretic peptide in detecting diastolic dysfunction: Comparison with Doppler velocity recordings. Circulation **105**, 595–601 (2002)

353. Lubsen, J., Pool, J., van der Does, E.: A practical device for the application of a diagnostic or prognostic function. Methods of Information in Medicine **17**, 127–129 (1978)

354. Lughezzani, G., Briganti, A., Karakiewicz, P.I., et al.: Predictive and prognostic models in radical prostatectomy candidates: A critical analysis of the literature. European Urology **58**, 687–700 (2010)

355. Luijken, K., Groenwold, R. H. H., van Calster, B., Steyerberg, E. W., van Smeden, M. Impact of predictor measurement heterogeneity across settings on performance of prediction models: A measurement error perspective. Stat Med (2019)

356. Lynch, H.T., de la Chapelle, A.: Genetic susceptibility to non-polyposis colorectal cancer. Journal of Medical Genetics **36**, 801–818 (1999)

357. Maas, A.I., Marmarou, A., Murray, G.D., Teasdale, S.G., Steyerberg, E.W.: Prognosis and clinical trial design in traumatic brain injury: The IMPACT study. Journal of Neurotrauma **24**, 232–238 (2007)

358. Maas, A.I., Murray, G.D., Roozenbeek, B., et al.: Advancing care for traumatic brain injury: Findings from the IMPACT studies and perspectives on future research. The Lancet Neurology **12**, 1200–1210 (2013)

359. Maas, A.I., Steyerberg, E.W., Butcher, I., et al.: Prognostic value of computerized tomography scan characteristics in traumatic brain injury: Results from the IMPACT study. Journal of Neurotrauma **24**, 303–314 (2007)

360. Maas, C.J.M., Hox, J.J.: Robustness issues in multilevel regression analysis. Statistica Neerlandica **58**, 127–137 (2004)

361. Maggioni, A. P., Maseri, A., Fresco, C., et al.: Age-related increase in mortality among patients with first myocardial infarctions treated with thrombolysis. New England Journal of Medicine **329**, 1442–1448 (1993)

362. Malek, M.H., Berger, D.E., Coburn, J.W.: On the inappropriateness of stepwise regression analysis for model building and testing. European Journal of Applied Physiology **101**, 263–264 (2007)

363. Marcus, R., Eric, P., Gabriel, K.R.: On closed testing procedures with special reference to ordered analysis of variance. Biometrika **63**, 655–660 (1976)
364. Marmarou, A., Lu, J., Butcher, I., et al.: Prognostic value of the Glasgow Coma Scale and pupil reactivity in traumatic brain injury assessed pre-hospital and on enrollment: An IMPACT analysis. Journal of Neurotrauma **24**, 270–280 (2007)
365. Marmot, M.G., Altman, D.G., Cameron, D.A., Dewar, J.A., Thompson, S.G., Wilcox, M.: The benefits and harms of breast cancer screening: An independent review. British Journal of Cancer **108**, 2205 (2013)
366. Marquand, A., Hanon, O., Fauvel, J.P., Mounier-Vehier, C., Equine, O., Girerd, X.: Validity of the clinical prediction rule for the diagnosis of renal arterial stenosis in hypertensive patients resistant to treatment. Archives des maladies du coeur et des vaisseaux **93**, 1041–1045 (2000)
367. Marshall, E.C., Spiegelhalter, D.J.: Reliability of league tables of in vitro fertilisation clinics: Retrospective analysis of live birth rates. BMJ **316**, 1701–1704 (1998)
368. Marshall, L.F., Marshall, S.B., Klauber, M.R., et al.: The diagnosis of head injury requires a classification based on computed axial tomography. Journal of Neurotrauma **9**(Suppl 1), S287–S292 (1992)
369. Mauff, K., Steyerberg, E.W., Nijpels, G., van der Heijden, A., Rizopoulos, D.: Extension of the association structure in joint models to include weighted cumulative effects. Statistics in Medicine **36**, 3746–3759 (2017)
370. McCormick, T.H., Raftery, A.E., Madigan, D., Burd, R.S.: Dynamic logistic regression and dynamic model averaging for binary classification. Biometrics **68**, 23–30 (2012)
371. McHugh, G.S., Butcher, I., Steyerberg, E.W., et al.: Statistical approaches to the univariate prognostic analysis of the IMPACT database on traumatic brain injury. Journal of Neurotrauma **24**, 251–258 (2007)
372. McHugh, G.S., Engel, D.C., Butcher, I., et al.: Prognostic value of secondary insults in traumatic brain injury: Results from the IMPACT study. Journal of Neurotrauma **24**, 287–293 (2007)
373. McShane, L.M., Altman, D.G., Sauerbrei, W., Taube, S.E., Gion, M., Clark, G.M.: Reporting recommendations for tumor marker prognostic studies (REMARK). Journal of the National Cancer Institute **97**, 1180–1184 (2005)
374. Menon, D.K., Maas, A.I.R.: Progress, failures and new approaches for TBI research. Nature Reviews Neurology **11**, 71 (2015)
375. Michel, P., Domecq, S., Salmi, L.R., Roques, F., Nashef, S.A.M.: Confidence intervals for the prediction of mortality in the logistic EuroSCORE. European Journal of Cardio-Thoracic Surgery **27**, 1129–1132 (2005)
376. Michel, P., Roques, F., Nashef, S A : Logistic or additive EuroSCORE for high-risk patients? European Journal of Cardio-Thoracic Surgery **23**, 684–687 (2003)
377. Michie, D., Spiegelhalter, D.J., Taylor, C.C.: *Machine learning, neural and statistical classification*. Ellis Horwood, New York (1994)
378. Mihaylova, B., Briggs, A., O'Hagan, A., Thompson, S.G.: Review of statistical methods for analysing healthcare resources and costs. Health Economics **20**, 897–916 (2011)
379. Miller, M.E., Hui, S.L., Tierney, W.M.: Validation techniques for logistic regression models. Statistics in Medicine **10**, 1213–1226 (1991)
380. Miller, M.E., Langefeld, C.D., Tierney, W.M., Hui, S.L., McDonald, C.J.: Validation of probabilistic predictions. Medical Decision Making **13**, 49–58 (1993)
381. Moineddin, R., Matheson, F.I., Glazier, R.H.: A simulation study of sample size for multilevel logistic regression models. BMC Medical Research Methodology **7**, 34 (2007)
382. Molinaro, A.M., Simon, R., Pfeiffer, R.M.: Prediction error estimation: A comparison of resampling methods. Bioinformatics **21**, 3301–3307 (2005)
383. Moons, K.G., Altman, D.G., Reitsma, J.B., et al.: Transparent Reporting of a multivariable prediction model for Individual Prognosis or Diagnosis (TRIPOD): Explanation and elaboration. Annals of Internal Medicine **162**, W1–W73 (2015)

384. Moons, K.G., de Groot, J.A., Bouwmeester, W., et al.: Critical appraisal and data extraction for systematic reviews of prediction modelling studies: The CHARMS checklist. PLoS Medicine **11**, e1001744 (2014)
385. Moons, K.G., Donders, R.A., Stijnen, T., Harrell Jr., F.E.: Using the outcome for imputation of missing predictor values was preferred. Journal of Clinical Epidemiology **59**, 1092–1101 (2006)
386. Moons, K.G., Grobbee, D.E.: Diagnostic studies as multivariable, prediction research. Journal of Epidemiology & Community Health **56**, 337–338 (2002)
387. Moons, K.G., Grobbee, D.E.: When should we remain blind and when should our eyes remain open in diagnostic studies? Journal of Clinical Epidemiology **55**, 633–636 (2002)
388. Moons, K.G., Harrell, F.E., Steyerberg, E.W.: Should scoring rules be based on odds ratios or regression coefficients? Journal of Clinical Epidemiology **55**, 1054–1055 (2002)
389. Moons, K.G.M., Wolff, R.F., Riley, R.D., et al.: PROBAST: A tool to assess risk of bias and applicability of prediction model studies: Explanation and elaboration. Annals of Internal Medicine **170**, W1–w33 (2019)
390. Moons, K.M., Altman, D.G., Reitsma, J.B., et al.: Transparent reporting of a multivariable prediction model for individual prognosis or diagnosis (tripod): Explanation and elaboration. Annals of Internal Medicine **162**, W1–W73 (2015)
391. Morgan, T.M., Elashoff, R.M.: Effect of categorizing a continuous covariate on the comparison of survival time. JASA **81**, 917–921 (1986)
392. Morise, A.P., Diamond, G.A., Detrano, R., Bobbio, M., Gunel, E.: The effect of disease-prevalence adjustments on the accuracy of a logistic prediction model. Medical Decision Making **16**, 133–142 (1996)
393. Morris, C.N.: Parametric Empirical Bayes inference: Theory and applications. JASA **78**, 47–55 (1983)
394. Morton, V., Torgerson, D.J.: Effect of regression to the mean on decision making in health care. BMJ **326**, 1083–1084 (2003)
395. Mueller, H. S., Cohen, L. S., Braunwald, E., et al.: Predictors of early morbidity and mortality after thrombolytic therapy of acute myocardial infarction. Circulation **85**, 1254–1264 (1992)
396. Murphy, A.H.: A new vector partition of the probability score. Journal of Applied Meteorology **12**, 595–600 (1973)
397. Murray, G.D., Barer, D., Choi, S., et al.: Design and analysis of phase III trials with ordered outcome scales: The concept of the sliding dichotomy. Journal of Neurotrauma **22**, 511–517 (2005)
398. Murray, G.D., Butcher, I., McHugh, G.S., et al.: Multivariable prognostic analysis in traumatic brain injury: Results from the IMPACT study. Journal of Neurotrauma **24**, 329–337 (2007)
399. Mushkudiani, N.A., Engel, D.C., Steyerberg, E.W., et al.: Prognostic value of demographic characteristics in traumatic brain injury: Results from the IMPACT study. Journal of Neurotrauma **24**, 259–269 (2007)
400. Mushkudiani, N.A., Hukkelhoven, C.W., Hernandez, A.V., et al.: A systematic review finds methodological improvements necessary for prognostic models in determining traumatic brain injury outcomes. Journal of Clinical Epidemiology **61**, 331–343 (2008)
401. Musoro, J.Z., Zwinderman, A.H., Puhan, M.A., ter Riet, G., Geskus, R.B.: Validation of prediction models based on lasso regression with multiply imputed data. BMC Medical Research Methodology **14**, 116 (2014)
402. Nab, H.W., Hop, W.C., Crommelin, M.A., Kluck, H.M., van der Heijden, L.H., Coebergh, J.W.: Changes in long term prognosis for breast cancer in a Dutch cancer registry. BMJ **309**, 83–86 (1994)
403. Nagelkerke, N. J.: A note on a general definition of the coefficient of determination. Biometrika, **78**, 691–692 (1991)

404. Nashef, S.A., Roques, F., Michel, P., Gauducheau, E., Lemeshow, S., Salamon, R.: European system for cardiac operative risk evaluation (EuroSCORE). European Journal of Cardio-Thoracic Surgery **16**, 9–13 (1999)

405. Nieboer, D., Vergouwe, Y., Ankerst, D.P., Roobol, M.J., Steyerberg, E.W.: Improving prediction models with new markers: A comparison of updating strategies. BMC Medical Research Methodology **16**, 128 (2016)

406. Nieboer, D., Vergouwe, Y., Roobol, M.J., et al.: Nonlinear modeling was applied thoughtfully for risk prediction: The Prostate Biopsy Collaborative Group. Journal of Clinical Epidemiology **68**, 426–434 (2015)

407. Normand, S.-L. T., Ash, A. S., Fienberg, S. E., Stukel, T. A., Utts, J., Louis, T. A.: League tables for hospital comparisons. Annual Review of Statistics and Its Application **3**, 21–50 (2016)

408. Normand, S.L., Glickman, M.E., Gatsonis, C.A.: Statistical methods for profiling providers of medical care: Issues and applications. JASA **92**, 803–814 (1997)

409. Normand, S.L., Wolf, R.E., Ayanian, J.Z., McNeil, B.J.: Assessing the accuracy of hospital clinical performance measures. Medical Decision Making **27**, 9–20 (2007)

410. Ogundimu, E.O., Altman, D.G., Collins, G.S.: Adequate sample size for developing prediction models is not simply related to events per variable. Journal of Clinical Epidemiology **76**, 175–182 (2016)

411. Oostenbrink, R., Moons, K.G., Bleeker, S.E., Moll, H.A., Grobbee, D.E.: Diagnostic research on routine care data: Prospects and problems. Journal of Clinical Epidemiology **56**, 501–506 (2003)

412. Ormsby, A.H., Petras, R.E., Henricks, W.H., et al.: Observer variation in the diagnosis of superficial oesophageal adenocarcinoma. Gut **51**, 671–676 (2002)

413. Oxford Center for Evidence-Based Medicine. *Glossary of terms in Evidence-Based Medicine.* https://www.cebm.net/2014/06/glossary/ (2019)

414. Pajouheshnia, R., van Smeden, M., Peelen, L.M., Groenwold, R.H.H.: How variation in predictor measurement affects the discriminative ability and transportability of a prediction model. Journal of Clinical Epidemiology **105**, 136–141 (2019)

415. Pal Choudhury, P., Wilcox, A., Brook, M., et al.: Comparative validation of breast cancer risk prediction models and projections for future risk stratification. bioRxiv 440347 (2018)

416. Palazon-Bru, A., Folgado-de la Rosa, D. M., Cortes-Castell, E., Lopez-Cascales, M. T., Gil-Guillen, V. F.: Sample size calculation to externally validate scoring systems based on logistic regression models. PLoS One **12**, e0176726 (2017)

417. Papworth, D.G., Lloyd, R.A.: Cancer survival in the USA, 1973–1990: A statistical analysis. British Journal of Cancer **78**, 1514–1515 (1998)

418. Parmigiani, G., Berry, D., Aguilar, O.: Determining carrier probabilities for breast cancer-susceptibility genes BRCA1 and BRCA2. The American Journal of Human Genetics **62**, 145–158 (1998)

419. Pauker, S.G., Kassirer, J.P.: Therapeutic decision making: A cost-benefit analysis. New England Journal of Medicine **293**, 229–234 (1975)

420. Pauker, S.G., Kassirer, J.P.: The threshold approach to clinical decision making. New England Journal of Medicine **302**, 1109–1117 (1980)

421. Peduzzi, P., Concato, J., Feinstein, A. R., Holford, T. R.: Importance of events per independent variable in proportional hazards regression analysis. II. Accuracy and precision of regression estimates. Journal of Clinical Epidemiology **48**, 1503–1510 (1995)

422. Peduzzi, P., Concato, J., Kemper, E., Holford, T.R., Feinstein, A.R.: A simulation study of the number of events per variable in logistic regression analysis. Journal of Clinical Epidemiology **49**, 1373–1379 (1996)

423. Peek, N., Arts, D.G., Bosman, R.J., van der Voort, P.H., de Keizer, N.F.: External validation of prognostic models for critically ill patients required substantial sample sizes. Journal of Clinical Epidemiology **60**, 491–501 (2007)

424. Peirce, C.S.: The numerical measure of success of predictions. Science **4**, 453–454 (1884)

425. Pencina, M.J., D'Agostino, R.B., Pencina, K.M., Janssens, A.C.J.W., Greenland, P.: Interpreting incremental value of markers added to risk prediction models. American Journal of Epidemiology **176**, 473–481 (2012)

426. Pencina, M. J., D'Agostino, Sr., R. B., D'Agostino, Jr., R. B., Vasan, R. S.: Evaluating the added predictive ability of a new marker: From area under the ROC curve to reclassification and beyond. Statistics in Medicine **27**, 157–172 (2008)

427. Pencina, M.J., D'Agostino Sr., R.B., Steyerberg, E.W.: Extensions of net reclassification improvement calculations to measure usefulness of new biomarkers. Statistics in Medicine **30**, 11–21 (2011)

428. Pencina, M.J., Fine, J.P., D'Agostino Sr., R.B.: Discrimination slope and integrated discrimination improvement - properties, relationships and impact of calibration. Statistics in Medicine **36**, 4482–4490 (2017)

429. Pencina, M.J., Steyerberg, E.W., D'Agostino Sr., R.B.: Net reclassification index at event rate: Properties and relationships. Statistics in Medicine **36**, 4455–4467 (2017)

430. Pepe, M.S.: *The statistical evaluation of medical tests for classification and prediction.* Oxford University Press, Oxford (2003)

431. Pepe, M.S.: Evaluating technologies for classification and prediction in medicine. Stat Med **24**, 3687–3696 (2005)

432. Pepe, M.S., Feng, Z., Huang, Y., et al.: Integrating the predictiveness of a marker with its performance as a classifier. American Journal of Epidemiology **167**, 362–368 (2008)

433. Pepe, M.S., Janes, H., Longton, G., Leisenring, W., Newcomb, P.: Limitations of the odds ratio in gauging the performance of a diagnostic, prognostic, or screening marker. American Journal of Epidemiology **159**, 882–890 (2004)

434. Pepe, M.S., Kerr, K.F., Longton, G., Wang, Z.: Testing for improvement in prediction model performance. Statistics in Medicine **32**, 1467–1482 (2013)

435. Perel, P., Arango, M., Clayton, T., et al.: Predicting outcome after traumatic brain injury: Practical prognostic models based on large cohort of international patients. BMJ **336**, 425–429 (2008)

436. Perel, P., Edwards, P., Wentz, R., Roberts, I.: Systematic review of prognostic models in traumatic brain injury. BMC Medical Informatics and Decision Making **6**, 38 (2006)

437. Perry, J.J., Stiell, I.G.: Impact of clinical decision rules on clinical care of traumatic injuries to the foot and ankle, knee, cervical spine, and head. Injury **37**, 1157–1165 (2006)

438. Picard, R.R., Cook, R.D.: Cross-validation of regression models. JASA **79**, 575–583 (1984)

439. Piccirillo, J.F., Tierney, R.M., Costas, I., Grove, L., Spitznagel Jr., E.L.: Prognostic importance of comorbidity in a hospital-based cancer registry. JAMA **291**, 2441–2447 (2004)

440. Piccirillo, J.F., Vlahiotis, A., Barrett, L.B., Flood, K.L., Spitznagel, E.L., Steyerberg, E.W.: The changing prevalence of comorbidity across the age spectrum. Critical Reviews in Oncology/Hematology **67**, 124–132 (2008)

441. Pocock, S.J., Assmann, S.E., Enos, L.E., Kasten, L.E.: Subgroup analysis, covariate adjustment and baseline comparisons in clinical trial reporting: Current practice and problems. Statistics in Medicine **21**, 2917–2930 (2002)

442. Poldermans, D., Bax, J.J., Kertai, M.D., et al.: Statins are associated with a reduced incidence of perioperative mortality in patients undergoing major noncardiac vascular surgery. Circulation **107**, 1848–1851 (2003)

443. Powers, C.A., Meyer, C.M., Roebuck, M.C., Vaziri, B.: Predictive modeling of total healthcare costs using pharmacy claims data: A comparison of alternative econometric cost modeling techniques. Medical Care **43**, 1065–1072 (2005)

444. Price, W. N.: Big data and black-box medical algorithms. Science Translational Medicine **10** eaao5333 (2018)

445. Putter, H., Fiocco, M., Geskus, R.B.: Tutorial in biostatistics: Competing risks and multi-state models. Statistics in Medicine **26**, 2389–2430 (2007)

446. Puvimanasinghe, J.P., Steyerberg, E.W., Takkenberg, J.J., et al.: Prognosis after aortic valve replacement with a bioprosthesis: Predictions based on meta-analysis and microsimulation. Circulation **103**, 1535–1541 (2001)

447. Raftery, A.E., Kárný, M., Ettler, P.: Online prediction under model uncertainty via dynamic model averaging: Application to a cold rolling mill. Technometrics **52**, 52–66 (2010)

448. Raftery, A.E., Madigan, D., Hoeting, J.: Bayesian model averaging for linear regression models. JASA **92**, 179–191 (1997)

449. Raghupathi, W., Raghupathi, V.: Big data analytics in healthcare: Promise and potential. Health Information Science and Systems **2**, 3 (2014)

450. Ransohoff, D.F., Feinstein, A.R.: Problems of spectrum and bias in evaluating the efficacy of diagnostic tests. New England Journal of Medicine **299**, 926–930 (1978)

451. Reilly, B.M., Evans, A.T.: Translating clinical research into clinical practice: Impact of using prediction rules to make decisions. Annals of Internal Medicine **144**, 201–209 (2006)

452. Reps, J.M., Schuemie, M.J., Suchard, M.A., Ryan, P.B., Rijnbeek, P.R.: Design and implementation of a standardized framework to generate and evaluate patient-level prediction models using observational healthcare data. Journal of the American Medical Informatics Association **25**, 969–975 (2018)

453. Resche-Rigon, M., White, I.R.: Multiple imputation by chained equations for systematically and sporadically missing multilevel data. Statistical Methods in Medical Research **27**, 1634–1649 (2018)

454. Rietveld, E., De Jonge, H.C., Polder, J.J., et al.: Anticipated costs of hospitalization for respiratory syncytial virus infection in young children at risk. The Pediatric Infectious Disease Journal **23**, 523–529 (2004)

455. Rietveld, E., Vergouwe, Y., Steyerberg, E.W., Huysman, M.W., de Groot, R., Moll, H.A.: Hospitalization for respiratory syncytial virus infection in young children: Development of a clinical prediction rule. The Pediatric Infectious Disease Journal **25**, 201–207 (2006)

456. Rigatelli, G.: Assessing the appropriateness and increasing the yield of renal angiography in patients undergoing coronary angiography: A scoring system. The International Journal of Cardiovascular Imaging **22**, 135–139 (2006)

457. Riley, R.D., Ensor, J., Snell, K.I., et al.: External validation of clinical prediction models using big datasets from e-health records or IPD meta-analysis: Opportunities and challenges. BMJ **353**, i3140 (2016)

458. Riley, R.D., Hayden, J.A., Steyerberg, E.W., et al.: Prognosis Research Strategy (PROGRESS) 2: Prognostic factor research. PLoS Medicine **10**, e1001380 (2013)

459. Riley, R.D., Moons, K.G.M., Snell, K.I.E., et al.: A guide to systematic review and meta-analysis of prognostic factor studies. BMJ **364**, k4597 (2019)

460. Riley, R. D., Snell, K. I., Ensor, J., et al.: Minimum sample size for developing a multivariable prediction model: PART II - binary and time-to-event outcomes. Statistics in Medicine **38**, 1276–1296 (2019)

461. Rizopoulos, D.: Dynamic predictions and prospective accuracy in joint models for longitudinal and time-to-event data. Biometrics **67**, 819–829 (2011)

462. Rizopoulos, D.: *Joint models for longitudinal and time-to-event data*. Chapman and Hall/CRC, New York (2012)

463. Robinson, L.D., Jewell, N.P.: Some surprising results about covariate adjustment in logistic regression models. International Statistical Review **59**, 227–240 (1991)

464. Roozenbeek, B., Lingsma, H.F., Perel, P., et al.: The added value of ordinal analysis in clinical trials: An example in traumatic brain injury. Critical Care **15**, R127 (2011)

465. Roozenbeek, B., Maas, A.I., Marmarou, A., et al.: The influence of enrollment criteria on recruitment and outcome distribution in traumatic brain injury studies: Results from the impact study. Journal of Neurotrauma **26**, 1069–1075 (2009)

466. Rosenbaum, P.R., Rubin, D.B.: The central role of the propensity score in observational studies for causal effects. Biometrika **70**, 41–55 (1983)

467. Ross, P.L., Scardino, P.T., Kattan, M.W.: A catalog of prostate cancer nomograms. The Journal of Urology **165**, 1562–1568 (2001)

468. Rothwell, P.M.: External validity of randomised controlled trials: To whom do the results of this trial apply? The Lancet **365**, 82–93 (2005)

469. Roukema, J., van Loenhout, R.B., Steyerberg, E.W., Moons, K.G., Bleeker, S.E., Moll, H. A.: Polytomous regression did not outperform dichotomous logistic regression in diagnosing serious bacterial infections in febrile children. Journal of Clinical Epidemiology **61**, 135–141 (2008)

470. Royston, P.: A strategy for modelling the effect of a continuous covariate in medicine and epidemiology. Statistics in Medicine **19**, 1831–1847 (2000)

471. Royston, P., Altman, D.G.: External validation of a Cox prognostic model: Principles and methods. BMC Medical Research Methodology **13**, 33 (2013)

472. Royston, P., Altman, D.G., Sauerbrei, W.: Dichotomizing continuous predictors in multiple regression: A bad idea. Statistics in Medicine **25**, 127–141 (2006)

473. Royston, P., Parmar, M.K., Sylvester, R.: Construction and validation of a prognostic model across several studies, with an application in superficial bladder cancer. Statistics in Medicine **23**, 907–926 (2004)

474. Royston, P., Parmar, M.K.B.: The use of restricted mean survival time to estimate the treatment effect in randomized clinical trials when the proportional hazards assumption is in doubt. Statistics in Medicine **30**, 2409–2421 (2011)

475. Royston, P., Sauerbrei, W.: A new measure of prognostic separation in survival data. Statistics in Medicine **23**, 723–748 (2004)

476. Royston, P., Sauerbrei, W.: Improving the robustness of fractional polynomial models by preliminary covariate transformation: A pragmatic approach. Computational Statistics & Data Analysis **51**, 4240–4253 (2007)

477. Royston, P., Sauerbrei, W.: *Multivariable model-building: A pragmatic approach to regression analysis based on fractional polynomials for modelling continuous variables.* Chichester: Wiley (2008)

478. Rubin, D.B.: Inference and missing data. Biometrika **63**, 581–592 (1976)

479. Rubin, D.B.: Estimating causal effects from large data sets using propensity scores. Annals of Internal Medicine **127**, 757–763 (1997)

480. Rutjes, A.W., Reitsma, J.B., Di Nisio, M., Smidt, N., van Rijn, J.C., Bossuyt, P.M.: Evidence of bias and variation in diagnostic accuracy studies. CMAJ **174**, 469–476 (2006)

481. Sackett, D.L., Rosenberg, W.M.: On the need for evidence-based medicine. Journal of Public Health **17**, 330–334 (1995)

482. Sanada, H., Sugama, J., Kitagawa, A., Thigpen, B., Kinosita, S., Murayama, S.: Risk factors in the development of pressure ulcers in an intensive care unit in Pontianak, Indonesia. International Wound Journal **4**, 208–215 (2007)

483. Sargent, D.J., Conley, B.A., Allegra, C., Collette, L.: Clinical trial designs for predictive marker validation in cancer treatment trials. Journal of Clinical Oncology **23**, 2020–2027 (2005)

484. Sauerbrei, W.: The use of resampling methods to simplify regression models in medical statistics. Journal of the Royal Statistical Society: Series C **48**, 313–329 (1999)

485. Sauerbrei, W., Meier-Hirmer, C., Benner, A., Royston, P.: Multivariable regression model building by using fractional polynomials: Description of SAS, STATA and R programs. Computational Statistics & Data Analysis **50**, 3464–3485 (2006)

486. Sauerbrei, W., Royston, P.: Building multivariable prognostic and diagnostic models: Transformation of the predictors by using fractional polynomials. Journal of the Royal Statistical Society: Series A **162**, 71–94 (1999)

487. Sauerbrei, W., Schumacher, M.: A bootstrap resampling procedure for model building: Application to the Cox regression model. Statistics in Medicine **11**, 2093–2109 (1992)

488. Scarvelis, D., Wells, P.S.: Diagnosis and treatment of deep-vein thrombosis. CMAJ **175**, 1087–1092 (2006)

489. Schafer, J.L.: Analysis of incomplete multivariate data. Chapman & Hall, London (1997)
490. Schapire, R.E.: The strength of weak learnability. Machine Learning **5**, 197–227 (1990)
491. Schemper, M.: Predictive accuracy and explained variation. Statistics in Medicine **22**, 2299–2308 (2003)
492. Schleidgen, S., Klingler, C., Bertram, T., Rogowski, W.H., Marckmann, G.: What is personalized medicine: Sharpening a vague term based on a systematic literature review. BMC Medical Ethics **14**, 55 (2013)
493. Schomaker, M., Heumann, C.: Bootstrap inference when using multiple imputation. Statistics in Medicine **37**, 2252–2266 (2018)
494. Schumacher, M., Binder, H., Gerds, T.: Assessment of survival prediction models based on microarray data. Bioinformatics **23**, 1768–1774 (2007)
495. Schumacher, M., Graf, E., Gerds, T.: How to assess prognostic models for survival data: A case study in oncology. Methods of Information in Medicine **42**, 564–571 (2003)
496. Schwarzer, G., Schumacher, M.: Artificial neural networks for diagnosis and prognosis in prostate cancer. Seminars in Urologic Oncology **20**, 89–95 (2002)
497. Schwarzer, G., Vach, W., Schumacher, M.: On the misuses of artificial neural networks for prognostic and diagnostic classification in oncology. Statistics in Medicine **19**, 541–561 (2000)
498. Seaton, S.E., Barker, L., Lingsma, H.F., Steyerberg, E.W., Manktelow, B.N.: What is the probability of detecting poorly performing hospitals using funnel plots? BMJ Quality & Safety **22**, 870–876 (2013)
499. Seeger, J.D., Walker, A.M., Williams, P.L., Saperia, G.M., Sacks, F.M.: A propensity score-matched cohort study of the effect of statins, mainly fluvastatin, on the occurrence of acute myocardial infarction. The American Journal of Cardiology **92**, 1447–1451 (2003)
500. Segaar, R.W., Wilson, J.H., Habbema, J.D., Malchow-Moller, A., Hilden, J., van der Maas, P.J.: Transferring a diagnostic decision aid for jaundice. The Netherlands Journal of Medicine **33**, 5–15 (1988)
501. Senn, S.: Testing for baseline balance in clinical trials. Statistics in Medicine **13**, 1715–1726 (1994)
502. Senn, S., Julious, S.: Measurement in clinical trials: A neglected issue for statisticians? Statistics in Medicine **28**, 3189–3209 (2009)
503. Shah, B.R., Laupacis, A., Hux, J.E., Austin, P.C.: Propensity score methods gave similar results to traditional regression modeling in observational studies: A systematic review. Journal of Clinical Epidemiology **58**, 550–559 (2005)
504. Shah, N.D., Steyerberg, E.W., Kent, D.M.: Big data and predictive analytics: Recalibrating expectations. JAMA **320**, 27–28 (2018)
505. Shahian, D.M., Normand, S.L., Torchiana, D.F., et al.: Cardiac surgery report cards: Comprehensive review and statistical critique. The Annals of Thoracic Surgery **72**, 2155–2168 (2001)
506. Shahian, D.M., Silverstein, T., Lovett, A.F., Wolf, R.E., Normand, S.L.: Comparison of clinical and administrative data sources for hospital coronary artery bypass graft surgery report cards. Circulation **115**, 1518–1527 (2007)
507. Shahian, D.M., Torchiana, D.F., Shemin, R.J., Rawn, J.D., Normand, S.L.: Massachusetts cardiac surgery report card: Implications of statistical methodology. The Annals of Thoracic Surgery **80**, 2106–2113 (2005)
508. Shmueli, G.: To explain or to predict? Statistical Science **25**, 289–310 (2010)
509. Silberzahn, R., Uhlmann, E.L., Martin, D.P., et al.: Many analysts, one data set: Making transparent how variations in analytic choices affect results. Advances in Methods and Practices in Psychological Science **1**, 337–356 (2018)
510. Simon, R., Altman, D.G.: Statistical aspects of prognostic factor studies in oncology. British Journal of Cancer **69**, 979–985 (1994)
511. Simon, R., Korn, E., McShane, L., Radmacher, M., Wright, G. Y. Z.: *Design and analysis of DNA microarray investigations*. New York: Springer (2003)

512. Simons, P.C., Algra, A., van de Laak, M.F., Grobbee, D.E., van der Graaf, Y.: Second manifestations of ARTerial disease (SMART) study: Rationale and design. European Journal of Epidemiology **15**, 773–781 (1999)

513. Siontis, G.C., Tzoulaki, I., Castaldi, P.J., Ioannidis, J.P.: External validation of new risk prediction models is infrequent and reveals worse prognostic discrimination. Journal of Clinical Epidemiology **68**, 25–34 (2015)

514. Siregar, S., Nieboer, D., Vergouwe, Y., et al.: Improved prediction by dynamic modeling: An exploratory study in the adult cardiac surgery database of the Netherlands association for cardio-thoracic surgery. Circulation: Cardiovascular Quality and Outcomes **9**, 171–181 (2016)

515. Siregar, S., Nieboer, D., Versteegh, M. I. M., Steyerberg, E. W., Takkenberg, J. J. M.: Methods for updating a risk prediction model for cardiac surgery: A statistical primer. Interactive Cardiovascular and Thoracic Surgery **28**, 333–338 (2019)

516. Skacel, M., Petras, R.E., Gramlich, T.L., Sigel, J.E., Richter, J.E., Goldblum, J.R.: The diagnosis of low-grade dysplasia in Barrett's esophagus and its implications for disease progression. The American Journal of Gastroenterology **95**, 3383–3387 (2000)

517. Smedinga, H., Steyerberg, E.W., Beukers, W., van Klaveren, D., Zwarthoff, E.C., Vergouwe, Y.: Prediction of multiple recurrent events: A comparison of extended cox models in bladder cancer. American Journal of Epidemiology **186**, 612–623 (2017)

518. Smits, J.M., De Meester, J., Deng, M.C., et al.: Mortality rates after heart transplantation: How to compare center-specific outcome data? Transplantation **75**, 90–96 (2003)

519. Smits, M., Dippel, D.W., Steyerberg, E.W., et al.: Predicting intracranial traumatic findings on computed tomography in patients with minor head injury: The CHIP prediction rule. Annals of Internal Medicine **146**, 397–405 (2007)

520. Snee, R.D.: Validation of regression models: Methods and examples. Technometrics **19**, 415–428 (1977)

521. Snell, K.I., Ensor, J., Debray, T.P., Moons, K.G., Riley, R.D.: Meta-analysis of prediction model performance across multiple studies: Which scale helps ensure between-study normality for the C-statistic and calibration measures? Statistical Methods in Medical Research **27**, 3505–3522 (2018)

522. Snijders, T.A.B., Bosker, R.J.: *Multilevel analysis: An introduction to basic and advanced multilevel modeling*, 2nd edn. Sage Publishers, London (2012)

523. Solomon, D.H., Chibnik, L.B., Losina, E., et al.: Development of a preliminary index that predicts adverse events after total knee replacement. Arthritis Rheum **54**, 1536–1542 (2006)

524. Sparano, J.A., Gray, R.J., Makower, D.F., et al.: Adjuvant chemotherapy guided by a 21-gene expression assay in breast cancer. New England Journal of Medicine **379**, 111–121 (2018)

525. Spiegelhalter, D.J.: Probabilistic prediction in patient management and clinical trials. Statistics in Medicine **5**, 421–433 (1986)

526. Spiegelhalter, D.J.: Funnel plots for comparing institutional performance. Statistics in Medicine **24**, 1185–1202 (2005)

527. Spiegelhalter, D.J.: Understanding uncertainty. Annals of Family Medicine **6**, 196–197 (2008)

528. Spiegelhalter, D.J., Crean, G.P., Holden, R., Knill-Jones, R.P.: Taking a calculated risk: Predictive scoring systems in dyspepsia. Scandinavian Journal of Gastroenterology **128**, 152–160 (1987)

529. Stahel, W. A.: *On strategies in regression analysis* (Vol. 100). Seminar für Statistik, Eidgenössische Technische Hochschule (2001)

530. Stein, C.M.: Estimation of the mean of a multivariate normal distribution. The Annals of Statistics **9**, 1135–1151 (1981)

531. Stephenson, A.J., Smith, A., Kattan, M.W., et al.: Integration of gene expression profiling and clinical variables to predict prostate carcinoma recurrence after radical prostatectomy. Cancer **104**, 290–298 (2005)

532. Sterne, J.A.C., White, I.R., Carlin, J.B., et al.: Multiple imputation for missing data in epidemiological and clinical research: Potential and pitfalls. BMJ **338**, b2393 (2009)

533. Steyerberg, E.W.: Validation in prediction research: The waste by data splitting. Journal of Clinical Epidemiology **103**, 131–133 (2018)

534. Steyerberg, E.W., Balmana, J., Stockwell, D.H., Syngal, S.: Data reduction for prediction: Robust coding of age and family history for the risk of having a genetic mutation. Statistics in Medicine **26**, 5545–5556 (2007)

535. Steyerberg, E.W., Bleeker, S.E., Moll, H.A., Grobbee, D.E., Moons, K.G.: Internal and external validation of predictive models: A simulation study of bias and precision in small samples. Journal of Clinical Epidemiology **56**, 441–447 (2003)

536. Steyerberg, E.W., Borsboom, G.J., van Houwelingen, H.C., Eijkemans, M.J., Habbema, J. D.: Validation and updating of predictive logistic regression models: A study on sample size and shrinkage. Statistics in Medicine **23**, 2567–2586 (2004)

537. Steyerberg, E.W., Bossuyt, P.M., Lee, K.L.: Clinical trials in acute myocardial infarction: Should we adjust for baseline characteristics? American Heart Journal **139**, 745–751 (2000)

538. Steyerberg, E.W., Earle, C.C., Neville, B.A., Weeks, J.C.: Racial differences in surgical evaluation, treatment, and outcome of locoregional esophageal cancer: A population-based analysis of elderly patients. Journal of Clinical Oncology **23**, 510–517 (2005)

539. Steyerberg, E.W., Eijkemans, M.J., Boersma, E., Habbema, J.D.: Applicability of clinical prediction models in acute myocardial infarction: A comparison of traditional and empirical Bayes adjustment methods. American Heart Journal **150**, 920 (2005)

540. Steyerberg, E.W., Eijkemans, M.J., Boersma, E., Habbema, J.D.: Equally valid models gave divergent predictions for mortality in acute myocardial infarction patients in a comparison of logistic regression models. Journal of Clinical Epidemiology **58**, 383–390 (2005)

541. Steyerberg, E.W., Eijkemans, M.J., Habbema, J.D.: Stepwise selection in small data sets: A simulation study of bias in logistic regression analysis. Journal of Clinical Epidemiology **52**, 935–942 (1999)

542. Steyerberg, E.W., Eijkemans, M.J., Harrell Jr., F.E., Habbema, J.D.: Prognostic modelling with logistic regression analysis: A comparison of selection and estimation methods in small data sets. Statistics in Medicine **19**, 1059–1079 (2000)

543. Steyerberg, E.W., Eijkemans, M.J., Harrell Jr., F.E., Habbema, J.D.: Prognostic modeling with logistic regression analysis: In search of a sensible strategy in small data sets. Medical Decision Making **21**, 45–56 (2001)

544. Steyerberg, E.W., Eijkemans, M.J., van Houwelingen, J.C., Lee, K.L., Habbema, J.D.: Prognostic models based on literature and individual patient data in logistic regression analysis. Statistics in Medicine **19**, 141–160 (2000)

545. Steyerberg, E.W., Gerl, A., Fossa, S.D., et al.: Validity of predictions of residual retroperitoneal mass histology in nonseminomatous testicular cancer. Journal of Clinical Oncology **16**, 269–274 (1998)

546. Steyerberg, E.W., Harrell Jr., F.E.: Prediction models need appropriate internal, internal-external, and external validation. Journal of Clinical Epidemiology **69**, 245–247 (2016)

547. Steyerberg, E.W., Harrell Jr., F.E., Borsboom, G.J., Eijkemans, M.J., Vergouwe, Y., Habbema, J.D.: Internal validation of predictive models: Efficiency of some procedures for logistic regression analysis. Journal of Clinical Epidemiology **54**, 774–781 (2001)

548. Steyerberg, E.W., Homs, M.Y., Stokvis, A., Essink-Bot, M.L., Siersema, P.D.: Stent placement or brachytherapy for palliation of dysphagia from esophageal cancer: A prognostic model to guide treatment selection. Gastrointestinal Endoscopy **62**, 333–340 (2005)

549. Steyerberg, E.W., Kallewaard, M., van der Graaf, Y., van Herwerden, L.A., Habbema, J.D.: Decision analyses for prophylactic replacement of the Bjork-Shiley convexo-concave heart valve: An evaluation of assumptions and estimates. Medical Decision Making **20**, 20–32 (2000)

550. Steyerberg, E. W., Keizer, H. J., Fossa, S. D., et al.: Resection of residual retroperitoneal masses in testicular cancer: Evaluation and improvement of selection criteria. The ReHiT study group. Re-analysis of histology in testicular cancer. British Journal of Cancer **74**, 1492–1498 (1996)

551. Steyerberg, E.W., Keizer, H.J., Fossa, S.D., et al.: Prediction of residual retroperitoneal mass histology after chemotherapy for metastatic nonseminomatous germ cell tumor: Multivariate analysis of individual patient data from six study groups. Journal of Clinical Oncology **13**, 1177–1187 (1995)

552. Steyerberg, E.W., Keizer, H.J., Habbema, J.D.: Prediction models for the histology of residual masses after chemotherapy for metastatic testicular cancer. ReHiT Study Group. International Journal of Cancer **83**, 856–859 (1999)

553. Steyerberg, E.W., Keizer, H.J., Sleijfer, D.T., et al.: Retroperitoneal metastases in testicular cancer: Role of CT measurements of residual masses in decision making for resection after chemotherapy. Radiology **215**, 437–444 (2000)

554. Steyerberg, E.W., Keizer, H.J., Stoter, G., Habbema, J.D.: Predictors of residual mass histology following chemotherapy for metastatic non-seminomatous testicular cancer: A quantitative overview of 996 resections. European Journal of Cancer **30A**, 1231–1239 (1994)

555. Steyerberg, E. W., Kievit, J., de Mol Van Otterloo, J. C., van Bockel, J. H., Eijkemans, M. J., Habbema, J. D.: Perioperative mortality of elective abdominal aortic aneurysm surgery. A clinical prediction rule based on literature and individual patient data. Archives of internal medicine **155**, 1998–2004 (1995)

556. Steyerberg, E.W., Lingsma, H.F.: Complexities in quality-of-care information. Medical Decision Making **30**, 529–530 (2010)

557. Steyerberg, E.W., Marshall, P.B., Keizer, H.J., Habbema, J.D.: Resection of small, residual retroperitoneal masses after chemotherapy for nonseminomatous testicular cancer: A decision analysis. Cancer **85**, 1331–1341 (1999)

558. Steyerberg, E.W., Moons, K.G., van der Windt, D.A., et al.: Prognosis research strategy (PROGRESS) 3: Prognostic model research. PLoS Medicine **10**, e1001381 (2013)

559. Steyerberg, E. W., Mushkudiani, N., Perel, P., et al. Predicting outcome after traumatic brain injury: Development and international validation of prognostic scores based on admission characteristics. PLoS medicine **5**, e165 (2008)

560. Steyerberg, E.W., Neville, B.A., Koppert, L.B., et al.: Surgical mortality in patients with esophageal cancer: Development and validation of a simple risk score. Journal of Clinical Oncology **24**, 4277–4284 (2006)

561. Steyerberg, E.W., Pencina, M.J., Lingsma, H.F., Kattan, M.W., Vickers, A.J., Van Calster, B.: Assessing the incremental value of diagnostic and prognostic markers: A review and illustration. European Journal of Clinical Investigation **42**, 216–228 (2012)

562. Steyerberg, E.W., Roobol, M.J., Kattan, M.W., van der Kwast, T.H., de Koning, H.J., Schroder, F.H.: Prediction of indolent prostate cancer: Validation and updating of a prognostic nomogram. The Journal of Urology **177**, 107–112 (2007)

563. Steyerberg, E.W., Uno, H., Ioannidis, J.P.A., van Calster, B.: Poor performance of clinical prediction models: The harm of commonly applied methods. Journal of Clinical Epidemiology **98**, 133–143 (2018)

564. Steyerberg, E.W., Van Calster, B., Pencina, M.J.: Performance measures for prediction models and markers: Evaluation of predictions and classifications. Revista Española de Cardiología **64**, 788–794 (2011)

565. Steyerberg, E.W., Vergouwe, Y.: Towards better clinical prediction models: Seven steps for development and an ABCD for validation. European Heart Journal **35**, 1925–1931 (2014)

566. Steyerberg, E.W., Vergouwe, Y., Keizer, H.J., Habbema, J.D.: Residual mass histology in testicular cancer: Development and validation of a clinical prediction rule. Statistics in Medicine **20**, 3847–3859 (2001)
567. Steyerberg, E.W., Vickers, A.J.: Decision curve analysis: A discussion. Medical Decision Making **28**, 146–149 (2008)
568. Steyerberg, E.W., Vickers, A.J., Cook, N.R., et al.: Assessing the performance of prediction models: A framework for traditional and novel measures. Epidemiology **21**, 128–138 (2010)
569. Stiell, I., Wells, G., Laupacis, A., et al.: Multicentre trial to introduce the Ottawa ankle rules for use of radiography in acute ankle injuries. Multicentre Ankle Rule Study Group. BMJ **311**, 594–597 (1995)
570. Stiggelbout, A.M., Pieterse, A.H., De Haes, J.C.J.M.: Shared decision making: Concepts, evidence, and practice. Patient Education and Counseling **98**, 1172–1179 (2015)
571. Strandberg, T.E., Pitkala, K.: What is the most important component of blood pressure: Systolic, diastolic or pulse pressure? Current Opinion in Nephrology and Hypertension **12**, 293–297 (2003)
572. Strasak, A.M., Umlauf, N., Pfeiffer, R.M., Lang, S.: Comparing penalized splines and fractional polynomials for flexible modelling of the effects of continuous predictor variables. Computational Statistics & Data Analysis **55**, 1540–1551 (2011)
573. Strobl, A.N., Vickers, A.J., Van Calster, B., et al.: Improving patient prostate cancer risk assessment: Moving from static, globally-applied to dynamic, practice-specific risk calculators. Journal of Biomedical Informatics **56**, 87–93 (2015)
574. Sturmer, T., Joshi, M., Glynn, R.J., Avorn, J., Rothman, K.J., Schneeweiss, S.: A review of the application of propensity score methods yielded increasing use, advantages in specific settings, but not substantially different estimates compared with conventional multivariable methods. Journal of Clinical Epidemiology **59**, 437–447 (2006)
575. Su, T.L., Jaki, T., Hickey, G.L., Buchan, I., Sperrin, M.: A review of statistical updating methods for clinical prediction models. Statistical Methods in Medical Research **27**, 185–197 (2018)
576. Tantithamthavorn, C., McIntosh, S., Hassan, A.E., Matsumoto, K.: An empirical comparison of model validation techniques for defect prediction models. IEEE Transactions on Software Engineering **43**, 1–18 (2017)
577. Teasdale, G., Jennett, B.: Assessment and prognosis of coma after head injury. Acta Neurochirurgica **34**, 45–55 (1976)
578. Terrin, N., Schmid, C.H., Griffith, J.L., D'Agostino, R.B., Selker, H.P.: External validity of predictive models: A comparison of logistic regression, classification trees, and neural networks. Journal of Clinical Epidemiology **56**, 721–729 (2003)
579. Therneau, T.M., Grambsch, P.M.: *Modeling survival data: Extending the Cox model.* Springer, New York (2013)
580. Thompson, K. M.: *Risk in perspective: Insight and humor in the age of risk management.* AORM (Newton Centre, MA) (2004)
581. Tibshirani, R.: Regression and shrinkage via the Lasso. Journal of the Royal Statistical Society: Series B **58**, 267–288 (1996)
582. Tibshirani, R.: The lasso method for variable selection in the Cox model. Statistics in Medicine **16**, 385–395 (1997)
583. TIMI-II Study Group: Comparison of invasive and conservative strategies after treatment with intravenous tissue plasminogen activator in acute myocardial infarction. Results of the thrombolysis in myocardial infarction (TIMI) phase II trial. New England Journal of Medicine **320**, 618–627 (1989)
584. Toll, D.B., Janssen, K.J., Vergouwe, Y., Moons, K.G.: Validation, updating and impact of clinical prediction rules: A review. Journal of Clinical Epidemiology **61**, 1085–1094 (2008)

585. Tomer, A., Nieboer, D., Roobol, M. J., Steyerberg, E. W., Rizopoulos, D.: Personalized schedules for surveillance of low-risk prostate cancer patients. Biometrics **75**, 153–162 (2019)

586. Torkamani, A., Wineinger, N.E., Topol, E.J.: The personal and clinical utility of polygenic risk scores. Nature Reviews Genetics **19**, 581–590 (2018)

587. Tu, J.V.: Advantages and disadvantages of using artificial neural networks versus logistic regression for predicting medical outcomes. Journal of Clinical Epidemiology **49**, 1225–1231 (1996)

588. Tu, J.V., Weinstein, M.C., McNeil, B.J., Naylor, C.D.: Predicting mortality after coronary artery bypass surgery: What do artificial neural networks learn? The steering committee of the cardiac care network of Ontario. Medical Decision Making **18**, 229–235 (1998)

589. Turner, E.L., Perel, P., Clayton, T., et al.: Covariate adjustment increased power in randomized controlled trials: An example in traumatic brain injury. Journal of Clinical Epidemiology **65**, 474–481 (2012)

590. Ulmer, H., Kollerits, B., Kelleher, C., Diem, G., Concin, H.: Predictive accuracy of the SCORE risk function for cardiovascular disease in clinical practice: A prospective evaluation of 44 649 Austrian men and women. European Journal of Cardiovascular Prevention & Rehabilitation **12**, 433–441 (2005)

591. Uno, H., Cai, T., Pencina, M.J., D'Agostino, R.B., Wei, L.J.: On the C-statistics for evaluating overall adequacy of risk prediction procedures with censored survival data. Statistics in Medicine **30**, 1105–1117 (2011)

592. Uno, H., Cai, T., Tian, L., Wei, L.J.: Evaluating prediction rules for t-year survivors with censored regression models. JASA **102**, 527–537 (2007)

593. Uno, H., Claggett, B., Tian, L., et al.: Moving beyond the hazard ratio in quantifying the between-group difference in survival analysis. Journal of Clinical Oncology **32**, 2380–2385 (2014)

594. Vach, W., Blettner, M.: Missing data in epidemiologic studies. *Encyclopedia of Biostatistics*, 2641–2654. New York: Wiley (1998)

595. van Beek, J.G., Mushkudiani, N.A., Steyerberg, E.W., et al.: Prognostic value of admission laboratory parameters in traumatic brain injury: Results from the IMPACT study. Journal of Neurotrauma **24**, 315–328 (2007)

596. Van Belle, V., Van Calster, B.: Visualizing risk prediction models. PLoS One **10**, e0132614 (2015)

597. Van Belle, V., Van Calster, B., Van Huffel, S., Suykens, J.A.K., Lisboa, P.: Explaining support vector machines: A color based nomogram. PLoS One **11**, e0164568 (2016)

598. Van Belle, V.M., Van Calster, B., Timmerman, D., et al.: A mathematical model for interpretable clinical decision support with applications in gynecology. PLoS One **7**, e34312 (2012)

599. van Buuren, S., Groothuis-oudshoorn, K.: mice: Multivariate Imputation by Chained Equations in R. Journal of Statistical Software **45**, 1–67 (2011)

600. van Buuren, S.: *Flexible imputation of missing data*. New York: CRC Press LLC (2018)

601. van Buuren, S., Boshuizen, H.C., Knook, D.L.: Multiple imputation of missing blood pressure covariates in survival analysis. Statistics in Medicine **18**, 681–694 (1999)

602. Van Calster, B., Nieboer, D., Vergouwe, Y., De Cock, B., Pencina, M.J., Steyerberg, E.W.: A calibration hierarchy for risk models was defined: From utopia to empirical data. Journal of Clinical Epidemiology **74**, 167–176 (2016)

603. Van Calster, B., Steyerberg, E.W., D'Agostino Sr., R.B., Pencina, M.J.: Sensitivity and specificity can change in opposite directions when new predictive markers are added to risk models. Medical Decision Making **34**, 513–522 (2014)

604. Van Calster, B., Van Belle, V., Vergouwe, Y., Timmerman, D., Van Huffel, S., Steyerberg, E.W.: Extending the c-statistic to nominal polytomous outcomes: The Polytomous Discrimination Index. Statistics in Medicine **31**, 2610–2626 (2012)

605. Van Calster, B., Van Hoorde, K., Valentin, L., et al.: Evaluating the risk of ovarian cancer before surgery using the ADNEX model to differentiate between benign, borderline, early and advanced stage invasive, and secondary metastatic tumours: Prospective multicentre diagnostic study. BMJ **349**, g5920 (2014)

606. Van Calster, B., Vickers, A.J.: Calibration of risk prediction models: Impact on decision-analytic performance. Medical Decision Making **35**, 162–169 (2015)

607. Van Calster, B., Vickers, A.J., Pencina, M.J., Baker, S.G., Timmerman, D., Steyerberg, E. W.: Evaluation of markers and risk prediction models: Overview of relationships between NRI and decision-analytic measures. Medical Decision Making **33**, 490–501 (2013)

608. Van Calster, B., Wynants, L., Verbeek, J.F.M., et al.: Reporting and interpreting decision curve analysis: A guide for investigators. European Urology **74**, 796–804 (2018)

609. van den Berg, M.J., Bhatt, D.L., Kappelle, L.J., et al.: Identification of vascular patients at very high risk for recurrent cardiovascular events: Validation of the current ACC/AHA very high risk criteria. European Heart Journal **38**, 3211–3218 (2017)

610. van der Graaf, Y., de Waard, F., van Herwerden, L.A., Defauw, J.: Risk of strut fracture of Bjork-Shiley valves. The Lancet **339**, 257–261 (1992)

611. van der Meulen, J.H., Steyerberg, E.W., van der Graaf, Y., et al.: Age thresholds for prophylactic replacement of Bjork-Shiley convexo-concave heart valves. A clinical and economic evaluation. Circulation **88**, 156–164 (1993)

612. van der Ploeg, T., Austin, P.C., Steyerberg, E.W.: Modern modelling techniques are data hungry: A simulation study for predicting dichotomous end points. BMC Medical Research Methodology **14**, 137 (2014)

613. van der Ploeg, T., Nieboer, D., Steyerberg, E.W.: Modern modeling techniques had limited external validity in predicting mortality from traumatic brain injury. Journal of Clinical Epidemiology **78**, 83–89 (2016)

614. van der Vaart, A.W., Dudoit, S., van der Laan, M.J.: Oracle inequalities for multi-fold cross-validation. Statistics & Decisions **24**, 351–371 (2006)

615. van Dijk, M.R., Steyerberg, E.W., Habbema, J.D.: A decision-analytic approach to define poor prognosis patients: A case study for non-seminomatous germ cell cancer patients. BMC Medical Informatics and Decision Making **8**, 1 (2008)

616. van Dijk, M.R., Steyerberg, E.W., Stenning, S.P., Habbema, J.D.: Identifying subgroups among poor prognosis patients with nonseminomatous germ cell cancer by tree modelling: A validation study. Annals of Oncology **15**, 1400–1405 (2004)

617. van Dijk, M.R., Steyerberg, E.W., Stenning, S.P., Habbema, J.D.: Survival estimates of a prognostic classification depended more on year of treatment than on imputation of missing values. Journal of Clinical Epidemiology **59**, 246–253 (2006)

618. van Dishoeck, A. M., Lingsma, H. F., Mackenbach, J.P., Steyerberg, E. W.: Random variation and rankability of hospitals using outcome indicators. BMJ Quality & Safety **20**, 869–74 (2011)

619. van Gorp, M.J., Steyerberg, E.W., Kallewaard, M., van der Graaf, Y.: Clinical prediction rule for 30-day mortality in Bjork-Shiley convexo-concave valve replacement. Journal of Clinical Epidemiology **56**, 1006–1012 (2003)

620. van Gorp, M.J., Steyerberg, E.W., van der Graaf, Y.: Decision guidelines for prophylactic replacement of Bjork-Shiley convexo-concave heart valves: Impact on clinical practice. Circulation **109**, 2092–2096 (2004)

621. Van Hoorde, K., Van Huffel, S., Timmerman, D., Bourne, T., Van Calster, B.: A spline-based tool to assess and visualize the calibration of multiclass risk predictions. Journal of Biomedical Informatics **54**, 283–293 (2015)

622. van Houwelingen, H., Putter, H.: *Dynamic prediction in clinical survival analysis.* CRC Press, Boca Raton (2012)

623. van Houwelingen, H. C.: Validation. calibration, revision and combination of prognostic survival models. Statistics in Medicine **19**, 3401–3415 (2009)

624. van Houwelingen, H. C., Brand, R., Louis, T. A.: Empirical Bayes methods for monitoring health care quality. https://www.lumc.nl/sub/3020/att/EmpiricalBayes.pdf (2006)

625. van Houwelingen, H.C., Putter, H.: Dynamic predicting by landmarking as an alternative for multi-state modeling: An application to acute lymphoid leukemia data. Lifetime Data Analysis **14**, 447 (2008)

626. van Houwelingen, H.C., Thorogood, J.: Construction, validation and updating of a prognostic model for kidney graft survival. Statistics in Medicine **14**, 1999–2008 (1995)

627. van Houwelingen, J.C., Le Cessie, S.: Predictive value of statistical models. Statistics in Medicine **9**, 1303–1325 (1990)

628. van Jaarsveld, B. C., Krijnen, P., Pieterman, H., et al. The effect of balloon angioplasty on hypertension in atherosclerotic renal-artery stenosis. Dutch Renal Artery Stenosis Intervention Cooperative Study Group. New England Journal of Medicine **342**, 1007–1014 (2000)

629. van Klaveren, D., Gonen, M., Steyerberg, E.W., Vergouwe, Y.: A new concordance measure for risk prediction models in external validation settings. Statistics in Medicine **35**, 4136–4152 (2016)

630. van Klaveren, D., Vergouwe, Y., Farooq, V., Serruys, P.W., Steyerberg, E.W.: Estimates of absolute treatment benefit for individual patients required careful modeling of statistical interactions. Journal of Clinical Epidemiology **68**, 1366–1374 (2015)

631. van Koningsveld, R., Steyerberg, E.W., Hughes, R.A., Swan, A.V., van Doorn, P.A., Jacobs, B.C.: A clinical prognostic scoring system for Guillain-Barre syndrome. The Lancet Neurology **6**, 589–594 (2007)

632. van Lier, M.G., Leenen, C.H., Wagner, A., et al.: Yield of routine molecular analyses in colorectal cancer patients ≤ 70 years to detect underlying Lynch syndrome. The Journal of Pathology **226**, 764–774 (2012)

633. van Smeden, M.: Should a risk prediction model be developed? https://twitter.com/MaartenvSmeden/status/1025315100796899328 (2018)

634. van Smeden, M., de Groot, J.A.H., Moons, K.G.M., et al.: No rationale for 1 variable per 10 events criterion for binary logistic regression analysis. BMC Medical Research Methodology **16**, 163 (2016)

635. van Smeden, M., Moons, K. G., de Groot, J. A., et al.: Sample size for binary logistic prediction models: Beyond events per variable criteria. Statistical Methods in Medical Research (2018)

636. van Smeden, M., Naaktgeboren, C.A., Reitsma, J.B., Moons, K.G.M., de Groot, J.A.H.: Latent class models in diagnostic studies when there is no reference standard—a systematic review. American Journal of Epidemiology **179**, 423–431 (2014)

637. van Westreenen, H.L., Westerterp, M., Sloof, G.W., et al.: Limited additional value of positron emission tomography in staging oesophageal cancer. British Journal of Surgery **94**, 1515–1520 (2007)

638. Vandenbroucke, J.P.: Prospective or retrospective: What's in a name? BMJ **302**, 249–250 (1991)

639. Vapnik, V.N.: *The nature of statistical learning theory*. Springer, New York (1995)

640. Vergouwe, Y., Nieboer, D., Oostenbrink, R., et al.: A closed testing procedure to select an appropriate method for updating prediction models. Statistics in Medicine **36**, 4529–4539 (2017)

641. Vergouwe, Y., Royston, P., Moons, K.G., Altman, D.G.: Development and validation of a prediction model with missing predictor data: A practical approach. Journal of Clinical Epidemiology **63**, 205–214 (2010)

642. Vergouwe, Y., Steyerberg, E.W., Eijkemans, M.J., Habbema, J.D.: Validity of prognostic models: When is a model clinically useful? Seminars in Urologic Oncology **20**, 96–107 (2002)

643. Vergouwe, Y., Steyerberg, E.W., Eijkemans, M.J., Habbema, J.D.: Substantial effective sample sizes were required for external validation studies of predictive logistic regression models. Journal of Clinical Epidemiology **58**, 475–483 (2005)

644. Vergouwe, Y., Steyerberg, E.W., Foster, R.S., Habbema, J.D., Donohue, J.P.: Validation of a prediction model and its predictors for the histology of residual masses in nonseminomatous testicular cancer. The Journal of Urology **165**, 84–88 (2001)

645. Vergouwe, Y., Steyerberg, E.W., Foster, R.S., et al.: Predicting retroperitoneal histology in postchemotherapy testicular germ cell cancer: A model update and multicentre validation with more than 1000 patients. European Urology **51**, 424–432 (2007)

646. Verweij, P.J., van Houwelingen, H.C.: Penalized likelihood in Cox regression. Statistics in Medicine **13**, 2427–2436 (1994)

647. Vickers, A.J., Cronin, A.M., Begg, C.B.: One statistical test is sufficient for assessing new predictive markers. BMC Medical Research Methodology **11**, 13 (2011)

648. Vickers, A.J., Elkin, E.B.: Decision curve analysis: A novel method for evaluating prediction models. Medical Decision Making **26**, 565–574 (2006)

649. Vickers, A.J., Kramer, B.S., Baker, S.G.: Selecting patients for randomized trials: A systematic approach based on risk group. Trials **7**, 30 (2006)

650. Vickers, A.J., Pepe, M.: Does the net reclassification improvement help us evaluate models and markers? Annals of Internal Medicine **160**, 136–137 (2014)

651. Vickers, A.J., Van Calster, B., Steyerberg, E.W.: Net benefit approaches to the evaluation of prediction models, molecular markers, and diagnostic tests. BMJ **352**, i6 (2016)

652. Virnig, B. A., Warren, J. L., Cooper, G. S., Klabunde, C. N., Schussler, N., Freeman, J. Studying radiation therapy using SEER-Medicare-linked data. Medical care **40**, IV-49–54 (2002)

653. Vittinghoff, E.: *Regression methods in biostatistics: Linear, logistic, survival, and repeated measures models*. Springer, New York (2005)

654. Vittinghoff, E., McCulloch, C.E.: Relaxing the rule of ten events per variable in logistic and Cox regression. American Journal of Epidemiology **165**, 710–718 (2007)

655. Volinsky, C.T., Raftery, A.E.: Bayesian information criterion for censored survival models. Biometrics **56**, 256–262 (2000)

656. von Hippel, P. T.: 4. Regression with missing Ys: An improved strategy for analyzing multiply imputed data. Sociological Methodology **37**, 83–117 (2007)

657. von Hippel, P. T.: 8. How to impute interactions, squares, and other transformed variables. Sociological Methodology **39**, 265–291 (2009)

658. Wallach, J.D., Sullivan, P.G., Trepanowski, J.F., Sainani, K.L., Steyerberg, E.W., Ioannidis, J.A.: Evaluation of evidence of statistical support and corroboration of subgroup claims in randomized clinical trials. JAMA Internal Medicine **177**, 554–560 (2017)

659. Wallach, J.D., Sullivan, P.G., Trepanowski, J.F., Steyerberg, E.W., Ioannidis, J.P.: Sex based subgroup differences in randomized controlled trials: Empirical evidence from Cochrane meta-analyses. BMJ **355**, i5826 (2016)

660. Wang, O.J., Wang, Y., Lichtman, J.H., Bradley, E.H., Normand, S.L., Krumholz, H.M.: "America's Best Hospitals" in the treatment of acute myocardial infarction. Archives of Internal Medicine **167**, 1345–1351 (2007)

661. Warren, J. L., Harlan, L. C., Fahey, A., et al.: Utility of the SEER-Medicare data to identify chemotherapy use. Medical Care **40**, IV-55–61 (2002)

662. Wehberg, S., Schumacher, M.: A comparison of nonparametric error rate estimation methods in classification problems. Biometrical Journal **46**, 35–47 (2004)

663. Wells, P.S., Anderson, D.R., Bormanis, J., et al.: Value of assessment of pretest probability of deep-vein thrombosis in clinical management. The Lancet **350**, 1795–1798 (1997)

664. Wells, P.S., Hirsh, J., Anderson, D.R., et al.: Accuracy of clinical assessment of deep-vein thrombosis. The Lancet **345**, 1326–1330 (1995)

665. Wells, P.S., Ihaddadene, R., Reilly, A., Forgie, M.: Diagnosis of venous thromboembolism: 20 years of progress. Annals of Internal Medicine **168**, 131–140 (2018)

666. Wessler, B. S., YH, L. L., Kramer, W., et al.: Clinical prediction models for cardiovascular disease. Circulation: Cardiovascular Quality and Outcomes **8**, 368–375 (2015)

667. White, I.R., Carlin, J.B.: Bias and efficiency of multiple imputation compared with complete-case analysis for missing covariate values. Statistics in Medicine **29**, 2920–2931 (2010)

668. White, I. R., Horton, N. J., Carpenter, J., Pocock, S. J.: Strategy for intention to treat analysis in randomised trials with missing outcome data. BMJ **342**, d40 (2011)

669. White, I.R., Royston, P., Wood, A.M.: Multiple imputation using chained equations: Issues and guidance for practice. Statistics in Medicine **30**, 377–399 (2011)

670. Whiting, P., Rutjes, A.S., Reitsma, J.B., Glas, A.S., Bossuyt, P.M., Kleijnen, J.: Sources of variation and bias in studies of diagnostic accuracy: A systematic review. Annals of Internal Medicine **140**, 189–202 (2004)

671. Wijesinha, A., Begg, C. B., Funkenstein, H. H., McNeil, B. J.: Methodology for the differential diagnosis of a complex data set. A case study using data from routine CT scan examinations. Medical Decision Making **3**, 133–154 (1983)

672. Wijnen, J.T., Vasen, H.F., Khan, P.M., et al.: Clinical findings with implications for genetic testing in families with clustering of colorectal cancer. New England Journal of Medicine **339**, 511–518 (1998)

673. Wikipedia contributors. Bootstrapping. https://en.wikipedia.org/wiki/Bootstrapping (2019)

674. Wilson, P.W., D'Agostino, R.B., Levy, D., Belanger, A.M., Silbershatz, H., Kannel, W.B.: Prediction of coronary heart disease using risk factor categories. Circulation **97**, 1837–1847 (1998)

675. Wolbers, M., Blanche, P., Koller, M.T., Witteman, J.C., Gerds, T.A.: Concordance for prognostic models with competing risks. Biostatistics **15**, 526–539 (2014)

676. Wolbers, M., Koller, M.T., Witteman, J.C., Steyerberg, E.W.: Prognostic models with competing risks: Methods and application to coronary risk prediction. Epidemiology **20**, 555–561 (2009)

677. Wood, A.M., Royston, P., White, I.R.: The estimation and use of predictions for the assessment of model performance using large samples with multiply imputed data. Biometrical Journal **57**, 614–632 (2015)

678. Wood, A.M., White, I.R., Royston, P.: How should variable selection be performed with multiply imputed data? Statistics in Medicine **27**, 3227–3246 (2008)

679. Wood, L., Egger, M., Gluud, L.L., et al.: Empirical evidence of bias in treatment effect estimates in controlled trials with different interventions and outcomes: Meta-epidemiological study. BMJ **336**, 601–605 (2008)

680. Wood, S.N.: *Generalized additive models: An introduction with R.* Chapman and Hall/CRC, Boca Raton (2006)

681. Wynne, R.: Variable definitions· Implications for the prediction of pulmonary complications after adult cardiac surgery. European Journal of Cardiovascular Nursing **3**, 43–52 (2004)

682. Xanthakis, V., Sullivan, L.M., Vasan, R.S., et al.: Assessing the incremental predictive performance of novel biomarkers over standard predictors. Statistics in Medicine **33**, 2577–2584 (2014)

683. Yang, Y.: Consistency of cross validation for comparing regression procedures. The Annals of Statistics **35**, 2450–2473 (2007)

684. Yates, J.F.: External correspondence: Decomposition of the mean probability score. Organizational Behavior and Human Performance **30**, 132–156 (1982)

685. Ye, J.: On measuring and correcting the effects of data mining and model selection. JASA **93**, 120–131 (1998)

686. Yue, J.K., Vassar, M.J., Lingsma, H.F., et al.: Transforming research and clinical knowledge in traumatic brain injury pilot: Multicenter implementation of the common data elements for traumatic brain injury. Journal of Neurotrauma **30**, 1831–1844 (2013)

687. Zelen, M.: The randomization and stratification of patients to clinical trials. Journal of Chronic Diseases **27**, 365–375 (1974)
688. Zhou, X.H.: Effect of verification bias on positive and negative predictive values. Statistics in Medicine **13**, 1737–1745 (1994)
689. Zou, H., Hastie, T.: Regularization and variable selection via the elastic net. Journal of the Royal Statistical Society: Series B **67**, 301–320 (2005)

Index

Printed in the United States
By Bookmasters